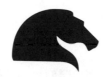

The Illustrated
VETERINARY
ENCYCLOPEDIA
for Horsemen

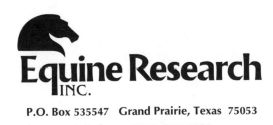

Equine Research
INC.

P.O. Box 535547   Grand Prairie, Texas 75053

Telephone (800) 848-0225

WRITTEN BY:

the research staff of Equine Research Publications

VETERINARY RESEARCH EDITOR:

M. M. Vale, D.V.M.

EDITOR/PUBLISHER:

Don M. Wagoner

ACKNOWLEDGEMENT

We wish to express our sincere appreciation to:

W. L. Anderson, D.V.M.
R. G. Greeley, D.V.M.
M. L. Ward, D.V.M.
G. E. White, D.V.M.

for their invaluable assistance to the research and writing staff of Equine Research Publications in the writing of this book.

CONTENTS

18. THE RESPIRATORY SYSTEM

23. THE REPRODUCTIVE SYSTEM

24. SYSTEMIC DISORDERS

INTRODUCTION

This book has been designed to fill the gap in equine literature between the highly technical books intended for use only by the veterinarian and the non-technical, less informative ones that are commonly available to the horseman.

A major objective of this book is to aid in increasing communication between the horseman and the veterinarian. For this reason, the book does not shy away from the use of medical terms for which there is no common name. Of course, common names are given where possible as an aid in simplifying the material. Frequent definitions, explanations, photographs and illustrations are also used throughout the text, and both a glossary and an index are provided.

For ease in reading, a format was used dividing the material into questions and answers. The text poses important questions about the subject matter much like the horseman might ask, then gives immediate answers to those questions.

In essence, every effort has been made to offer scientifically accurate data in a form that will be of optimum usefulness to the horseman. This was done because the single most important purpose of this book is to aid the horseman in giving his horses the very best care possible.

GUIDE TO THE USE OF
THE ILLUSTRATED VETERINARY
ENCYCLOPEDIA FOR HORSEMEN

Organization

This book is organized by parts of the horse's body in which signs of a disorder appear. For instance, although the source of Laminitis may originate in the digestive system, it is found in the chapter entitled "Foot" because that is where the signs of the disorder are observed. Only a few exceptions to the basic rule of organization will be found and they were made to direct the reader's attention to matters that are important to general understanding.

General Understanding

The first chapter "Disease Process" has been included to help the horseman understand and recognize the various signs and processes of disease. Fever, shock, inflammation and other syndromes are given in-depth coverage in this chapter. This should add to the horseman's understanding of all of the disorders discussed throughout the book.

"Wounds, Drugs and Treatments" is a brief, highly-illustrated chapter which has been included to increase the horseman's understanding of the medications and treatments that are frequently prescribed by the veterinarian. This knowledge too is vital to a general understanding of horse care.

Index

Although this book provides interesting and enjoyable reading, it is also intended as a useful reference. For this reason, the detailed index, in the yellow pages at the back of the book, has been carefully compiled to list subjects only on the pages where they are most thoroughly discussed. Listing pages which merely mention the word being indexed has been avoided since this type of reference is of little value to most readers. Both common names and scientific names have been indexed, and page numbers appear after every entry.

Glossary

The glossary in the blue pages at the back of the book contains definitions of unfamiliar words and medical terms which are likely to be encountered throughout the book. Adding to the horseman's vocabulary of veterinary terms is one important goal of this book, as a means of improving communication between the horseman and the veterinarian.

DISEASE PROCESS

SHOCK

What is shock?

Shock is the term used to describe an acute and progressive failure of the peripheral circulation (blood circulation to the outer body parts—legs, head, etc.).

What are the signs of shock?

There are many indicators of shock: apathy, prostration, rapid shallow pulse, rapid breathing, subnormal temperature, cool skin, sweating, low or falling blood pressure, and the mucous membranes will be pale and slightly blue.

What causes this condition?

The specific causes are unknown, but it appears to follow events which affect the peripheral circulatory system. This occurs after most major injuries including severe trauma, massive hemorrhage, internal obstructions, anemia, major infections, burns, cardiac failure, dehydration and anaphylaxis (allergic-like sensitization).

What happens when a horse is in shock?

Whether it is caused by massive blood loss, tissue toxins (from damaged tissues) or fluid loss from the vascular system into the tissues, the peripheral circulatory system begins to fail. In the mind form of shock, the body can compensate automatically by constricting the dilated vessels in the peripheral system. This gives the heart sufficient back pressure to work against which is necessary for it to maintain circulation to major organs. It is when damage or trauma is severe or extensive that this mechanism is not sufficient to maintain effective blood pressure. When lowered pressure deprives the heart, the nerves that stimulate construction of the blood vessels, and vaso constrictor muscles, of blood and oxygen, the heart weakens and cannot keep the vessels constructed. This allows them to dilate, further lowering blood pressure. This further reduces flow, and the body's ability to maintain critical systems is reduced. It should be understood that this tissue

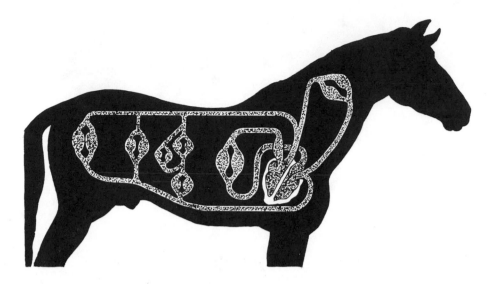

Fig. 1-1. Representation of normal circulation. The major organs are supplied with circulating blood, which removes metabolic wastes and provides oxygen for tissue metabolism.

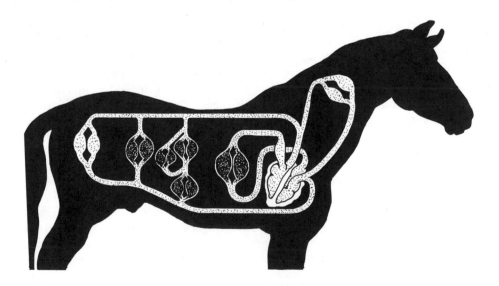

Fig. 1-2. Representation of shock mechanism. The blood pools in the extremities and major organs, but circulation of the blood is very poor. Oxygen is not supplied to the tissues and metabolic wastes accumulate when the peripheral circulatory system fails.

deprivation includes the major organs of the body. Inadequate circulating blood results in cellular damage to the liver and kidneys which sometimes cannot be repaired. Past a certain point, this tissue deprivation becomes irreversible and death soon follows.

What is the treatment for shock?

Primary treatment must be administered by a veterinarian because it involves massive replacement of fluids to restore both blood pressure and volume. Whole blood, plasma, plasma extenders or saline (salt) solution will be used, depending on the need of the collapsing system. Hemorrhage should be controlled immediately and pain should be relieved because it aggravates shock. Antibiotics and corticosteroids are of great value and are used frequently. The animal should be kept warm, but if the temperature is raised, the peripheral vessels will dilate, lowering blood pressure even more. All of these treatments should be balanced by a veterinarian.

Can shock be prevented?

Shock can be avoided or lessened by preventative treatment. Avoiding dehydration of animals and calling a veterinarian before mild shock becomes irreversible are the best preventative measures. Shock treatment should be closely supervised because animals that appear to be responding well can quickly and unexplainably relapse and become critical once again.

THE PROCESS OF INFLAMMATION AND HEALING

What is inflammation?

Inflammation is a dynamic process in which the body responds to a sublethal injury by attempting to destroy, dilute, or wall off an irritating agent. This defense process ends in healing, which is the resolution of the offensive response and includes the repair of damaged tissue. Healing is the direct result of the process of inflammation.

What are the signs of inflammation?

The five primary signs of inflammation are: (1) redness; (2) swelling; (3) heat; (4) pain; and (5) loss of function in the inflamed area. Redness is caused by an increased flow of blood to the irritated part of the body. This increase of blood results in swelling due to seepage of the fluid portions of the blood from the blood vessels into the tissues surrounding the irritated site. The heat that accompanies the inflammatory reaction is radiant heat from the increased blood supply. Blood from internal organs is supplied to the inflamed area, where it gives up the greater heat generated within the body. Pain at the site of inflammation may be from increased pressure on pain receptors, or it may be due to the nerve irritation caused by toxic substances involved in the inflammatory process. Many inflammations result in a loss of function because of associated pain, swelling, the formation of fibrous adhesions or destruction of tissue.

Is the process of inflammation beneficial?

Inflammation is the body's defense against disease-causing organisms and injury. The leukocytes of the blood are the most important elements in the defense. An increase in the flow of blood to an affected part delivers the leukocytes and

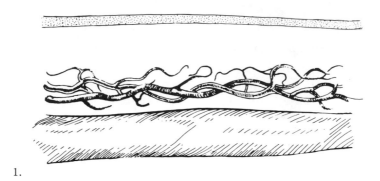

1.

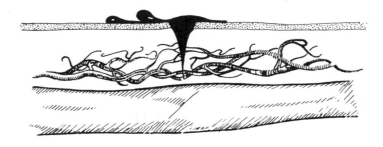

2.

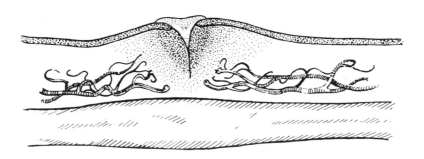

3.

Fig. 1-3.

Fig. 1-3. The process of inflammation and healing
1. Normal tissue, skin unbroken.
2. Trauma to tissue, skin is broken and bleeding begins.
3. From the engorged blood vessels, exudates enter the area, causing redness and swelling.
The swelling helps to stop the bleeding and permit the lymphocytes to "police" the wound.

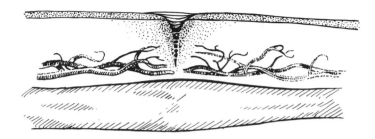

4.

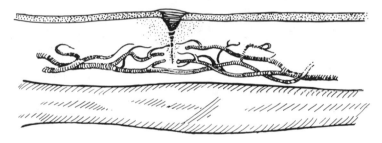

5.

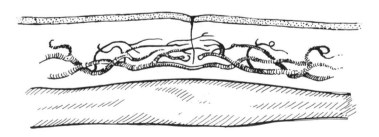

6.

4. The wound is past the acute phase and a scab is beginning to form. From the exudate, fibrous adhesions are forming.
5. The tissues are returning to normal and the exudate is being absorbed by the body.
6. A scar has formed from the fibrous adhesions, leaving the tissue area slightly contracted. Notice the poor blood supply of the scar tissue.

antibodies to the site of an irritant substance or to injured cells. Inflammation attempts to confine and destroy an irritant with the only weapons available to the body. It may not seem so, but inflammation is a beneficial process.

What are the causes of inflammation?

Inflammation is the reaction of tissues to an irritant. Irritants may be disease-causing organisms (pathogens) and their toxins, chemical poisons, burns, mechanical injuries, venoms and antigens (like pollen) against which the tissues possess antibodies.

What is the process of inflammation?

The inflammatory process is primarily a function of the circulatory system which involves changes in the amount and quality of blood reaching the affected area. At first, histamine (released from damaged cells) causes dilation of the blood vessels and accounts for the reddening of the tissues. This initial dilation slows the flow of blood and stretches the walls of the vessels, making the escape of fluid contents and elements easier. The leukocytes, erythrocytes, globin, serum and other cells pass easily through the gaps in the stretched capillaries, carrying antibodies and enzymes to the site of inflammation. Other chemicals (bradykinin and kallidin) maintain the state of capillary dilatation begun by histamine and block the action of inflammation inhibitors like epinephrine and norepinephrine. At this time, the leukocytes have the ability to travel to areas of inflammation by independent movement, which is assisted by the increased blood supply. Following the release of histamine, swelling in the surrounding tissues is due to the leaky capillary walls which permit the inflammatory cells to reach the irritated area. The exudate from the vascular system attempts to dilute the irritating substance in addition to the infection-fighting function it performs in carrying antibodies and bringing heat to the area. During this process, fever is one defense the blood utilizes to weaken the infectious organism, since many bacteria are destroyed by increased heat (the principle behind sterilization).

When the leukocytes arrive in the inflamed area, they attempt to remove the irritant. If it is an invading bacteria or particle, they have the ability to phagocytize (eat and digest) many types of organisms. Powerful enzymes and antibodies destroy and remove cells and the resulting debris. The presence of the infection fighting elements begins the healing process which is the result of inflammation. Many cells participate in the process; each will be discussed separately.

What are the types of inflammatory reactions?

The eight types of inflammatory reactions (explained below) are: (1) a serous, exudative inflammation; (2) a fibrous, exudative inflammation; (3) a purulent, exudative inflammation; (4) a hemorrhagic, exudative inflammation; (5) a mucous, exudative inflammation; (6) a lymphocytic inflammation; (7) an alterative inflammation; and (8) a proliferative inflammation.

What is an exudate?

An exudate is a material (such as fluid, cells and cellular debris) which has escaped from blood vessels and been deposited in tissues or on the surface of tissues. The escaped material may be blood, mucus, serum, fibrin or pus and often forms a "scab" in cases of inflammation.

What are the characteristics of the various types of inflammation?

(1) SEROUS. A serous inflammation is characterized by the exudation of blood serum which may be caused by an infection or trauma especially in a cavity or joint.

It is most commonly associated with simple skin abrasions, swellings in joint capsules and brief irritations of the skin (as in a bee sting). The purpose of the serous exudate is dilution of the poison or irritating substance. Most serous inflammations are relatively mild.

(2) FIBRINOUS. The fibrinous inflammation is characterized by an exudation of fibrin, the clotting factor in the blood. Fibrinous exudates clot, forming a detachable sheath or cast over the inflamed tissues. This reaction is frequent in bronchial and intestinal mucous membranes, where it prevents loss of blood and protects the tissues from further irritation. In some cases, the fibrin may undergo organization, forming permanent adhesions (connections) which inhibit function and movement in the affected area (as in bowed tendon).

(3) PURULENT. Purulent inflammations are characterized by the exudation of pus (white blood cells and fluids) which may be thick and semi-solid or thin and watery. When pus is diffused through the inflamed tissues without definite boundaries or ridges, cellulitis is said to be present. Such inflammation may also be called phlegmonous and is frequent when a wound becomes infected with bacteria. A suppurative inflammation indicates that the pus runs from a surface or fills cavities. If the pus is enclosed in a fibrous capsule, an abscess has formed. Most purulent inflammations are caused by pyogenic (disease-producing) bacteria which are found in large numbers in the purulent material. Confined pus (as in an abscess) may allow the bacteria to enter the bloodstream, where they may travel to various parts of the body. This migration through the blood (metastasis) can be prevented by providing an abscess with an exterior drainage channel, if at all possible, once it is completely formed.

(4) HEMORRHAGIC. Characteristically, a hemorrhagic exudate contains large numbers of erythrocytes (red blood cells). The red blood cells leave the capillaries and make the exudate look like whole blood. This type of exudate is an indication of a violent reaction by the body to chemical poisons or to a highly virulent micro-organism. Enteritis (inflammation of the intestines) is frequently associated with a hemorrhagic exudate, which usually causes the mucous membranes to appear a deep red color in addition to the presence of the bloody exudate.

(5) MUCOUS. A mucous inflammation produces excessive amounts of mucus in the epithelial (surface) cells which are found on mucous membranes. Similar to the flow of tears or saliva, the exudate attempts to reduce the irritation of the sensitive membranes caused by low virulence bacteria, irritating chemicals, poor quality food, dust or allergic substances. While a mucous inflammation is not serious in most cases, it can develop into a more severe reaction. A runny nose is a common example of a mucous inflammation.

(6) LYMPHOCYTIC. Lymphocytic inflammation is characterized by an increased blood supply to the irritated site and the accumulation of lymphocytes in the tissues. This is a frequent sign in inflammations of the central nervous system (rabies), liver, mucous membranes and kidneys. Lymphocytes are found throughout the tissues and lined up outside the walls of blood vessels, giving the appearance of a "cuff" or sleeve in the vessel.

(7) ALTERATIVE. Alterative inflammations cause changes in the cells which lead to necrosis (tissue death). These degenerative changes are due to the action of irritants or toxins from bacteria which are not severe enough to cause a more serious

form of inflammation. Liver damage (as in hepatitis) which results in tissue death is a type of alterative inflammation.

(8) PROLIFERATIVE. Proliferation (the production of new tissue) is the characteristic of a proliferative inflammation. Inflammatory proliferation of fibrous tissue is beyond what is required to repair tissue damage; in some cases, it may cause additional damage. Fibrous connective tissue, bone, cartilage, reticulo-endothelial tissue and epithelium are susceptible to the formation of "proud flesh." This new tissue often appears ulcerated and bloody, bulging above the wound in irregular clumps of knobs or granules. Granulation is caused by infectious, toxic, mechanical or radiational irritants which act with moderate severity for a long period of time. Often, granulation is present because the pathogen lacks the virulence to kill the host (the horse) and the host is not able to produce sufficient antibodies or fever to kill the pathogen. Granulation tissue is the body's attempt to wall off or isolate the irritant. Surface irritations may cause the skin to produce corns to reduce the irritation caused by pressure or rubbing. Strongyle migrations cause fibrous granulation tissue when they damage the delicate arteries and veins, which may result in the formation of obstructions in the blood vessels.

What are the reactive elements in the inflammatory process?

There are three major types of cells involved in the inflammatory process; the reticulo-endothelial cells, leukocytes and plasma cells.

How do the reticulo-endothelial cells participate in inflammation?

Reticulo-endothelial cells have been mentioned in connection with the proliferative inflammation. These cells are notably phagocytic, that is, they absorb and digest foreign particles in the body. They destroy and remove irritants from the scene of infection and are found in the framework of the tissues.

What is the function of the leukocytes?

There are several kinds of leukocytes: neutrophils, basophils, eosinophils, lymphocytes and monocytes. Each performs a slightly different function, although this is not completely understood.

Neutrophils are the most potent of the leukocytes, although they are not capable of reproduction and must be constantly replenished by the bone marrow. Their function is to ingest foreign material, remove dead bacteria and body cells, secrete substances that promote the inflammatory reaction and release a pyrogen (a substance that initiates and maintains fever).

Basophils are not frequently found in the circulating blood. They contain chemicals that cause dilatation of the blood vessels, but their function in the inflammatory process is not understood.

Eosinophils are usually stored in the bone marrow and in the intestinal, lung, skin and vagina walls. They are not present at the start of inflammation, but they have ameboid (independent) movement and appear frequently in allergic inflammations. It is assumed that they limit the inflammatory response because they oppose (are antagonistic) and are drawn to histamine. Eosinophils are phagocytic, so they also serve to reduce the level of irritating substances or bacteria. Corticosteroids greatly reduce the number of eosinophils available at the site of an infection, which is why anti-inflammatory drugs must be used very carefully.

Lymphocytes are the most numerous of the circulating leukocytes and can reproduce to further increase their numbers. It is known that lymphocytes tend to be involved in inflammation of delicate tissues such as liver and brain, but the mechanism of their function is unknown. These cells can also become plasma cells to participate in the immune reaction.

What do plasma cells do in inflammatory reactions?

Plasma cells are not found in the blood, but function most frequently in the tissues of the intestines and the reproductive organs. The plasma cell produces antibodies at the site of the inflammation to combat the invading organisms. They function best in chronic inflammations where they are formed from small lymphocytes.

Do any other cells participate in the inflammatory response?

Most tissue cells may also function in the inflammatory reaction since they contain granules of enzymes that are released when the body responds to irritants.

How long does inflammation last?

An acute inflammation arises suddenly, is characterized by hyperemia, exudative and alterative changes without proliferation, and progresses promptly to either recovery or death. Chronic inflammations begin slowly and indefinitely and continue for long periods of time. Proliferation and the presence of immature new tissue cause an acute inflammation to be called subacute. The presence of any mature granulation tissue classifies an inflammation as chronic. If only mature, proliferated fibrous tissue is present, the inflammatory reaction is considered complete—a scar has formed.

How is the degree of inflammation judged?

Inflammations may be adequate, producing just enough new tissue to heal and close the wound; or they may be inadequate, unable to defeat the infection and repair the damaged tissue. In some cases, inflammation is excessive, causing proud flesh and the obstruction or limitation of function in the affected area. Inflammation can cause damage in certain areas of the body. When inflammation occurs in the foot (Laminitis, page 59), the location of the swelling causes great pressure leading to destruction and pain, possibly resulting in loss of the hoof.

When does healing begin?

Healing begins when the injurious agent is overcome by the inflammatory defenses and the clean-up operation starts. Dead tissues are liquefied by their own enzymes, and the remaining fluid is absorbed into the lymph and blood. The damaged tissue repairs itself by proliferation of fibrous tissue, which can then be replaced by normal tissue. Regeneration is the term for final replacement of inflammation-produced fibrin with tissue of the appropriate kind.

How does tissue regenerate?

Epithelium (skin and mucous membrane tissue) and *mesothelium* (body cavity lining tissue, e.g., peritoneum) regenerate rather easily, but they cannot replace specialized structures (glands, nephrons, hair follicles). Lack of hair development or pigmentation is characteristic of regenerated skin tissue.

Muscle tissues unite by the formation of a scar which enables them to function normally again. Many types of muscles do not replace the fibrous scar tissue with true muscle tissue, however. Tendons and ligaments regenerate slowly, but perfectly, although fibrous adhesions may remain to impair function of the structures.

When *nerves* are damaged, the severed portion (branch of each neuron) dies and may be regenerated by the surviving nerve cell body (or neuron). If the nerve cell body dies, the neuron cannot be replaced. Alternate nerve routes are often developed to carry the motor messages to various parts of the body, thereby restoring at least partial use of a part whose nerve supply was destroyed. This is the goal of physical therapy.

Connective tissue proliferates readily, replacing almost any other kind of tissue easily with scar tissue. Scars eventually lose their rich blood supply and fade to a pale, glossy finish.

Cartilage and bone are first repaired by fibrous connective tissue, formed when the periosteum or bone membrane is irritated, which is then "organized" and converted to imperfect bone. The imperfect tissue is eventually broken down and replaced by more perfect bone.

Blood vessels (capillaries) organize easily in the subacute phase of an inflammatory reaction, but they never develop a muscular wall which is characteristic of arteries or the one-way valves that are common to veins.

Can inflammation be controlled?

Attempts to control inflammation should be made only with the advice and supervision of a veterinarian. Anti-inflammatory drugs may permit any invading organism to destroy delicate structures that cannot be replaced. If there is any possibility of infection, corticosteroids should never be used by non-medical personnel because they are very long lasting in their effects upon the body. Corticosteroids block all aspects of the inflammatory reaction and remove the normal body defenses. Wounds cannot heal properly if inflammation does not take place or is excessive due to added irritation of strong antiseptics. Under the management of a veterinarian, inflammation will be carefully aided or mediated, but will always be respected as the dynamic process of defense and repair. A veterinarian may use corticosteroids to modify the inflammation, in rare cases, but always with the knowledge of their specific actions upon the inflammatory mechanism. Properly managed, drugs can be used to modify or promote the natural process of inflammation and healing.

FEVER

What causes fever in a horse?

The word fever is usually taken to mean an abnormal rise in body temperature, which is not the direct result of diet, exercise or environment. This means, then, that the heightened temperature is usually due to toxins that accompany an infection. Fever may also result when the destruction of tissue causes toxins in the blood. This may happen, for instance, when large parts of a tumor are undergoing necrosis (tissue death), or when burned tissue is being sloughed.

What happens internally to bring on fever?

The temperature of the horse (normally 99.0° to 100.5° F) is controlled by the hypothalamus, which is at the base of the brain. The hypothalamus causes fever by bringing into action a cold defense mechanism and inhibiting the heat loss mechanism. This occurs when it is stimulated by endopyrogen, a substance released from infection-fighting cells of the body. This entire chain may be set into motion by endotoxins, which are produced by infectious bacteria. Endopyrogens may also be released without the presence of infection, such as when a fever accompanies surgical recovery.

What are the external signs of fever?

In the initial stages of fever, constriction of the vessels near the surface of the skin brings on "chills" and the skin feels cold. In spite of this, body temperature, taken through the rectum, is higher, and the pulse is faster (than the normal 44 beats per minute). The activity of shivering caused by the chills results in a further increase in temperature, and it is at this stage that sweating begins. The vessels in the skin dilate, and the skin itself feels warm to the touch. At the peak of the fever, sweating may stop entirely. After the fever has "broken," muscles go limp, sweating begins again and body temperature falls.

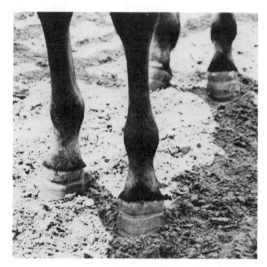

Fig. 1-4. Fever rings are visible on this colt's feet following a severe illness which was accompanied by a prolonged fever.

During this process, the horse may feel the same sort of discomfort common to fever in humans. General weakness, sensitivity to touch and irritability may be expected.

Is fever harmful?

Beyond an increase in temperature of about 10°, the body is not capable of sustaining life. Even before this point is reached, there may be damage to tissue, and severe loss of fluids through sweating can lead to dehydration. However, many organisms that are dangerous to the health can only grow slowly and with great difficulty where a fever exists. Phagocytes and antibodies, the cells that fight infection in the body, can carry on their activities at a stepped-up pace during periods of fever. In other words, a fever is actually a beneficial body process.

How is a fever treated?

Since fever can accompany most infections, a veterinarian should be called to determine the exact cause. When this is done, the fever is best controlled by removing the source of the inflammation. Antibacterial drugs may be used against infection, or if dead tissue is the cause, it should be removed. If the temperature becomes high enough to be dangerous to the horse, drugs are available, through the veterinarian, which act directly on the temperature control mechanism. (Aspirin has this effect on humans.) These are generally not administered, though, until it is established that all sources of inflammation are removed.

NON-INFLAMMATORY EDEMA

What is non-inflammatory edema?

Edema is a disorder of the fluid-regulating mechanism of the body. Non-inflammatory edema is characterized by the presence of excess fluid between the cells within the body tissues.

What causes edema?

There are several causes of edema in the horse, all of them involving a dysfunction (breakdown) of the fluid regulating system. Parasite infections, poor nutrition and heart and kidney disorders are the primary causes of failure of the body to maintain a balance of fluid between the circulation and tissues.

Where does the edema fluid come from?

The fluid found within the body tissues in non-inflammatory edema comes from the blood and lymph circulation (See Anatomy of Blood, page 447). Normal pressure in the arteries causes much of the fluid to escape from the circulation before the capillaries return the blood to the veins. Low pressure in the veins allows fluid to filter back into the capillaries as the blood cells continue to move slowly toward the venous circulation. Abnormal protein or salt content in the blood alters its chemical balance, and the pressure of the tissue outside the blood vessels allows more fluid to filter through the capillary walls out into the tissue spaces. This abnormal protein or salt content may be caused by disorders of the kidneys or imbalances in the diet. Lack of blood pressure from heart disorders can also cause the blood pressure to be inadequate for efficient fluid circulation. Parasites affect the fluid circulation by blocking arteries and veins, causing hemorrhages and drawing fluid and proteins from the blood circulation.

What are the signs of edema?

Unlike inflammatory edema, non-inflammatory edema is not accompanied by pain and heat. Non-inflammatory edematous swellings are cool and painless and retain pressure marks when they are pressed. Swellings which retain the imprint of a finger are said to "pit" on pressure.

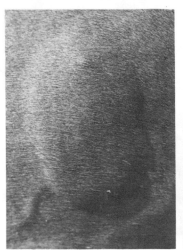 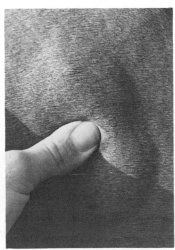 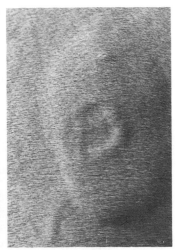

Fig. 1-5. Example of the "pitting" in non-inflammatory edema.

Where is edema found?

Depending on the cause, edema may occur in all parts of the body. Generalized edema (not caused by a local blockage or circulatory failure) tends to sink to the lowest part of the body. Most frequently, it forms "ventral or midline edema," along the lower side of the abdomen and sternum. There is usually a well-defined ridge

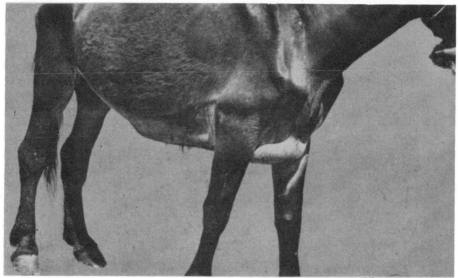

Courtesy of CLINICAL DIAGNOSIS OF DISEASES OF LARGE ANIMALS, Lea and Febiger Publishing Co., Philadelphia, Pa., W. J. Gibbons, D.V.M.

Fig. 1-6. An example of ventral edema in an aged mule.

along the side of the belly where the edema stops. In some cases, it even involves the skin of the sheath in male horses. A frequent location of edema is the hind legs. Lack of exercise (in stalled horses) can cause the lower legs to "stock up" or swell with edema. This type of edema can also affect the front legs, if exercise and muscular movement are greatly limited.

What are the effects of edema?

Most non-inflammatory edemas do not remain in the area after the cause is removed. In some cases, the edema may organize, or form adhesions between the tissue spaces, leaving the tissues permanently separated and swollen. Because non-inflammatory edema does not specifically attempt to heal or transport materials (see inflammation), it is not as likely to form adhesions as is the exudate in inflammatory edema.

How may edema be treated?

Since edema is usually a secondary disorder, most veterinarians look for (and treat) the cause. Diuretics may be used to give temporary relief in some cases of severe local edema, but the judgment of the veterinarian is important to insure that an essential underlying problem is not being ignored. Protein and chemical balance of the blood may be checked by a laboratory, and the veterinarian may wish to send a fecal or urine sample if he suspects parasite or kidney disorders. Edema due to lack of exercise can be prevented by supportive elastic bandages, but it usually disappears quickly when the horse is exercised.

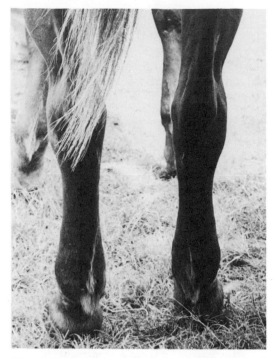

Fig. 1-7. Back view of stocked-up hind legs.

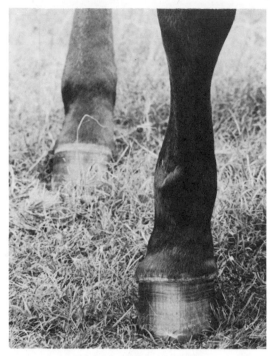

Fig. 1-8. Front view of stocked-up legs. Notice the "filling" in the front legs.

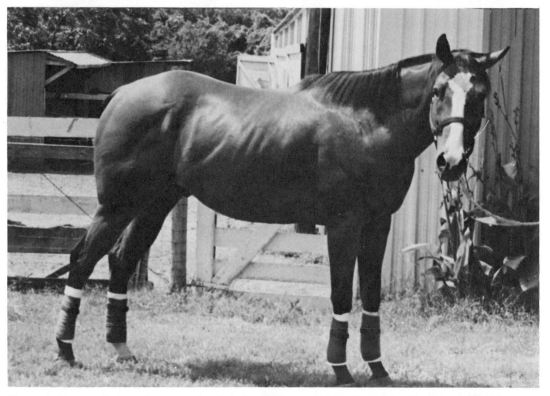

Fig. 1-9. Protective and supportive bandaging can reduce "stocking-up" in stalled horses that receive limited exercise.

ARTHRITIS

What is arthritis?

There are many different types of arthritis, characterized by the cause and effect of the disability. Generally speaking, arthritis is any inflammation of the tissues associated with a joint. The importance of early diagnosis and differential treatment makes the condition difficult to deal with as a single disorder. For more complete coverage, refer to joint ill (septicemia), spavin, salmonellosis, etc., and their disease processes.

What are the various types of arthritis?

The most common form of arthritis is chronic osteoarthritis, characterized by deterioration of the articular cartilages and joint surfaces. This type of arthritis includes ringbone, spavin, osselets and various other stress injuries. Perhaps the next frequently occurring form is acute serous arthritis resulting from trauma to the joint. Purulent (infectious) arthritis is the most common form in foals, and is involved in navel ill or lacerations of a joint capsule. Characterized by the formation of pus following infection, erosion of bone and articular cartilage is very likely in this form of arthritis.

What are the causes of arthritis?

Arthritis may be caused by a blow to the joint, concussion, blood-borne infections, and punctures or tears of the joint sac. Some horses are more susceptible to various forms or locations of inflammation. Faulty conformation or poor nutrition resulting in bone deficiencies can predispose a horse to chronic osteoarthritis. Foals are most susceptible to blood-borne infections (septicemia) which settle in joints. Severe joint injury is usually due to destruction of the lubricating properties of the synovial joint fluid, if the initial infection does not destroy the joint cartilages first. Arthritic inflammations accompany many infections and are fully explained in the respective disorders.

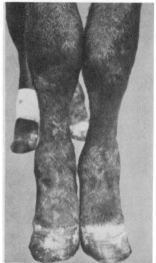 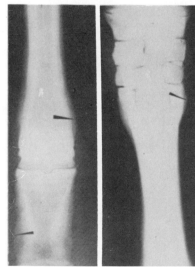

Courtesy of LAMENESS IN HORSES, Edition III, O. R. Adams, Lea and Febiger Publishing Co., Philadelphia, Pa.

Fig. 1-10. Swelling and bone growth due to pulmonary osteoarthropathy. This rare disorder is thought to be caused by a lung infection which produces toxins that inflame the bones. In some cases, the bones grow to twice their normal size.

What are the signs of arthritis?

Most forms of arthritis involve severe pain in the affected joint and great reluctance to bend or use the limb. If the inflammation of the joint is an active or recent process, there will be a swelling or distension of the joint capsule and the surrounding tissues. Heat and swelling will be present in the joint area and movement will be very painful. If the condition is chronic (of long standing), there

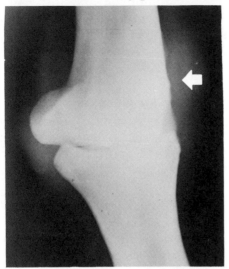

Fig. 1-11. This x-ray shows the soft tissue swelling that accompanies arthritis.

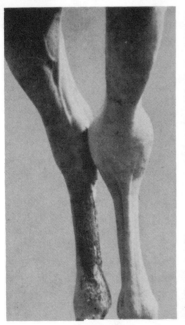
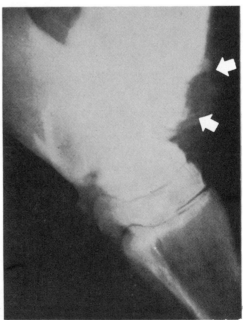

Courtesy of LAMENESS IN HORSES, Edition III, O. R. Adams, Lea and Febiger Publishing Co., Philadelphia, Pa.

Fig. 1-12. Periarticular arthritis of infectious origin. The picture of the clinical case on the left shows involvement of the left hock. The disease starts with diffuse swelling of the periarticular structures and eventually works its way into the joint, leaving either a severe osteoarthritis or ankylosis of the joint. The radiograph on the right shows the same hock. Note the extensive bone changes on the distal end of the tibia and tibial tarsal bone. There are also periosteal changes on the cranial aspect of the central and third tarsal bones.

may be greatly reduced movement in the joint due to fibrous adhesions and degeneration of the articular surfaces. Severe or prolonged arthritis involves solidification of the joint by new bone growth.

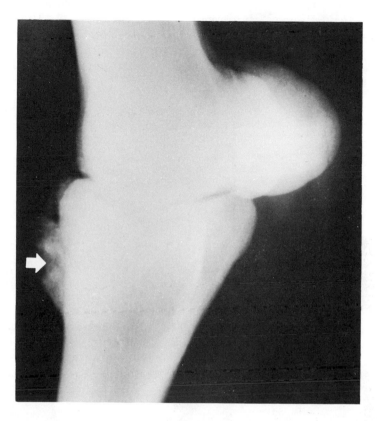

Fig. 1-13. X-ray of the fetlock showing new bone growths.

What treatment should be given?

The treatment depends on the type of arthritis involved. Chronic osteoarthritis is usually treated with X-ray therapy, counterirritants, blisters, pin-firing, ultrasonic therapy, or surgical fusion, depending on how early in the course of the disease it is diagnosed. Following any of the treatments, a period of six months' rest is required. During this period, corticosteroids may be administered to relieve joint discomfort and encourage use of the limb. If movement is too restricted, the joint may lose a great deal of movement from the formation of adhesions and mineral deposits.

Purulent arthritis is best treated with systemic antibiotics to control the infection. The joint contents may be aspirated (withdrawn) and antibiotics injected directly into the joint capsule. Phenylbutazone helps to relieve pain and allow movement of the limb to prevent adhesions until the joint returns to normal.

When the arthritis involves only one joint, as does serous arthritis, rest and application of cold water or ice to relieve pain are very effective. As with purulent arthritis, the fluid contents of the joint may be aspirated and the joint injected with corticosteroids. In treatment of arthritis, the absolute rest and relief of pain in the affected limb are very important. Moderate use as in stall rest and very light exercise in hand, but no riding or work, will prevent restriction of movement when the worst inflammation has been reduced.

Can arthritis be prevented?

To some extent, arthritis can be prevented. Proper shoeing of horses with faulty conformation can remove some stress from overworked joints. Navel stump disinfection and antibiotic treatment of newborn foals can minimize navel ill and joint ill. Prevention of recurring arthritic episodes in older horses is difficult, but corticosteroids have been found to be helpful. The most meaningful prevention consists of rapid treatment before the joint surfaces are worn away and joint movement is restricted. Prompt veterinary diagnosis and treatment can accomplish this best.

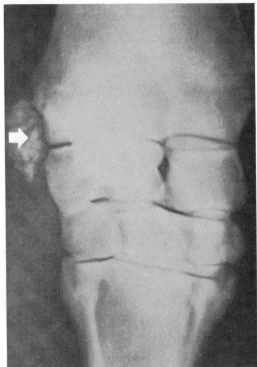

Courtesy of LAMENESS IN HORSES, Edition III, O. R. Adams, Lea and Febiger Publishing Co., Philadelphia, Pa.

Fig. 1-14. Calcified hematoma resulting from injection of the carpus with a corticoid. When passing the needle into a joint there is a danger of hitting blood vessels. In some cases the resulting hemorrhage will calcify as shown. A small needle, and an attempt to miss all skin vessels when passing the needle, will help in preventing such a complication. Calcification is sometimes caused by the long-acting corticoids when injected into soft tissue, presumably by the chemicals used to delay absorption.

NECROSIS AND GANGRENE

What is necrosis?

Necrosis is the death of cells or body tissue while the body is still alive. This tissue death may affect the body systemically, or the body may function normally while this process is going on. Necrosis is frequently involved in inflammation.

What causes necrosis?

There are many causes of necrosis. Any kind of poison (chemicals, plants, tissue toxins) may cause tissue death, either directly or indirectly. Poisons (like insecticides) may cause direct tissue damage when they come in contact with the mucous membranes of the intestines or they may cause liver damage, if they have been diluted and are absorbed by the body. Mechanical injuries and burns frequently cause immediate necrosis and inflammation. If cells are deprived of blood or nerves, they usually die. Sweeney is a good example of tissue death caused by nerve damage (see Sweeney, page 253). Prolonged or severe pressure also results in necrosis.

What are the results of necrosis?

During the course of inflammation, the body attacks foreign bacteria and toxins, and loses many cells that have been damaged by the irritating substance that initiated the process. The death of these body cells (necrosis) is followed by break-down of the dead cells by their own cell enzymes and those of the leukocytes. This is called liquefaction, the most common result of necrosis. In some cases, however, the dead cell products may be walled off in cyst-like accumulations or abscesses. Sometimes the tissue is sloughed off (as in photosensitization) or is replaced by scar tissue (as in liver or kidney damage). Death of bone periosteum can result in calcification as is the case with splints, or regeneration of perfect tissue (replacement of fibrous proliferation with good bone). One of the unfortunate results of necrosis is gangrene.

Does necrosis cause gangrene?

Necrosis does not cause gangrene, but it must occur before gangrene can develop. Gangrene is the invasion of dead tissue by saprophytic bacteria (bacteria that can only live on dead tissue). They produce strong toxins that are very irritating and damaging to the surrounding living tissues.

How does the body react to these toxins?

The body reacts to the saphrophytic bacteria with inflammation. In cases of gangrene, a line of inflammation can be seen between the dead tissue and the healthy tissue. When skin or tissue is sloughed, it is an attempt by the body to get rid of an overwhelming amount of toxic or gangrenous material. Infarctions of the intestine frequently develop gangrene in long segments of the intestine due to the availability of saprophytic bacteria in the intestinal contents. Also, peritonitis may be associated with gangrene.

How is gangrene recognized?

Gangrene is characterized by a foul smell, if the gangrenous tissue is open to the surface of the body. Necrotic tissue often appears pale, but it may be very black if it contains a great deal of coagulated blood. There usually is no heat or pain in the affected area. Moist, swollen, black or dark tissue may be affected with moist gangrene. If the affected tissues have a limited supply of blood, they may appear light colored, shriveled, dry and leather-like. These are characteristics of dry gangrene.

What is the result of gangrene?

In most cases, the gangrenous limb or tissues are separated from the body (sloughed). If this process is not rapid enough, the horse may develop septicemia or other serious infections. Any suspected cases of gangrene should be treated by a veterinarian to avoid the spread of bacteria throughout the body. The usual mode of treatment is surgical removal of the gangrenous tissue.

SEPTICEMIA (BLOOD POISONING)

What is septicemia?

Septicemia is a systemic disease state caused by the presence and persistence of large numbers of pathogenic (disease-causing) microorganisms or their toxins in the blood. These organisms or toxins cause fever, a rapid pulse rate and marked prostration which is frequently followed by death.

What causes septicemia?

There are many organisms that cause septicemia. It is frequently the cause of death in neonatal infections of *Streptococcus zooepidemicus, Escherichia coli, Actinobacillus equuli, Salmonella, Listeria monocytogenes, Staphylococcus aureus* and *Klebsiella*.

How does septicemia affect the body?

The metabolism of pathogenic bacteria produces toxins which act as poisons in the body of the horse. Toxins interfere in carbohydrate metabolism, resulting in a fall in the blood sugar level (hypoglycemia). Other damage to enzyme systems and endocrine glands combines with the hypoglycemia to reduce the functions of most tissues. In septicemia, the infection may localize in a joint or an organ, causing direct tissue damage which releases more toxic substances that are by-products of the tissue damage. The systemic reaction of shock tends to magnify any imbalance, causing the circulation to suffer when the heart muscle loses tone (see Shock, p. 1), which deprives vital organs of the blood necessary to carry out their functions. Dysfunction of the liver and kidneys, due to poor circulation, leads to a buildup of the normal body wastes which are usually excreted, increasing the toxic rate. Loss of tone in skeletal and digestive muscles adds to the general weakening of the body which is expressed by dullness, depression and coma. If these reactions are not reversed, death follows.

What are the signs of septicemia?

The signs of septicemia are fever, hemorrhages under the skin or mucous membranes, depression, lethargy, a weak, rapid pulse and eventual collapse. Signs of localization vary with the area infected, which may be the joints, heart valves, nerves, eyes or various internal organs. In foals, localization in the eyes (blindness) and joints (pyoarthritis) is a frequent effect of septicemia. Systemic reactions are not easily reversed, which makes early attention by a veterinarian most important.

How is septicemia treated?

Treatment with antibacterial drugs and antitoxins must be provided quickly to stop the septic progression. In young foals, treatment is often too late because they have no defenses against even the common bacteria found in most stalls or foaling areas. Prevention is the best treatment for foals. Most horses require intravenous administration of fluids and electrolytes to maintain their circulation, in addition to stimulants given by the veterinarian to support respiration. Usually, the veterinarian will use adrenocortical hormones to reduce inflammation and aid in healing.

Can septicemia be prevented?

In many cases septicemia can be prevented. It is highly fatal in foals which suggests that hygiene in foaling is frequently poor. Prompt treatment of the navel stump with iodine prevents many infections from entering the body. Colostrum should always be provided as soon as possible, since it is the only source of antibodies that a foal can utilize.

Older horses develop septicemia primarily from neglect of wounds and infections. All infected wounds should receive treatment and infection should be prevented whenever possible. Sensible care and nursing will usually prevent mild infections from becoming septic.

DEHYDRATION

What is dehydration?

Dehydration is a state of the body in which more fluid (water) is lost than is absorbed.

What causes dehydration?

Excessive fluid loss may be caused by fever, diseases accompanied by diarrhea, severe hemorrhage and increased sweating or urination. Lack of fluid intake frequently occurs when animals are sick, but may also be caused by the absence of available water.

What are the signs of dehydration?

Dehydration may cause a slight rise in body temperature, an increased respiratory rate and a small, weak pulse. As dehydration advances, the skin loses its pliability and appears dry and wrinkled. The skin may seem too large for the body, hanging in loose folds and wrinkles. Fat recedes from around the eyeballs allowing them to sink into the skull, and the rest of the body drops weight rapidly. Muscular weakness, lack of appetite and increased thirst are seen until the animal becomes depressed and goes into a coma. Circulatory collapse and muscle tremors are terminal signs.

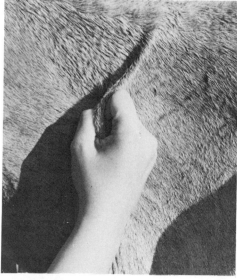

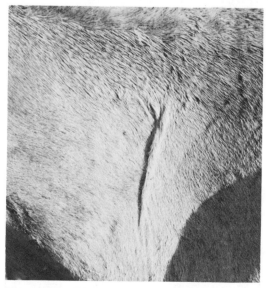

Fig. 1-15. When the skin is grasped, it wrinkles easily due to the loss of muscle tone.

Fig. 1-16. When the skin is released, it returns to its original position very slowly, if at all.

What are the effects of dehydration?

When sufficient fluid is not absorbed, the body first draws upon available water between and in the tissues. Essential organs and systems contribute little fluid, the majority of which is drawn from the connective tissue, muscles and the skin.

If fluid is still needed, the body draws fluid from the circulating blood, which causes the blood to become thicker and less effective in circulation. Fluid drawn from the tissues disturbs tissue metabolism and causes chemical imbalances in the body (electrolyte imbalance).

How is dehydration treated?

When dehydration is due to lack of available water, treatment consists of allowing the horse to drink small quantities at frequent intervals. Dehydration due to excessive fluid losses must be treated by a veterinarian. Since body chemicals (electrolytes) are also lost in dehydration, the veterinarian must determine the proper solution and rate of administration. Many cases of dehydration are associated with digestive disorders, so fluids are not usually given by stomach tube. Intravenous administration of electrolyte solutions is usually continued until some effect is visible. Potassium salts promote the restoration of fluid within the tissues and are usually included in fluid therapy. Care must be taken to regulate the fluid flow to prevent overload of the stressed circulatory system or cardiac failure might occur.

HEMORRHAGE

What is hemorrhage?

Hemorrhage is the uncontrolled escape of blood from a vessel. This may allow blood to travel outside the body, into a body cavity or into surrounding tissue spaces.

What causes hemorrhage?

Hemorrhage may be caused by: (1) a mechanical break or cut in the wall of a blood vessel, (2) death or destruction of a vessel by an ulcer or tumor, (3) rupture of a vessel wall when it is weakened or partially destroyed by parasites or larvae, (4) injuries to the vessel wall from toxins or poisons, (5) disorders of the clotting mechanism, or (6) rupture of vessels from increased pressure due to excitement or exercise (stress).

What are the effects of hemorrhage?

If the hemorrhage is acute, the major effects are loss of blood volume, plasma proteins and red blood cells. Rapid blood loss may cause failure of the peripheral circulation and shock. Tissue death may occur due to lack of oxygen and the buildup of tissue waste products. Less rapid blood loss may be replaced temporarily by blood stored in the spleen and liver and the withdrawal of fluid from the tissue spaces. This sometimes causes chemical imbalances in the body which result in edema, dehydration and anemia.

What are the signs of hemorrhage?

Visible signs of hemorrhage include pallor of the mucous membranes, weakness, staggering and recumbency (lying down), rapid heart rate and a subnormal temperature. Most animals with a considerable amount of hemorrhage are very thirsty. Various types of lesions may be noticed, depending on the type of bleeding.

Seepage of blood from damaged tissues may be slow (one cell at a time, turning serous exudates light pink), or rapid, pulsating or flowing in a stream from breaks in the skin. Tiny, pinpoint hemorrhages are called petechiae and are seen most frequently on mucous membranes. Larger spots are called ecchymoses but large areas are termed extravasations. Hematomas are formed when blood escapes into the tissues and produces a tumor-like enlargement. This is the "blood blister" that forms when the skin is severely pinched.

How are hemorrhages treated?

The first concern in the treatment of hemorrhage is the control of bleeding and the replacement of all portions of the blood. Volume as well as cellular components must be restored in order to prevent peripheral circulatory failure. Whole blood is the best replacement, especially if blood-matched donors are available. At least one-fourth to one-third of the total blood volume must be lost to cause death. When fluid loss is replaced with plasma, plasma expanders or saline solutions, the body requires one to two weeks to replace white blood cells and four to six weeks to replace red blood cells.

ANEMIA

What is anemia?

Anemia is not a disease, but a condition of the blood characterized by a deficiency in the quality or quantity of the erythrocytes (circulating red blood cells) and hemoglobin (oxygen-carrying element of the red blood cells).

What are the causes of anemia?

There are four major causes of anemia in the horse. They are: (1) decreased production of erythrocytes, (2) decreased production of hemoglobin, (3) increased destruction of erythrocytes, and (4) the loss of large amounts of blood.

What causes a decreased production of red blood cells?

Normal production and replacement of red blood cells depends heavily on good nutrition and physical health. The most common causes of low red cell count are heavy parasite infestations by strongyles and poor quality feed. This failure to supply proper nutrition and ensure its proper assimilation is the principal cause of anemia in the horse.

Decreased production of red blood cells also accompanies bacterial and viral infections, and can be caused by a suppurative (pus-forming) condition. These anemias are usually reversible by removing the cause.

What causes insufficient hemoglobin production?

Improper nutrition is a major cause of hemoglobin deficiency in horses. The lack of copper, vitamin E and iron in a balanced diet will result in pale erythrocytes, which are normal in number but deficient in hemoglobin. Since hemoglobin is the element which combines with oxygen for transport to the tissues, a deficiency in the amount or quality of hemoglobin can be as serious as a reduction in the number of circulating red blood cells.

What causes increased red cell destruction?

In some horses, exposure to oxidant drugs (such as phenothiazine) can shorten the life span of older red blood cells, especially if the animal is in a weakened condition from some ongoing disease process. Red cells may also be coated by antibodies and removed by the spleen, or pathogenic organisms may become attached to red blood cells, causing hemolysis (rupture) and further stress to the system with the released toxins. Piroplasmosis and equine infectious anemia (EIA) are always accompanied by hemolysis. Incompatibility of blood types between a mare and a stallion may result in antibody coating and hemolysis of red blood cells in the foal, if the mare has been sensitized by the pregnancy. This condition is called neonatal isoerythrolysis (see page 474).

Can defective erythrocytes cause a loss of red blood cells?

Yes. General poor nutrition is the primary cause of fragile or misshapen red cells. Deficiency of a certain enzyme (G6PD) within a red blood cell can make it more fragile and subject to removal by the spleen. Though it happens rarely, high levels of radiation can cause defects in the bone marrow which impair the mechanism of red blood cell production. This results in immature and defective red blood cells being released into the blood stream, where they may cause blockages (thrombosis) before the spleen can remove them.

Can anemias be rapid and temporary?

Yes. A temporary state of anemia can be caused by severe or recurring hemorrhage following serious wounds or episodes of epistaxis (nosebleed). These anemias are easily reversed if the overall body condition is not lowered by massive infection or continued blood loss. Since hemorrhages involve the loss of red blood cells, white blood cells, and plasma (the transporting fluid), transfusions of plasma or whole blood are usually required when the loss is severe. If whole blood is not transfused, the red blood cell numbers will rise slowly because the body replaces plasma proteins and restores volume to the circulation much more quickly than it can increase the production and replace all of the red and white blood cells. Anemia associated with hemorrhage is usually overlooked because shock is generally present. In these cases, restoration of the body fluid levels is the most immediately important aspect of treatment. Due to the great number of white blood cells lost in severe hemorrhage, the animal is open to severe infection, so antibiotics should probably be administered.

What are the signs of anemia?

The general signs of anemia are poor hair coat, pallor of the mucous membranes, muscular weakness, depression, lack of appetite, and an increased heart rate. Conditions that may accompany anemia are edema, jaundice, and hemoglobinuria (the presence of hemoglobin in the urine). Hemoglobinemia (the presence of free hemoglobin in the blood plasma) accompanies the hemolytic anemias in which red blood cells rupture while still in circulation. Clinical signs of anemia may not be apparent until the level of hemoglobin in the blood falls to as low as 50 percent of normal.

What is the treatment for anemia?

Anemia is usually treated by treating its source first. Poor nutrition, parasitic infestations, viral and bacterial infections and severe hemorrhages must be dealt with before the anemia can be corrected. In many cases, removal of the associated condition (infection, infestation, etc.) takes enough pressure off the sytem to allow it to spontaneously return to normal within a month or two. If immediate treatment is required, however, iron is usually given in the feed or water and vitamin B12 has been proven an effective non-specific hematinic (hemoglobin booster). If the horse has ever received a transfusion before, subsequent transfusions should be attempted only after careful cross-matching of blood types to prevent hemolytic reactions. In the case of a newborn foal with isoerythrolysis, this cross-matching is an absolute necessity unless the sire is immediately available as a blood donor. The sire's blood is known to be compatible with the blood of his foal in an isoerythrolysis case.

Can anemia be prevented?

In most cases, anemia can be prevented quite easily. Good sanitary management, regular worming schedules, and good quality feed are the best preventatives. Anemias associated with disease processes usually respond to successful treatment of the disease or deficiency. Mineral supplements may be required for horses in some areas. (For detailed information on equine nutritional requirements refer to the text FEEDING TO WIN.)

NEOPLASMS

What is a neoplasm?

The word "tumor" is generally used to describe a neoplasm. Although there are many different kinds of neoplasms, they all have several basic characteristics in common. First of all, they multiply and grow continuously, seemingly with no limit. Although the individual cells are quite similar to the healthy cells where the neoplasm started, they are not arranged in an orderly manner. They serve no useful purpose, and their cause is not well understood.

Are neoplasms harmful?

A benign neoplasm is one which grows slowly, looks much like the tissue in which it is growing, and has a definite "border." Unless this kind of tumor interferes with the functions of the body, it is not particularly dangerous.

Malignant neoplasms are called cancerous in human beings, a term not popularly applied to horses. In all species they grow quite rapidly, infiltrating the body through a process called metastasis. If metastasis occurs through the lymph glands, malignant cells may break off and be carried by the lymph vessels to surrounding areas, where they grow again. This process is called embolism. If the cells simply grow along the vessel walls and pass through the walls to surrounding tissue, the process is called permeation. The cells may also be metastasized through the bloodstream, which carries the malignancy to the lungs. The process of metastasis makes the tumors very difficult to isolate and potentially fatal.

What makes this growth potentially fatal?

Malignant cells have the quality of hardiness, and seem to be able to survive with little oxygen. Healthy cells cannot compete with malignant ones for available space, and everything in the path of the unhealthy cells, including bone, is destroyed. Often the simple pressure of the runaway growth stops a vital function, and brings death in this manner.

Are some neoplasms more malignant than others?

At present, there are not even solid boundaries between the terms "benign" and "malignant." Sometimes there are obvious differences: a tumor attached by a slender "neck," for instance, is not likely to be malignant. An ulcerated tumor, or one that "spreads out" is malignant more often. Tumors that have been benign, though, for long periods of time, may suddenly begin to act malignant. An obviously malignant growth may have an unexplained slowdown.

The judgment concerning a tumor's malignancy is partially based on microscopic evidence about the number, size, and normality of the tissue cells. Also considered important is the manner of growth. If a tumor has metastasized, it is undoubtedly malignant. The basic determining factor, though, is the degree of "anaplasia" that the growth shows. By definition, the more "anaplastic" a cell is, the less it resembles its original "parent" (normal) cell in form, function and manner of growth.

Why is anaplasia important?

The degree of anaplasia of a growth is commonly measured in grades. Grade 1 most closely resembles the original cells; grade 4 cells are hardly recognizable. Since grade 1 cells do not grow as quickly, surgical removal of the tumor may be successful. Grade 3 and 4 tumors, however, are much more susceptible to radiation treatment than are the others. Of course, more than one degree of anaplasia may be present at once, but knowing the degree of malignancy does help in assessing the situation.

Where can a neoplasm occur?

Any part of the body can be subject to a neoplastic growth. The body contains many different kinds of cells, and nearly every one of them is subject to a distinct kind of neoplasm with a distinct appearance and behavior. There are several general groupings of neoplasms, however, based on the similarity of the tissue in each group. There are four separate groups as follows: (1) supporting tissue, (2) epithelium (covering tissue), (3) pigment tissue, and (4) teratomas.

What kind of neoplasms occur in supporting tissue?

The term "supporting tissue" refers to connective tissue, muscle, blood and lymph tissue. The name of a neoplasm in this group gives considerable information about its nature and location. A name ending in "-oma" indicates that the tumor is benign. A word ending in "-sarcoma" indicates malignancy. "Blastoma" is usually reserved for tumors involving immature or embryonic cells.

Supporting tissue appears in nearly every part of the body, but the first syllables of the name of the neoplasm indicate the type of tissue involved. As an example, the most common neoplasm of the blood-forming tissues is the lymphosarcoma; a malignant tumor of the lymph system. Even under this classification there are several types of neoplasms, each of which progresses differently. As with other neoplasms in this group, if metastasis spreads the disorder throughout the body, secondary kinds of neoplasms may occur. In brief, the supportive tissue is capable of all degrees of malignancy, which may affect nearly any area of the body.

What kind of neoplasms occur in the epithelium?

The epithelium is subject to four basic types of neoplasms. The papilloma is benign, and consists of a group of small projections (papillae) which may sometimes be considered warts (see Warts, page 401). Although they occur most frequently on the skin, they have also appeared in the intestines and in the pancreas.

The glands are affected by adenomas, which are benign, and carcinomas, which are malignant. Their interference with the functioning of those glands may produce astonishing results. A tumor of the adrenal cortex, for instance, where a masculine hormone is manufactured, may cause a mare to develop a stallion's crest and voice.

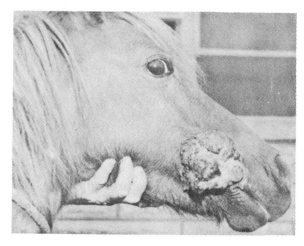
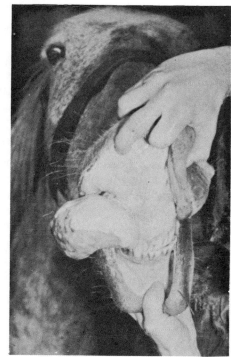

Photos this page courtesy of VETERINARY SURGERY, Edition VI, E. R. Frank, Burgess Publishing Co., Minneapolis, Minn.

Fig. 1-17. An example of a fibrosarcoma. Growths of this type frequently recur if they are surgically removed.

Fig. 1-18. Osteoma of the premaxilla.

Other epithelial structures are also affected by carcinomas which are malignant. The most frequent site of these growths is the eye, but any mucous membrane is highly susceptible.

What kind of neoplasms affect the nervous system?

Tumors of the nervous system begin in the supportive tissue (neuroglia), and are called "gliomas." There are six kinds of supporting tissue, but only five produce gliomas. Tumors originating in the nervous system do not often metastasize to other parts of the body, but the more malignant ones may spread very rapidly through the brain and spinal cord.

What neoplasms occur in pigment tissue?

Melanomas are neoplasms of pigmented (melanin-forming) cells. They are most

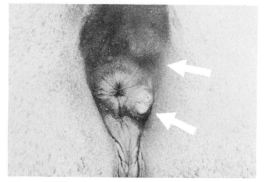
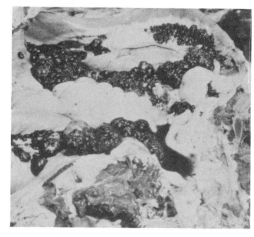

Fig. 1-19. A melanoma of the ventral surface of the tail has metastasized, involving the tissues of the abdominal cavity.

common in grey horses, and are usually found in the area just under the tail (see Skin and Hair, page 404).

What are teratomas?

Teratomas are distinctive because of their origins. They usually appear near the body midline, and evidence suggests that they exist before birth. They begin in one of the "layers" of the fetus, and usually show up during young life. A good example of this is a dentigerous cyst, which contains a jumbled mass of fluid, cartilage and bone (see Dentigerous Cyst, page 343).

Are there any suspected causes of neoplasms?

Several theories have been proposed regarding the origin of neoplasms, none of which offer a wholly adequate explanation. Chronic irritation, for instance, seems to have a high coincidence with cancer in humans. Horses, however, irritated and injured constantly by collars, had virtually no neoplasms where contact with the collar took place. On the other hand, it is accepted that the constant irritation of parasites may "set up" the conditions for neoplasms to start.

In areas of constant and intense sunlight, it is fairly well established that constant exposure to the sun greatly increases the risk of neoplasms. Exposure to radiation and chemicals (such as the chemicals in cigarette smoke) have been proven to produce neoplasms under laboratory conditions.

Causation by viruses has been examined, along with the presence of excess hormones, and the possibility that the tendency toward neoplasms is inherited. In each case, the conclusions are incomplete.

In general, two statements may be safely made. First of all, the affected tissue of a neoplasm was probably disturbed in its early life. Secondly, there is usually a "lag" between the time of exposure and the time when growth begins. This encourages the belief that the causes may "accumulate," and must reach a certain level before a neoplasm occurs.

How are neoplasms treated?

At present, surgical removal of the neoplasm is most favored, but some success has been obtained with radiation treatment. The outcome of such treatments depends on a wide variety of factors, the most important being the degree of malignancy at the time of treatment. Even this is not a dependable measure, though, since a benign tumor may be "stimulated" into malignancy by surgery. In general, the prognosis is fair if a removed growth does not grow back.

2

FOOT

ANATOMY AND PHYSIOLOGY

Do the words "foot" and "hoof" mean the same thing?

No. Foot refers to the hoof and all its internal structures. The hoof is only the cornified epithelium (horny covering) of the foot including the wall, the sole and the frog. It is nonvascular (does not have a blood supply) and has no nerve supply.

What are the major structures of the foot?

The four major structures of the foot are: (1) the bones; (2) the sensitive structure; (3) the insensitive structure; and (4) the elastic structure. (Discussion of each to follow.)

Which bones are in the foot?

The foot contains the coffin bone, the navicular bone and the lower portion of the short pastern bone.

What is the structure and location of these bones?

The short pastern bone extends downward from the long pastern bone to just below the coronet. Therefore, half of the short pastern bone is considered part of the pastern region, while the other half is contained within the foot, where it articulates with the coffin bone and the navicular bone.

The coffin bone is shaped much like the hoof. The bottom part, called the sole surface (because it faces the sole of the foot), is shaped somewhat like a half-moon.

The distal sesamoid bone (also called the shuttle or navicular bone, and for purposes of this text referred to as the navicular bone) is wedge-shaped and lies behind the short pastern bone and the coffin bone in the coffin joint. It has a pulley-like action which changes the direction of pull of the deep digital flexor tendon on the coffin bone. The deep digital flexor tendon passes over the back of the navicular bone, holding it firmly in the joint. The sides of this bone are enclosed by the wings of the coffin bone.

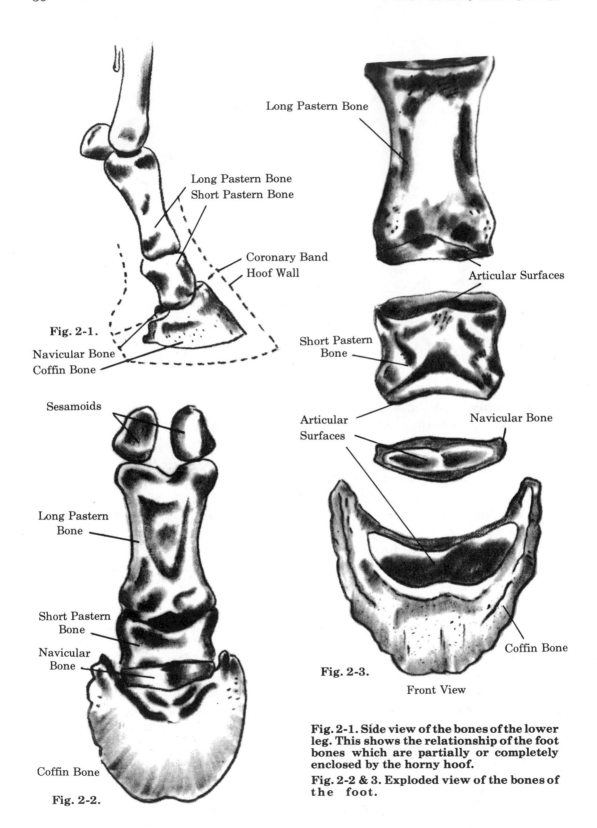

Fig. 2-1.

Long Pastern Bone
Short Pastern Bone

Coronary Band
Hoof Wall

Navicular Bone
Coffin Bone

Sesamoids

Long Pastern
Bone

Short Pastern
Bone

Navicular
Bone

Coffin Bone

Fig. 2-2.

Long Pastern Bone

Articular Surfaces

Short Pastern
Bone

Articular
Surfaces

Navicular Bone

Coffin Bone

Fig. 2-3.

Front View

Fig. 2-1. Side view of the bones of the lower leg. This shows the relationship of the foot bones which are partially or completely enclosed by the horny hoof.

Fig. 2-2 & 3. Exploded view of the bones of the foot.

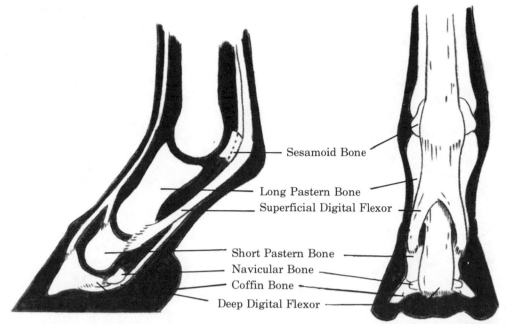

Fig. 2-4. Side and back views showing attachments of extensor, superficial and deep flexor tendons. Notice the pulley action over the navicular and sesamoid bones.

What are the wings of the coffin bone?

The wings of the coffin bone are small extensions of bone on each side of the coffin bone, located inside the heel of the hoof wall. On their upper surface, the wings give attachment to the lateral cartilages. These cartilages can be easily felt above the coronet as they form the contour of the heel above the foot.

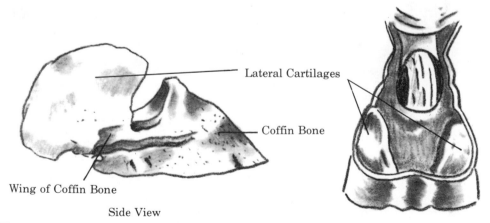

Fig. 2-5. Side view of the coffin bone showing attachment of the lateral cartilages to the wings of the coffin bone. The back view of the foot shows the shape of the lateral cartilages which shape the bulbs of the heel.

Do these bones have any unique characteristics?

Yes. The coffin bone is so perforated it resembles a hard sponge. These holes allow tiny branches of large arteries, veins and nerves deep within the foot to pass through the bone to the active structures (corium) nearer the surface.

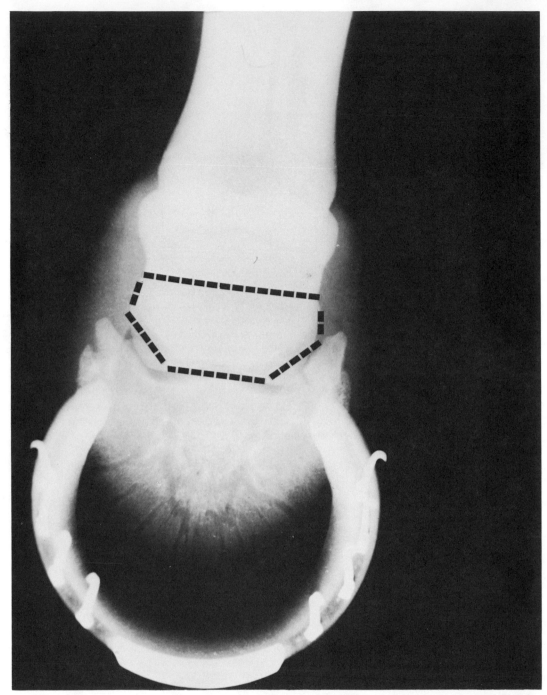

Fig. 2-6. Radiograph of the foot showing extensive vascular channels through the coffin bone, the perforated "hard sponge" appearance. The navicular bone is outlined with dotted lines.

What is the sensitive structure of the foot?

The sensitive structure of the foot is the corium, the modified skin tissue within the foot. The corium lines the hoof with each of its parts named according to the insensitive structure it underlies and produces.

In other words: (1) the perioplic corium (perioplic ring) lies just under the wall of the hoof at the coronet and produces the periople; (2) the coronary corium (coronary band) encircles the foot at the coronet and produces the wall of the hoof; (3) the laminar corium (sensitive laminae) lines the hoof wall from the coronary band to the sole; (4) the sole corium (sensitive sole) lies on the under surface of the coffin bone, for the most part, and produces the horn of the sole; and (5) the frog corium (sensitive frog) lies below and produces the horny frog.

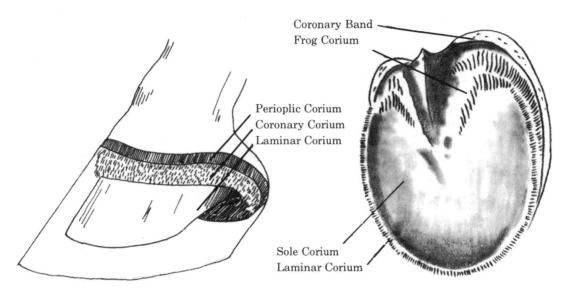

Fig. 2-7. View of foot with hoof layer removed showing relative location of the coronary and perioplic coriums. The laminar corium is also shown covering the coffin bone.

Fig. 2-8. Sole view of foot with hoof removed shows location of the various corium layers.

What is the function of the sensitive structure?

The sensitive structure (corium) is a highly vascular inner layer of tissue which carries blood to keep the foot warm and to nourish the horn-producing structures of the foot. Growth of all portions of the hoof originates in the corium. Its complex structure serves to attach the hoof wall firmly to the rest of the foot. The corium also dissipates excess heat and concussion.

What is the coronary corium?

The coronary corium is a band of highly specialized skin tissue which lies just under the hoof wall near the coronet. Its outer surface is covered with villiform papillae (tiny hairlike extensions) which produce the tubular layer of the hoof wall. Since the coronary corium is quite vascular, lacerations of this area may bleed profusely. Injuries to the coronary corium may result in a permanent scar or malformation of the part of the hoof wall that grows from the injured site.

What is the perioplic corium?

The perioplic corium is a narrow ring of skin located within the extreme upper limit of the hoof wall. It produces a narrow band of skin called the periople that grows over the upper edge of the hoof, turns down, and forms and encircles the surface of the wall near the coronet.

What is the laminar corium?

The laminar corium is attached to the wall surface of the coffin bone and the lower edges of the lateral cartilages by a membrane of connective tissue. It provides nourishment for the sensitive laminae, insensitive laminae of the wall and the extralaminar horn (white line).

The laminar corium has hundreds of primary, secondary and tertiary sensitive laminae projecting outward (similar to the plush of velvet). The insensitive laminae firmly mesh with the sensitive laminae forming a secure attachment between the hoof wall and the bones. Together these laminae bear most of the weight of the horse since this is the only structural attachment of the hoof wall to the rest of the foot.

What is the sole corium?

The unit of specialized skin tissue known as the sensitive structure turns under the coffin bone where it becomes known as the "corium of the sole." Here the corium is practically indistinguishable from the periosteum (bone covering) of the coffin bone. Numerous microscopic papillae on the sole corium produce the horn of the sole and attach the horny sole to the foot.

What is the frog corium?

The sensitive structure that lies below the frog is called the frog corium. Its papillae produce the insensitive frog. This corium of the frog is similar in structure to that of the sole.

What is the insensitive structure of the foot?

The insensitive laminae, the periople, wall, bars, sole and frog of the foot are all produced by a corresponding sensitive structure. All sensitive structures produce some type of insensitive horn. The insensitive laminae can be seen on the outside of the hoof as a white line where the sole meets the walls.

What makes up the hoof wall?

The wall consists of three layers: the periople and tectorial layer on the outermost surface; the tubular layer, which makes up the bulk of the wall; and the laminar layer on the inner surface of the wall that connects the hoof to the sensitive laminae.

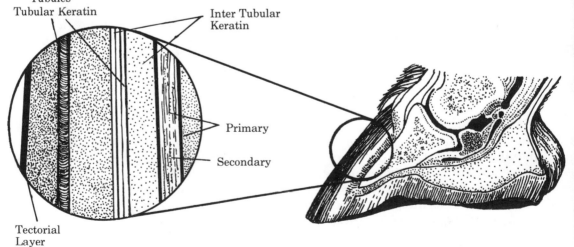

Fig. 2-9. Cross section of the hoof showing the arrangement of the structures within the layers of the hoof wall.

What is the periople?

The perioplic band is a narrow band above the hoof wall running around the hoof above the coronary band. It is about one-fourth inch wide at the toe and quarter. At the heels it widens to cover the bulbs. The periople is similar to the human cuticle in its function. The perioplic band produces a waxy substance which migrates down the surface of the hoof forming a protective coating. This coating is called the tectorial layer which functions to maintain moisture in the wall of the hoof.

What is the tectorial layer of the hoof wall?

The tectorial layer is a thin coating of soft keratinized cells which covers the outer hoof wall much like a furniture polish. Keratin is a strong, glue-like substance between the cells, which may be elastic or brittle depending upon the amount of moisture it contains. It gives a glossy look to the hoof and seals in moisture. Together the periople and tectorial layer make up the outermost layer of the hoof.

What is the tubular layer of the hoof wall?

The major portion of the horny wall consists of tubules formed around, and growing down from, the papillae of the coronary corium. These tubules, formed by hard keratin material, are the fibers of the wall and run parallel to each other as they grow down from the coronary band to the bearing surface of the wall. The center of each tubule is hollow and contains its share of the moisture which is so vital to the health of the hoof wall.

What is the laminar layer of the hoof wall?

The laminar layer fastens the hoof wall to the coffin bone by the interlocking of the insensitive and sensitive laminae. This layer is composed of fine, leaf-like ridges and is often called the insensitive laminae since, like the rest of the horn, it contains no nerve endings. The laminar layer has about 600 thin primary laminae with 100 or more secondary laminae on each primary surface.

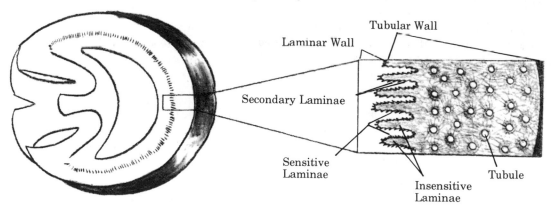

Fig. 2-10. Cross section of the foot and hoof wall showing the composition and arrangement of the layers of the hoof wall.

What are the bars of the hoof?

The bars of the hoof are formed by the wall as it turns forward and inward at the heels. The bars run on each side of the frog and converge toward one another, helping to preserve the width of the heel and prevent excessive expansion or contraction of the heel. When bars are cut away too much, contracted heels may be the consequence.

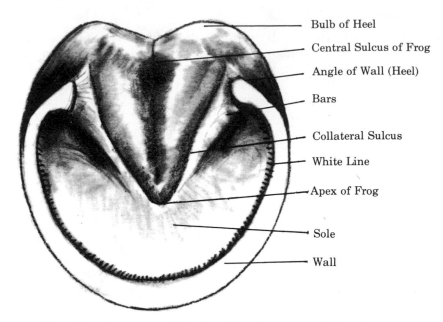

Bulb of Heel

Central Sulcus of Frog

Angle of Wall (Heel)

Bars

Collateral Sulcus

White Line

Apex of Frog

Sole

Wall

Fig. 2-11. Anatomy of the foot showing external structures.

What is the sole?

The sole has a tubular structure similar to that of the wall, although the keratin is softer. The tubules are produced by the corium of the sole. They run vertically, but curl near the surface of the ground. This results in self-limiting growth by the constant shedding of bits of dead horn, making the horny sole tough and irregular.

What is the function of the sole?

The sole is the largest section of the bottom of the hoof. However, it is not intended to bear weight from the ground surface. It is arched upward slightly and bears only a little internal weight. A primary function of the tough sole is to protect the sensitive inner foot parts from injury by hard objects on the ground. If the sole is actually allowed to touch the ground, lameness from bruises or corns can occur.

What is the frog?

The frog, a V-shaped cushion of soft keratin material, is located in the ground surface of the hoof. The grooves on each side of the frog are called the collateral sulci and separate the frog from the bars and the sole. This allows lateral yielding when weight is placed on the frog.

What is the purpose of the frog?

The frog has several purposes. One is to give the foot a firmer grip in stopping and turning. It also stores moisture for the rest of the hoof and its elasticity helps it act as a shock absorber.

Which parts of the hoof bear the horse's weight?

The wall bears most of the weight of the horse. The bars and frog are also weight-bearing structures of the hoof in its normal unshod condition. The sole bears a little weight, but only along a strip about one-fourth inch wide inside the white line. The bars should bear weight, and in shoeing should be lowered only enough to allow fitting of the shoe. The bearing surface of the wall should be level with the frog to distribute the weight evenly.

How does the horny wall grow?

The horn grows about one-fourth to one-half inch per month. It grows evenly downward from the coronary band so that the youngest weight-bearing portion of the wall (in contact with the ground) is at the heel, because the foot is shortest there. Since this is the youngest wall, it is also the most elastic, which aids in heel expansion during movement. The wall is thickest at the toe and gradually reduces in thickness so that the thinnest portion is at the heel. It thickens slightly, however, at the angles where the bars are formed. This portion of the wall and bar is commonly called the "buttress" of the hoof.

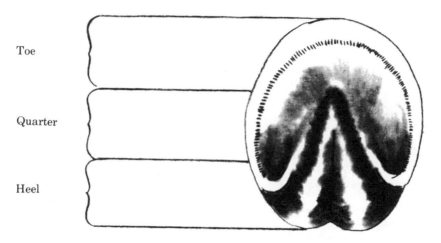

Fig. 2-12. For purposes of description, the regions of the foot are called the toe, quarter and heel. These are names for sections of the foot, not of specific structures.

What is the elastic structure of the foot?

The elastic structure of the foot refers to the ability of the hoof wall, the lateral cartilages, the digital cushion and the frog to absorb concussion. In other words, the foot is not entirely rigid. The frog can flatten when bearing weight by exerting pressure on the internal elastic structures of the foot (digital cushion and lateral cartilages). The frog indirectly forces the heels to expand.

What is the digital cushion?

This is a fibrous, elastic, fatty, wedge-shaped pad in the posterior one-half of the foot. It is avascular (without blood supply) and lies above the frog, between the lateral cartilages and below the short pastern bone and the deep digital flexor tendon. The back part of the digital cushion lies inside the lateral cartilages and forms the bulbs of the heels. It functions primarily to absorb concussion.

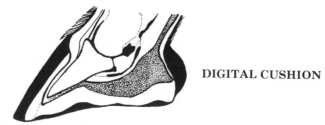

DIGITAL CUSHION

Fig. 2-13. Sole view of the digital cushion. The function of the digital cushion is to reduce concussion to the foot.

What is the function of the elastic structure?

As weight is placed on the foot, the frog and the digital cushion are compressed between the coffin bone and the ground, causing them to spread out and become thinner. The normally concave sole flattens and will spread the heels when pressure is put on the bars, wall and lateral cartilages. This forces blood out of the vascular bed of the foot and up into the veins of the leg. This pumping action of the foot is an important means of returning venous blood from the foot to the general circulation. These movements occur almost simultaneously, causing the over-all height of the hoof to decrease and the heel to expand about one-sixteenth inch on each side of the foot.

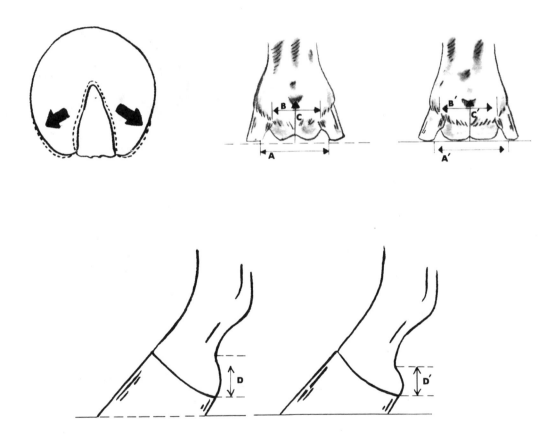

Fig. 2-14. This illustration shows the weight-bearing and elastic structure of the hoof. The ability of the foot to expand as pressure is exerted on the limb aids in distribution of concussion.

Is elasticity of the hoof related to moisture content of the horn material?

Yes. It has been proven that the frog contains more moisture than either the sole or the wall, and it is also more elastic. From this it is deduced that moisture content and elasticity are related.

CONFORMATION

Why is conformation of the foot important?

Conformation of the foot is closely related to the way it functions and to the form of the limb itself. Malformations of the foot may cause actual injury (breakdown of the foot structures, concussion ailments), or may simply predispose an animal to injury (brushing, forging). The shape and composition of the foot are indexes to the health and general soundness of the whole horse.

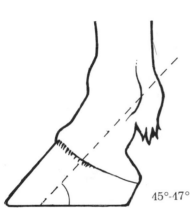

Fig. 2-15. View of ideal foot and pastern angle of the front and hind feet. This angle best minimizes the strain and concussion on the various structures.

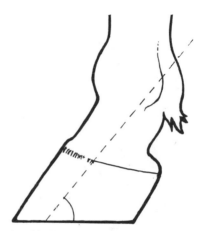

Fig. 2-15A. Front foot is 45°-47°. Fig. 2-15B. Hind foot is 50°-55°.

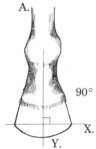 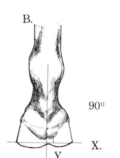 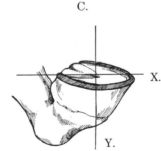

Fig. 2-16. A. and B. Views of the foot, showing the ideal pastern angle as seen from in front and from behind. Line Y should be straight, with no deviation of the limb from the fetlock down. Line X is drawn at ground level, which should form a 90° angle, if the hoof has been trimmed level. C. When the foot has been picked up the same line should be projected down the foot and pastern. This should form a 90° angle with another imaginary line projected at ground level across the quarters, if the foot is level.

What is "ideal" conformation of the foot?

The ideal foot is one in which the axis through the pastern and front of the foot forms an angle of 45°-50° with the ground line. The sole sould be concave to prevent undue shock to sensitive inner structures and permit the majority of weight to be borne by the wall, and lesser amounts by the bars and frog. The bottom of the foot should be divided by the frog into two equal halves, with the point of the frog aimed directly at the toe of the hoof wall. The horny wall should not be too dry and brittle, but should have sufficient moisture content to allow for expansion as the foot bears weight.

Is the conformation of the forefoot the same as that of the hindfoot?

No. The forefoot should have a rounded toe and broad heel, while the hindfoot should be slightly narrower and more pointed at the toe. The sole of the hindfoot is normally more concave and the foot axis should slope more than the forefoot. The axis in the forefoot is best in the 45°-50° range but the hindfoot should slope more, 50°-55° being considered ideal.

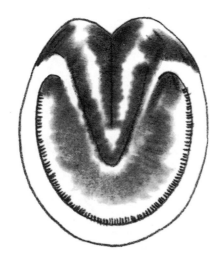 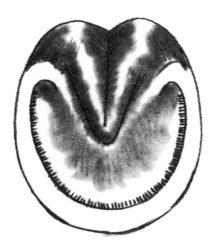

Fig. 2-17. Relative shape of front and hind feet. The hind foot (left) is more elongated, while the front foot (right) is more rounded.

What is the basis for the different shapes of the fore and hindfeet?

The rounded toe of the front foot makes it easier for the foot to break over and travel straight ahead easily. The elongated back foot encourages the hind leg to act as a power source, while the front legs absorb most of the concussion.

Should the foot be level?

Yes, unless the upper leg conformation of the horse dictates some change from the usual practice of leveling the foot to ensure weight distribution through the middle of the limb. If feet remain level when shoes are checked, it is a good indication of soundness of conformation and freedom from injury.

Do all breeds of horses have the same foot conformation?

No. Man, in his desire for a pleasing appearance and soft ride, has tampered with the natural shape and conformation of the horse's foot. Noticeably, the foot on Quarter Horses and Thoroughbreds has been reduced in size, increasing the concussion by distributing the shock over a smaller area. In like manner, the feet of Walking Horses and American Saddlebreds are grown to extreme length of hoof wall and plastic platforms are added to obtain increased flashy action of the show stock. This promotes contraction of the heels from lack of frog pressure. Even draft horses have had their feet altered since the very large foot is thought stylish in show circles, but this practice encourages dropped soles and flat feet.

If the feet are not formed properly, should they be changed?

No. If a horse is coon-footed, or has a buttress foot and the axis through the foot is correct, change will only increase the strain on the limb from the malformation. Whether the cause is improper shoeing or heredity, interference will compound the problem.

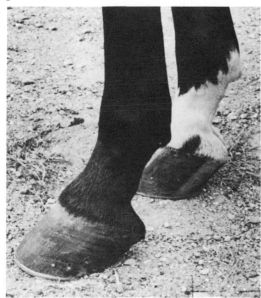

Fig. 2-18A.
An Arabian Horse's foot.

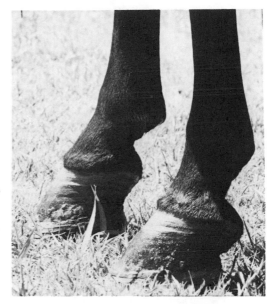

Fig. 2-18B.
A Tennessee Walking Horse's foot.

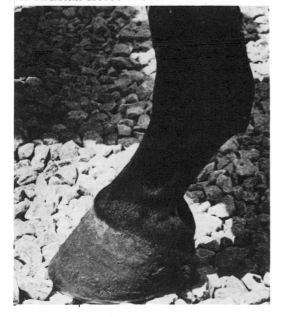

Fig. 2-18C. A Thoroughbred Horse's foot.

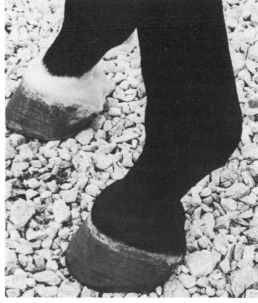

Fig. 2-18D. A Quarter Horse's foot.

What about acquired foot faults?

Faults in foot conformation caused by man can be more easily handled. If contracted heels or dry, brittle hooves are caused by neglect or improper care, they can, in large numbers, be corrected by proper foot care and diet.

How long does it take to correct a foot problem?

Contracted heels may take a year or so to correct, but only one or two months to create. The growth nature of the hoof favors this correction, however. The toe grows more slowly than the quarters or the heel. More rapid heel growth encourages modification of the frog pressure and heel spread.

What is the effect of foot conformation on stride and way of going?

The flight of the foot (travel in the air) should be such that the foot passes its opposite member at the height of the arc of travel. Abnormal foot conformation, an upright foot with a short toe and high heel or a long toe and low heel, will cause the foot to reach its peak too late or too early in the arc. Longer toe length causes greater strain on the flexor tendons, suspensory ligament, and proximal sesamoid bones, but gives a smoother ride. Short toes and high heels come to the ground abruptly, giving a short, choppy ride.

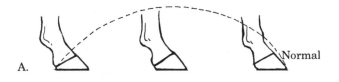

A.   Normal

Fig. 2-19. Example of foot flight. The line X marks the location of the opposite foot. A. Flight of a foot with normal foot and pastern axis. The peak of the arc occurs as the foot passes the opposite supporting foot. B. Flight of foot with less than normal foot and pastern axis. The peak of this arc occurs too early, before the foot reaches the opposite supporting foot. C. Flight of foot with greater than normal foot and pastern axis. The arc occurs too late, after the foot has passed the opposite supporting foot.

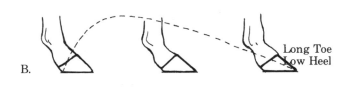

B.   Long Toe / Low Heel

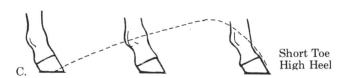

C.   Short Toe / High Heel

What about color of the hoof?

No firm evidence has been provided to support the idea that a "white" or unpigmented hoof is drier or of poorer quality than a "blue" or black pigmented hoof. Proper care of the feet results in healthy, well-formed pigmented and unpigmented hooves.

CONTRACTED HEELS

What are contracted heels?

This is a condition where the foot is narrower than normal, literally contracted, especially at the heel. The name "contracted heels" is misleading because in many cases the whole foot is involved.

Does a horse usually get this in all four feet?

No. Ordinarily only the front feet are affected. Many times only one foot will be contracted.

What causes a foot to contract?

The causes are considered to be a lack of frog pressure and a lack of moisture in the hoof. The lack of frog pressure can be due to a variety of factors.

What are some of the factors that interfere with normal frog pressure?

There are a number of things which may interfere with normal frog pressure. One such factor is trimming or shoeing in such a manner that eliminates pressure on the frog when the foot is on the ground. This can be done by: (1) leaving the hoof wall too long; (2) trimming away too much frog tissue; (3) trimming too much (even all) of the bars; (4) leaving the toe of the hoof wall too long which allows the wall to slope in under the foot rather than out.

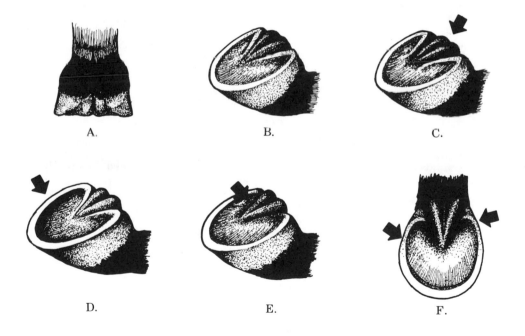

Fig. 2-20. Trimming errors may eliminate frog pressure. A. & B. Hoof properly trimmed. Frog pressure maintained when the foot is on level ground. C. Trimming off too much frog. D. Leaving wall or toe too long, leaving frog off ground and possibly even causing hoof to slope inward. E. & F. Trimming off too much or all of the bars.

Sometimes a horse will keep the heel of his foot off the ground because of pain resulting from navicular disease, sole or frog abscess, sesamoid fracture or inflammation, flexor tendon inflammation, or suspensory apparatus damage; or because of mechanical problems such as contracted deep digital flexor tendon and moderate to severe bucked knees.

In a few cases, genetics or a congenital malformation will result in a heel that is narrow and appears contracted.

What are the signs of contracted heels?

The actual appearance of the foot is the main factor in diagnosis. The foot will be narrow, especially at the heel, and the frog will be shrunken and recessed in the foot. In severe cases the bars may actually touch. There may be heat and pain in the area of the heels and quarters. If only one foot is affected, it will be noticeably smaller than the others.

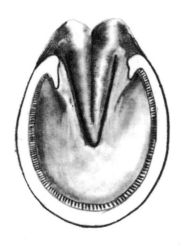

Fig. 2-21A. Sole view of contracted heels. Notice the narrowing of the heels and quarters compared with normal foot, page 37.

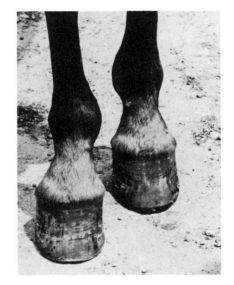

Fig. 2-21B. Front view of contracted foot. Note hoof wall actually growing inward from coronet downward toward bearing surface.

Will the horse be lame?

Lameness is not always a symptom of contracted heels. The horse may not be lame or he may possibly exhibit only a shortened stride. Other possibilities are lameness at fast speeds or a slight lameness that disappears with exercise.

Chances are that if the contracted condition was induced by improper shoeing over a period of time, the animal won't be lame. When lameness accompanies contracted heels, it is frequently the result of some condition that caused the horse to keep his heel off the ground, as listed above.

How are contracted heels treated?

Restoring normal frog pressure and restoring moisture to the hoof wall are the only ways to treat primary contracted heels. If contraction is secondary to another problem as listed above, the correction of that problem will automatically result in the resolution of the contraction. Veterinary assistance is recommended to correctly determine the primary cause and establish the best means of treatment.

What methods are used to re-establish normal frog pressure?

Most therapy for contracted heels involves corrective trimming and shoeing. In mild cases, corrective trimming and allowing the horse to go unshod will permit enough hoof wall expansion to restore frog pressure. Popular methods of corrective trimming include grooving the hoof wall over the heels and quarters to promote expansion and carefully thinning the wall over the quarters with a rasp. The quarters can be very thin near the coronet, but must be tapered so that the weight-bearing surface (bottom edge) of the wall has normal thickness.

There are a variety of corrective shoeing methods commonly used. Slipper shoes are sometimes employed. With this type of shoe the web (width) of the shoe is slanted behind the quarters (thicker on the inside edge) so that the weight of the horse forces the heels to expand. Bar shoes and T-bar shoes are both designed to apply constant pressure to the frog. Devices such as the Chadwick spring are used in severe cases of contracted heels. The Chadwick spring is a V-shaped steel spring, fitted to the bottom of the foot, which keeps constant pressure on the bars of the foot. The tension of the spring can be adjusted. Hoof compounds should be applied consistently when treating contracted heels.

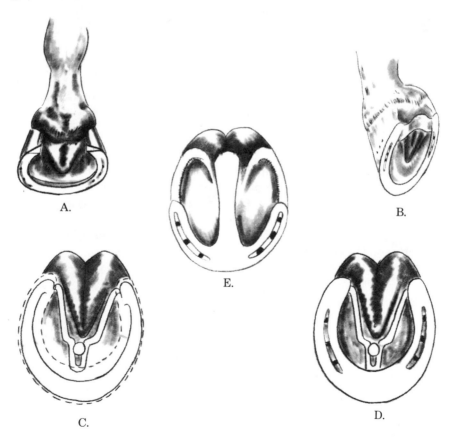

Fig. 2-22. Shoeing methods used to correct contracted heels. A. Slipper shoe is thicker on the inside at the quarters, causing the heels to expand when weight is placed on the foot. B. The bar shoe can be used to increase frog pressure if the bar is bent upward toward the frog. C. Spring in place. The adjustable Chadwick Spring applies constant pressure on the bars of the foot, causing them to expand. D. Shoe placed over spring. E. T-bar shoes are designed to apply constant pressure on the frog.

Why are hoof compounds an important part of therapy?

These dressings and compounds will keep the hoof soft and contribute directly to the more normal shaping of the hoof wall. This is necessary to prevent cracking of the hoof wall during treatment to expand the foot.

Can a horse be completely cured of contracted heels?

Yes, except for congenital cases. However, depending upon the severity of contraction, it can take a year or longer to restore the foot to its normal condition. During this period corrective shoeing must be repeated as the hoof grows out until it is normally expanded.

Naturally, if the contracted condition is secondary, its cure depends entirely upon the alleviation of the primary problem.

CORNS AND BRUISED SOLE

Are corns and bruises of the hoof the same thing?

No. Corns are caused by constant small repeated pressures to a part of the foot. These pressures cause a lesion to develop over a period of time. This happens when a horse is poorly shod or properly shod but left for too long a time without resetting or re-shoeing.

A bruise is caused by a single traumatic blow to some part of the foot. Corns and bruises are both the result of damage to the live inner parts of the foot.

Are corns and bruises caused by the same things?

They are contributed to by very similar practices of shoeing and trimming the feet; otherwise, no.

A foot trimmed with removal of a lot of sole and frog tissue also removes the protective cover over the sensitive part of the foot, thus contributing to possible bruising. A foot trimmed for shoeing this way and then shod with a shoe that fits "close" at the quarter and heel is likely to develop corns. A horse properly shod, but whose shoes are not reset or replaced soon enough, will possibly have a hoof wall that will overgrow the shoe at the heels and develop a corn.

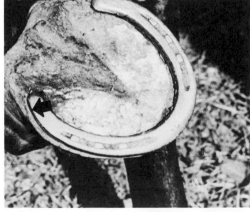

Fig. 2-23. Horse shod too close, allowing bearing surface of the heel to overgrow the shoe. This can result in the development of corns.

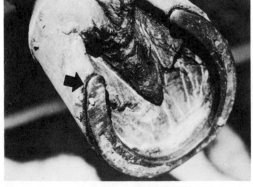

Fig. 2-24. Faulty shoeing leading to formation of corns. When shoes are not reset or replaced frequently enough, the heels may overgrow the shoe causing excessive pressure on the sole at the heels which leads to corns.

How will the veterinarian diagnose bruises and corns?

The veterinarian's diagnosis is usually clinical, i.e., without laboratory or X-ray aids. Lameness is probably the first sign noted. When a hoof tester is used by the veterinarian to examine the foot, localized pressure sensitivity will be found. Then he will use a hoof knife to cut down on the sensitive area until visual evidence is found. A red or reddish-yellow discoloration and, in some cases, clear yellowish fluid may be present. This would be diagnostic for bruising of the foot or a corn. A pus-filled abscess in this area can be sterile, if caused by a bruise, or infected, if caused by a puncture wound. However, if the cause is unknown, it should be treated as an infected abscess.

What is meant by dry, moist and suppurating?

Dry—A hemorrhage on the inner surface of the horn resulting from bruising of sensitive tissue which usually causes red stains in the involved area.

Moist—This is caused by a severe injury which results in serum beneath the injured horn.

Suppurating—An abscess resulting in necrosis (death) of the sensitive sole or the digital cushion and subsequent drainage of pus.

How are bruised sole and corns treated?

If improper shoeing or overgrown feet are the cause, simply taking off the shoe and trimming will alleviate the problem. However, veterinary advice is required for all phases of treatment. For dry corns, relieving the pressure from the affected area and promoting frog pressure is the answer. If it is suppurating, drainage should be provided by removing the undermined part of the sole. A tetanus injection is needed. Daily antiseptic soaks or topical antibiotic application and bandaging follow. After the infection is controlled, an antiseptic pack should be placed in the cavity and a metal or leather sole placed between the shoe and the foot. A wide-webbed shoe may be helpful with corns to protect the area without exerting pressure on it.

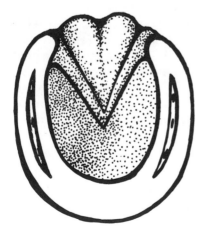

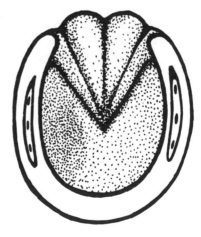

Fig. 2-25. Wide webbed shoe set full to protect corns.

Fig. 2-26. Normal web shoe.

What is the prognosis in cases of corns and bruised sole?

The prognosis is good if the condition can be corrected before any permanent damage or bone involvement occurs. However, some cases do tend to become chronic which can lead to osteitis (inflammation) of the coffin bone. Indeed, this should be suspected if bruised sole does not respond to treatment.

THRUSH

What is thrush?

Thrush is usually an almost inapparent disease of the hoof that responds well to treatment in early stages. The condition primarily involves the sulci in the center and along the sides of the frog. It is characterized by a putrid dark, often black, discharge that usually is associated with poor growth and disintegration of the horn of the frog. An occasional case becomes complicated, however, with deep involvement of the corium of the frog, inflammation of the digital cushion, and even destruction of the tendons. Such cases are hard to distinguish from canker.

What causes thrush?

Poor sanitation, atrophy of the frog as found in contracted heels, and lack of frog pressure resulting from poor shoeing or poor trimming predispose the foot to thrush. *Spherophorus necrophorus* is the organism most commonly involved. This organism is an anaerobe (a micro-organism that lives without oxygen) that is present in the digestive tract of horses and other animals in wide distribution throughout the world. *S. necrophorus* also exists in the soil, but only grows actively and produces necrotizing (death causing) toxin in unsanitary surroundings in the absence of air and presence of decaying matter. Because of this, a foot that is not kept clean so that air gets to all its external structures, becomes an ideal growth medium for *S. necrophorus*. It has all the needs of an anaerobe for growth, multiplication, toxin production and invasion of the tissues of the frog.

How is thrush detected?

The foul odor and blackish discharge of the frog are characteristic. The sulci of the frog may be deeper than normal when cleaned and, in advanced cases, the sensitive tissues of the foot may be exposed. The foot will be tender in these areas causing the horse to resist having the hoof cleaned. In these cases, the horse may be lame due to the involvement of the sensitive tissues. If thrush has invaded the sensitive area, the horse may show signs of infection similar to those of a puncture wound. The frog will be undermined and large areas of it may require removal because of the loss of continuity with the underlying sensitive frog and invasion of the area by infection.

What can be done to treat thrush?

The horse should be stabled on a dry surface. The foot should be cleaned thoroughly to assure exposure of all the affected areas of the foot. Affected portions of the frog should be trimmed to achieve drainage. Daily cleaning and packing with medication is required until exudation (pus formation) can no longer be detected. Recommended medications for early cases include drying agents such as 10% formalin, equal parts of phenol and iodine, or of tincture of iodine—applied to the infected area.

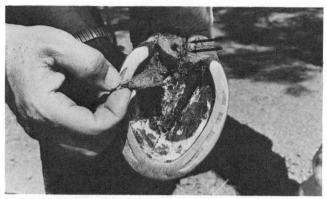

Fig. 2-27. A foot with advanced thrush. Frog material is just falling away. Note deep cleft at heel that goes to sensitive tissue indicated by arrows and the very deep sulci between the frog and sole.

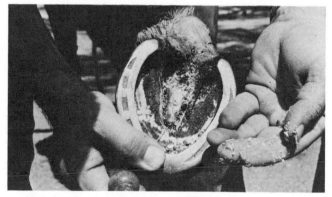

Fig. 2-28. The same foot after very little scraping with a hoof pick. The granular looking black and white material is the consistency of soft putty.

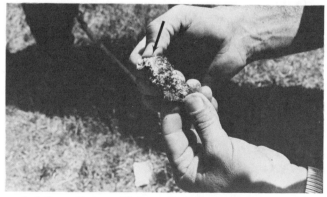

Fig. 2-29. Degenerated frog tissue. Note soft formless texture of material indicated by mashed appearance at arrow after slight finger pressure. The black part of the material is the discharge characteristic of thrush that is old and "set up"

What can be done to remedy advanced thrush?

The advice and care of a veterinarian will be required. He will probably administer tetanus antitoxin as a protective measure. When the condition is advanced, he will radically remove hoof tissue to expose all undermined areas as necessary to assure that applied medication will contact all of the infected area. After the tissue removal, an antibiotic, or sodium sulfapyridine, or other medication will be applied and the foot bandaged to keep the lesion clean and in contact with the medication. Retreatment and bandaging should be a daily procedure for three to five days. Then topical treatment with a drying agent, recommended by the veterinarian, should be used daily for several days. Once the lesion is clean and dry, the frequency of treatment may be reduced to once or twice a week. This protects the sensitive areas until new frog and sole tissue have grown to the extent that the foot is essentially normal. Once some new frog tissue has formed over the area that had been surgically denuded, a bar shoe may be applied, if it is deemed necessary by the veterinarian, to encourage frog regeneration.

Are the chances of recovery for a horse with thrush good?

Yes, provided it was treated early and proper care continued. If the sensitive structures were extensively involved, then the prognosis is guarded.

How can thrush be prevented?

This condition is best prevented by keeping stables and turnout pens clean and dry, and by providing proper care of the feet, such as cleaning them daily and trimming them every four to six weeks.

CANKER

What is canker?

Canker is a chronic hypertrophy (overgrowth) of the horn-producing tissues of the foot. It begins in the frog and slowly progresses to the sole and sometimes to the wall. It may involve one or all feet, although it is most common in the hindfeet. It is a rare condition in modern times, probably because of better husbandry than in the past.

How does canker start?

Canker is found in unhygienic stables where the horses have to stand in urine, feces, or mud soaked bedding. A specific bacterial cause is unknown. Lack of proper frog pressure may also be a factor.

Is canker easily detected?

Lameness is usually not present in early stages and, since neglect is a contributing cause of the disease, canker may not be detected until the disease is well advanced. When the foot is examined it usually has a foul odor and the frog, which may appear intact, has a ragged, oiled appearance. The horn tissue of the frog loosens easily and when removed reveals a foul smelling, swollen corium covered with a caseous (curdled), white discharge. The corium shows chronic vegetative growth. The disease may extend to the sole or even to the wall of the foot. It has little tendency, if any, to heal and the tissues bleed easily.

How is the diagnosis of canker different from thrush?

The diagnosis is made on the basis of odor and foot appearance which are similar to that of thrush (refer to thrush and canker descriptions). However, canker, unlike thrush, may involve the entire foot and may result in separation of the horn of the foot from the sensitive laminae. The degree of lameness is related to the extent of involvement.

How is canker treated?

First of all, the horse should be moved into a very clean, dry stall or, preferably, a dry pasture to remove predisposing conditions.

In order to allow for new, healthy tissue growth and to assure that topically applied antibiotics actually come into contact with the disease causing organisms, the veterinarian will cut away diseased tissue fairly extensively. Bandaging the whole foot is indicated in the early stages of treatment to keep the lesions clean and medicated. In advanced cases, systemic antibiotics are indicated.

Is the prognosis favorable for horses with canker?

If treatment is given early and persistently, the prognosis is fair. However, if canker is allowed to reach an advanced stage, the prognosis is poor.

SAND CRACKS

What are sand cracks?

This is a general name for cracks in the hoof wall. The cracks can either start at the bearing surface and progress up the foot or start at the coronet and go down. The front and hind feet can both be affected. The cracks are classified by their location. They are termed toe cracks, quarter cracks and heel cracks. Cracks in the hoof wall vary in severity. Quarter and heel cracks are the most serious because they frequently involve the sensitive laminae.

What causes the hoof wall to crack?

Cracks that begin at the top of the foot are the result of disturbances in hoof growth due to coronet injuries, such as wire cuts or interfering. Those cracks initiating at the bearing surface of the hoof wall are caused by excessively dry hoof walls, thin walls and improper trimming (such as excessively long hoof walls). All of these factors reduce the strength of the hoof wall making it susceptible to cracking upon concussion.

Heel cracks are usually caused when the horse steps on or kicks sharp objects that tear away a part of the back of the hoof wall.

What are the signs of sand cracks?

The split in the hoof wall is obvious. Depending upon the depth of the crack the horse may or may not be lame. If the crack bleeds after the horse has exercised, it is an indication that the crack goes down into the sensitive laminae. Infections in these cracks occur frequently and are marked by a discharge of blood or pus and warmth in the hoof wall around the crack. The lesion is usually quite apparent when an injury of the coronary band causes a crack in the horny wall.

How are these cracks treated?

The treatment of a crack in the horny wall will vary according to the location and

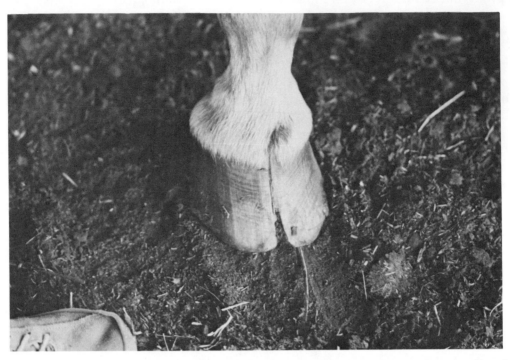

Fig. 2-30. Toe crack originating at coronet. Cracks which begin at the coronet are often due to injury of the coronary band causing defective hoof growth.

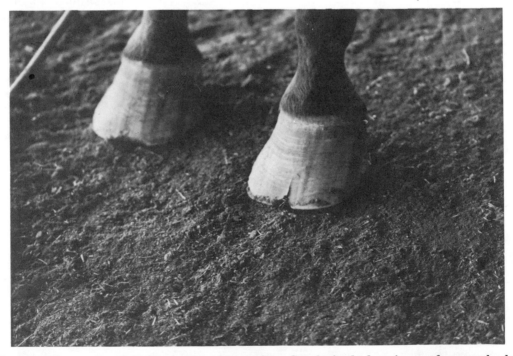

Fig. 2-31. Toe crack originating at bearing surface. Cracks in the bearing surface may be due to poor quality hoof, dryness or lack of trimming and excessive growth of the hoof wall.

severity of the crack, as determined by the veterinarian. Most therapy consists of corrective trimming and shoeing to prevent the portion of the hoof wall around the crack from bearing weight and to limit the progress of the crack.

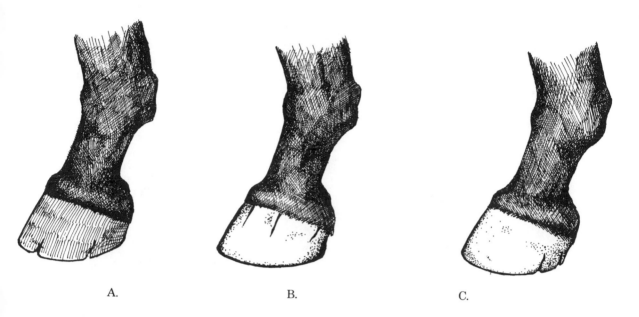

A.   B.   C.

Fig. 2-32. Diagrams of various sand cracks. (A) Toe crack and quarter crack originating at bearing surface. (B) Toe, quarter and heel cracks originating at coronet. (C) Quarter crack and heel crack originating at bearing surface.

When a crack does not extend into the sensitive laminae, a notch or groove is cut into the hoof wall at the leading end of the crack. Whether the crack originates at the coronet or bearing surface, this treatment is aimed at preventing the hoof from splitting up or down its entire length. For cracks originating at the bearing surface, the wall on either side of the crack is shortened to help prevent expansion by removing weight from this portion of the wall. Shoes with clips positioned on either side of the crack are frequently used as another measure to prevent expansion of the crack.

Cracks that extend the entire length of the foot, go down into the sensitive laminae, or are accompanied by infection, usually cause lameness. Cracks that are this severe require more extensive treatment. Patching the hoof wall is commonly done to seal the crack and prevent infection of the sensitive structures.

The general procedure is to strip out the crack and fill it with some type of plastic material, epoxy glue, fiberglass, etc. In more severe situations, the crack is drilled out dovetail fashion, with tiny holes drilled on either side of the crack. The crack is laced with stainless steel wire to further hold it together and serve as reinforcement for the plastic material. Then the crack is filled with a plastic.

Heel cracks may require different treatments. Frequently the hoof wall behind the crack is shortened so that it does not touch either the ground or the shoe. A deep heel crack with accompanying bleeding or exudation will demand relatively radical treatment. The procedure is to remove the segment of horny wall behind the crack down to the sensitive laminae, apply antibiotic powder or ointment to the lesion, and bandage the foot with a pressure bandage for several days. The lesion is then treated with a drying agent such as 10% formalin or 7% tincture of iodine. A bar shoe may be used to protect the heel until this portion of the hoof wall grows out again.

It is important to pay close attention to any crack in the foot until it has completely grown out since it has a degree of weakness that can be likened to a split board. An important adjunct in all foot crack treatment is the liberal use of moisturizing hoof dressing on a regular basis.

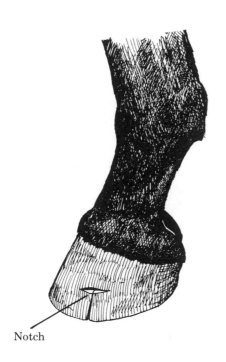

Notch

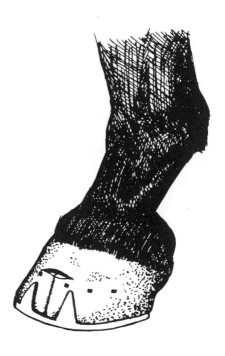

Fig. 2-33. Treatment of toe crack originating at bearing surface. The hoof wall is grooved or notched to prevent further cracking and the edge of the crack is trimmed short to prevent pressure from the shoe. Toe clips are used on either side of the crack to support the wall and prevent expansion of the crack under pressure.

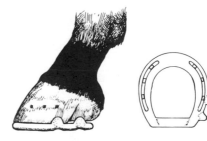

Fig. 2-34. View of bar shoe with clips applied to immobilize a bearing surface heel crack.

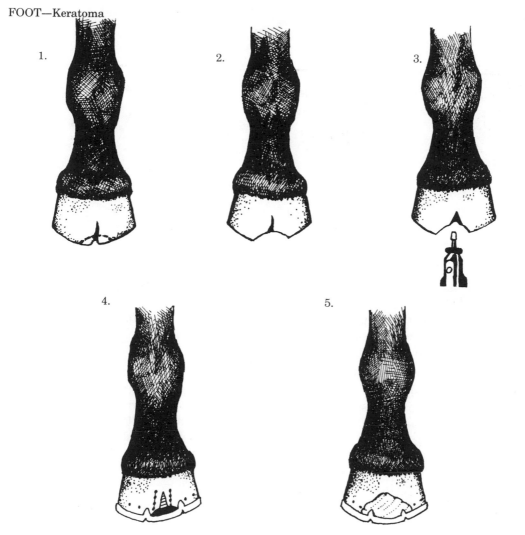

Fig. 2-35. Views of procedure for repair of a hoof wall crack using plastic and lacing for immobilization.

KERATOMA

What is keratoma?

This term applies to an abnormal growth of horn on the inner surface of the hoof wall.

What causes the hoof wall to grow like this?

The actual cause is not known. However, keratoma is often associated with a chronic inflammatory process of the laminar structures. This can be brought about by puncture wounds and other mechanical injuries of the hoof wall or coronet. In some instances, hoof grooving procedures have been incriminated as a cause of keratoma.

What are the signs of keratoma?

The horse may or may not be lame. Often the condition is not noticeable until it is quite advanced. The abnormal growth, most likely at the toe region of the foot, is cylindrical in shape. The bulge begins at the coronet and gradually advances down

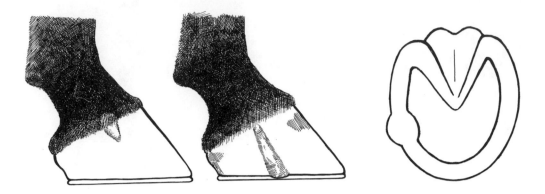

Fig. 2-36. Advancing keratoma. This cylindrical growth begins at the coronet and advances down the hoof as the wall grows. Sole view shows pressure upon the white line and sensitive structures of the hoof.

the hoof wall as the hoof wall grows. This growth pushes the white line in toward the center of the sole, thus pressing on the sensitive laminae which occasionally causes the horse to be lame.

How is this condition treated?

Surgical removal of the abnormal growth by a veterinarian seems to be the only treatment for advanced cases of keratoma. After surgical removal, the hole in the hoof wall is ordinarily filled with plastic to protect the sensitive structures until new horn growth covers the site of removal. However, this treatment is not always successful because the abnormal growth can recur. In mild cases temporary relief may possibly be achieved by corrective shoeing.

Does a horse fully recover from keratoma?

This depends on how severe the condition is and whether surgical removal is followed by normal or keratomatus growth of hoof wall. If the case is not severe and no lameness is apparent, nothing may need to be done except for cosmetic purposes.

If lameness is present, the prognosis is guarded when surgery is performed, and unfavorable if regrowth of the keratoma occurs. The prognosis is also poor if the keratoma is extensive enough that there is pressure necrosis of the underlying sensitive laminae.

GRAVEL

What is a gravel?

This refers to an infection resulting from a penetration of the white line. The infection travels up the white line and drains at the coronet. People call it a gravel because they associate it with a piece of gravel getting into the bottom of the foot and erupting at the coronet.

What causes a gravel?

A gravel can develop from any injury at the white line that allows infection to enter and separate the insensitive and sensitive laminae. Common causes include bruises, puncture wounds, cracks, thrush, chronic laminitis, etc.

How can a gravel be detected?

The foot will be hot and the area above the coronet may be swollen. Before the wound erupts at the coronet, the puncture or break at the white line can easily be seen because the lesion turns black. A cut down into this black area usually leads to an abscess, or pocket of pus. Until the abscess erupts and drains at the coronet, the pressure of the abscess against the sensitive laminae will make the horse lame. After drainage of the lesion begins, lameness disappears in most cases.

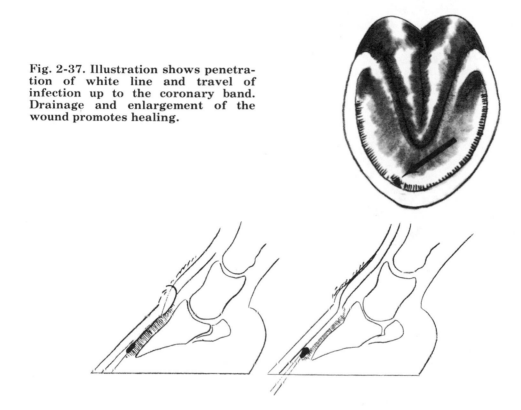

Fig. 2-37. Illustration shows penetration of white line and travel of infection up to the coronary band. Drainage and enlargement of the wound promotes healing.

How is a gravel treated?

The pus must be drained by the veterinarian from the site of the wound at the white line. In severe cases the wound at the coronet will also need to be enlarged for drainage. If the infection has not erupted at the coronet, soaking the foot in epsom salts will help reduce the swelling and promote drainage. Tetanus antitoxin must be administered. The foot should be bandaged until the drainage stops. At this point, shoes with full pads can be used to prevent debris from entering the wound and reinfecting the foot.

Does gravel cause a horse to be permanently unsound?

Unless gravel is brought about by an ever-present condition such as chronic laminitis, it usually heals quickly.

How can gravel be prevented?

Gravel can be prevented by consistent, careful inspection of the bottom of the foot for any discolorations or cracks large enough to allow foreign material entry into the sensitive layers.

SEEDY TOE

What is seedy toe?

This is a disease of the hoof wall in the toe region in which the hoof wall is separated from the white line. There is a characteristic change in the consistency of the horn that results in the "crumbling" of the inner wall. This causes a separation of the hoof wall and the sensitive laminae.

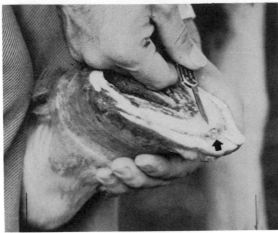

Fig. 2-38. Seedy toe secondary to dropped sole. Knife blade and arrow point to the lesion.

What causes seedy toe?

Negligent foot care is a major cause of seedy toe. It can easily occur when the wall is allowed to grow too long. In this situation, the weight of the horse itself can push the hoof wall away from the sensitive structures. Frequently, debris packs into the hollow space and enlarges the hole.

Seedy toe commonly occurs with chronic laminitis, due to the separation of the sensitive and insensitive laminae. A slight crack or injury between the sole and wall can also bring about this condition. Shoes with close-fitting toe clips have been known to cause a chronic inflammation of the laminae, resulting in seedy toe.

What are the signs of seedy toe?

The outer surface of the horny wall will look sound, but the inner surface is mealy or "seedy." When the hoof wall is tapped over this region it may make a hollow sound, due to the dead space. Seedy toe may appear in only a small area, or through the entire width of the wall at the toe. The horse may or may not be lame, depending upon the severity of the condition. A veterinarian will be able to diagnose whether the condition is primary, or secondary to chronic laminitis; a fact that is of importance in determining the prognosis in the case.

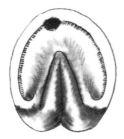 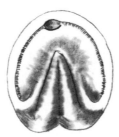 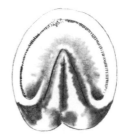

Fig. 2-39. Illustration of seedy toe repair. Affected area is hollowed out and packed.

How is this condition treated?

The diseased portion of the foot is hollowed out, making a cavity between the horny wall and sensitive laminae. This cavity is then packed to keep it clean with a mixture such as gauze soaked in pine or juniper tar, or with cotton soaked with 7% tincture of iodine or an antibiotic preparation. In many cases, the veterinarian may find it helpful to shoe the affected foot with a wide-webbed shoe which covers the packed area and protects the thin inner wall. Unless seedy toe is the result of chronic laminitis, the chances of a complete recovery are good. Proper healing will be a matter of good management of the lesion until it has completely grown out leaving a normal wall, white line-sole relationship, i.e., a normal foot.

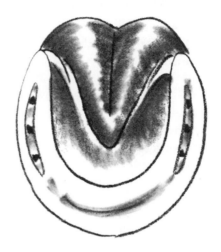

Fig. 2-40. Illustration of wide-webbed shoe applied to protect the packed area and the thinned wall.

LAMINITIS

What is laminitis?

Laminitis (founder) is defined as an inflammation of the sensitive laminae of the foot. In light of recent studies, however, it seems that this is not exactly the case. This recent work indicates that there is inflammation in the foot region but not in the laminae themselves. The inflammatory region is now theorized to severely restrict the blood supply to the laminar structures thereby causing keratin synthesis to be limited and the strength of the keratin that is formed to be drastically reduced. This mal keratin synthesis during acute laminitis results in a "founder ring."

The cause of acute founder seems to be due to a toxic condition in the bloodstream in almost all cases. The originating seat of the toxemia can be the digestive tract in horses and also the reproductive tract in mares. It is known that the toxic incidents result in the formation of histamine, a chemical which finds its way into the bloodstream and causes constriction of the small arteries. Histamine is thought to be the causative substance of acute laminitis.

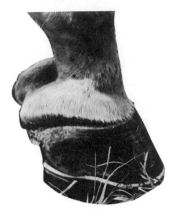 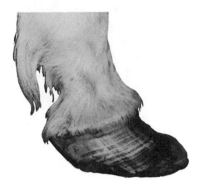

Fig. 2-41 & 2-42. Examples of founder rings.

Does laminitis affect all four feet?

Laminitis may affect one or all four feet. Most commonly it affects the two forefeet.

What is the difference between acute founder and chronic founder?

Acute laminitis is the inflammatory reaction and suppression of keratin formation described above. Chronic founder is the name given to the resultant tissue damage and associated complications following one or a series of acute attacks of laminitis. It could be said that a horse has a chronic tendency toward laminitis if his feet show founder rings. Each ring is the result of an acute laminitis attack.

A horse may or may not suffer complications such as rotation of the coffin bone following acute laminitis.

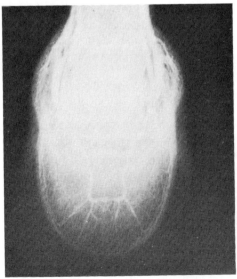 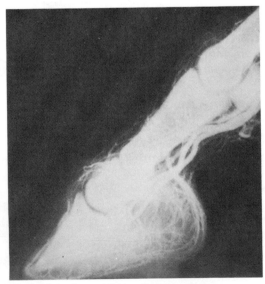

Courtesy of LAMENESS IN HORSES, Edition III, O. R. Adams, Lea and Febiger Publishing Co., Philadelphia, Pa.

Fig. 2-43. X-ray of arterial system of equine foot after injection with radiopaque material to show extensive blood supply in normal circumstances.

What causes laminitis?

Laminitis has been noted to occur as a result of the following:

Grain Founder—caused by ingestion of greater quantities of grain than can be tolerated by the horse. This founder is associated with enterotoxemia, the presence in the blood of toxins produced in the intestines.

Water Founder—caused by ingestion of large amounts of water by an overheated horse—possibly an enterotoxic effect.

Road Founder—the result of concussion to the feet from hard or fast work on a hard surface or standing too long on a hard surface. This is possibly just sore foot syndrome but it may be that a toxemic condition develops in these cases, too.

Foal (postparturient) Founder—the result of retaining portions of fetal membranes (afterbirth) or a uterine infection resulting in a systemic toxic condition.

Grass Founder—common among horses grazed on lush pasture, particularly clover and alfalfa. This type of founder more often affects fat horses. It can also occur in winter when feeding legume hays. This is probably an enterotoxic effect.

Other predisposing factors include hormonal difficulties in mares, viral respiratory diseases, colic, and the administration of strong purgatives.

How can one tell if a horse has acute laminitis?

The onset of acute laminitis is very sudden. There will be an increased temperature of the sole, the wall and the coronary band. The digital artery, located over the fetlock joint, will have a pounding pulse. Diarrhea or constipation may develop. The horse may show anxiety and visible trembling of small muscles from the severe pain. This is accompanied by increased respiration, sweating and an elevated temperature. If forced to walk, the horse will shuffle and occasionally stumble. Use of a hoof tester will indicate a uniform tenderness over the entire sole. This tenderness makes the horse reluctant to move. In fact, he will assume a characteristic "founder stance" to try to minimize the pain. It should be noted that these signs can be quite variable from almost nothing to any or all of these signs, depending upon the severity of the syndrome.

What is a "founder stance"?

The horse will assume a stance that will decrease weight on the affected feet. If just the two front feet are affected, the horse will stand with its hind feet well up under the body and the front feet placed forward, with the weight on the heel of the foot. If laminitis occurs in all four feet, the horse tends to lie down for extended periods and may refuse to get up. When standing, the horse tries to pull his hind feet and fore feet in toward each other under the center of his body, which will more evenly distribute body weight over the feet. These positions are typical of foundered horses.

What happens with chronic laminitis?

Recurrent acute attacks of laminitis may result in severe damage which is referred to as chronic laminitis. Mild cases of chronic laminitis may not be discovered if there is no visible hoof deformity.

Periodic acute attacks can leave severe multiple ring formations on the hoof, one ring with each attack. If an acute attack is severe enough and lasts long enough, or

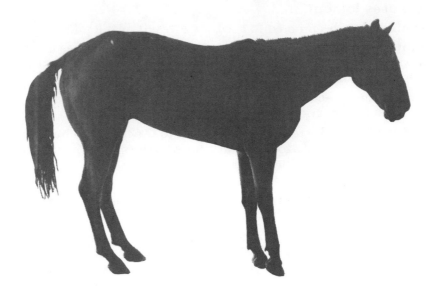

if attacks recur, permanent damage to the laminae can result, depriving the horse of his normal attachment of coffin bone to hoof wall. This attachment is almost the sole means of physical support, through the hoof, of the entire animal. When this attachment is destroyed, the weight of the horse pushes down on the coffin bone. The posterior aspect of the coffin bone is supported from beneath by the plantar (digital) cushion and frog which is supported by the ground. The anterior aspect of the coffin bone has no support from below. The result is rotation of the coffin bone which shows up on the outside of the foot as "dropped sole." In severe rotation, the coffin bone can even be pushed right through the sole to the ground.

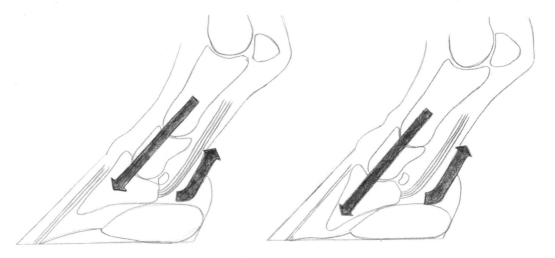

Fig. 2-45. Diagram of rotation of the coffin bone. Severe founder destroys the attachment by laminae of the coffin bone to the hoof wall, allowing the coffin bone to drop down toward the sole.

The white line at the toe may become wider than at the heel because of the separation of the laminae. This is further indication that rotation has taken place. Early or slight rotation of the coffin bone may show up only on X-ray. Depending upon the stage of the syndrome, the horse may or may not be lame. In travelling, he may tend to land on his heel in an exaggerated motion. The severe rotation will leave the horse prone to seedy toe (Seedy Toe, see page 58) and infection entering through the white line.

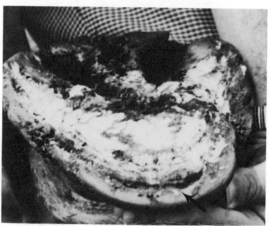

Fig. 2-46. Separation of the laminae from the wall following severe founder. The separation may be clearly seen at the toe.

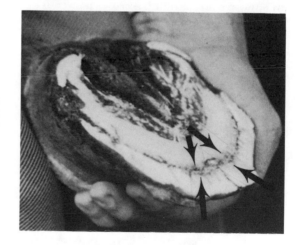

Fig. 2-46A. Dropped sole. Notice the width of the area that has been rasped flat. Arrows indicate the widened white line.

How does one treat laminitis?

There are a multitude of suggested treatments for acute laminitis. Treatment is given by the veterinarian for two purposes: (1) to reduce inflammation so as to relieve pressure and restore blood circulation to the laminae, and (2) to counteract the specific cause of the toxemic condition.

To reduce inflammation, anti-inflammatory drugs, anti-histamine drugs, hot or cold packs to the feet, forced exercise and a low volar nerve block can be administered. (Caution: Forced exercise in limited amounts—only as prescribed by the veterinarian.) Cold packs and anti-inflammatory drugs both aid in reducing inflammation. The rationale of the low volar nerve block, forced exercise and hot packs is to help re-establish the blood supply to the foot and relieve pain.

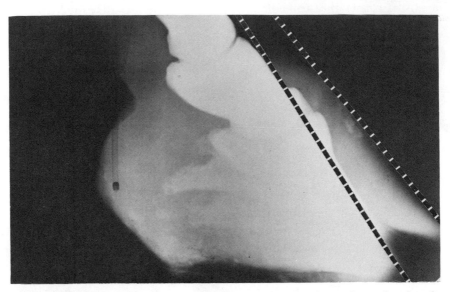

Fig. 2-47. X-ray of moderate rotation of coffin bone. Dotted lines show that hoof wall and bone are not parallel as in normal foot.

Fig. 2-47A. X-ray of severe rotation of the coffin bone. Dotted lines show that hoof wall and coffin bone are not parallel. Arrows point out actual line of hoof wall which is curved due to rotation mechanism.

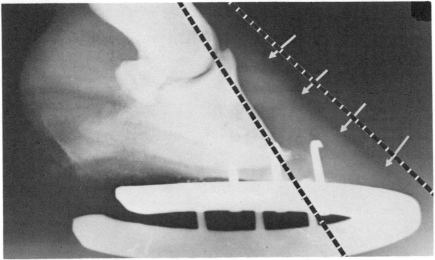

For grass, grain and water founder, the important thing is to remove as much of the offending substance as possible. Therefore, mineral oil administered by stomach tube is used as a laxative and to coat the intestinal wall, thereby preventing histamine absorption into the bloodstream. This may need to be followed by intravenous dextrose and electrolytes to replace body fluids if excessive diarrhea results from the laxative treatments.

To treat foal founder, the retained fetal membranes must be removed by the veterinarian and antibiotics administered parenterally and directly into the uterus to control the uterine infection.

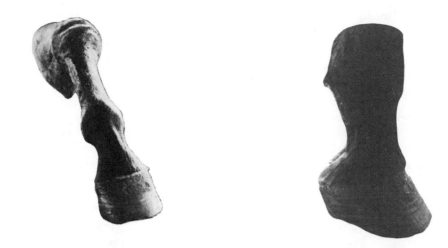

Fig. 2-48. Sloughing or shedding of the hoof due to extensive damage to the laminae following founder.

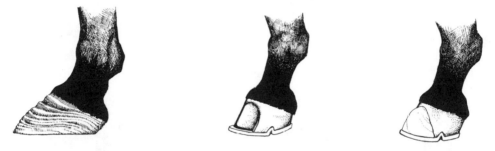

Fig. 2-49. One treatment for rotation of the coffin bone. The toe of the hoof wall is rasped away and filled with plastic to prevent rotation of the coffin bone. A disadvantage of this treatment is the possibility of destroying the hoof, since the temperature of the plastic may reach 280° while it sets up.

Is there any special feeding program for a horse with acute laminitis?

In any founder case, the management of feed for the convalescent horse, prescribed by the veterinarian, is of utmost importance. Some veterinarians feel the horse should be kept completely off feed for one or two days, and some suggest bringing the horse back onto feed immediately. Fresh water should be made available immediately, and at all times. In any case, once the feeding schedule is begun, it should be started out gradually, beginning with the offering of a small amount of grass hay only. The hay should be offered just a very few pounds at a time, two or three times a day, while observing the horse carefully for signs of relapse. After the first 24 hours of hay feeding, grain can be offered the horse in small amounts, several times a day. On the first day it is offered, the feeding should be in quantities amounting to no more than a fourth of his usual ration. This quantity can be doubled on the second day, if the horse eats well and shows no signs of relapsing into laminitis or other distress. From this point on, the feeding schedule can be programmed toward a more normal routine over a five day period.

What can be done for the horse with chronic laminitis?

Corrective trimming, shaping and shoeing of the hoof is recommended at frequent intervals. The hoof should be trimmed to as normal a shape as possible. Gradually lowering the heels, removing excess toe and protecting the dropped sole, will help to restore normal alignment of the rotated coffin bone. Leather pads, steel plates and acrylic plastics are all popularly used. Preventative treatment is necessary to avoid secondary infection, which may accompany radical cutting away of hoof wall down to the sensitive structures.

Can a horse be made sound again after having laminitis?

Some horses with acute laminitis respond to therapy without developing complications. However, if the disease is not treated immediately, the laminar structures may be permanently damaged, and the blood supply will not be entirely restored. Occasionally, infection will enter the sensitive tissues of the foot, as a result of separation of the sensitive and insensitive laminae (seedy toe), or through the sole, making the prognosis unfavorable. If a crack appears all the way around the coronary band with purulent-looking material in it, the hoof is beginning to slough off. This usually leaves no alternative but to destroy the horse. Chronic cases can be kept reasonably sound by proper trimming and shoeing and a sensible feeding program. However, if rotation of the coffin bone has occurred, the outlook is poor.

SIDEBONES

What is a sidebone?

In each foot there are two lateral cartilages attached to the wings of the coffin bone. These cartilages are positioned along the sides of the foot, extending above the coronary band toward the bulbs of the heel. When the lateral cartilages ossify (change into bone) they are called sidebones.

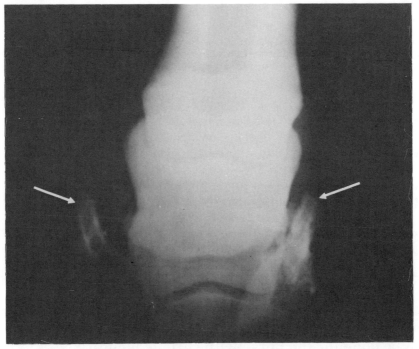

Fig. 2-50. Radiograph of coffin bone of horse with sidebones (arrows). Compare with same view of normal foot on page 32. Another good X-ray of side bone is Fig. 2-55 on page 70.

What causes the cartilages to ossify?

The exact factor causing the cartilage to change into bone is not known, but there are several factors that certainly can lead to ossification. Concussion is thought to be the primary factor in the development of sidebones, especially when it is increased by faulty conformation. Improper shoeing can predispose a horse to sidebones. Injuries, such as wirecuts which damage the cartilage, can also lead to sidebones.

Does this happen in all four feet?

Sidebones can occur in both the front and rear feet, but are much more common in the front feet.

What are the signs of sidebones?

Only in rare cases, do sidebones cause lameness. Appearing as bulges on the sides of the feet, sidebones can be felt on the outside of the foot as hard protrusions. Normally the cartilage is resilient, but in the case of sidebones, the ossified cartilage does not "give" when pressed. This is especially noticeable when pressure is applied to the heel right above the hairline. Sidebones also show up clearly on X-rays.

Are sidebones serious?

Because they do not usually cause lameness, sidebones are not considered too serious. However, the ossified cartilage has no flexibility, so the foot cannot expand normally. This condition might be a predisposing factor to corns and contracted heels. In some cases, the sidebones become so large that they cause lameness by mechanical interference with movement between the foot and the short pastern bone, rather than pain.

What kind of treatment does sidebone require?

Treatment is not needed unless the horse is lame. If the horse is lame, the usual treatment is corrective shoeing to allow the quarters to expand. Thinning the quarters and grooving the quarters are two methods commonly used. To decrease the action of the coffin joint, full roller motion shoes can be used.

Fig. 2-51. Corrective measures for sidebones. Quarters are grooved to permit expansion and a roller motion shoe is used.

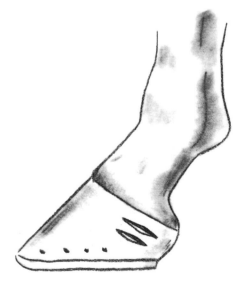

On occasion, firing or blistering is used, but they are thought to be of little value. In severe cases, where the bulbs of the heel are grossly enlarged, sidebones can be surgically removed. This is sometimes done for cosmetic reasons.

QUITTOR

What is quittor?

Quittor is a chronic, deep-seated inflammation of the lateral cartilages, characterized by necrosis (death) of the inflamed part of the cartilage and drainage of pus through the coronary band.

How is it caused?

Quittor usually results from an injury over the coronet in the region of the lateral cartilages. Wounds near the coronary band and deep, penetrating injuries of the sole are common causes. Interfering, wire cuts and bruises which damage the lateral cartilage are also frequent causes of quittor.

When a part of the cartilage dies as a result of injury, characteristic sinus drainage follows. A small, narrow channel forms, with an opening near the coronary band for the discharge of pus. This channel leads directly down to the area of necrotic cartilage.

What are the signs of quittor?

There is swelling, heat and pain over the coronary band in the area of the lateral cartilages when quittor is acute. Sores which periodically break open, drain and heal over, only to break open again are found in the quarter region of the coronet.

Does quittor cause the animal to be lame?

Generally, the horse is lame when quittor is acute. Pressure builds up over the dead cartilage, followed by the rupture and drainage of the sinuses. When the sinuses drain, the lameness usually disappears until pressure again builds up, forcing recurrent rupture and drainage. This normally proceeds in cycles lasting about a month.

How is quittor treated?

A veterinarian's services are necessary, since surgical removal of the necrotic cartilage is considered the only successful treatment.

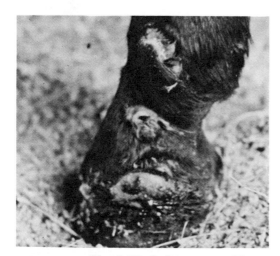 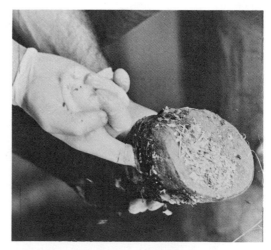

Fig. 2-52. Quittor caused by a wound near the lateral cartilage.

What are the chances of total recovery from quittor?

If quittor is diagnosed and treated early, the chances of total recovery are quite good. However, if the condition has been present for a long period of time, the nearby tendons and bones, especially the joint capsule of the coffin joint, may be involved. In such cases the prognosis is poor.

NAVICULAR DISEASE

What is navicular disease?

The term "navicular disease" covers a progressive series of degenerative changes involving the navicular bone, navicular bursa and deep flexor tendon.

On two sides, the navicular bone meets with the coffin bone and short pastern bone (much like a wedge) to form the coffin joint. This small bone is bound in the back by the deep flexor tendon. The navicular bursa lies between the navicular bone and the deep flexor tendon, and is simply a small sac filled with synovial fluid. The purpose of a bursa is to reduce friction between two surfaces that rub against each other; in this case, the opposing surfaces of the navicular bone and the deep flexor tendon.

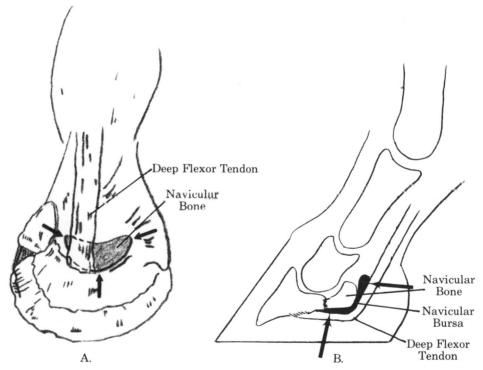

Fig. 2-53. (A & B) Diagrams showing location of navicular bone, deep flexor tendon, and the navicular bursa involved in the development of navicular disease.

What are the stages of the disease?

Bursitis of the navicular bursa is the beginning of navicular disease. This is an inflammation of the bursa which causes it to produce excess synovial fluid, resulting in swelling. As the disease progresses, the navicular bone erodes on the rear surface facing the tendon. In some cases, the small fibers of the tendon are torn by the roughened edges of the bone, causing progressive destruction of the tendon's

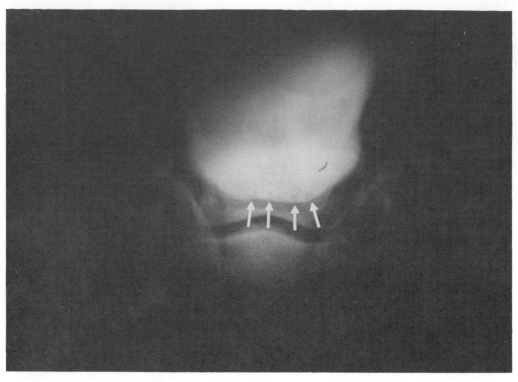

Fig. 2-54 & 2-55. Radiographs of navicular disease showing erosion and demineralization of the navicular bone. Arrows point to the affected part. Compare this radiograph to the same view of a normal foot, page 32. Fig. 2-55 also has sidebones indicated by smaller arrows.

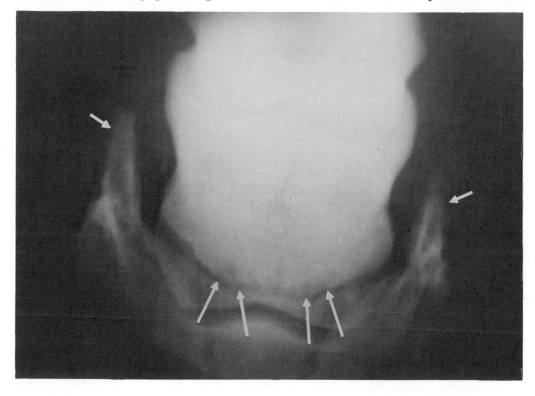

surface. Bone spurs may develop on the navicular bone. This entire process progresses very slowly.

What is the cause of navicular disease?

The exact cause of navicular disease is not known, but several factors can contribute to it. Faulty conformation (particularly small feet, straight pasterns and too straight shoulders) increases concussion on the navicular bone. By way of the coffin joint, weight is transmitted to the navicular bone, forcing it firmly against the deep flexor tendon. The intensified concussion causes excessive vibration of the navicular bone against the tendon, often resulting in navicular bursitis—the first stage of the disease.

Many types of improper trimming and shoeing have been blamed for the development of navicular disease. Examples are: (1) heels too high and heels too low (because they break the pastern axis), and (2) any sort of trimming and shoeing that interferes with the normal action of the frog and quarters (covered in Contracted Heels, p. 43).

Strenuous work such as racing, roping, cutting and barrel racing, especially when performed on hard surfaces, makes a horse more subject to navicular disease. Nutritional and hormonal influences are also thought to be contributing factors.

Does navicular disease affect all four feet?

The front feet support more of the weight of the horse than the hind feet, so they are subjected to greater amounts of concussion. Since concussion is a predisposing influence on navicular disease, the fore feet are more commonly affected; the hind feet are rarely involved.

What are the signs of navicular disease?

The signs vary depending upon the severity (or stage) of the disease. Navicular disease appears slowly, with lameness getting progressively worse. Many times, the horse will have an obscure history of intermittent lameness.

In the early stages of the disease, the horse will be lame after hard work but will return to normal after a rest period, or there may be a slight "cold" lameness that disappears with exercise.

As the disease progresses, the horse will try to land toe first when in motion, in an effort to avoid painful frog pressure and concussion on the heels. As a result, the stride of a horse with navicular disease is shortened and his gait is choppy. Also, the afflicted horse will wear the toes of his feet much more than the heels.

The continuous lameness at this stage results in the characteristic shuffling, stumbling, "navicular gait" which frequently causes the rider to think the horse is sore in his shoulders. When at rest, the horse will extend the most severely affected foot forward in a pointing manner, or alternately point the front feet, or stand with the feet extended forward; all efforts to reduce the pressure of the deep flexor tendon on the navicular bone. Continued attempts to relieve pressure cause the foot to gradually change shape. The heels contract and raise, so that the foot becomes narrow and upright, with a small frog.

What tests can a veterinarian use to tell if a horse has navicular disease?

The application of hoof testers will reveal pain at the central third of the frog and, to a lesser degree, over the ends of the navicular bone. Of course, the veterinarian will compare these reactions ("flinches" in most cases) to the reactions when hoof testers are applied to a normal foot. Radiographic examination (X-ray) in

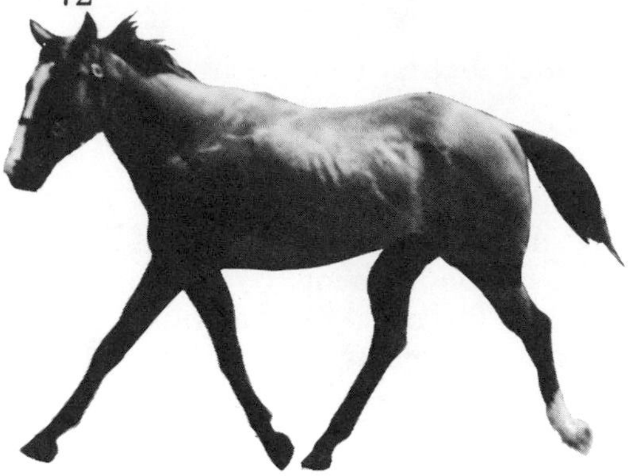

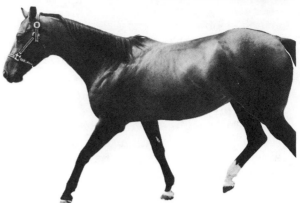

Fig. 2-56. Normal stride. Notice the extension of the foot, heel first.

Fig. 2-57. Navicular stride. Notice the toe-first placement of the front and hind feet.

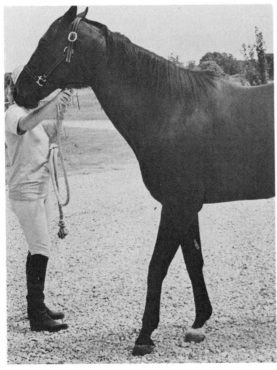

Fig. 2-58. "Navicular Point", typical position assumed at rest to relieve pressure on the navicular bursa.

the later stages of the disease will show degenerative changes of the navicular bone.

Also, the veterinarian may anesthetize the navicular bursa and the heel area of the foot to help diagnose this condition. This type of nerve block will alleviate pain to temporarily improve the gait of a horse afflicted with navicular disease.

Can navicular disease be cured?

No. Once the bone is eroded, it can never be restored to the normal condition. Therefore, treatment of navicular disease primarily concentrates on relieving pain to prolong the usefulness of the horse.

What kind of treatment does the veterinarian use?

In the early stages, the navicular bursa can be injected with corticosteroids to temporarily reduce inflammation. The results are varied.

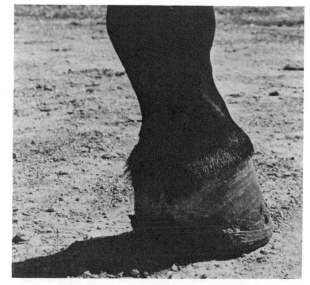

Fig. 2-59. Shoeing for navicular—Rolled toe and raised heel.

Corrective shoeing is used as a means of therapy throughout the course of the disease. The primary methods are to shorten the toe and elevate the heel, to reduce pain and pressure in the heel region. Roller shoes and rocker shoes are normally used to shorten the toe and help the foot break over faster. Heels are commonly raised with caulks, or the branches of the shoe are rolled back for more heel height. In advanced cases, a bar shoe may be used to protect the frog. However, the bar must be curved down to avoid pressing against the frog. Shoeing as a therapeutic measure has only temporary beneficial results, and much depends upon the severity of the disease.

Anti-inflammatory drugs are also used to help alleviate the pain. Phenylbutazone is an example.

Is there any way to achieve permanent relief of pain for the horse?

A posterior digital neurectomy is a surgical procedure to cut the nerves that give "feeling" to this part of the foot. (NOTE: After a posterior digital neurectomy the feet must be checked conscientiously for puncture wounds, cuts, bruises, etc., since there will no longer be pain or lameness to indicate these problems. Therefore, these could easily go unnoticed until the foot is seriously infected.) This operation is usually considered to be a last resort because there are possible serious side effects which can be even more painful than navicular disease itself.

What are some of the bad side effects known to occur as a result of a posterior digital neurectomy?

In some cases, there is the formation of a neuroma (tumor or mass growing of the nerves), which usually requires another surgical operation for removal. Although the exact cause of neuroma formation is not known, irritation from the surgery itself, or exercise too soon after surgery, is thought to be a major factor.

Fibrous attachment of the deep digital flexor tendon to the navicular bone, due to chronic irritation of the tendon, occurs in a number of long standing cases of navicular disease. The horse begins to use the foot normally following a neurectomy. Normal use of the foot tears the deep digital flexor tendon loose from the navicular bone and the weak tendon ruptures. There is no known treatment for this after effect.

Another possible side effect of a neurectomy is loss of the entire hoof wall. This occasionally happens when additional surgery to remove a neuroma is required. Current theories speculate that either the loss of nerve supply, or efforts of the nerve to regenerate, close off the blood supply to the foot, resulting in gangrene and subsequent sloughing of the hoof wall.

Some posterior digital neurectomies are only partially successful. One reason is that a number of horses have variations in nerve patterns, with small branches of other nerves also supplying the heel area. In some instances the posterior digital nerves will regenerate, again supplying sensation to the heel area. Both cases require another neurectomy to completely desensitize the heel.

FRACTURES

Which bones in the foot can fracture?

The coffin bone and the navicular bone are the two bones involved in fractures in the foot area.

How does a horse fracture a coffin bone?

There are many things that can cause a bone to break. A penetrating wound to the foot can easily fracture the coffin bone. Concussion, when violent enough, is responsible for many fractured coffin bones. This is especially true if the foot twists as it lands. Trauma to a large sidebone can also cause a coffin bone to fracture; in this situation, the bone usually fractures at the wing.

In many instances, coffin bone fractures can be attributed to pathological conditions in the bone (pedal osteitis, for example).

What are the symptoms of a fractured coffin bone?

The signs vary, depending upon the location of the fracture. When it is an articular fracture (a break involving the joint surface) there is a sudden, severe lameness. Often the horse will sweat and tremble. There is an increased pulse and heat in the foot region. When hoof testers are applied, pain is evident over the sole.

When the fracture involves the wings of the coffin bone, lameness is not as severe and it is most noticeable when the horse turns. The foot region will be warm and sensitive to pressure. However, diagnosis by a veterinarian is required to establish that a fracture has actually occurred.

How does the veterinarian determine a coffin fracture?

An X-ray is the only method of positive diagnosis.

How does the veterinarian treat fractures of the coffin bone?

The foot must be immobilized for the bone to heal properly. There are several ways to do this. One of the most popular is a full bar shoe with clips behind the quarters. When carefully fitted, this type of shoe will prevent frog pressure and limit expansion of the foot. This type of shoe is worn for three to six months and reset periodically, when needed.

A cast from the foot to just below the knee is another method for immobilizing the foot. Usually, there is not a great deal of bone displacement in a coffin fracture because of its enclosed position within the foot.

The horse should be rested from work for a period of six months to a year. If the fracture was caused by a puncture wound, the wound must be treated and tetanus antitoxin (tetanus toxin if the horse has been on a tetanus immunization program)

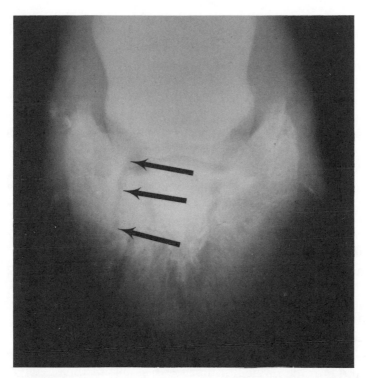

Fig. 2-60. Fracture of the coffin bone at arrows.
Fig. 2-61. Arrow indicates site of fracture of wing of coffin bone.

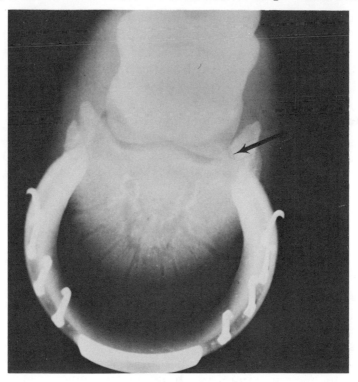

administered. In some cases, infection sets in or small splinters of bone break off and die. In both situations, surgery may be required to remove the infection or bone fragments so that lameness will not be prolonged unnecessarily.

A relatively new surgical method of treatment utilizes a compression screw to immobilize the bone segments and promote faster healing.

Do fractures of the coffin bone usually heal completely?

The age of the horse and the site of the fracture are major factors affecting the extent and speed of healing. When the wings of the coffin bone are fractured, the chances of complete healing are good. Three to nine months is the length of time normally required.

The prognosis for fractures involving the joint surface is not as favorable. However, if the treatment was instigated soon after the bone was fractured, the chances are improved. Chances of complete recovery are also better if the horse is less than three years old. Older horses exhibit a definite tendency toward chronic lameness following coffin bone fractures.

If a puncture wound caused the fracture, the extent of infection will have a bearing on the healing process. When fractures are due to pathological causes, such as pedal osteitis, the prognosis is extremely unfavorable since a diseased bone is rarely capable of healing completely.

What causes the navicular bone to fracture?

There are two major causes of navicular bone fractures. Violent concussion is one cause and chronic navicular disease, because of the degenerated condition of the bone, is the other. Fracture of the navicular bone is most common in race horses and aged horses.

What are the signs of a fractured navicular bone?

The signs can be very similar to navicular disease, especially if the fracture occurs as a result of chronic navicular disease. There is an acute lameness which is usually reduced after the horse has been confined to a stall for several days. The horse will be sensitive to pressure over the middle one-third of the frog. An X-ray is the only means to be certain that lameness is due to a fractured navicular bone.

What is the treatment for a fractured navicular bone?

Because fractures of the navicular bone almost never heal, a posterior digital neurectomy is the only means of treatment. This surgical procedure cuts the nerves that give this area of the foot sensitivity, relieving the pain and lameness in most cases.

PEDAL OSTEITIS

What is pedal osteitis?

The term pedal bone (os pedis) is another name for the coffin bone. Pedal osteitis means that the coffin bone is inflamed. This is a specific type of inflammation. The chronic stage is characterized by rarification of the bone.

What does "rarification" mean?

This means that the bone is demineralized; the inflammation "eats away" the minerals in the bone, making it rough, porous and much less dense than normal bone.

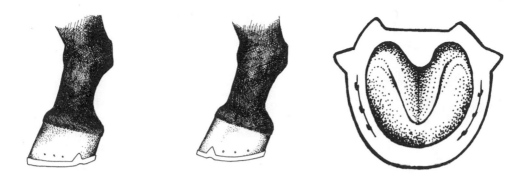

Fig. 2-62. Shoeing used to immobilize hoof for fracture of the coffin bone.

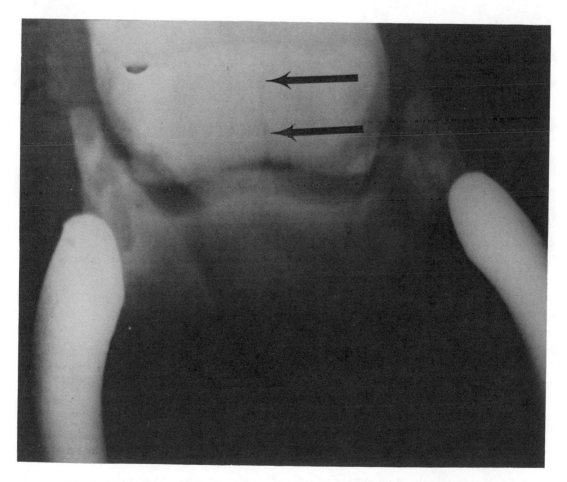

Fig. 2-63. Fracture of navicular bone. X-ray arrows point to fracture line.

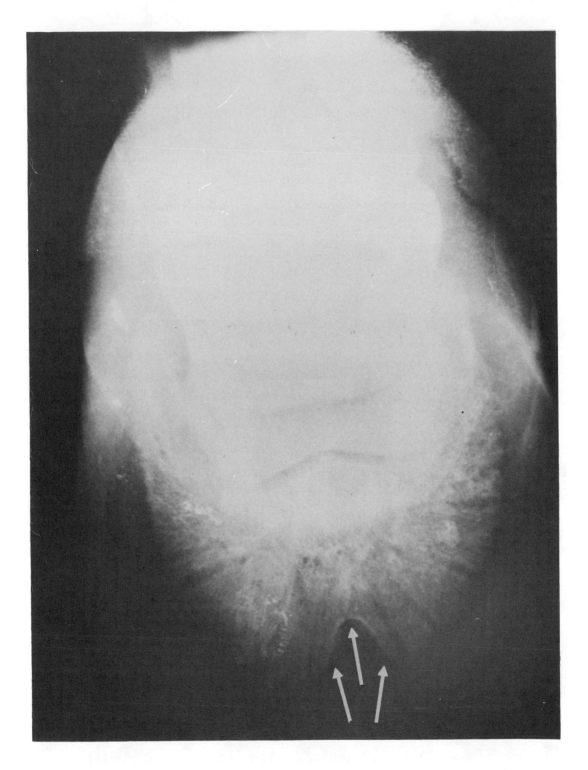

Fig. 2-64. Pedal osteitis. Rarification of the coffin bone. Notice the totally demineralized area along the margin of the coffin bone indicated by the arrows.

What causes this to happen to the coffin bone?

The inflammation is easily caused by repeated concussion, especially with a thin-soled foot on hard or uneven ground. Pedal osteitis often develops as a secondary complication of chronic laminitis.

Injuries of the foot, such as severe bruises, corns and puncture wounds, can lead to this type of chronic inflammation of the coffin bone.

Is it more common in the front feet?

Yes, because the front feet support more weight than the hind feet. If pedal osteitis is due to concussion, both feet will be affected. When it is due to an injury, ordinarily only one foot will be involved.

Are there specific signs of pedal osteitis?

A veterinarian is needed to positively diagnose pedal osteitis. The degree of lameness depends upon the seriousness of the condition, but the horse shows general discomfort in the foot area.

The application of hoof testers will cause pain at the bottom of the foot. Radiography (X-ray) is necessary to diagnose chronic pedal osteitis.

How is it treated?

The treatment depends on the cause. Any primary lesions (sole bruises, corns, puncture wounds, etc.) should be treated first, according to veterinary recommendations. Rest and corrective shoeing are the treatments commonly employed. The use of a full pad, of leather or neolite, between the shoe and the hoof helps keep the sole away from the ground in an attempt to alleviate painful pressure on the coffin bone.

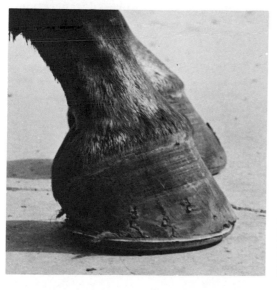 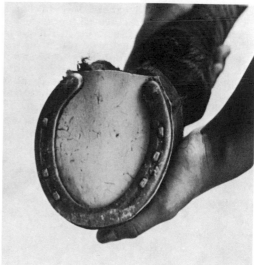

Fig. 2-65. Photographs show shoe with pad used to protect the sole of the foot from pressure.

What is the prognosis for pedal osteitis?

This again depends on the development and cause of the condition. In mild cases the corrective shoeing will give some relief. When the inflammation has been active for a period of time, the prognosis is guarded to poor. In chronic cases, treatment is usually not successful because the demineralization is essentially irreversible.

PYRAMIDAL DISEASE

Is pyramidal disease the same as buttress foot?

Buttress foot is also used to describe this lesion, because in the advanced stage of the disease, the foot looks like a buttress (a bulging structure). The term "pyramidal" disease is used because the "pyramidal," or extensor, process (upper front) of the

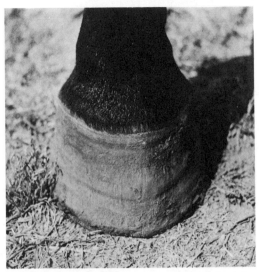

Fig. 2-66. Notice slight "pyramiding" of the front of the hoof. Also called low ringbone. This is a case of fracture of the extensor process of the coffin bone with little displacement and very mild effect on the outward shape of the foot. This horse's way of going changed to compensate for the lack of extensor action of the toe. He now has a somewhat exaggerated knee action to prevent stumbling.

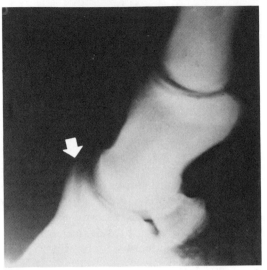

Fig. 2-67. Pyramidal process degeneration.

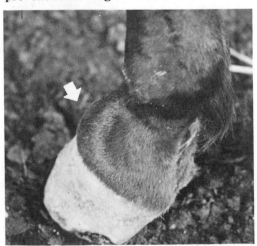

Fig. 2-68. Severe buttress foot, involving high and low ringbone.

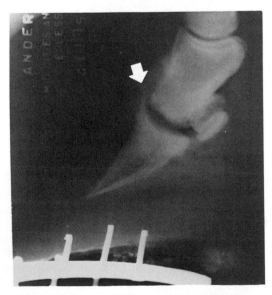

Fig. 2-69. Pyramidal process ossification.

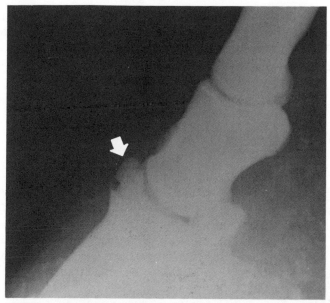

Fig. 2-70. Extensor process immediately after fracture.
Fig. 2-71. Extensor process two years "after."

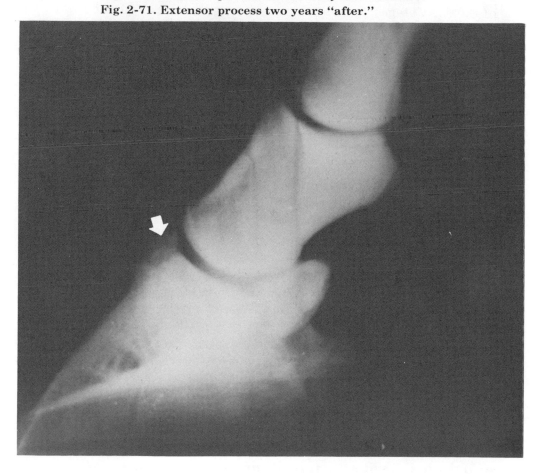

coffin bone is involved. Pyramidal disease is a form of low ringbone, a new abnormal bone growth which may be due to fracture or periostitis or osteitis of the extensor process of the coffin bone.

What are periostitis and osteitis?

Periostitis is an inflammation of the membrane of connective tissue that closely covers all bones except at the articular (joint) surfaces. Osteitis is an inflammation of bone.

As these inflammations heal, they often manufacture excessive bone growth. At the pyramidal process this is called pyramidal disease.

How do periostitis and osteitis develop?

The periostitis and osteitis that develop in pyramidal disease result from extensive strain or tearing of the common digital extensor tendon attachment to the extensor process of the coffin bone. This excessive pull of the tendons can also result in a fracture of the pyramidal process (literally pulls a fragment off the bone) which usually heals with a large callus. Therefore, a fracture of the pyramidal process looks identical to advanced pyramidal disease, so a fracture can either be confused with, or cause, the bony growth known as pyramidal disease.

How does one detect pyramidal disease?

In the early stages, heat, swelling and sensitivity are evident at the coronary band in the toe region. Signs of lameness vary, but the horse will tend to point the affected foot when at rest. The hair may stand upright at the center of the coronary band as in low ringbone. (See page 95.)

What are the effects of pyramidal disease?

Permanent arthritis of the coffin joint generally results. As the condition progresses, a change takes place in the shape of the hoof wall. A bulge will be evident at the coronary band, and in time the foot will contract.

What do X-rays show?

Radiographs reveal variable changes in the short pastern bone and in the coffin bone and joint. Radiographs enable the veterinarian to distinguish between a fracture of the pyramidal process and early pyramidal disease.

How is pyramidal disease treated?

There are a number of treatments which can be tried by the veterinarian, but none are particularly successful.

In the early stages, the veterinarian may choose one of two courses: simply rasping the hoof wall below the coronet to allow expansion at the toe, which may relieve pressure and be of temporary benefit; or injecting corticosteroids and immobilizing the part with a plaster cast.

X-ray therapy may help curtail excessive periostitis. Firing and blistering are also possible treatments, but experience shows them to have doubtful value.

Initially, alleviation of lameness can be attained through the use of anti-inflammatory drugs. However, this works only temporarily. Eventually the veterinarian will have to perform a neurectomy to desensitize the area, if the lameness is to be relieved and limited use of the horse achieved. A neurectomy could result in such complications as loss of the hoof wall. (See Navicular, page 73.)

What if there is a chip fracture of the pyramidal process?

In this case, surgical removal of the free fragment should be considered. In such a case recovery could be relatively complete.

Does corrective shoeing help?

Full roller motion shoes on the affected foot, to take as much motion as possible from the coffin joint, will give some relief and improve the horse's way of going.

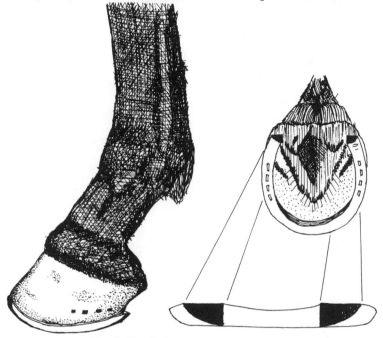

Fig. 2-72. Full roller motion shoe.

WOUNDS

What types of wounds can occur in the foot region?

Puncture wounds can happen to any part of the foot from any direction. They are most commonly found in the sole and frog region. "Stepping on a nail" is a classic method of incurring a puncture wound.

Incised wounds can easily happen across the coronet, especially in the area of the bulbs of the heel. A cut caused by a straight edge of a piece of sheet metal roofing material is a good example of this type of wound.

Lacerations are relatively common in the heel region of the foot and can also occur in the coronary region of any aspect of the foot. These wounds can be extensive enough to nearly or completely cut off the heel region of a foot as, for instance, with a horse that has kicked through the sheet metal side of a barn. A horse that has tangled a foot in barbed wire and fought it has surely caused foot lacerations. A very hard blow to the heel region of the foot by, or on, a blunt object can result in contused wounds of the less dense foot structures. Here the area is bruised so severely that necrosis and sloughing of the skin and subcutaneous tissue develop into a contused open wound.

Are there any common principles to keep in mind in the management of the above described wounds?

Yes. In all cases the wound should be cleaned and foreign objects mechanically

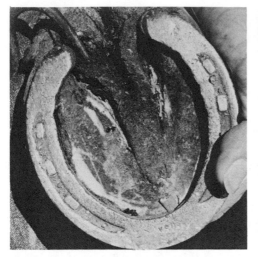

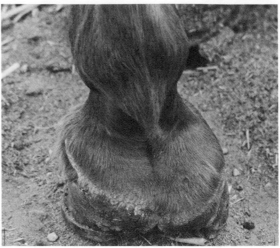

Fig. 2-73. As shown above, puncture wounds of the frog are often impossible to detect visually.

Fig. 2-74. Old wire cut. Severe scarring from lacerations can usually be prevented if pressure bandaging is used.

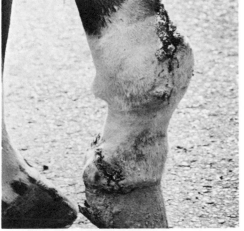

Fig. 2-75. Incised wound, caused by sharp edge.

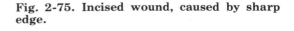

Fig. 2-76. Contusion, resulting in sloughing of the damaged tissues and open wound surface.

Fig. 2-75

Fig. 2-77. Frequent site of contusions. Notice swelling above coronary band.

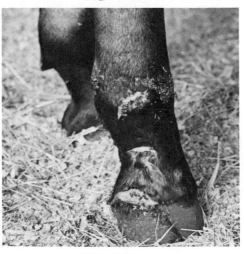

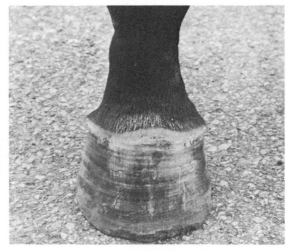

Fig. 2-76

Fig. 2-77

removed so that as much cause for pus formation as possible is removed. This is not easy to do in a wound that has hay, sand, hair, manure and any number of other contaminants in it, but is well worth the effort for quicker, better healing with less scar tissue. Once the wound is cleansed, measures should be taken to *keep it clean* by proper, careful bandaging.

Another thing that demands attention in the management of wounds is fly control. Flies can recontaminate wounds, lay eggs in them and cause irritation leading to "proud flesh" by feeding on the transudates and exudates, and by causing the horse to lick or chew the wound for relief from the irritation.

If the wound tends to gap open, it should be immobilized as much as possible with pressure bandaging or casting to encourage healing with less scar tissue.

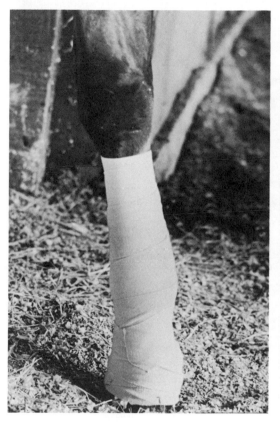 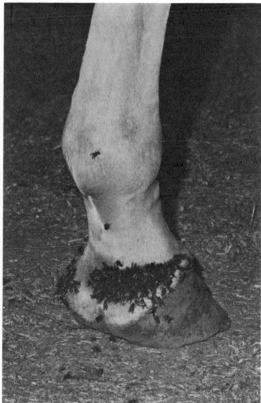

Fig. 2-78. Pressure bandaging to prevent formation of proud flesh.

Fig. 2-79. Fly control is necessary to prevent contamination of wounds.

Tetanus immunization is of uppermost importance in all wound cases for obvious reasons.

Suturing of wounds in the foot region is impractical because of the lack of soft subcuticular tissue and the great problem of contamination.

What are good medicines to use in the various wounds of the foot?

In most cases the use of an antibacterial agent is indicated, preferably something that is not very caustic. The veterinarian will be able to recommend a suitable preparation for routine use in minor wounds and will use treatments that have proven to be of value. He may recommend after-care involving the use of topical medicines, including some that are antibacterial, some that have enzymes to digest necrotic tissue, and if needed, some that actually eat away live tissue to be used in controlled situations such as when "proud flesh" has formed. ("Proud flesh" does not form in foot generating tissue but it can form immediately adjacent to it causing a misshapen foot and hoof to develop.)

Is there a particular method of treating puncture wounds of the foot?

Yes. If a puncture wound is known to have occurred, the site of entry of the foreign object should be found and marked, if possible. If the penetration of the object is known to be fairly deep, a veterinarian should be called to examine the wound in order to evaluate the structure damage and treat it most advantageously for uncomplicated recovery. He will cut down into the puncture site with a narrow hoof knife following the lesion to its deepest point, or to the sensitive tissues, whichever comes first. If sensitive tissues are penetrated, he will follow the penetration on down with other instruments to be sure no fragment remains in the wound. Then he will medicate it with 7% iodine or an antibiotic of his choice and pack the wound and bandage the foot for one or more days. Systemic antibiotics may be instituted. Retreating and rebandaging will probably be recommended for 7 to 14 days, followed by treatment with a drying agent and packing the wound with cotton and tar or other suitable material.

What is the prognosis in puncture wound cases?

The prognosis will be good if the wound is not too deep and proper treatment is immediate; fair if infection has been allowed to form before treatment; guarded to poor if there is bone or lateral cartilage involvement.

How are the incised wounds treated?

The incised, lacerated and contused wounds are treated in much the same way. If the wounds are not too extensive, all foreign objects can be extracted and the wounds cleaned, medicated and bandaged to prevent recontamination. Extensive wounds that are deep and gap a lot as the horse moves about, require pressure bandaging or the application of a cast to immobilize them. For this, the veterinarian should be called.

What is the prognosis in these cases?

The prognosis is good in the incised wound cases since there is not too much bruising to cause debilitation of the tissues that need to function in the healing process. Contamination and poor management can ruin this hopeful outlook.

The prognosis is fair to guarded in the lacerated and contused wound because the tissues are somewhat debilitated by bruising. The use of anti-inflammatory drugs, either topically or systemically, may be of value to combat excessive bruising in the early stages of treatment. It should be noted, however, that certain of these agents will tend to discourage the natural healing process; therefore, these agents should be used sparingly.

PASTERN

ANATOMY AND CONFORMATION

What is the pastern?

The pastern is the area between the fetlock joint and the coronary band. It is composed of the long pastern bone and the short pastern bone which are held together by two sets of paired ligaments to form a joint. This joint is capable of volar (backward or down) flexion only, contributing to the flexion of the whole limb in motion and permitting the dorsal (up or forward) flexion of the fetlock joint while the bottom face of the hoof is planted on the ground.

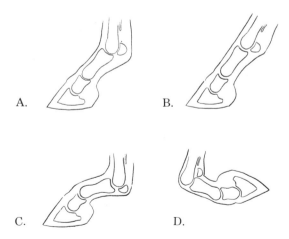

Fig. 3-1. Diagrams of the various flexions of the pastern. A. Normal dorsal flexion as when a horse is standing. B. Complete extension. The pastern is straight relative to the cannon. C. Severe dorsal flexion as in a horse running very hard or landing from a jump. D. Ventral or volar flexion as when the foot is off the ground.

What is "ideal" conformation of the pastern?

Good conformation of the pastern centers around the pastern axis. This is an imaginary line running through the core of the pastern. The pastern axis should be exactly the same angle, about 47°, as the foot axis. This results in a straight, unbroken line through the foot and pastern. When viewed from the side, the hoof wall and the pastern should have identical slopes, making a smooth continuous line.

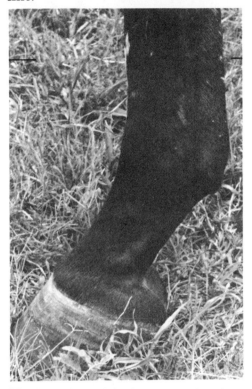

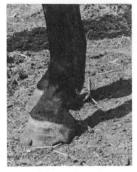

Fig. 3-3. An example of "broken" slopes of the hoof wall and pastern. The angle of the hoof axis is greater than that of the pastern axis, commonly referred to as "coon foot".

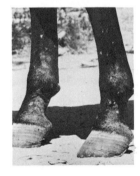

Fig. 3-4. An example of "broken" slopes in which the angle of the hoof is less than that of the pastern.

Fig. 3-2. View of the lower leg showing an ideal pastern angle.

If the slope is not smooth and unbroken, either the bones or the supporting structures (tendons and ligaments) are subjected to greater than normal stress. The pastern bones are relatively small, but function to absorb and distribute much of the force from concussion.

Why is a pastern that slopes too much considered poor conformation?

A pastern that slopes too much decreases concussion on the bones, but greatly increases strain on the flexor tendons, suspensory ligaments and proximal sesamoids. The result is a horse susceptible to tendon and ligament injuries in the lower leg.

What is undesirable about a too straight pastern?

This type of pastern conformation places less than normal strain on the flexor tendons and suspensory ligaments because of their straight position, but greatly increases concussion to the bones. This is because a straight pastern lacks the natural shock-absorbing quality ("springiness") of a sloping pastern. Therefore, a pastern that is too straight predisposes a horse to bone injuries of the lower leg such as ringbone, navicular disease and osselets.

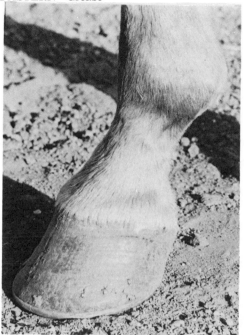 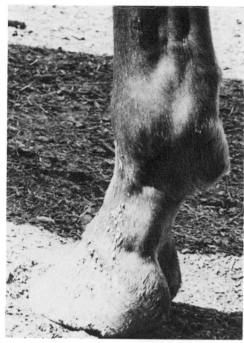

Fig. 3-5. Side view of a weak pastern, showing a low pastern angle.

Fig. 3-6. Side view showing upright or too straight pastern.

GREASE

What is grease?

Grease or grease-heel is a chronic dermatitis (skin disease) found on the back surface of the pastern. It affects hindlegs more often than forelegs. Heavy, coarse-legged horses seem most susceptible.

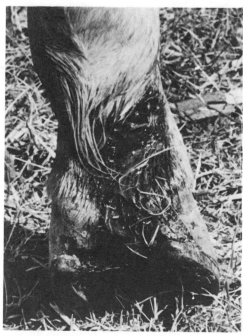

Fig. 3-7. View of grease heel as seen from behind. Notice the "grapes".

What causes grease?

Causes are unknown, although long hair in the pastern region, constant moisture and filthy bedding are thought to be predisposing factors.

How is grease detected?

Redness on the back of the pastern followed by oozing of serous fluid and crust formation are early signs. Grease often goes undetected until it is advanced. If left untreated, lesions spread. The skin is itchy, sensitive and swollen in acute cases. Eventually it becomes thickened, cracks open, and most of the hair is lost. The surface of the skin feels soft and mushy, and a grayish, foul-smelling exudate forms. In severe chronic cases, there is a thickening and hardening of the skin of the affected area. In a few cases, swelling can reach extremely large proportions. Cracks in the skin may be followed by formation of various sized masses of granulation tissue known as "grapes" (because the surface form of this "proud flesh" looks like a bunch of grapes). Lameness depends on the severity of the condition.

How is grease treated?

Treatment of early to moderate cases consists of clipping the area and washing with warm water and a mild soap (soaking to remove crusts if needed). In these cases, a topical astringent is then applied. In more advanced cases, the veterinarian should be consulted, since a topical antibiotic-corticosteroid ointment will be needed to cut down on the inflammatory reaction and combat infection. In severe cases, the veterinarian will need to use systemic administration of antibiotics. If "grapes" are present, the veterinarian will cauterize or excise them in order to allow for healing in the area just as would be done with "proud flesh" found anywhere else on the horse.

CONTRACTION OF THE DIGITAL FLEXOR TENDON

What is a contraction of the digital flexor tendon?

This may be either a congenital or an acquired condition. It involves the shortening of the deep or superficial digital flexor tendons. The degree of contraction is highly variable.

What are the causes of congenital and acquired contractions?

Congenital contractions are thought to result from inheritable characteristics, malposition of the fetus in the uterus, or nutritional deficiency of calcium, phosphorus, vitamin A or vitamin D. Acquired contractions are thought to be the result of a previous injury to the tendon, the sheath or a nutritional deficiency.

How are the tendons affected?

In congenital cases the contraction can occur in one or both hindlimbs, but usually occurs in the forelimbs. In severe cases there may be bony involvement. Contractions of the flexor tendon due to nutrition, heredity, or malposition of the fetus in the uterus are bilateral (affecting both left and right legs) while if due to injury, the contraction will be unilateral (affecting only one leg). In severe congenital cases the animal bears weight on the front of the fetlock. If not corrected, complications such as inflammation and infection of the fetlock joint can occur.

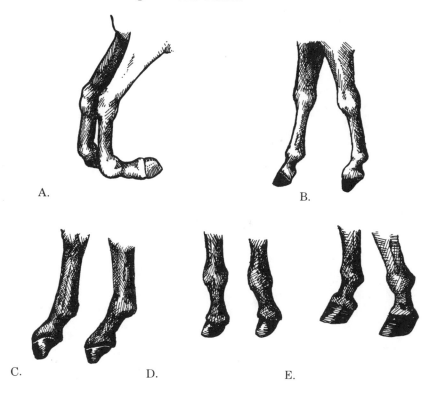

Fig. 3-8. Contraction of the digital flexor tendons. A. Severe congenital bilateral contraction of the flexor tendons, causing the colt to walk on the front of the fetlocks. B. Acquired and C. Congenital contraction of the deep digital flexor tendons, causing the heels to be raised. D. Moderate contraction of the flexor tendons. E. Leg on the right shows contraction of the deep digital flexor tendon, while the left leg is normal.

What is the appearance of this condition?

If this condition is present at birth, the foal might walk on the front of the fetlock joint. If it is an acquired condition, the foal will appear normal at birth, but as it grows older the fetlocks gradually straighten until they "knuckle" over. Any degree of contraction may develop, causing a corresponding interference with normal action of the lower leg.

How is this condition treated in congenital cases?

The important point in treating contracted tendons is a good understanding and "feel" of how the involved young tissues respond to treatments of varying intensity. The veterinarian is probably the only person who has seen enough of these cases to be able to make an accurate evaluation of the mode of treatment that will be appropriate in a given case. If the case is congenital, the treatment may need to be started within the first few hours after birth.

If the case is very mild, treatment may not be indicated. The most conservative treatment available to the veterinarian is to splint the leg from the foot to the elbow (or near the stifle if in the hindlimb). The limb should be well padded when the splint is applied and the splint removed and the leg massaged every 12 hours. The splint

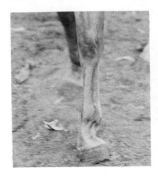
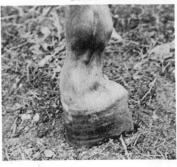

Fig. 3-9 & 3-10. Two side views of a forefoot with mild contraction of the digital flexor tendon.

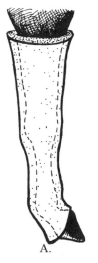
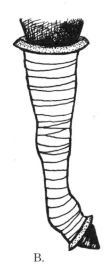
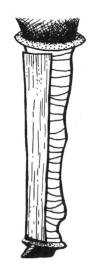
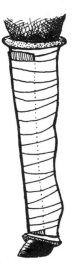

A.   B.   C.   D.

Fig. 3-11. Illustration of steps in applying a splint to a congenital case of deep digital flexor tendon contraction. A. Apply cotton padding. B. Wrap with gauze bandage. C. Apply piece of yucca board. D. Wrap tightly with more bandage material.

should be used as long as necessary and the animal allowed to exercise without the splint as soon as weight is borne on the feet.

A plaster cast may also be applied for 10-14 days, by which time the tendon will have relaxed enough to allow the animal to walk on the foot. If the tendon has not straightened sufficiently after one application of the cast, the cast can be reapplied.

A tenotomy of the involved tendon (surgical cutting of the tendon) may be necessary when splinting or casting is unsuccessful.

If contraction in the newborn is not too severe, the tendon may stretch as the foal grows and treatment may not be required. If the foot can be placed flat on the ground, correction is usually not advised by the veterinarian as long as progress continues.

What treatment will the veterinarian recommend in acquired cases?

In the early stages, the animal should have its hooves trimmed correctly, be dewormed and have any dietary imbalance corrected. In advanced cases, the veterinarian will ordinarily recommend a tenotomy.

What are the chances of recovery in these cases?

For congenital contractions, the prognosis depends on the extent of contraction

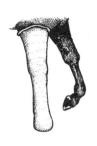 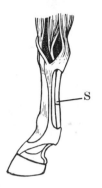 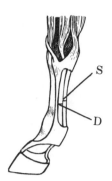

Fig. 3-12. Bilateral contraction of the digital flexor tendons, with a cast applied to one foreleg.

Fig. 3-13. Diagram to show site of tendon cutting in surgery for contracted tendons. S—superficial digital flexor tendon. D—deep digital flexor tendon.

and the age of the foal. The outlook is good if treatment was begun at an early stage and the contraction was slight. If a tenotomy was performed, the prognosis is guarded, particularly if the tendon cannot be pulled into a normal position afterwards. The prognosis is unfavorable if there was injury or infection to the fetlock joint capsule.

RINGBONE

What is ringbone?

Ringbone is a general term that applies to bony enlargements (any new bone growths) below the fetlock. It is classified as being high (pastern joint area) or low (coffin joint area) ringbone and is commonly divided into either "true" or "false,"

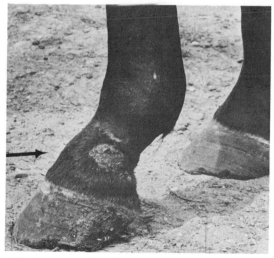

Fig. 3-14. Side view of the lower leg showing a high ringbone (arrow).

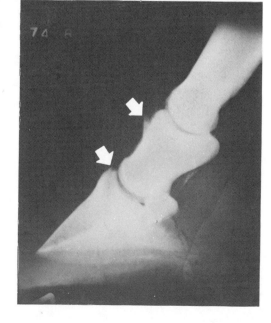

Fig. 3-15. Radiograph of high and low periarticular ringbone (arrows).

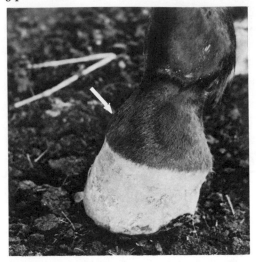

Fig. 3-16. Side view showing high and low articular ringbone. Complete fusing of the pastern and coffin joints has occurred.

depending on its relationship to a joint. "True" and "false" are common terms for articular and periarticular, with articular meaning on the joint surface and periarticular meaning around the joint but not actually involving the joint surface. It is better to use the terms articular and periarticular than "true" and "false" because "false" is also applied to uncalcified ringbone-like enlargements due to mineral imbalances of nutritional or hormonal origin. X-rays are required to differentiate between articular and periarticular ringbone.

Ringbone can affect either the fore or hindlegs, but it is most common in the forelegs. Ringbone can occur in horses of any age.

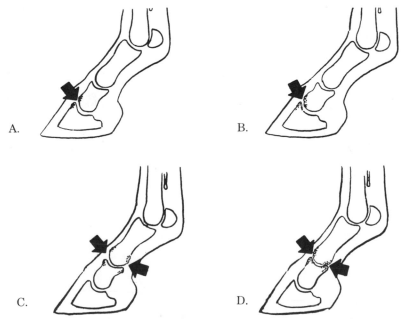

Fig. 3-17. Side view of the bones of the lower leg showing the location of various types of ringbone (arrows). A. Low periarticular. B. Low articular. C. High periarticular. D. High articular.

What causes ringbone?

Direct injury, such as pulling and tearing of tendons, ligaments and joint

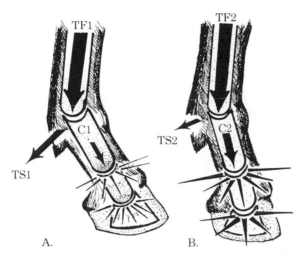

Fig. 3-18. Diagrammatic representation of increased stress due to concussion on pastern and coffin joints when pastern angle is too straight. TF1 and TF2, representing equal total force, are indicated by arrows. Tendon strain, TS1, is greater than TS2, but is well within its normal limits. Concussion, C1, is much less than C2, hence damage to the joint is much less likely in Case A than in Case B.

capsule attachments to bone, is the cause of the majority of cases. Blows and cuts are also examples of causative trauma. Any type of injury that disturbs the bone covering (periosteum) of the coffin bone, short pastern bone or long pastern bone can result in ringbone.

Poor conformation can predispose a horse to ringbone by increasing stress in this region. Base wide, base narrow, toe-in and toe-out conformation all increase stress on the joints and associated structures. Constant concussion on hard surfaces will have the same effect.

What are the signs of ringbone?

Ringbone is a condition in which there is usually a long period of time between the cause and the actual lesion. This is due to the nature of the disease, in which new bone growth occurs slowly.

Lameness will also develop gradually when conformation is the cause. Of course, when trauma is the cause, lameness usually appears suddenly but is related to the trauma, not the new bony growths.

In most cases of low ringbone there is swelling, heat and pain just above the coronary band. In fact, the hair on the coronary band will stand out at the front of the foot when extensive new bone growth is underlying this area.

With high ringbone, the enlargement will be in the pastern region. The initial signs, in most cases, are a generalized soreness and possibly heat in the area of the affected bone or joint.

How is ringbone treated?

The veterinarian will recommend complete rest. Sometimes firing, blistering and radiation therapy are employed, but the results are extremely variable.

Corticosteroid injections into the joint and phenylbutazone given systemically are also commonly used to control inflammation and thus relieve pain. However, with articular ringbone, treatment by intra-articular injection may lead to further joint destruction.

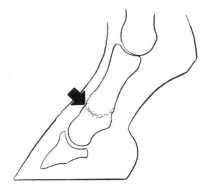

Fig. 3-19. A high articular ringbone, causing a fusing of the pastern joint (arrow).

Neurectomies (severing nerves to desensitize the area) are sometimes performed by the veterinarian to alleviate pain in chronic cases.

Casting of the limb is also used. With periarticular ringbone this treatment is designed to immobilize the joint until the inflammation subsides. In cases of high articular ringbone, articular cartilage is often surgically removed before the cast is applied. The object of this treatment is to ankylose (fuse) the joint, in hopes of prolonging limited usefulness of the animal. Corrective shoeing aimed at reducing the action of the joints may be advised by the veterinarian. Roller motion shoes to shorten the animal's stride, and make an easier break-over, are an example.

What is the prognosis in cases of ringbone?

An animal affected with periarticular ringbone may be returned to serviceability if new bone growth is arrested early and there is no interference with joint action. Periarticular ringbone, therefore, has a guarded prognosis.

The prognosis is poor in cases of articular ringbone because of the joint involvement. The goal of treatment for articular ringbone is simply to alleviate pain. This might be accomplished by surgical fusion of the bones of the joint as described in the modes of treatment above.

RACHITIC RINGBONE

What are the characteristics of rachitic ringbone?

Rachitic ringbone is a fibrous tissue enlargement of the pastern area of young horses (under two years of age, usually six to twelve months). The fibrous tissue swelling resembles new bone growth caused by true ringbone, but actually there are no bone or joint changes so it is not true ringbone.

What causes rachitic ringbone?

This condition is due to a deficiency of calcium, phosphorus, vitamin A, vitamin D, or possibly vitamin C, either singularly or in combination.

What are the signs of rachitic ringbone?

More than one foot is usually involved and all four feet can be affected. There is generally some evidence of lameness and joint soreness in the pastern area. Enlargement of the carpal joints, bog spavin and contraction of flexor tendons are other symptoms which may be evident. X-rays show soft tissue swelling which feels hard when palpated.

How is rachitic ringbone treated?

Correction of dietary deficiencies is the proper treatment. The veterinarian will be able to accomplish this by a study of the diet, and blood chemistry tests of the affected horse, in order to correctly determine what deficiency or excess is causing the problem. If corrected early enough, the swellings will not be evident as the horse grows older. However, other changes which may accompany rachitic ringbone can leave permanent damage. Four to six weeks are required after the dietary correction before a judgment can be made as to the future soundness of the horse.

FRACTURES OF THE PASTERN

What causes fractures of the pastern?

There are two kinds of pastern fractures, each of which is caused differently. Chip fractures occur primarily to the first phalanx or long pastern bone, and seem to be caused by overextension of the joint. More extensive fractures often result from hard turns accompanied by a twisting action. Barrel racers, cutting horses and horses shod with heel calks run a particularly high risk of pastern fracture.

Fig. 3-20. Fractures of the pastern (arrows).

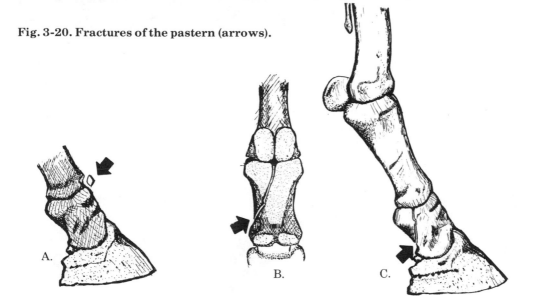

A. Side view showing a chip fracture on the long pastern bone.

B. Back view showing a single line fractures of the long pastern bone.

C. Side view showing a single line fracture of the short pastern bone.

How are fractures of the pastern diagnosed?

A chip fracture causes arthritis in the joint, and a small amount of swelling. The major indicator of chip fracture is lameness in the trot, and increased lameness after a workout. These signs are also typical of osselets, however, so proper diagnosis can only be made by X-ray.

More extensive fractures will cause severe lameness, swelling in the pastern area, pain, and reluctance of the horse to put weight on the limb. Crepitation (sounds of bone fragments being rubbed against one another) may be very obvious, but it is difficult to produce when there is only one fracture line. Since all of these signs are very similar to luxation (dislocation), X-ray is necessary for diagnosis here as well.

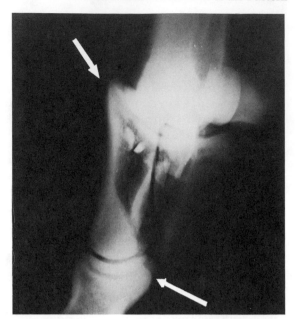

Fig. 3-21. X-ray showing a comminuted fracture of the long pastern bone.

How are fractures of the pastern treated?

Any indication of pastern fracture calls for immediate consultation with a veterinarian. The most frequently used treatment for small bone chips is surgical removal. Once the chip has been removed, the foot is placed in a cast or strong wrap for six to eight days. When the wrap or cast is removed, pressure bandages are applied for two weeks and the horse is confined for 30 days. It is recommended that the horse be allowed six month's rest before training is resumed.

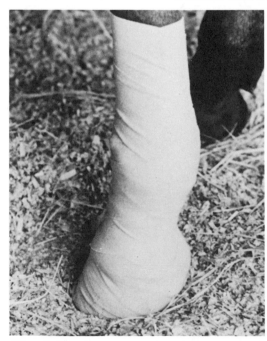

Fig. 3-22. A pressure bandage, applied after surgical treatment of a pastern fracture.

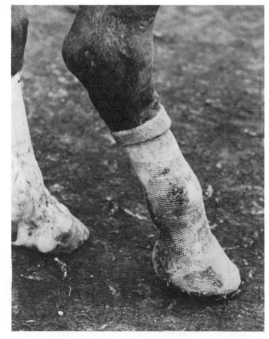

Fig. 3-23. A hard cast, used to immobilize the lower leg after treatment of a pastern fracture.

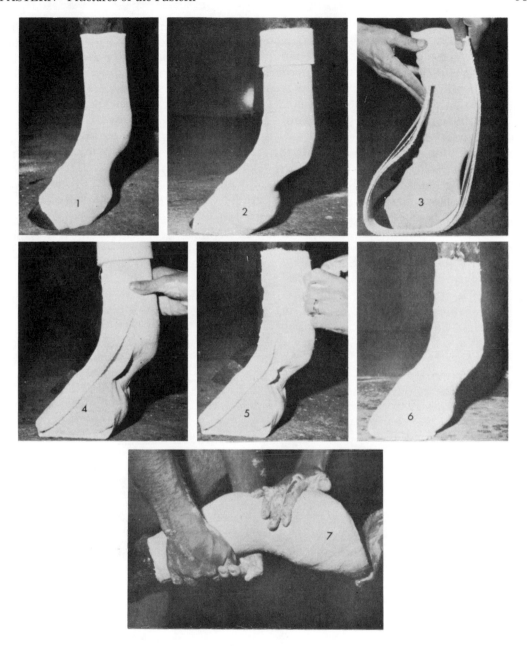

Courtesy of LAMENESS IN HORSES, Edition III, O. R. Adams,
Lea and Febiger Publishing Co., Philadelphia, Pa.

Fig. 3-24. Application of a standing plaster cast. 1, After the leg is cleaned, dried, and powdered, a double layer of stockinette is applied. 2, A piece of ¼" orthopedic felt is applied just below the carpus or tarsus. 3, A plaster splint is applied. 4, The plaster splint is moistened and contoured to the limb. 5, Four-inch plaster of paris rolls are then applied firmly over the plaster splint. Extra pressure must be applied over the orthopedic felt at the top to keep the cast from being loose at this point. The plaster is applied more snugly than when the cast is applied in the recumbent position, because the plaster splint is applied later in a recumbent cast. 6, The horse is allowed to stand a few minutes to allow forming of the cast without complete drying. The cast is then moistened and the limb is picked up and the cast is finished with the limb in the flexed position. 7, The limb has been picked up and the cast is finished in this position. If the plaster is moistened beforehand, the layers will form a bond. This allows complete normal positioning of the foot.

A single line fracture may sometimes be repaired by the use of one or more bone screws. Compound fractures, in which the bone pierces soft tissue, or comminuted fractures, in which the bone is crushed, require the careful application of a plaster cast by a veterinarian. The case may require changing several times over an eight- to ten-week period. When the cast is removed, the horse should be confined for 30 days.

The removal of bone chips usually is quite successful. Fractures with greater damage are frequently treated effectively, but ankylosis resulting in immobility of the pastern joint is often expected. This may pose a problem with the front legs. The rear legs seem to be only slightly affected. The major difficulty in successful treatment of pastern fracture is that the weight of the horse compresses the healing leg, making it shorter than the others. In addition, there is considerable danger of necrosis (death of bone tissue), sequestration (dead bone fragments), osteomyelitis (inflammation of the bone marrow) and other complications. For these reasons, prognosis is guarded to poor.

FETLOCK

ANATOMY AND CONFORMATION

What is the fetlock?

The fetlock is the joint formed by the pastern bone and the cannon bone. Located at the back of this joint are the proximal sesamoid bones.

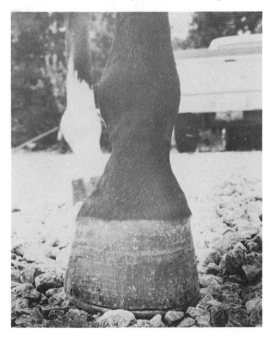

Fig. 4-1A. Front view of normal fetlock joint.

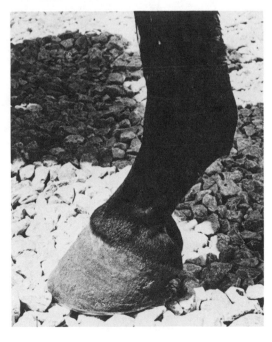

Fig. 4-1B. Side view of normal fetlock joint.

What type of joint is the fetlock?

The fetlock is a hinge joint, one which moves from front to back in dorsal (up or forward) flexion and volar (backward or down) flexion. In a normal standing position, the fetlock is partially flexed dorsally, which allows the pastern to assume a slope equal to that of a well-shaped hoof.

Fig. 4-2A, B, C. Fetlock joint.

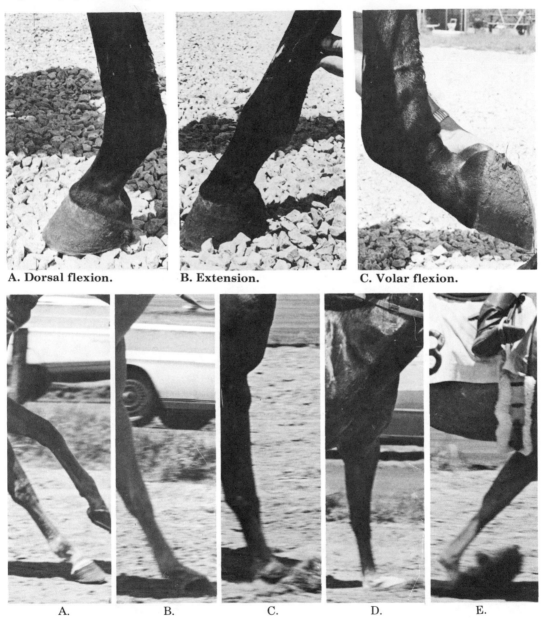

A. Dorsal flexion.   B. Extension.   C. Volar flexion.

A.   B.   C.   D.   E.

Fig. 4-3. These photographs show the phases of the stride. Notice the position of the fetlock joint in shock absorption (A-D) and propulsion (E).

What is the role of the fetlock joint?

The role of the fetlock joint is equally divided between shock absorption and locomotion. At times the entire body weight may be carried by one fetlock joint. Weight and concussion come from the cannon bone changing the position of the fetlock from extreme extension through its total dorsal flexion. This sends the concussion through the pastern into the shock absorbing structures of the hoof.

What ligaments and tendons are involved in this joint?

The ligaments and tendons of the fetlock hold it together, support its shock-absorbing movements, and provide its locomotor function. The collateral ligaments of the sesamoids and the fetlock joint proper hold the bones of the joint together. Its supporting ligaments begin at the knee (carpus) in the forelimb, and the hock (tarsus) in the hindlimb. This group is called the suspensory apparatus and consists

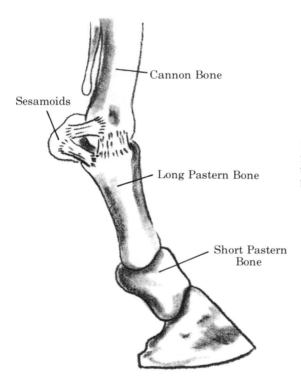

Fig. 4-4. Side view of the ligaments of the fetlock joint, showing the attachments of the sesamoids, cannon bone and long pastern bone.

of: (1) the suspensory ligament; (2) the intersesamoidean ligament; (3) the distal sesamoidean ligaments (superficial, middle, deep); (4) the short sesamoidean ligaments (this complex of ligaments includes the proximal sesamoid bones) and (5) the superficial and deep flexor tendons.

What are the proximal sesamoid bones?

The proximal sesamoid bones are two roughly pyramidal-shaped bones on the back of the fetlock joint. They are considered to be ossified parts of the suspensory apparatus. Weight from the cannon is received and transmitted to the long pastern bone directly via the suspensory apparatus functioning through the sesamoids like a pulley.

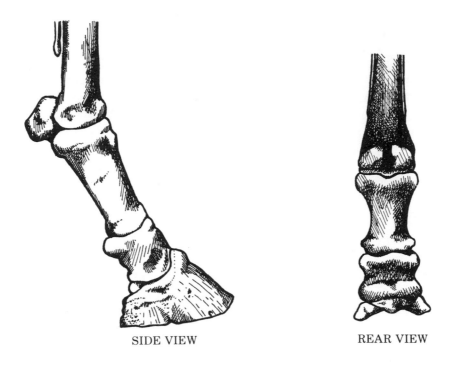

SIDE VIEW   REAR VIEW

Fig. 4-5. Placement of the proximal sesamoid bones on the fetlock joint.

What is the importance of the suspensory apparatus?

Although the suspensory apparatus has no muscular function, it is an important shock absorber for the leg. It is one of the main supporting structures of the horse's leg and is the largest structure in the stay apparatus of the limbs. Its main function is to support the fetlock.

What is the stay apparatus?

The stay apparatus is a system of check ligaments which branches off the flexor tendons and works together with the suspensory apparatus to allow the horse to "lock" his lower legs in extension with no muscular effort. This mechanism makes it possible for the horse to sleep while standing (check ligaments are explained and illustrated on page 126.)

What is the structure of the suspensory ligament?

The suspensory ligament lies in the metacarpal groove in a wide, thick band. It attaches above to the lower posterior surface of the large metacarpal (cannon of foreleg) or metatarsal (cannon of hindleg) bone and to the lower row of carpal (knee) or tarsal (hock) bones. At the lower quarter of the cannon bone it divides into two branches. Each branch passes to the outside face of the corresponding sesamoid, to which a large segment of the ligament actually attaches, nearly encasing the bone. The rest of the ligament passes obliquely downward and forward to the front surface of the long pastern bone where it joins the digital extensor tendon. There is a bursa (lubricating sac) between the extensor branch and the proximal (upper) end of the long pastern bone. This ligament is elastic and consists mainly of tendinous

Fig. 4-6. Side view showing the way the suspensory ligament functions over the sesamoids like a pulley. The suspensory ligament attaches at the top of the cannon bone and at the lower front edge of the short pastern bone.

Fig. 4-7. View of the suspensory ligament as seen from behind.

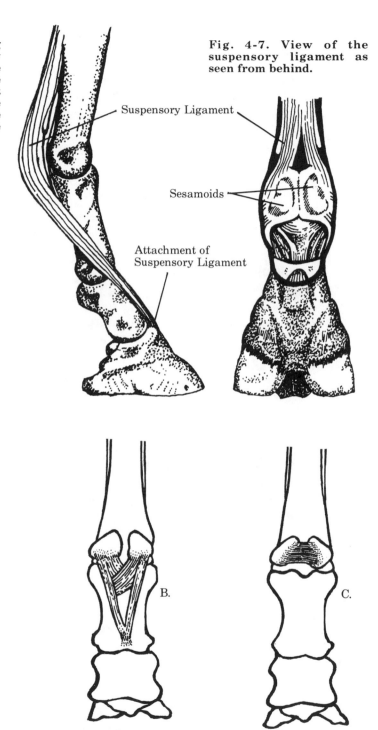

Suspensory Ligament

Sesamoids

Attachment of Suspensory Ligament

A. Superficial sesamoidean ligament.

B. Middle and deep (crossing each other) sesamoidean ligaments.

C. Intersesamoidean ligament.

Fig. 4-8. View of the fetlock joint from behind showing the sesamoidean ligaments.

tissue, with a small amount of muscular tissue in its deep part in young horses. Its primary function is to support the fetlock, guarding against excessive flexion of the joint when it bears weight. Those branches which join the extensor tendon prevent extreme forward flexion of the pastern joint.

What is the intersesamoidean ligament?

The intersesamoidean ligament fills the space between the proximal sesamoid bones and forms a groove for the flexor tendons to slide across.

What are the distal sesamoidean ligaments?

The distal sesamoidean ligaments are the superficial sesamoidean ligament, the middle sesamoidean ligament and the deep sesamoidean ligament.

The superficial sesamoidean ligament attaches above to the bases of the sesamoid bones and to the intersesamoidean ligament, and below to the overhanging lip of the upper end of the back surface of the short pastern bone.

The middle sesamoidean ligament attaches above to the base of the sesamoid bones and the intersesamoidean ligament, and below to the back surface of the long pastern bone.

The deep sesamoidean ligaments are composed of two layers of fibers arising from the base of the sesamoid bones, crossing each other, and ending on the opposite upper end of the back side of the long pastern bone.

What are the short sesamoidean ligaments?

They are short bands which extend from the anterior (front) part of the base of the sesamoid bones outward and inward to the posterior (back) margin of the articular surface of the long pastern bone.

Where are the superficial and deep flexor tendons and how do they assist in supporting the fetlock joint?

The superficial and deep flexor tendons are found on the back of the leg. Via their respective muscles, they have multiple attachments in the region of the elbow and pass behind the fetlock joint on their way to insertion on the back of the pastern bones and on the coffin bone. These tendons pass through annular (ring-shaped) ligaments at the knee and fetlock. It is necessary to sever both of them, in addition to the suspensory ligament, to cause the fetlock system to collapse completely to the ground.

What is "good" conformation of the fetlock?

The fetlock should be wide and flat to allow for strong attachments of the ligaments forming the joint and have sufficient room for the tendons to pass around and through the sesamoids at the back of the joint. The fetlock should angle adequately to provide for maximum use of tendons and ligaments in propulsion, support, shock absorption, and weight bearing.

A slope of 47^0 in the forefoot and 55^0 in the hindfoot is considered ideal. Too upright pasterns result in increased concussion which is conducive to ringbone, navicular disease, and arthritis of the fetlock. Pasterns which are too sloping increase the strain on the flexor tendons, suspensory ligaments, and the proximal sesamoid bones.

Fig. 4-9A, B. Location of the suspensory ligament and flexor tendons of the lower leg.

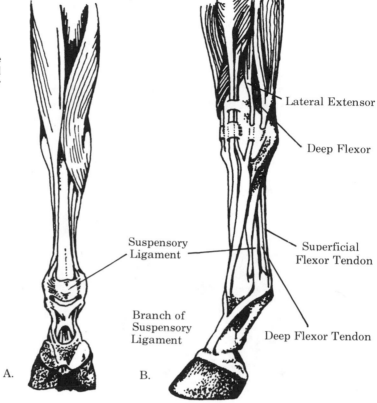

Lateral Extensor

Deep Flexor

Suspensory Ligament

Superficial Flexor Tendon

Branch of Suspensory Ligament

Deep Flexor Tendon

A.   B.

A. Rear view.   B. Side view.

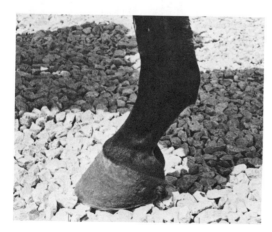

Fig. 4-10. Good fetlock showing good attachment of the sesamoids and a good pastern angle.

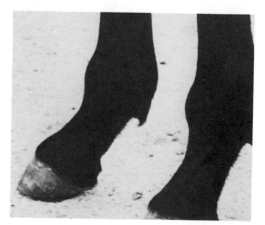

Fig. 4-11. Poor fetlocks showing weak placement of the sesamoids and weak pasterns.

WINDPUFFS

What are windpuffs?

Windpuffs (windgalls) are a distension (overfilling) of the synovial sheath (lubricating sac) between the suspensory ligament and the cannon bone, or of the synovial sheath between the long pastern and the middle inferior sesamoidean ligament.

What kind of trauma causes windpuffs?

Horses subjected to heavy work tend to develop windpuffs. A horse that is in full training and then suddenly does not get any exercise will frequently show windpuffs. In young horses, windpuffs can also be the result of poor nutrition.

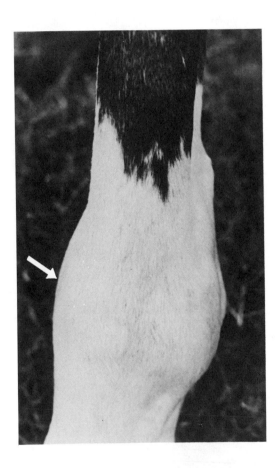 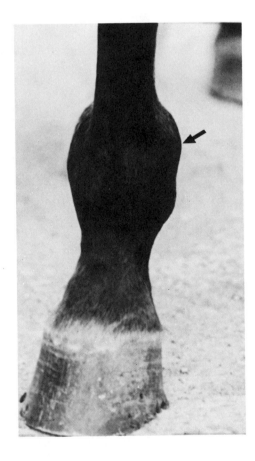

Fig. 4-12. Front view of windpuff of hind leg, most common site of windpuffs.

Fig. 4-13. Front view of severe windpuffs of the front leg.

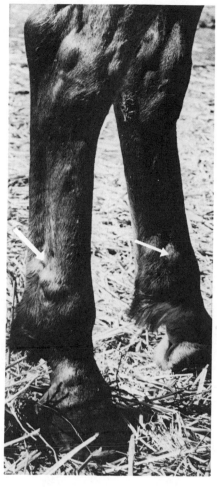

Fig. 4-14. Side view of windpuffs which are probably the result of poor nutrition.

What are the signs of windpuffs?

Joint capsule distension (without concurrent lameness) and a firm, fluid swelling in the area of the fetlock are the common signs of windpuffs. A longstanding case may harden and become a permanent blemish as a result of the replacement of fluid swelling by scar tissue.

How are windpuffs normally treated?

Treatment is usually not effective or required if no lameness is involved. Decreased work for the horse normally will suffice. If there is lameness, veterinarians generally prescribe enforced rest in addition to local heat, draining of the excess synovial fluid and local injection of corticosteroids. Elastic wraps after injection may be used. To reduce the swelling, applying an elastic wrap over a sweat, such as equal parts of glycerin and alcohol, will work temporarily because some lesions apparently result from improper venous drainage.

Draining the joint capsule and injecting a corticosteroid may provide temporary improvement, but if lameness is not involved, veterinary treatment will probably be conservative. If lameness is involved, it may be a sign of arthritis, bursitis or tenosynovitis and should be treated as such. If the windpuffs are due to inadequate nutrition, the ration should be adjusted according to the nutritional needs of the animal.

OSSELETS

What are osselets?

There are two types of osselets. The term "green osselets" refers to an inflammation of the joint capsule of the fetlock joint. When abnormal new bone growth appears and the condition has become chronic, the condition is called "true osselets." Since concussion is a causative factor, osselets rarely occur in the hindlimbs of horses.

How are osselets caused?

Any type of injury resulting in tearing, stretching and/or straining of the joint capsule and its attachments can cause osselets. Strain and repeated trauma from excessively hard training are considered primary causes of osselets. Repeated concussion is also a major factor in their development. Upright pastern conformation predisposes a horse to osselets because it increases concussion on the fetlock. When young horses are raced too frequently osselets often develop.

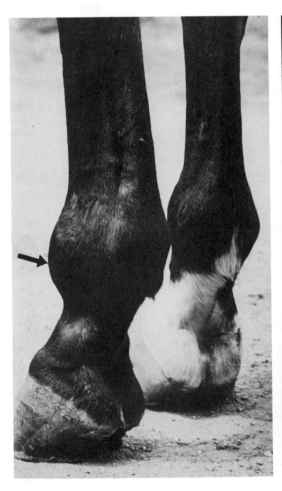

Fig. 4-15. Photograph of true osselets.

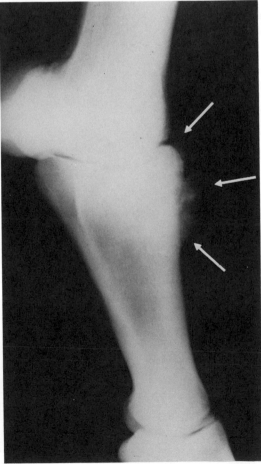

Fig. 4-16. X-ray of true osselets (arrows).

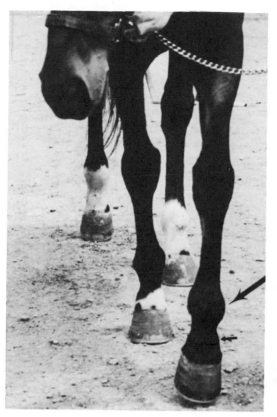
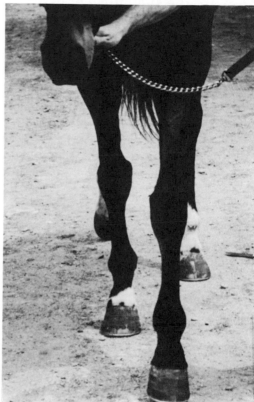

Fig. 4-17. Above, on the left and right, notice the travel and plant of the horses's left foot, which lands on the outside edge. This causes increased stress to the lateral fetlock and pastern joints, resulting in periarticular ringbone (small arrow) and osselets (large arrow).

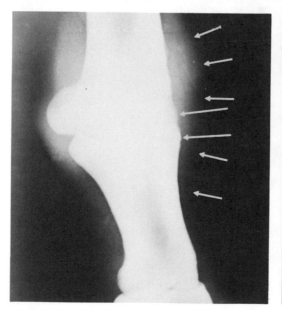
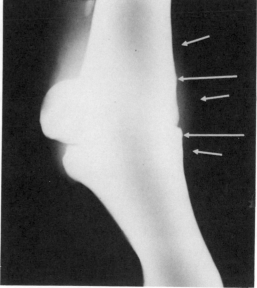

Fig. 4-18A, B. Two x-rays of green osselets, progressing to true osselets (large arrows). Notice the areas of inflammation of the soft tissues (small arrows).

What are the symptoms of osselets?

A shortened stride is characteristic of both green and true osselets. In the acute stage there will be a soft, warm swelling over the frog and possibly over the sides of the fetlock. Pressure on these areas will cause the horse to flinch. Also, he will avoid extreme dorsal or volar flexion of the fetlock joint. Lameness is usually readily apparent.

In advanced stages, characterized by new bone growth (true osselets), the symptoms are similar except that the swellings are of a bony nature. A short, choppy gait is characteristic of osselets.

When there is new bone growth, a small fragment can chip off and remain enclosed in the joint capsule. This piece of bone in the joint capsule is called a joint mouse. A veterinarian can detect joint mice by X-ray examination.

What is the usual treatment for osselets?

Absolute rest accompanied by treatment to reduce the inflammation is mandatory. Specific veterinary care depends upon the individual case. Commonly used treatments include the following: antiphlogistic packs, ice packs, cold water bandages, corticosteroid injections, phenylbutazone, poultices and sweats. When the inflammation has subsided it is a common veterinary practice to fire or blister the affected area in the hope of strengthening the joint capsule.

Firing and blistering along with radiation therapy are the usual treatments

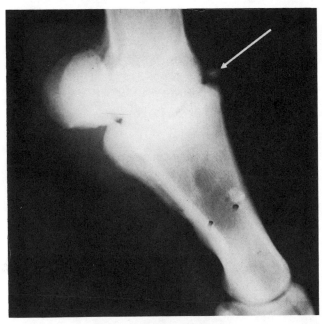

Fig. 4-19. X-ray showing joint mouse (arrow).

when the inflammation is chronic. Joint mice should normally be surgically removed to prevent constant irritation in the joint capsule.

Is a horse able to recover completely from osselets?

Yes. When osselets are treated in the "green" stage the horse will regain soundness if rested until the inflammation totally subsides. The prognosis for true osselets is also favorable if the new bone growth is not on the actual joint surface. The chance of total recovery is lessened if upright pastern conformation is a predisposing factor because the possibility of recurrent injury is much greater.

SESAMOIDITIS

What is sesamoiditis?

This is an inflammation of the proximal sesamoid bones, usually involving both osteitis and periostitis (inflammation of the bone and its covering). The associated ligaments may also become involved eventually showing calcified areas due to chronic inflammation. It more commonly affects the front legs because they carry more weight, hence more stress, and because they are subject to direct trauma from the toe of the hindfoot hitting the sesamoid region of the front foot.

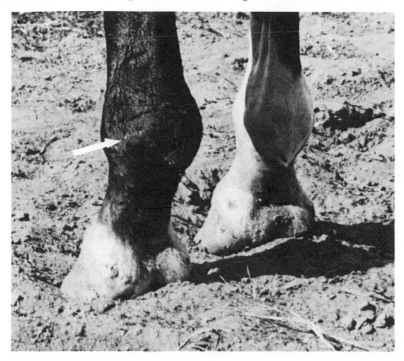

Fig. 4-20. Sesamoiditis of the front legs. Notice the "jewelry" marks of pin firing on the fetlock area.

How is sesamoiditis caused?

Sesamoiditis can be caused by any unusual strain in the area of the fetlock joint. Bruising and injuries to the bones themselves have also been known to cause sesamoiditis. This is most common in race horses, hunters and jumpers, all of whom place great stress on their front legs in competition. Sesamoiditis usually occurs in both of the paired bones in any one fetlock joint, but occasionally only one bone will be affected.

Some types of poor conformation make a horse especially susceptible to sesamoiditis. For example, long sloping pasterns decrease concussion but they greatly increase strain on the ligaments surrounding the fetlock joint and the suspensory apparatus, therefore predisposing the horse to inflammation in the fetlock area.

What are the signs of sesamoiditis?

Pain and swelling of the fetlock joint, with the area of the sesamoids being particularly tender, are the major symptoms. Lameness may be present in varying degrees. It is most evident when a horse is in motion.

Ordinarily, X-ray is used to differentiate sesamoiditis from a fracture of the proximal sesamoids which has very similar signs. If the disease is long standing, new bone growth on the back of the sesamoids and calcification of the ligaments will show up on the X-ray. In addition, sesamoiditis may occur in conjunction with tendon injuries, fracture of the sesamoid bones and suspensory ligament injuries.

What treatment is used for sesamoiditis?

The serious nature of sesamoiditis requires that the veterinarian be called in to make a positive diagnosis and to administer subsequent treatment.

The inflammation must be reduced. Methods frequently used by the veterinarian include alternating hot and cold packs, local injections of corticosteroids, antiphlogistic packs and phenylbutazone therapy. In cases of severe lameness the joint should be immobilized with either a cast or a tight support bandage. Corrective shoeing (shortening the toe and elevating the heel) can be used to relieve tension on the sesamoids.

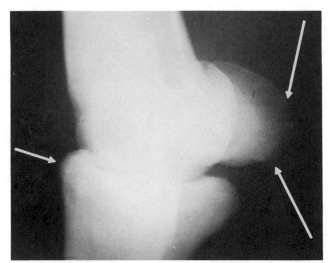

Fig. 4-21. X-ray of sesamoiditis. Large arrows indicate the area of inflammation. Small arrow indicates a true osselet.

Fig. 4-22. Hard fiberglass cast applied to the hindleg to immobilize the fetlock.

Fig. 4-23. A support bandage applied to the fetlock.

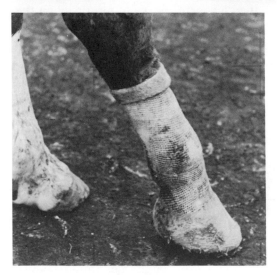

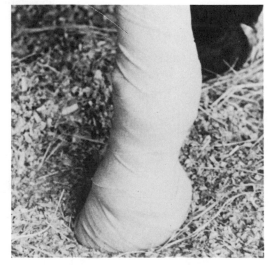

Firing and blistering are occasionally used to treat chronic sesamoiditis but the results usually are not very successful. Radiation therapy can also be employed by the veterinarian. As a last resort, he may perform a volar neurectomy to alleviate pain. This surgical procedure cuts the nerves giving sensation to the portion of the limb from the fetlock down.

What is the prognosis for this disease?

The prognosis is not very favorable and depends greatly upon the extent of damage and new bone growth. Many times an animal will regain soundness and go back into training, only to have sesamoiditis recur. This is because the sesamoids have a less than normal ability to heal, due to a very limited blood supply and periosteum development. Naturally, any partial healing is easily aggravated by the normal stress and strain of work. Extended periods of rest even up to one to two years are the best hope of a horse returning to true soundness.

SUSPENSORY LIGAMENT INJURIES

What are the types of injuries which can occur to the suspensory ligament?

The suspensory ligament can be strained, sprained or ruptured. A strain is a stress on the ligament which results in soreness and inflammation of the ligament. A sprain also involves stress and inflammation, but goes on to incur actual tearing of some fibers of the ligament. A rupture is a complete tearing of a section of the fibers of the ligament. The involved inflammation of the ligament related to all three type of injuries is called "Desmitis."

Fig. 4-24. This diagram shows the different types of injury and the degree of damage to the tendons and ligaments.

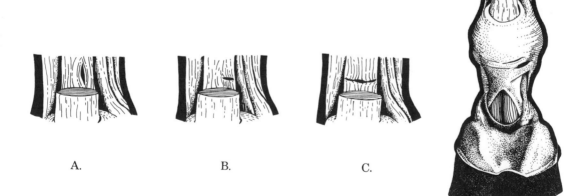

A.   B.   C.

A. Damage to the ligament in a strain injury. Some hemorrhage and stretching occurs.

B. Damage to the ligament in sprain injury. Stretching and hemorrhage are accompanied by actual tearing of some of the tissue fibers.

C. Damage to the ligament when it is rputured involves separation of the ends of the fibers and serious amounts of hemorrhage. This includes loss of function of the ligament.

How is a suspensory ligament strained or sprained?

Strains can occur in the branches, at the point of branching (bifurcation), or in the middle or at the top of the suspensory ligament.

Branch strains result from the medial (inward) or lateral (outward) twisting of the lower limb that occurs when a horse lands on uneven ground or an improperly leveled shoe.

Fig. 4-25. Views of the suspensory ligament.

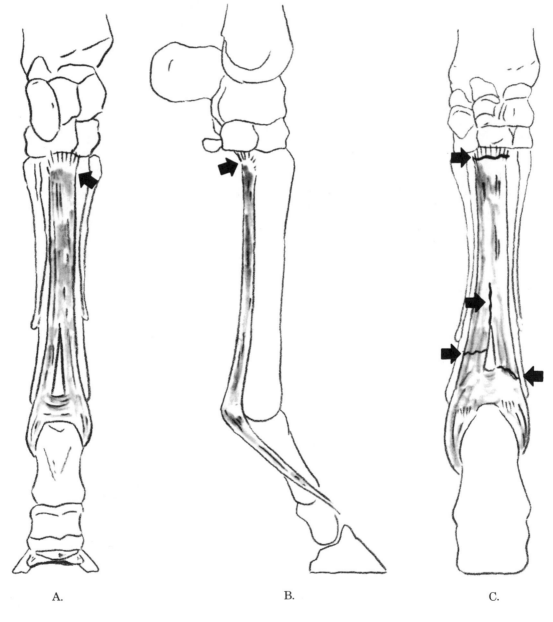

A.

B.

C.

A. Rear view

B. side view showing the upper attachment of the suspensory ligament.

C. rear view showing the locations of tears in the suspensory ligament (arrows).

Extensive dorsal flexion of the fetlock joint can result in injury to the bifurcation area. This usually happens at the end of a long race when the horse is fatigued. It is a very painful condition since every time the leg hits the ground and the fetlock sinks down, the two branches of the suspensory ligament are spread. The action is like trying to pry two fingers apart. Obviously, movement prolongs the injury and prevents healing.

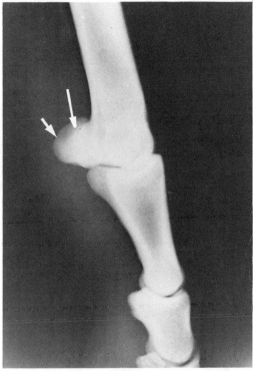

Fig. 4-26. X-ray showing a case of a sprained branch of the suspensory ligament below the sesamoid, causing that sesamoid to be higher than the other. (arrows point out tops of both sesamoids).

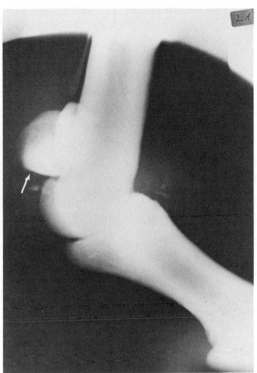

Fig. 4-27. X-ray showing displacement of the sesamoids (arrow) caused by a rupture of both branches of the suspensory ligament below the sesamoids.

In the fetlock area, suspensory sprains or enlargements heal fairly well unless the proximal sesamoid bones are involved. Unfortunately, the sesamoid bones are affected in most cases causing periostitis (inflammation of the bone covering), sesamoiditis and new bone growth on the sesamoids.

Below the fetlock, suspensory injuries heal easily although there may be some bony growth in the area of attachment to the pastern.

Injuries occurring to the suspensory ligament at its upper attachment to the cannon bone are very serious. This is because the fine fibers of the ligament fit into tiny holes on the surface of the bone. If these fibers are torn loose, they do not go back into the holes upon healing but adhere to the bone surface. This is a very weak attachment which easily comes loose again. Horses with such a condition often remain lame for months.

Splints or calcification of the splint bone are associated with pressure on the middle portion of the suspensory ligament which results in strain of this area.

Fatigue, and placing more weight on one leg than another, may lead to suspensory ligament injuries. Suspensory ligament lamenesses occur most frequently in the forelegs of the horse except for the harness racing Standardbred. Trotters and pacers are affected more in the hindleg because of the form of their racing gait.

What are the signs of suspensory ligament strains?

If the suspensory ligament is merely strained, several slight injuries may be suffered before the problem is evident. Inflammation of the affected area accompanied by a cold lameness will be noticed first. Eventually the lameness will be constant.

Strains of the body of the suspensory ligament result in acute signs which eventually, like chronic cases of other ligament strains, make the area thick, hard and sometimes calcified.

Inflammation and thickening also occur with various fractures of bones in the suspensory ligament area and with sesamoiditis. Strains may or may not be present at the same time. X-ray examination by a veterinarian can determine the damage to the horse.

What are the signs of a sprained suspensory ligament?

Sprains result in acute lameness and swelling in the early stages. The horse will hold his knee and fetlock forward and raise the heel slightly off the ground. In moving, the fetlock will not be lowered all the way. The horse will get off the affected leg as quickly as possible. In the chronic stage, there is extensive fibrosis (scar tissue) and swelling at the bifurcation or the attachment to the sesamoid bones. Palpation and observation of the affected limb by the veterinarian will indicate the area and extent of injury.

How are strains treated?

Treatment for strains of the suspensory ligament depends on the severity of the injury. For acute strains, complete rest and anti-inflammatory treatments are required.

The veterinarian may treat chronic strains with corticosteroid injections followed by a cast from the hoof wall to just below the carpal joint which is worn for two to four weeks. Then an elastic bandage is worn for a month. Six to twelve months of rest will normally be prescribed for the horse.

There is little successful treatment for chronic strains because of the decreased elasticity of the area. Firing, blistering, X- and gamma ray therapy are all possibilities, but a satisfactory result is doubtful. Rest will be required for about a year. If the horse is trained again after that, he should run with supporting bandages.

What is the prognosis for strains?

The prognosis is extremely variable depending on the location and severity of injury. Branch strains heal fairly well, but strains of the body of the ligament or strains which result in a sinking of the fetlock have a poor prognosis. Suspensory ligament strains associated with sesamoiditis or strains of the flexor tendons have about a 20 percent recovery rate.

What is the prognosis for sprains?

In nearly all cases of sprains the prognosis is unfavorable. This is because tendosynovitis of the flexor tendons (bowed tendon) commonly occurs with suspensory ligament injuries. However, if treated properly in the acute stage, some horses can return to work, even racing.

In all types of suspensory ligament injuries, whether a strain, sprain or rupture, a considerable amount of time must be allowed for healing because this ligament does not have a large blood supply. A simple strain of the ligament could require only six weeks to heal, which is still much longer than most ailments caused by stress. A tear could take a year to heal, and injuries to the upper area of the ligament might never heal satisfactorily.

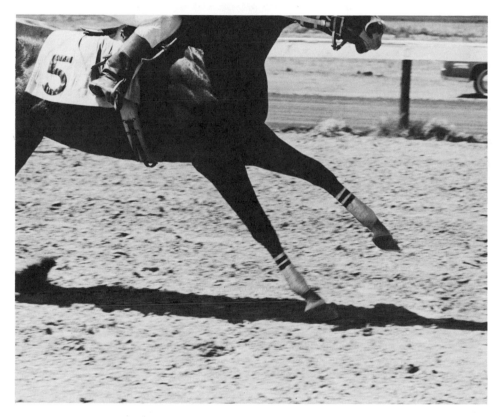

Fig. 4-28. A horse running in exercise bandages which are applied for support and protection of the leg.

What part of the suspensory ligament is most prone to ruptures?

Ruptures involve the branches of the suspensory ligament, rarely the body. Sometimes though, the body will tear longitudinally at its bifurcation.

How do ruptures occur in the suspensory ligament?

Landing on uneven ground and twisting the foot violently to one side or the other is the usual cause of branch ruptures. If the branches are chronically inflamed due to splint bone or proximal sesamoid bone fractures, this is especially likely to happen.

How is a rupture treated?

The veterinarian will probably restrict movement of the leg in a cast and prescribe stall rest for at least two months. Confinement will continue after that for another four to six months in a stall or small paddock.

What are the chances of recovery with a rupture?

A rupture of a branch can heal if at least a year's rest is given. It must be remembered, however, that this is such a severe injury the horse will probably not work soundly again.

Other problems arise from this type of injury. A tear may result in a thickening of the suspensory ligament. This puts pressure on the adjoining splint bone to the point of pushing it out of place where the bottom inch or two of the bone will snap off. Further complications result. In other words, there is somewhat of a vicious circle here: a fractured splint bone can cause a thickening of the suspensory ligament through inflammation and a thickened suspensory ligament can cause a fracture of a splint bone.

FRACTURES

How does a fracture of the proximal sesamoids occur?

This injury is often the result of stress accompanied by fatigue from a long race. Normally, the leg moves backward at about the same speed at which the body moves forward. If the leg movement is slower than that of the body, the hoof will strike the ground in a more forward position than normal, putting the sesamoid bones higher up so they no longer articulate completely with the cannon bone and are more susceptible to a break near the top. If the leg moves faster than the body, the hoof will impact further back than normal. This pulls the sesamoid bones down out of the usual articulation track with the cannon bone, subjecting them to possible fractures near their base.

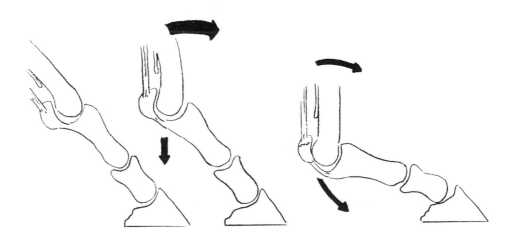

Fig. 4-29. This figure shows the position of the foreleg when the foot strikes the ground in an extreme forward stride. The sesamoids are more subject to fracture at the top.

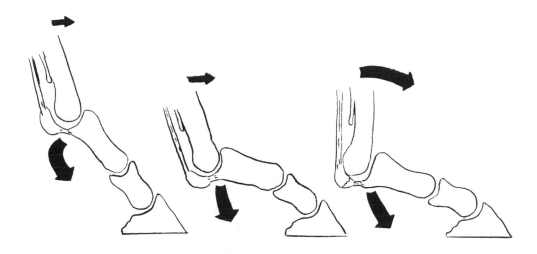

Fig. 4-30. Position of the foreleg when it strikes the ground further beneath the horse. This applies more stress to the lower attachment of the sesamoids.

In other words, top and bottom sesamoid breaks are simple bending fractures that result from improper timing of the leg and body movements. Extreme lack of coordination may even allow the fetlock joint to touch the ground. Although these stresses more commonly result in top fractures of the outermost sesamoid bone and bottom fractures of the innermost sesamoid bone, the breaks may be in multiple areas of one or both sesamoid bones.

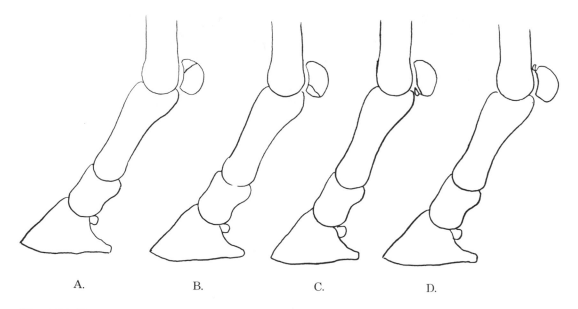

A.   B.   C.   D.

Fig. 4-31. These drawings illustrate locations of chips and fractures of the sesamoid bones. A. Apical fracture. B. Distal fracture. C. Distal chip. D. Apical chip.

How is a fracture detected?

Chip fractures may produce no signs until the animal is cooling out, at which time swelling of the fetlock with accompanying lameness may be noticed. Severe fractures involving the proximal sesamoids usually result in immediate swelling and severe supporting lameness. In this case the horse will try to support the weight on the affected leg on tiptoe or will not even put his foot to the ground. Exact diagnosis as to extent and location of the break can only be made upon X-ray examination.

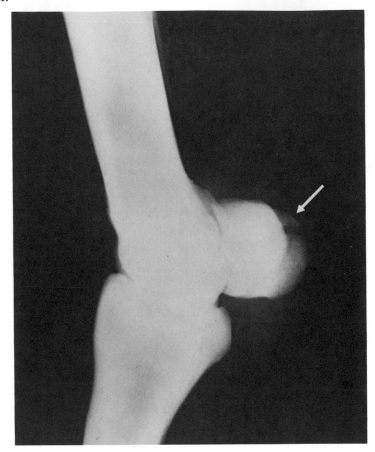

Fig. 4-32. X-ray showing an apical fracture of the sesamoid bone (arrow).

What can be done to treat a fracture or chip?

Treatment will be either surgical or a casting of the leg, depending on the size and type of fracture and the discretion of the veterinarian.

A cast will probably be applied in those cases that: (1) have bone fragments close together with little displacement; (2) have separation of the bone fragments, but the horse will not be used for racing; or (3) have a bone fragment that is larger than one-third of the whole bone.

The veterinarian will cast the leg in as normal a position as possible and will leave the cast on 12-16 weeks with periodic changes. Sesamoid bone fractures heal very slowly. Care must be taken to confine an injured horse to prevent reinjury. Applied immediately after injury, casting can produce excellent improvement.

If the bone fragment is less than one-third of the whole sesamoid bone in cases of fragment displacement, or if it is an old injury that has not healed, the veterinarian will normally remove the fragment surgically. A cast or supporting bandages will follow surgery for about ten days, followed by supporting wraps and rest with daily short walks for another thirty days.

If the fracture is incomplete or if the fragment is small, the horse may be walking relatively soundly in seven to ten days after simple anti-inflammatory treatment. However, lameness will recur with strenuous work. For this reason, the veterinarian will probably recommend casting or surgery.

What is the prognosis in cases of sesamoid bone fractures?

If the injury was slight and treated immediately, the horse could possibly be returned to work after an extended rest. Otherwise, the prognosis is always guarded to unfavorable, with lameness often recurring.

What are bipartite sesamoids?

This is the name given to a condition found in some horses where X-rays show fractures of the upper part of both sesamoid bones in both front ankles. It seems to be congenital since, in the cases that have been found, there was no heat, swelling or sign of lameness.

CANNON

ANATOMY AND CONFORMATION

Which bone is the cannon bone?

This is the bone which is part of the knee joint at its top and part of the fetlock joint at its bottom. Starting at the upper end on each posterior corner of the cannon bone are the two splint bones. They articulate with the lower row of carpal (knee) bones. Together the three bones are known as the metacarpals in the foreleg and metatarsals in the hindleg. The cannon bone is the large or third metacarpal (metatarsal) and the splint bones are called the second and fourth, or medial and lateral metacarpals (metatarsals), respectively. The central bone of the cannon region is very dense and strong, so fractures are less common than one might think they would be.

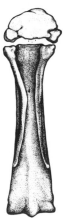 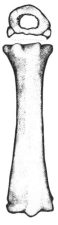

Fig. 5-1. On the left, a rear view of the metacarpal bones and a top view of their articular surfaces. To the right, front view and cross-section of the same bones.

What is the position and purpose of the splint bones?

The splint bones articulate with another bone only at their upper ends. They are tapered in shape as they run down the inside (medial) and outside (lateral) borders of the cannon bone to about three inches above the fetlock. The triangular shape of a splint bone narrows from nearly an inch wide to as little as one-sixteenth inch just above its end where there is a small bony knob which may be visible through the skin. The lower end does not have any direct support, but is in contact with the cannon bone and attached to it by a ligament. Irritation of this ligament results in the condition known as "splints." (See section on Splints, page 129.)In older horses this ligament usually ossifies, fusing the splint bone to the cannon bone.

Splint bones have little useful value other than providing a channel for the suspensory ligaments.

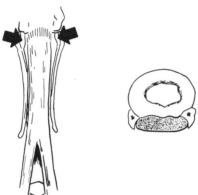

Fig. 5-2. On the left, a rear view of the metacarpals, showing the channels in the splint bones for the suspensory ligament (arrows). Right, a cross-section of the bones, showing the ligament in place.

Which muscles, ligaments and tendons are in the cannon area?

The superficial digital flexor tendon, the deep digital flexor tendon, the inferior check ligament and the suspensory ligament of the fetlock (interosseous medius) all run along the back of the cannon bone. The check ligament is between the suspensory ligament and the flexor tendons.

Passing over the front of the cannon bone are the flat tendons of the lateral digital extensor and long digital extensor muscles.

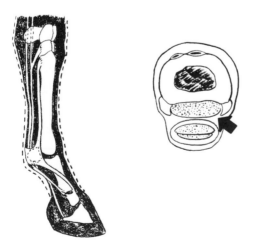

Fig. 5-3. On the left, side view of the cannon bone and pastern bones, showing attachment of the superficial and deep digital flexor tendons, check ligament and suspensory ligament. Right, cross-section of the cannon area, showing suspensory ligament (arrow), superfical and deep digital flexor tendons.

The tendons in the cannon region are particularly susceptible to injury from excessive strain. This results in the inflammation known as bowed tendon if the flexor tendons are affected. If the extensor tendons are affected, the common term for the disorder is bucked shins.

What is the correct conformation for the cannon area?

From a front view the cannon looks very narrow, but from the side the cannon looks flat and wide due to the tendons, which are well defined. The superficial digital flexor is actually set well away from the bone. Thin skin and sparse connective tissue leave the bone, the ligaments, the tendons and the blood vessels visible in detail.

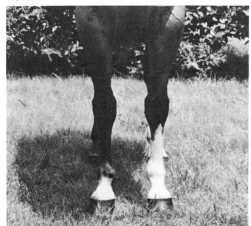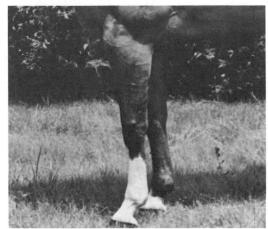

Fig. 5-4. Front and side views of the cannon area.

BUCKED SHINS (SHIN BUCK)

How are bucked shins (sore shin, skinbuck) defined?

Bucked shins are a periostitis (inflammation of the bone covering) of the front side of the cannon bone. They are common in the forelimb, but rare in the hindlimb. The condition is most often seen in the forelegs of young horses that have been subjected to strenuous physical activity.

How do they occur?

In milder cases, bucked shins are from stretching or tearing of the periosteum adjacent to the extensor tendons, although trauma of the periosteum from other causes may be involved (generally caused by concussion in immature horses). They rarely occur in horses over three years old unless from direct trauma. When the attachment of the periosteum to the bone is torn, a hematoma (blood collection) forms between the periosteum and the bone. This hematoma then forms into fibrous scar tissue which will contract as it heals if rest is allowed. Fibrous tissue can become ossified, leaving permanent bony enlargements called "calcium deposits," which tend to interfere with the smooth action of the extensor tendons. Bucked shins can also result from many micro-fractures, which are very tiny pieces of bone that are broken off of the cannon in the region of the injury.

What are the signs of bucked shins?

This condition is easily diagnosed since a painful swelling appears on the front of the cannon bone which is warm to the touch. Lameness will increase with exercise and the gait will be choppy. If only one limb is involved, the horse will tend to rest the affected limb, but if both limbs are involved, he will shift his weight from one to the other.

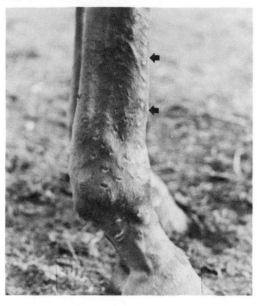
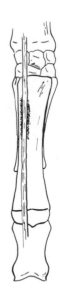

Fig. 5-5. Swelling typical of bucked shins.
Fig. 5-6. The bones of the shin, showing inflammation of the periosteum (darkened area).

In longstanding cases there is active periostitis and a thickening of the bone at the injury site.

X-rays can differentiate this condition from saucershaped or "march" fractures (a wedge-shaped fracture of the front of the cannon bone). This is due to the same causes as shinbuck but is a more severe manifestation of those causes.

How are bucked shins treated?

A minimum of one month of rest is the most effective therapy. The veterinarian may relieve the acute inflammation with antiphlogistic packs, poultices or cold water bandgages, phenylbutazone or corticosteroids. Firing after the inflammation has subsided may be used to enhance the healing process and improve the chance of

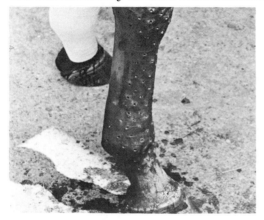

Fig. 5-7. This horse has been pin-fired to "prevent" bucked shins.

a return to training after rest (without recurrent periostitis). This is a common practice with race horses. If there is a relapse during training, probably the rest period was not long enough or the return to training was too abrupt.

Is recovery complete with bucked shins?

The prognosis is good in all cases if enough rest is given. This condition will be recurrent if the rest is not sufficient. Permanent new bone growth results if the periostitis is severe or recurs several times, or if a "saucer" fracture is present.

SPLINTS

What is a "splint?"

A splint is usually a disorder of young horses that most often affects the forelimbs. Splint is a term used to describe any hard swelling (exostosis) that develops in the area of the splint bone and primarily involves the interosseous ligament which binds the splint bone to the cannon bone.

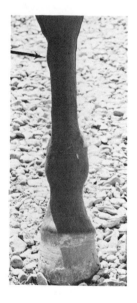

Fig. 5-8. Swelling that typically accompanies splints.

How are splints caused?

Trauma from concussion or direct trauma causes all splints. Most splints are due to strain from a training schedule that is excessive, especially in the horse that is three years old or younger. Faulty conformation such as bench knees (page 155), or improper shoeing (heel high and inside wall too high will increase concussion to the ligament of the splint) may contribute to the development of this condition. Nutritional bone disease associated with mineral imbalance of calcium, phosphorus, vitamin A or D, often seems to be a factor leading to splints in horses up to two years of age. It is thought that the nutritional deficiency has caused poor development of bone, hence weak attachment of periosteum (bone membrane) to bone in these young horses. Because of this, less concussion is necessary to cause the periosteum to tear loose from the bone which leads to inflammation and new bone growth.

What is a true splint?

Though the splint bones bear some weight, they are unopposed at their lower ends. The second metacarpal (inside splint bone) is affected more often because it supports more weight. The interosseous ligament between the cannon and the splint bones and adjacent periosteum is torn slightly in a "true splint" resulting in periostitis (inflammation of the bone covering) at the site of ligament damage. Trauma to the metacarpal bones can result in periostitis and enlargement of the splint bone other than at the site of the interosseous ligament. Some authorities differentiate between this and the "true" splint mentioned above because this does not include damage to the interosseous ligament.

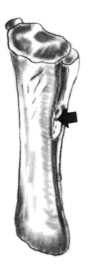 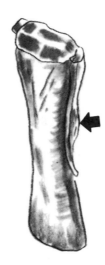

Fig. 5-9. On the left, "true" splint. On the right, enlargement of the periosteum, with no damage to the interosseous ligament.

What are the signs of splints?

Originally there will be heat, pain and swelling (often hard) along the side of the cannon bone, although the heat and pain may not be very apparent. This usually happens abruptly, which is why the phrase "popped a splint" is so descriptive. The horse will usually show lameness according to the degree of inflammation, although some cases of splints may never cause lameness. Eventually the swelling is reduced in size but becomes firmer due to ossification (bone formation). The bony growth itself does not get smaller, but remains as a small calcified growth. Reduction in size that is apparent to the observer is due to the subsiding of inflammation of the soft tissues involved. Following ossification, the lameness disappears, except in occasional cases where the growth encroaches on the suspensory ligament, flexor tendons or carpal joint.

What is the treatment for splints?

Various methods of treatment are available and in each case the veterinarian can best determine and administer the proper care. To help prevent the development of bone growth after the interosseous ligament has been torn, immediate rest and antiphlogistic packs or cold bandages are beneficial to minimize the inflammation. Then firing or internal blistering may be used to help arrest the periostitis. In the very early stages of treatment the veterinarian may choose to inject the area around

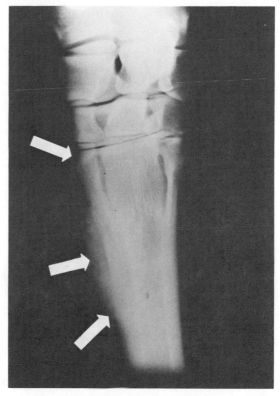

Fig. 5-10. X-ray showing new bone formation in a case of splints (arrows).

the splint with a corticosteroid to help reduce inflammation as this may help prevent excessive bone growth. This should be accompanied by pressure bandages. All treatments must include at least 30 days of complete rest, although the veterinarian may recommend a longer rest in a case where corticoid treatment is used.

In the case of bone growth (exostosis) which encroaches on the suspensory ligament, surgery may be recommended to remove the impinging growth.

Fig. 5-11. New bone growth impinging on the suspensory ligament (arrow).

Is the prognosis favorable in cases of splints?

In most cases the prognosis is good. A visible exostosis rarely causes lameness after the acute phase has passed, but the appearance of the limb may be undesirable due to the lump. If the original inflammatory reaction is treated immediately, it is possible that new bone growth may not take place. In this case the splint may disappear once the inflammatory reaction subsides, which may take from a few days to a few weeks.

An exostosis that impinges on the suspensory ligament and/or carpal joint has a guarded prognosis because it requires surgery for correction.

Is the rule of thumb true that a splint closer than two fingers' width to the knee will be likely to cause permanent lameness?

There is some validity to this rule but it is not because of the splint itself. If permanent lameness results, it is because the attachment of the suspensory apparatus to the back of the cannon and knee was damaged and did not heal completely.

BOWED TENDON

What is a bowed tendon?

Any damage to the tendon which causes inflammation may be referred to as a "bow." The terms tendinitis and tendosynovitis differentiate between an inflammation involving only the tendon and one which involves both the tendon and its sheath. Damage to the tendon may result in a high, middle or low bow in addition to the "classic" bow, which involves all three categories.

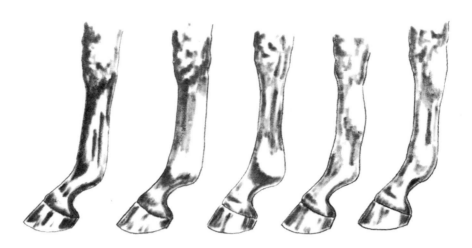

Fig. 5-12. From the left: normal tendon, "classic" bow, low bow, middle bow, high bow.

What structures are involved in a bowed tendon?

Both the deep flexor tendon and the superficial flexor tendon may be bowed, singly or in combination. Most frequently, the superficial flexor tendon in the foreleg is injured, although bows occur with equal frequency in the hindlimbs of harness racing horses.

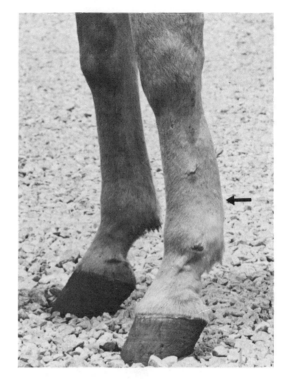

Fig. 5-13. Side view of a cannon with an extensive middle bow.

The tendon structures (paratenon, tendon sheath, annular ligaments) are important factors which limit the movements of the tendon when it is injured. Paratenon is a specialized loose tissue that fills the space between a tendon and the immovable fascial compartment through which the tendon moves. Elastic and pliable, with long fibers, the paratenon allows the tendon to move back and forth. Since the paratenon is attached to the tendon, it is not a true gliding mechanism (like a sheath). This loose tissue is simply dragged with the tendon while it remains attached at the other end to fascia or some other fixed structure.

Tendon sheaths are composed of two layers of synovia: a visceral layer which covers the tendon (epitenon) and a parietal layer (sheath) which lines the fascial tunnel through which the tendon glides. These two layers form a double thickness called the mesotenon. Blood vessels are carried by the mesotenon to the tendon at both the origin and the insertion. Vessels enter the tendon in the mesotenon on the nonfriction side, run longitudinally in the epitenon, and send branches at right angles along the endotenon septa. Normally, this loose, filmy layer does not limit motion of the tendon.

Endotenon septa are fibrous divisions which run from the epitenon to the tendon, dividing it into bundles. When the tendon sheath is injured the healing process causes these divisions to contract, resulting in a telescoping effect.

Tough, fibrous, thickened parts of the fascial sheath are called annular ligaments. These encircle the tendons at the top and the bottom to keep the tendons in the proper track. It is this involvement with firm tunnels and encircling ligaments that causes a great deal of the damange in a bowed tendon. The enclosure

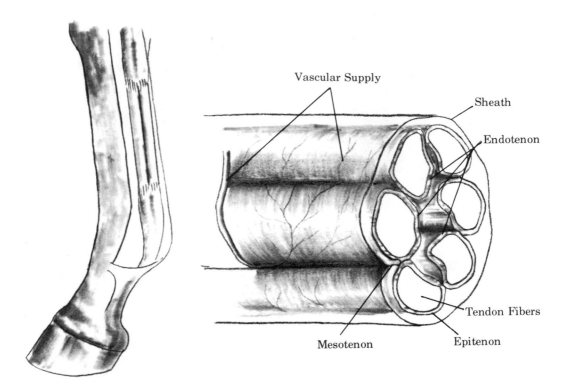

Fig. 5-14. Side view of a normal tendon.

Fig. 5-15. Cross-section diagram of the parts of a tendon.

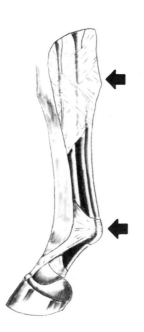

Fig. 5-16. Side view diagram showing annular ligaments (arrows).

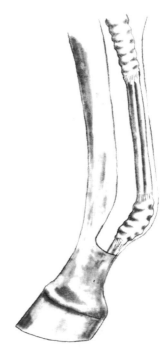

Fig. 5-17. Side view diagram showing "telescoped" tendon sheaths that result from bowed tendon.

causes pressure and damage when the injured tissues swell, resulting in tissue death and sloughing of the tendon. If the sloughed tendon is replaced by scar tissue that involves the sheath, the tendon sheath may flex and contract.

What happens when a tendon is bowed?

The bow may be caused by a number of factors, but the inflammation causes the tissue damage. When the tendon and the sheath are involved, the tendon sheath telescopes around the deep and superficial flexors. The attachment of the mesotenon may be torn from its position on the tendon which causes hemorrhage and inflammation. If the injury involves the central portion of the tendon where there is no sheath, adhesions may develop between the tendons, paratenon and the surrounding subcutaneous tissues. Adhesions may be formed all along the tendon, between the deep and superficial flexor tendons and may involve the sheath. Fibrous scar tissue may also develop between the tendon sheath and the surrounding connective tissue. Although it may not appear on the surface of the tendon, hemorrhage usually occurs within the tendon in addition to varying degrees of tendon fiber tearing. Necrosis may occur within the tendon as a result of torn fibers or due to crushing and bruising of the tendon.

What causes a bowed tendon?

A severe strain to the area of the flexor tendon is the major cause of bowed tendon. Long, weak pasterns are important causes of bowed tendons. In addition, forced training procedures, muscular fatigue, a misstep, speed and exertion and muddy footing are major contributors to injury of the tendons. Tight-fitting bandages or boots, improper shoeing and top-heavy conformation have also been cited as predisposing factors to tendon injury in the working horse.

Some authorities believe that degeneration of tendon cells begins before the acute lesion develops. This degeneration is evidenced by small swellings and heat in the tendon which can be detected by careful examination. If training were discontinued when these early lesions were discovered, it is believed that they would heal with rest. When tendons are partially severed or crushed and bruised, they swell and soften and may rupture from ordinary pull several days to three weeks later.

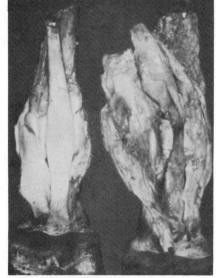

Fig. 5-18. (Left) A normal deep flexor tendon within the digital sheath of a hindlimb. (Right) Partial, primary rupture of a deep digital flexor tendon of the opposite hindlimb. The torn tendon has been overgrown with synovial membrane.

Photo courtesy of EQUINE MEDICINE and SURGERY, Second Edition, American Veterinary Publications, Inc. Wheaton, Illinois, 1972.

What are the signs of tendosynovitis?

Signs of acute tendosynovitis occur soon after the injury, causing the horse to pull up lame or to go lame shortly after the injury. If the bow is new, there will be swelling and heat throughout the involved area. There will be a rapidly forming swelling at the back of the cannon which is extremely painful. Characterized by severe lameness, this condition causes the horse to stand with the heel elevated to ease pressure on the flexor tendon area. The knee will usually be cocked forward at rest, and the horse will not allow the fetlock to drop during motion in order to avoid painful pressure.

Careful examination by a veterinarian is necessary to determine the extent of the injury. Injury to the suspensory ligament or to the sesamoid bones can occur with a bowed tendon.

Old or chronic bows are characterized by the presence of a firm, prominent swelling on the back of the cannon. This firm swelling is actually scar tissue in the tendon, caused by the invasion of lymph fluid at the time of the original injury. Often the horse with a chronic bowed tendon remains sound when walking or trotting, but "breaks down" under heavy work or training.

What is the treatment for acute bowed tendon?

Prompt attention can mean the difference between ability to return to work or retirement after a bowed tendon. If there is any indication that the horse might have bowed, a tight (very tight) bandage should be applied immediately. When the horse is some distance from the stable, this is even more important. The bandage is not primarily for support, but is used to cut down the massive hemorrhage and blood flow in the affected area. Any track bandage will work, but it should be wet down and applied directly to the leg, without cotton. The tourniquet-bandage should be left on no longer then 20 minutes, removed for a few minutes, then reapplied. This tourniquet serves to cut down the amount of lymph fluid that seeps out of the injured blood vessels. Presence of fluid in the surrounding tissues will form adhesions, which cause massive scar tissue in the affected area.

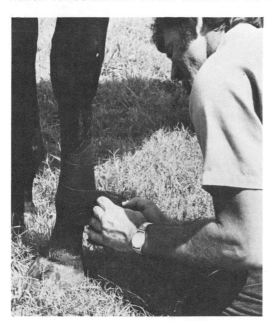

Fig. 5-19. Application of a wet wrap for an acute bowed tendon.

Once the horse is back in the stable, remove the bandage and put the leg in ice for several hours, overnight if possible. At this time, the veterinarian will start the horse on some anti-inflammatory drug which can be continued for ten days to two weeks. If the horse can't be iced overnight, a soft cast or tight bandage may be applied by the veterinarian.

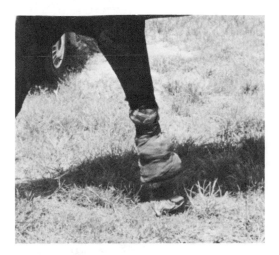

Fig. 5-20. Ice bandage, as applied to bowed tendon.

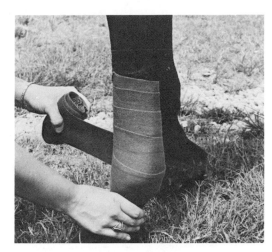

Fig. 5-21. A snug bandage for firm support.

Damage can usually be evaluated by the veterinarian the next morning. If the horse was iced overnight, a cast will normally be applied from the knee to the hoof to prevent further fluid swelling and support the limb. First casts usually remain in place for a week to ten days, at which time they are removed and replaced. A second cast is usually required for two or three weeks depending on the extent of the injury. If there is any period when the cast is off (if the horse tears it up or if it falls off), a snug bandage should be applied to prevent fluids rushing back into the injured vessels that have been constricted for some time. Until the veterinarian arrives to replace the cast, an elastic bandage placed snugly over a half sheet of cotton will prevent further stretching and tearing of the tissue fibers.

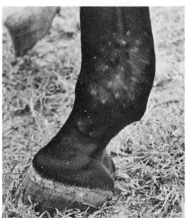

Fig. 5-22. An old bow that has been fired and carefully managed.

After a month or so has passed, the tendon will have reached a point of resolution. The ice, the steroids and the casts have accomplished as much as they can—healing is now up to nature. Since tendons heal very slowly, almost a year of rest will be required for complete healing. Light exercise in a supportive bandage will help prevent some adhesions in the limb. Leg braces or paints are effective from this point on, but time and lack of stress will promote the best healing. Care should be taken to prevent reinjuring the tendon before it is fully healed. Horses that tend to exercise too vigorously when turned out should be given very light exercise in hand or under saddle.

Light supportive bandages should be removed and left off for several hours a day, to prevent hair loss from constant pressure. Both front legs should be bandaged or the horse may overload the "good" leg and injure it.

Can corrective shoeing help bowed tendons?

Yes, corrective shoeing is important. If the suspensory ligament is not involved, the heel can be raised one to one and one-half inches for four to six weeks to take weight off the bow. This should be lowered gradually over a period of six to eight weeks. If the heel is raised longer than three months, the tendon may contract.

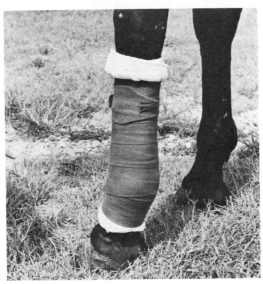 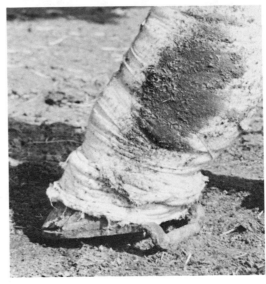

Fig. 5-23. Supportive bandages commonly used for bowed tendon.

Fig. 5-24. Corrective shoeing of the type used for bowed tendon.

How are chronic bows treated?

Since chronic bows usually involve a great deal of scar tissue, treatment to prevent this formation (as for new bows) is usually ineffective. Chronic bows are treated surgically or are blistered and fired. Surgical treatment attempts to either remove existing scar tissue or to stimulate increased circulation and healing. The theory behind causing damage to the tendon surgically is that by disturbing the tendon artificially, there will be an increased circulation in an attempt to heal the area. Hopefully, this will also benefit the healing process of the bowed tendon. Pin firing and blistering work on the same principles, although poor healing of the tendon fibers is thought to be due to the absence of collagen (a main supportive protein) which is not produced by tendon cells. Rest and limiting stress on the weakened tendon are necessary in the management of old bows.

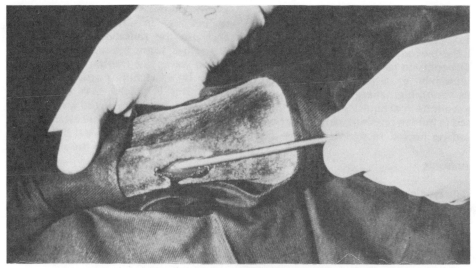

Courtesy of THE HORSE, by Peter Rossdale, M.A., F.R.C.V.S., published by The California Thoroughbred Breeders Association. Photo by Peter Rossdale.

Fig. 5-25. Tendon splitting surgery.

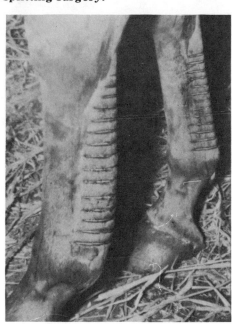

Courtesy of THE HORSE, by Peter Rossdale, M.A., F.R.C.V.S., published by The California Thoroughbred Breeders Association. Photo by Peter Rossdale.

Fig. 5-26. Bar firing, which may be used for treating chronic bowed tendons.

Do many horses recover from bows?

Yes. With proper management and treatment many horses can completely recover from a bowed tendon. *However,* even if the tendon is completely healed, it will never be as strong and elastic as a tendon that has never been injured. Therefore, cases which return to the stressful work which caused the bow are very likely to reinjure the tendon. Incidence of reoccurence of the bow in race horses is between 50 and 60 percent. The promptness of the initial treatment and only slight tendon damage permit perhaps ten percent of the horses to return to their former work at the level of past performance. In many cases, stakes horses become claimers and performance horses hold up only for pleasure use.

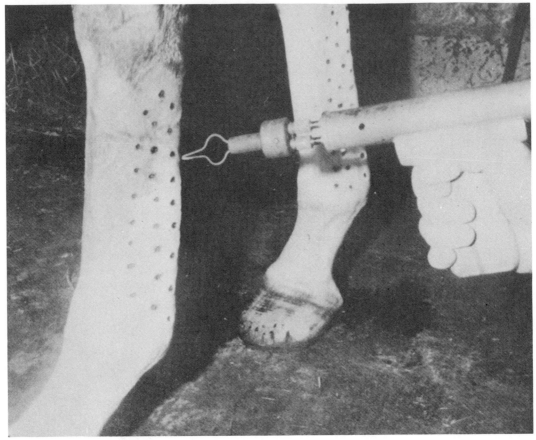

Courtesy of THE HORSE, by Peter Rossdale, M.A., F.R.C.V.S., published by The California Thoroughbred Breeders Association. Photo by Peter Rossdale.

Fig. 5-27. Pin firing, a method that was frequently used for treating bowed tendons, although research indicates that the inflammation may be too superficial to benefit the tendon itself.

CANNON AREA FRACTURES

Are fractures of the cannon bone very common?

No. They do occur, but not very often.

What causes them?

Fractures of the main bone (third metacarpal) are the result of severe trauma such as being kicked by another horse or a bad fall while the leg is caught in a hole or under a stout fence. Fractures of the splint bones can occur as a result of interference, wherein the splint bone is hit by another foot of the same horse while he is running or otherwise maneuvering.

Are fractures of the main bone curable?

Fissured (a longitudinal crack through only one surface of the bone) fractures can be successfully treated by merely casting the leg from just below the knee to and including the hoof. Oblique fractures of the lower end involving the fetlock joint can be treated by the application of a cast that includes the hoof if displacement of the

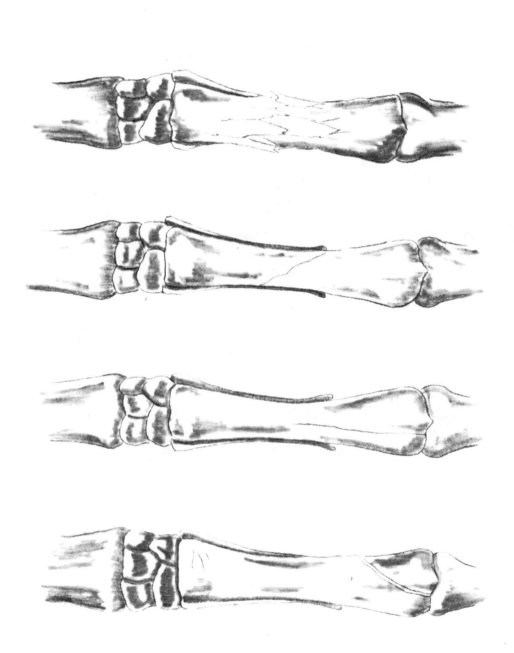

Fig. 5-28. From left to right: oblique fracture involving the fetlock joint, fissured longitudinal crack, fracture across the long axis of the bone, comminuted fracture.

fragment is minimal. Surgical treatment, using compression screws to fix the fragment, is indicated if displacement is appreciable. In either case the prognosis for oblique fractures healing successfully is fair.

If a fracture of the cannon bone is transverse or oblique, but goes entirely across the long axis of the bone, the chances of healing the break are not very good. The use of a surgically applied bone plate would be necessary and the horse would have to spend a long period of time in a sling during convalescence.

Treatment of compound or comminuted (crushed into small pieces) fractures of the cannon bone is not likely to be successful. The veterinarian will not recommend treatment of these cases as the mechanical aspects are so poor and the likelihood of bone infection is so great.

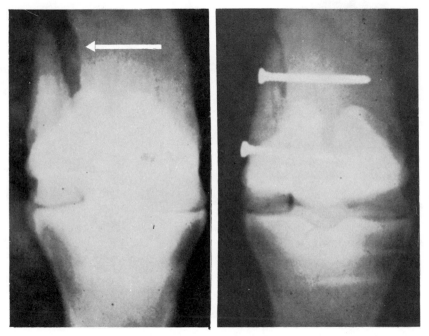

Courtesy of LAMENESS IN HORSES, Edition III, O. R. Adams, Lea and Febiger Publishing Co., Philadelphia, Pa.

Fig. 5-29. X-ray showing a longitudinal fracture of the cannon bone. On the left, the fractured bone before surgical treatment. On the right, the same fracture with two bone screws in place.

What about fractured splint bones?

Fractured splint bones are much more common in the front legs than full cannon fractures, and treatment of them is much more likely to be successful.

What are the signs of fractured splint bones?

The horse will be lame to a variable degree, depending upon the location and nature of the fracture. Fractures can occur anywhere along the length of the splint bone but are usually in the lower one-third of the bone. Splint bone fractures, close to the carpal joint or involving the suspensory ligament, are more serious than the lower ones. In most cases lameness is ordinarily most evident when the horse is exercised at a trot. The signs of lameness may diminish when the horse is rested.

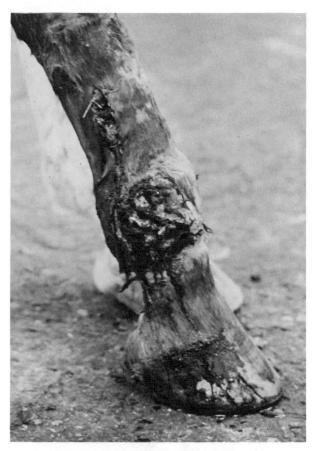

Fig. 5-30. The appearance of a hind leg that has had a fracture of the cannon bone, after the cast has been removed.

Swelling which may extend over the entire length of the splint bone will usually be present, accompanied by heat and pain. A veterinarian will be needed to differentiate between a fracture and a fresh splint because X-ray is the only means of positively identifying a fractured splint bone.

Fig. 5-31. On the left, fracture of the splint bone. Right, same splint bone with fragment removed.

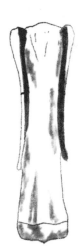
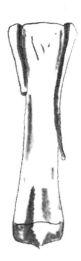

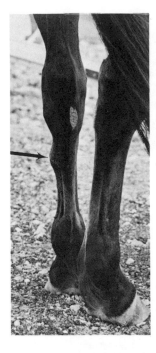 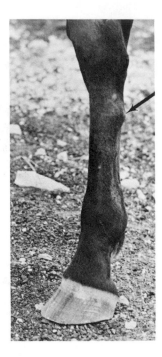 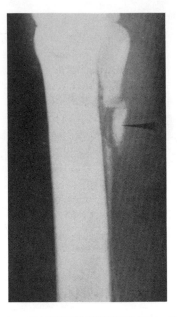

Courtesy of LAMENESS IN HORSES, Edition III, O. R. Adams, Lea and Febiger Publishing Co., Philadelphia, Pa.

Fig. 5-32 & Fig. 5-33. Views of the hindleg showing the swelling (arrow) that accompanies a fracture of the splint bone.

Fig. 5-34. X-ray showing a chip fracture (arrow) of the splint bone.

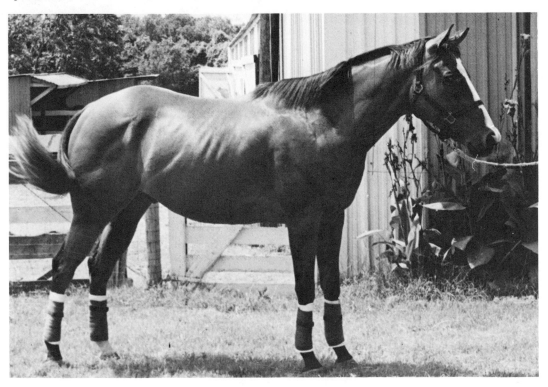

Fig. 5-35. All four legs are protected by heavy wraps to prevent injury to the cannon bones.

How are fractured splint bones treated?

The veterinarian's judgment, based on his past experience with cases of this type will be the best guide to treatment. If he finds the break is fairly low and that displacement of the fragment is minimal, he will probably recommend rest for four to eight weeks. After the rest period, another X-ray examination will determine whether healing has been sufficient to resume normal use of the horse.

If the fragment is large or displaced appreciably, surgical removal will probably be recommended. The surgery will involve the removal of the fragment including its periosteum (bone membrane) and the suturing shut of the remaining periosteum over the broken end of the major part of the bone that is left. The veterinarian will probably fix the upper portion of the splint bone to the cannon bone with one or two compression screws to aid in its weight-bearing function if the fracture site is in the upper third of the cannon bone. After surgery, rest will probably be recommended for at least four weeks.

Can complete recovery to full soundness from splint fractures be expected?

Yes. The prognosis in almost all splint fractures is good. Problems such as exostosis developing that impinges on the suspensory ligament or displacement of the upper fragment which would disturb the continuity of the knee (or hock if the hindleg is the site of the injury) are rare.

6

KNEE

ANATOMY AND CONFORMATION

Is the "knee" of a horse really a knee?

Although "knee" is the common term for this joint, the carpus (knee) of the horse actually corresponds anatomically to the human wrist.

What is the structure of the carpus?

This is a very complex joint composed of numerous small bones. Between the radius (long bone in the forearm) and the cannon bone there are two rows of small carpal bones. The upper row contains the radial, intermediate and ulnar carpal bones. The lower row is made up of the first, second, third and fourth carpal bones, although the first is sometimes missing. The larger accessory carpal bone projects backward from the inner side of the carpus. The projection is readily visible externally. Because of its projecting position, the accessory carpal bone forms a lever for the attachments of some of the muscles which bend the knee. A complex system of short, strong ligaments bind these seven or eight carpal bones together.

The entire joint actually consists of three major joints. The radiocarpal joint is formed between the lower end of the radius and the upper surface of the top row of carpal bones. This joint permits hingelike flexion and extension between the radius and carpal bones. The intercarpal joint is formed between the two rows of carpal bones and allows some hinge flexion and extension at this location. The third main joint, the carpometacarpal joint, is formed between the bottom surface of the lower row of carpal bones and the upper end of the cannon bone. This joint has very little movement, mainly slight sliding and gliding.

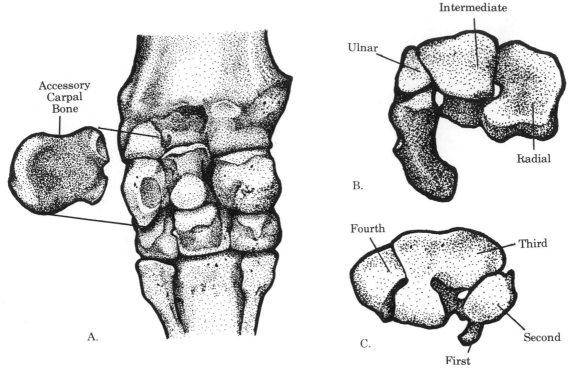

Fig. 6-1. A. View of the knee as seen from behind, with accessory carpal bone removed. B. Upper row of carpal bones. C. Lower row of carpal bones.

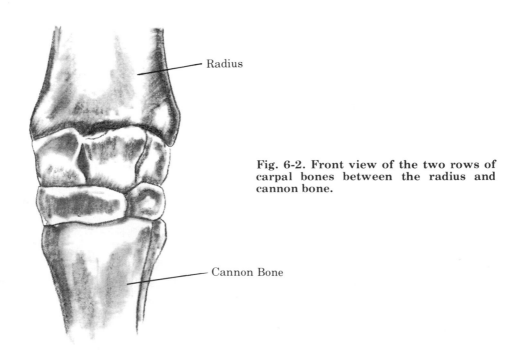

Fig. 6-2. Front view of the two rows of carpal bones between the radius and cannon bone.

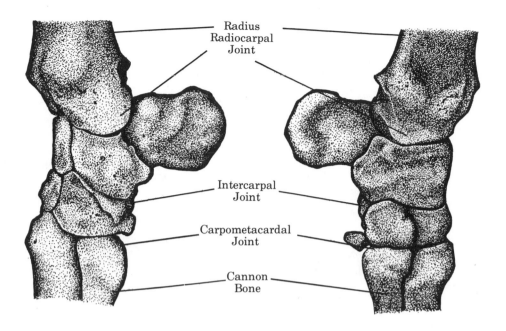

Fig. 6-3. Two side views showing the three major joints of the knee. Left, a lateral view of the left knee. Right, a medial view of the left knee.

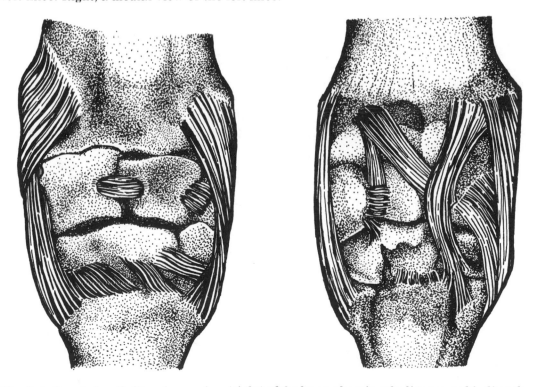

Fig. 6-4. Front view (left) and rear view (right) of the knee, showing the ligaments binding the carpal bones together.

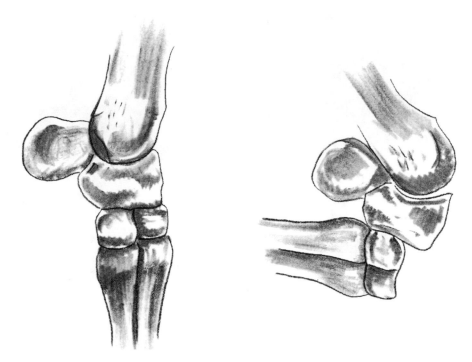

Fig. 6-5. To the left, a medial view of normal extension of the left knee, as when the horse is standing. To the right, volar flexion of the knee.

In addition, numerous small intracarpal joints are formed between adjacent carpal bones. Although these joints have very limited movement, they absorb a great deal of concussion and are a vitally important segment of the natural shock-absorbing system of the horse.

All the joints of the carpus are enclosed within a single, extensive joint capsule. The carpal joint capsule, much like a long sleeve, reaches from the radius to the cannon bone. Within the joint capsule, however, are three separate synovial sacs corresponding to each main joint. They are: (1) the radiocarpal sac, (2) the intercarpal sac and (3) the carpometacarpal sac.

Which muscles are associated with the carpus?

Because the carpus is a hinge joint, there are extensor muscles on the front leg and flexor muscles on the back. The most prominent muscle on the front of the forearm is the extensor carpi radialis. (Note: The radius and the ulna are the bones of the forearm; the ulna is relatively short and fused to the inner side of the radius. The descriptive terms "radialis" and "ulnaris" refer to the bone or the side of the forearm over which a muscle passes.) The extensor carpi radialis extends from the outer side of the upper portion of the elbow joint down the front of the leg to the upper front of the cannon bone. This muscle acts to extend (straighten and lift) the carpus.

The extensor carpi ulnaris also originates at the upper portion of the elbow joint, but passes down around the outside of the carpus, attaching to the outer splint bone. Although this muscle is called an extensor (because of its origin and the nerves supplying it), it acts to flex (bend) the carpus. Some of the tendons of the digital

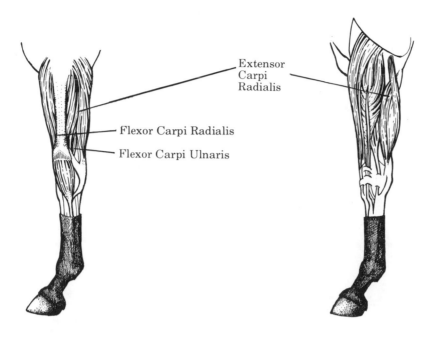

Extensor
Carpi
Radialis

Flexor Carpi Radialis

Flexor Carpi Ulnaris

Fig. 6-6. Left, a medial view of the right foreleg showing the extensor and flexor muscles of the knee. Right, a lateral view of the left foreleg.

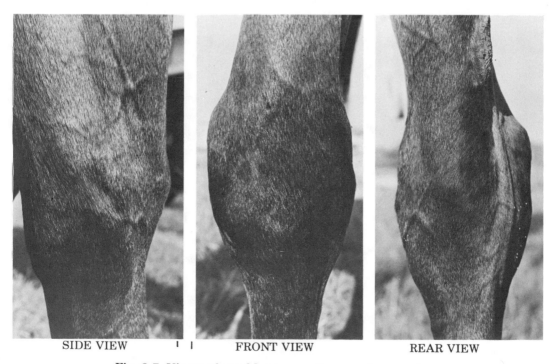

SIDE VIEW   FRONT VIEW   REAR VIEW

Fig. 6-7. Views of good knee seen from various angles.

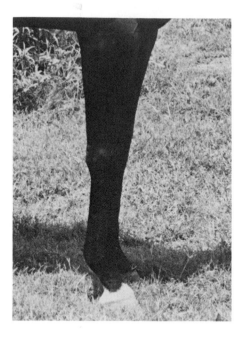

A. Desirable forearm muscling in a Thoroughbred-type horse.

B. Desirable forearm muscling in a Quarter horse. Notice that the Quarter horse muscling is shorter and heavier than that of the Thoroughbred.

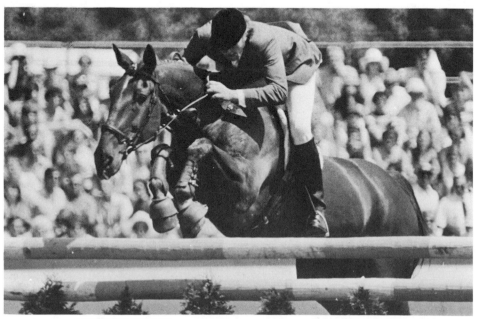

Photo Courtesy of FRUEN MILLING CO.

Fig. 6-9. View of horse taking a jump. Notice the use of the muscles of the knee.

flexor muscles pass over the back of the carpus and act secondarily to flex the carpus.

There are two major flexor muscles on the back of the leg. Extending from the upper surface of the elbow joint to the outside of the upper back surface of the cannon bone is the flexor carpi radialis. The flexor carpi ulnaris also originates at the upper surface of the elbow, but extends downward attaching to the accessory carpal bone. Both of these muscles act to flex the carpus.

What constitutes good conformation of the knee?

Viewed from every angle, the knee should be of adequate size in proportion with the size of the horse, well balanced and well defined. The knee should not be round-looking, especially at the front. A flattened front surface of the carpus provides a smooth surface for the up and down actions of the extensors.

Viewed from the side, the knee should be wide from front to back and exhibit a clean look. From all directions the knee should correspond with the line formed by the forearm and the cannon with no deviation in any direction.

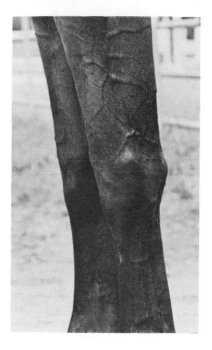

Fig. 6-10. Side view of calf knees.

What are some common conformation faults of the knee?

Viewed from the side, there are several conformation faults which may be present. "Calf knees" is a conformation fault in which the knees deviate toward the back or the front leg bends back at the knees. "Bucked knees" (knee sprung or over at the knees) is the opposite conformation fault.

A horse is said to be "tied in at the knees" when the flexor tendons appear to be too close to the cannon bone just below the knee. In this case the cannon bone is small and the tendons are not adequate to support the horse under stress. "Tied in knees" also inhibit free movement, however, the degree of movement lost depends upon the severity of the defect. "Cut out under the knees" means that there is a dent, or cut out appearance, just below the knee on the front of the cannon bone.

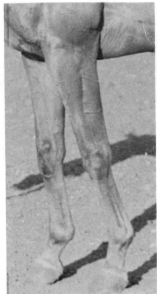

Fig. 6-11. Side view of bucked knees (Over at the knees).

Also apparent from the side is the conformation fault "open knees." In this situation, the profile of the knee is irregular due to the enlarged epiphysis of the lower end of the radius and the carpal bone deviation toward the back. This defect is usually the result of a mineral imbalance and frequently becomes less obvious as a horse matures.

Fig. 6-12. Conformation faults of the knee.

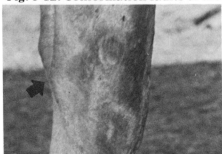

A. "Tied in" at the knees.

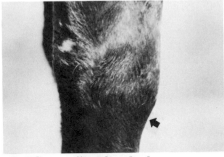

B. "Cut out" under the knees.

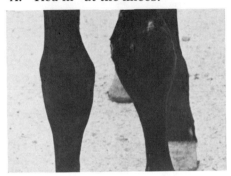

C. "Knock" knees.

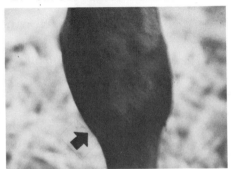

D. "Bench" knees.

What types of faulty knee conformation are apparent when viewing a horse from the front?

"Knock knees," or "in at the knees," is one example. In this case the knees deviate toward each other. The opposite condition is bow legs, where the knees deviate away from each other.

Also noticeable from the front is the defect "bench knees," or "offset knees." In this situation the leg does not follow a straight line through the radius and cannon bone. The cannon bone is offset to the outside of the knee. A horse with this fault is very prone to breaking down under hard work.

Why is conformation of the knees so important?

Poor conformation of the knee affects the weight-bearing efficiency of the entire leg. With any conformation defect of the knees, concussion is not spread equally over the bones of the limb. Therefore, some parts are subjected to greater stress while others receive lighter than normal stress. This naturally predisposes the horse with faulty knee conformation to a multitude of injuries involving the knee and lower leg, especially the fetlock joint.

X-RAYING KNEES

Why are the knees of young horses X-rayed?

This is a method to attempt to determine the maturity of young horses, and is usually employed to decide whether they can physically withstand the rigors of training without any harmful effects.

How can X-rays indicate whether or not a horse is mature?

An animal's body grows by slowly increasing the length and size of bones. Long bones increase in length near their ends where there is a layer of cartilage called the epiphysis which separates the ends of the bone from the shaft (diaphysis).

The epiphysis is often called the growth plate because this is the area where a bone increases in length. Growth takes place gradually as the cartilage at this location changes into bone. As long as the epiphyseal cartilage continues to grow, the bone will continue to grow in length. When the cartilage stops growing and changes into bone, growth ceases.

When interpreted by an experienced person, an X-ray of the growth plate or epiphysis of a bone will indicate whether or not the bone is still growing.

Is a specific bone used for making this determination?

Yes. The site most commonly used is the distal (lower) epiphysis of the radius (long bone in the forearm). This is near the top of the knee region.

There is a sound reason for using the lower epiphysis of the radius to determine skeletal maturity. Bones mature at different rates and this epiphysis closes (changes completely into bone) later than other epiphyses, such as the lower end of the cannon bone. This is due in part to the position of the individual bone and is under the influence of many complicated, interrelated nutritional and hormonal factors.

Does this closure take place gradually?

Yes. The lower epiphysis of the radius closes first in the center and then on the sides. This regularity of the closing process makes it possible for a veterinarian to

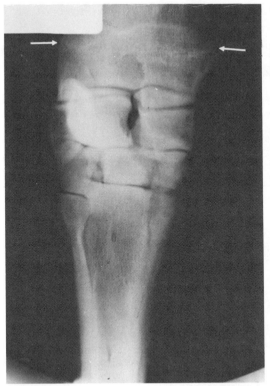

Fig. 6-13

Fig. 6-14

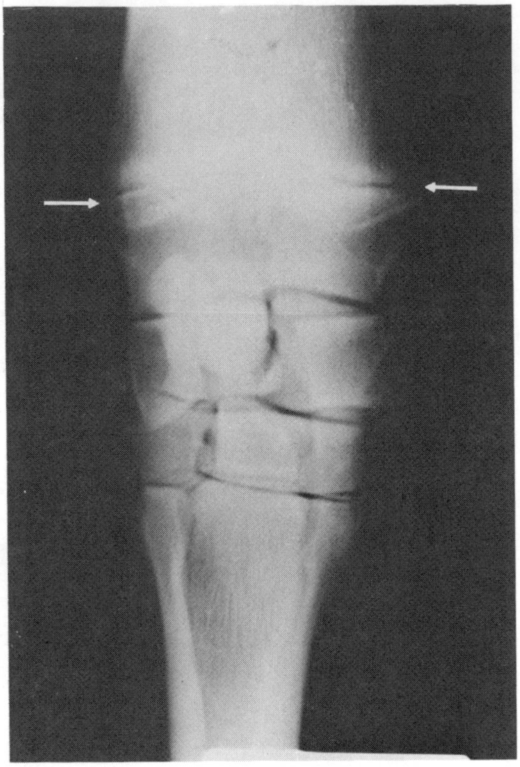

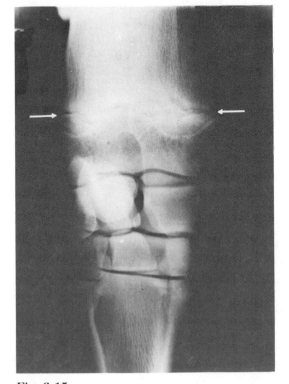

Fig. 6-15

Fig. 6-13. Radiograph of type A knee Arrows indicate epiphyseal line. "Closed".

Fig. 6-14. Radiograph of type B knee "Partially Open".

Fig. 6-15. Radiograph of type C knee "Open".

establish from X-ray evidence whether the epiphysis is just beginning to close, or is further along in the process.

As a result there are standardized grades for the states of the lower epiphysis of the radius. They are as follows:

Type A — Mature; completely closed.

Type B — In the process of closing, slightly open.

Type C — Open; immature.

How are these grades used?

Veterinarians generally agree that young horses with "type A knees" are adequately mature to withstand full training. Young horses with "type B knees" can withstand light training although they are still growing to a certain extent, while those with "type C knees" should be subjected to *no* training until they are more mature.

Since a major cause of unsoundnesses is racing before bone maturation has occurred, these veterinary recommendations should be heeded.

EPIPHYSITIS

What causes a young horse to develop "big knees" or "knock knees"?

The cause of the abnormal growth is epiphysitis.

What is epiphysitis?

It is an inflammation of the growth plate of the long bones, primarily found in the lower end of the radius above the knee. This epiphyseal area closes at around 24 to 27 months of age, which is why the problem appears only in young stock.

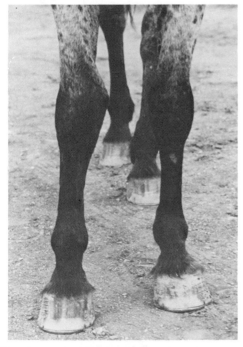

Fig. 6-16. Front view of forelegs showing epiphysitis (big knee) of the right knee.

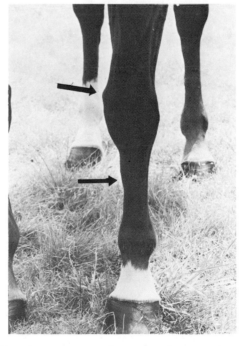

Fig. 6-17. Front view of a horse with epiphysitis (large arrow) and a splint (small arrow) of the left foreleg.

What causes epiphysitis?

The primary cause is believed to be successive pressure on the unclosed plates, as is the case when a young horse injures one leg and is forced to carry much weight on the other leg, developing epiphysitis in the sound leg. This can also be caused by diet deficiencies in foals (knock knees) and concussion in young racehorses (big knee).

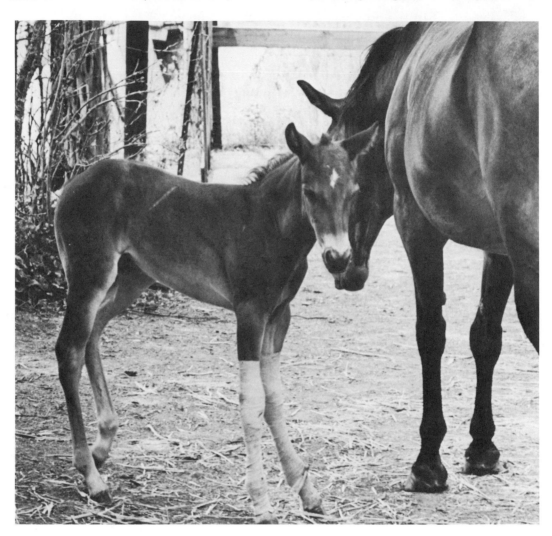

Fig. 6-18. Foal with epiphysitis (knock knees).

What are the signs of epiphysitis?

An enlargement or swelling over the knee that is firm and painful should be checked by a veterinarian to determine if the cause is epiphysitis. The horse may not be lame, but an X-ray showing open, inflamed epiphyses will confirm the veterinarian in his diagnosis of epiphysitis.

How is epiphysitis treated?

The veterinarian will determine the cause and treat the case accordingly. If it was caused by malnutrition, proper diet and rest may be all that is needed to correct the problem. If the deviation in the legs is severe, as is sometimes the case in very young foals, the veterinarian may staple the epiphyses or cast the legs to encourage even growth. In young racehorses, rest and postponement of training are necessary until the epiphyses close naturally.

Fig. 6-19. Illustration of the steps involved in stapling the epiphyses.

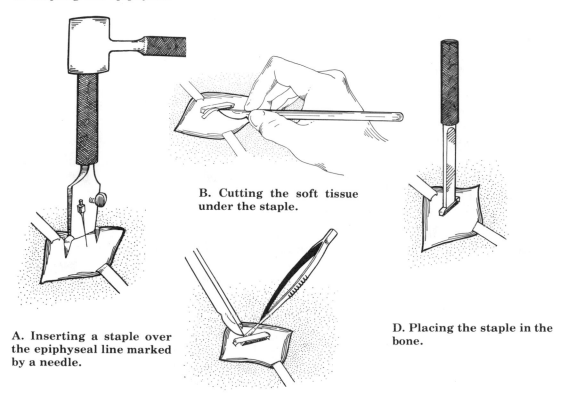

A. Inserting a staple over the epiphyseal line marked by a needle.

B. Cutting the soft tissue under the staple.

C. Removing the soft tissue.

D. Placing the staple in the bone.

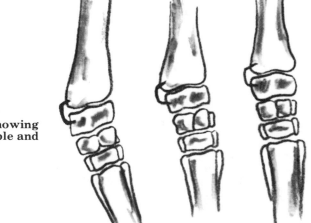

Fig. 6-20. Diagram of the knee, showing the placement of an epiphyseal staple and its effect in straightening the leg.

What is the prognosis for epiphysitis?

The prognosis is good if promptly treated because the condition occurs in young horses when there is opportunity for correction as the epiphyses continue to close. If the case of epiphysitis is not treated, the prognosis is good if the degree of deviation is mild, and guarded if the deviation is moderate to severe.

RUPTURE OF THE EXTENSOR CARPI RADIALIS

As the largest extensor of the carpus, what kind of injury can occur to the extensor carpi radialis?

The extensor carpi radialis, which extends from the outside epicondyle of the humerus to the front of the top end of the cannon bone, may rupture although this is comparatively rare.

What causes the extensor carpi radialis to rupture?

The general cause is trauma, but the specific cause is usually unknown. Overflexion of the knee while the elbow is extended may be cited as the incident most likely to result in a rupture.

What are the signs of this rupture?

The horse will be obviously lame. This is because with the resistance of the extensor carpi radialis gone, the flexor tendons are able to overflex the knee during movement. The limb can be extended by means of the common digital extensor and the lateral digital extensor at walking and trotting paces, but not as well as a

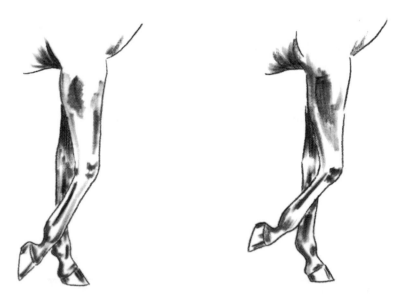

Fig. 6-21. On the left, the normal flexion of the knee at a walking pace. On the right, the extensor carpi radialis has ruptured, allowing the flexor tendons to overflex the knee because of the lack of resistance of this extensor muscle.

normal leg. The end of the ruptured tendon can be palpated. Atrophy (wasting away) of the muscular portion will begin after a short time, so that the muscle becomes smaller than the one in the opposite leg.

How can the rupture be treated?

The veterinarian may attempt to surgically reunite the ruptured ends of the tendon if the injury is discovered soon after its occurrence. The limb would then need to be immobilized in a cast for about six weeks.

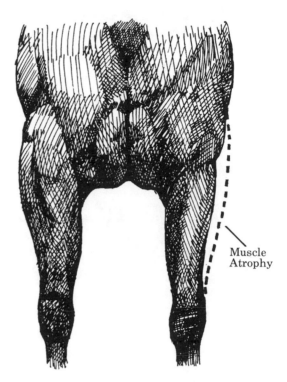

Fig. 6-22. Front view showing atrophy of the extensor carpi radialis. Notice the smaller size of the musculature of the horse's left forearm.

Muscle Atrophy

If the injury is longstanding, it is impossible to bring the ends together. The veterinarian might be able to repair the extensor carpi radialis by attaching it to the nearby extensor carpi obliquus tendon. However, since the prognosis for the successful healing of a rupture of this nature is poor, surgery is usually attempted only on those horses whose economic value merit it.

HYGROMA OF THE CARPUS, "CAPPED KNEE"

What is a hygroma?

A hygroma of the carpal joint (knee), also known as "capped knee," is any fluid filled swelling over the front surface of the knee. Most commonly it is an acquired bursitis as a result of trauma. It may, however, be free synovia outside a ruptured bursa or a serum pocket.

Is trauma always the cause?

Yes. Getting up and down, falling on a hard surface or pawing and hitting the carpus on a hard surface such as a wall, are the most common causes.

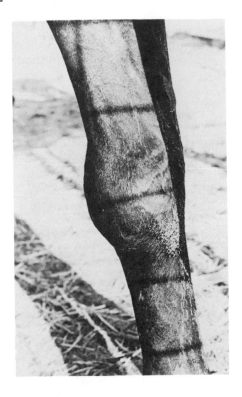

Fig. 6-23. Side view of capped knee.

How is hygroma diagnosed?

Following trauma there will be a sudden fluctuating swelling over the entire front of the knee, indicating a hygroma. If the swelling is large, it can interfere with movement. This condition should not be confused with carpitis (popped knee) since the swollen area is not as large with carpitis. (See page 163.)

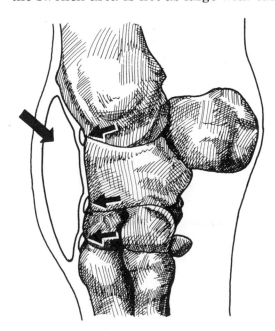

Fig. 6-24. Diagrammatic representation of hygroma. The enlarged bursa is not the same structure as the joint capsule. The large arrow points to the bursa. Small arrows point to parts of wall of joint capsule between each bone.

What is done to treat a hygroma?

In the case of an acute capped knee, the veterinarian will be required for treatment. Draining of the synovial fluid or serum followed by corticosteroid injections is the usual procedure. Counterpressure with an elastic bandage is most important. This will promote adhesions between the distended skin and underlying tissue and will help prevent the area from filling with fluid again.

With a chronic capped knee, a second possible treatment is to open and drain the hygroma and swab the cavity daily with tincture of iodine. This results in drainage over a long period of time. Extreme care must be taken in this procedure not to open the carpal joint capsule as this would be disastrous. In longstanding cases, surgical removal of the entire hygroma should be considered because of the amount of fibrin collected in the swelling.

Is the prognosis favorable in these cases?

The prognosis is favorable in acute cases. However, with chronic cases the outlook is guarded because the fibrous tissue may cause a permanent swelling over the knee, requiring surgical drainage or removal.

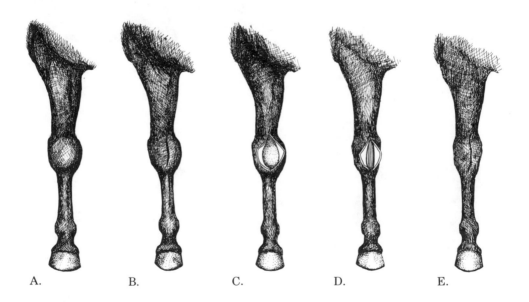

A. B. C. D. E.

Fig. 6-25. Illustration of steps involved in surgical removal of a chronic hygroma. A. Capped knee. B. An incision over the knee. C. Tissue layers pulled back to expose the hygroma. D. Removal of the entire hygroma. E. The sutured incision after surgery has been completed.

CARPITIS

What is carpitis?

Carpitis, commonly called "popped knee," is either an acute or chronic inflammation of the carpus (knee). It involves the joint capsule, ligaments and/or bones of the knee. When popped knee is not carefully treated, it can progress to an older, chronic form with exostoses (new bone growth) on the surfaces of the carpal bones.

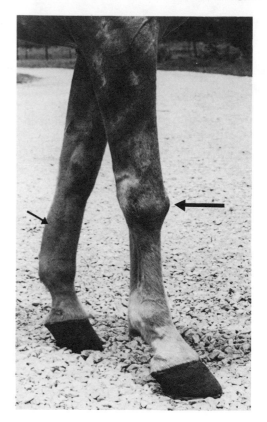

Fig. 6-26. Side view of carpitis (large arrow) of the right knee. The left cannon shows an extensive middle bow (small arrow) of the tendon.

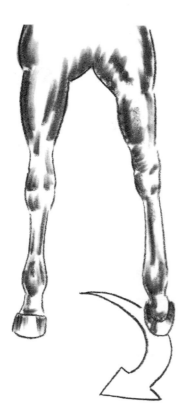

Fig. 6-27. Illustration of the "swinging leg" type of lameness characterisitic of popped knee. Due to the pain involved, the horse swings the leg out and around instead of bending the knee as he walks.

How is "popped knee" caused?

Concussion and trauma are the major causes of popped knee. This condition is most common in race horses in hard training, especially when they are not in condition or are tired (near the end of a hard workout, for example). Because of the fast gaits, the horses are prone to tearing the joint capsule and associated ligaments of the knee. Also, popped knee is frequently seen in hunters and jumpers as a result of knee injuries. Poor conformation, particularly those types involving improper alignment of the knees, can predispose a horse to popped knee.

In summary, the cause of popped knee is either a strain or sprain of some of the ligaments that hold the knee in position or damage to the joint capsule—both of which may be brought on by a variety of factors.

What are the signs of popped knee?

When the condition is acute, lameness comes on suddenly and is a "swinging leg" type. This means that the horse is reluctant to bend the knee because of the pain. Consequently, when the leg is moved forward he swings it out and around instead of flexing the knee in a normal stride. There will be a swelling of the joint capsule which is most evident on the front surface of the knee. These "swollen knee" cases should be examined and X-rayed by the veterinarian to make certain that there is no fracture present.

In chronic cases new bone growth may be present, caused by earlier injuries to the periosteum (bone covering) when the joint capsule or ligament attachments were pulled. Many times an animal with chronic carpitis will not show up lame until worked at a fast gait. An X-ray examination by the veterinarian can provide conclusive evidence of new bone growths on the front surface of the knee.

How is popped knee treated?

In the early, acute stages rest is the most important treatment. An adequate prolonged rest period is the most effective way to insure complete healing and avoid chronic inflammation. In conjunction with the rest period, the veterinarian may use corticosteroid injections into the joint to aid in reducing the inflammation. Mild blisters are used on occasion when the periosteum is also inflamed. Complete rest (six months or more) is extremely important to allow time for healing.

When new bone growth is present, it can possibly be removed by firing, blistering, radiation therapy or surgery. Phenylbutazone or corticosteroids are frequently used to relieve the pain.

Does the horse regain soundness?

In the early stages, if the horse was given an adequate rest, chances are good. New bone growths somewhat decrease the chances, but if the exostoses are not encroaching on the articular (moving) surfaces of the joint, there is still a fairly good chance for complete recovery. When the joint surfaces are involved, very seldom does the animal regain full working soundness. Surgical removal of the bony growths followed by adequate aftercare and rest has resulted in some full recoveries.

Another factor that influences recovery chances is conformation. Regardless of when treatment was instigated, poor conformation greatly increases the chances of carpitis recurring.

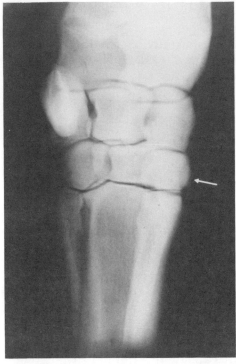

Fig. 6-28. Radiograph of the knee showing carpitis (arrow). This knee is also an example of a type A knee.

Fig. 6-29. Radiograph of the knee showing carpitis. The knee has been flexed to show the new bone growth (arrows) on the surfaces of the carpal bones.

Fig. 6-28.

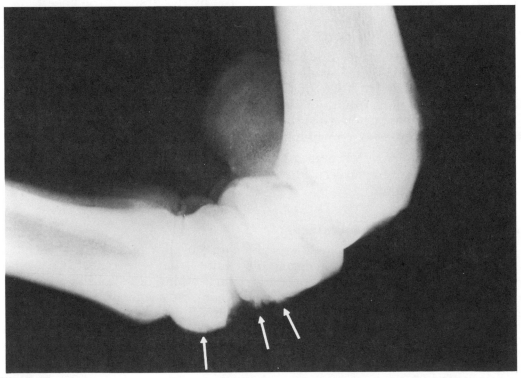

Fig. 6-29.

CARPAL FRACTURES

What are carpal fractures?

As previously explained in the "Anatomy of the Knee" section, the carpus is composed of eight bones arranged in two rows. The most common type of carpal fracture is a chip fracture. In this case a small piece breaks off of one or more of the bones. The larger accessory carpal bone at the back of the joint can also break.

How does this happen?

Carpal fractures occur most commonly in race horses and are almost solely due to trauma. Concussion is thought to be a contributing factor. Most carpal fractures happen near the end of a race when the horse is fatigued and most likely to overflex and overextend the knee. It is when the limb is overextended that most fractures take place. Any one or a combination of the eight bones may fracture.

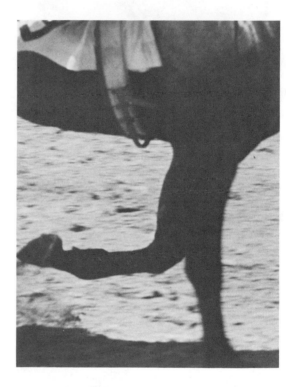

Fig. 6-30. Side view of running horse showing a frequent cause of injury. The right knee is overextended, due to fatigue, which may result in carpal fractures.

What are the signs of fractures in the knee area?

The animal will be lame although the degree of lameness can vary greatly. In some cases the horse may be lame only when exercised and in other cases he may be severely lame. Heat and swelling are also signs of carpal fractures. Pain is most evident when pressure is applied to the joint and when the joint is flexed. If the bone has been fractured for some length of time, there is usually a hard swelling on the front of the knee.

Since these signs are the same as those for carpitis, the veterinarian will use X-rays from several different angles to conclusively diagnose fractures.

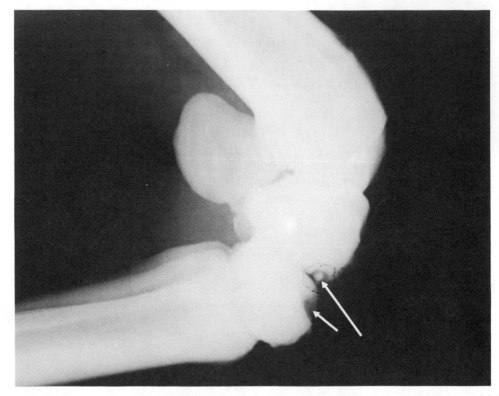

Fig. 6-31. Radiograph of the knee, which has been flexed to show a chip fracture (large arrow). The small arrow indicates an area of cartilage erosion on the third carpal bone.

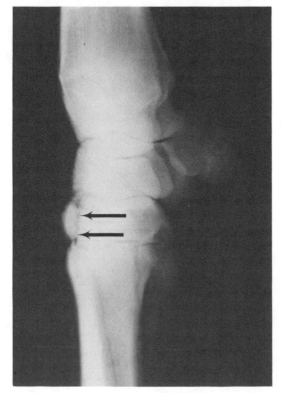

Fig. 6-32. Radiograph of the knee showing a slab fracture (arrows) and some exostosis.

How are carpal fractures treated?

When the bone chips are small, they are usually surgically removed by the veterinarian. Larger chips, which are usually of the "slab" type that could interfere with the action of the joint if removed, are often surgically fixed in place with bone screws. After either surgical procedure, the veterinarian will recommend that the horse be rested and hard work not resumed for at least six months.

Fractures of the accessory carpal bone require different treatment. These fractures are extremely difficult to treat for two reasons. First, the curve of the bone makes it impossible in many cases to insert a bone screw. Secondly, the pull of the carpal flexor tendons frequently keeps the bone segments separated. For these reasons, fractures of the accessory carpal bone are best left alone. They will eventually form a fibrous union. The usual veterinary procedure is to keep the horse relatively quiet and rested for a six-month period.

What is the prognosis for carpal bone fractures?

After surgery the prognosis for chip fractures is good, with many of the horses returning to racing. Slab fractures properly and promptly surgically treated have a hopeful outlook. However, for fractures of the accessory carpal bone the prognosis is guarded to unfavorable regarding future racing ability.

FOREARM

ANATOMY AND CONFORMATION

What is the forearm?

The forearm is that part of the horse's front limb between the elbow joint and the knee. The chestnuts are found in this area.

What are the chestnuts?

These are masses of horn on the inside of the forearm slightly above the knee. Because no two chestnuts are exactly alike, they may sometimes be used as "fingerprints." Some race tracks are considering the use of the shape of the chestnuts as positive identification for horses so that a "substitute" horse cannot be tattoed and represented as another horse.

Which bones make up the forearm?

The radius and the ulna are the two bones of the forearm. The radius is well developed and its ends enter into the elbow joint at the top and the carpus at the lower end. The ulna is a short bone fused to the upper end of the radius. The olecranon process of the ulna projects beyond the elbow joint to form the point of the elbow and serves as a lever of attachment for muscles which extend the elbow.

Compared with other animals, the ulna of the horse is very reduced in size. In combination with the fusion to the radius, this prevents the forearm from rotating backward and outward.

Which muscles are associated with this region?

The extensor carpi radialis is the most prominent muscle and forms the bulge on the front of the forearm. As presented in the "Anatomy and Conformation of the Knee" section, the extensor carpi ulnaris, flexor carpi radialis and flexor carpi ulnaris also extend the length of the forearm.

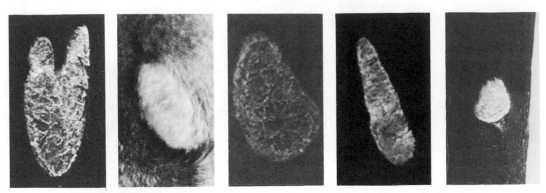

Fig. 7-1. Views of several forearms. Notice the various shapes of the chestnuts.

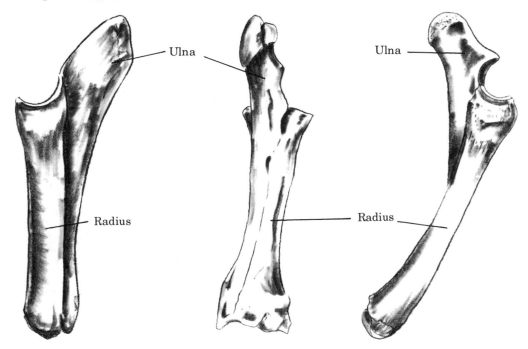

Fig. 7-2. Comparison of the fused radius and ulna of the cow (left and center) to those of the horse (right). In the cow, notice the attachment of the ulna along the length of the radius. In the horse, notice the smaller ulna and the smaller area of attachment.

Many of the strong muscles of the shoulder and chest attach to the upper portions of the radius and ulna. These include the triceps, biceps, brachialis and tensor fascia antebrachii muscles. Also present is the anconeus muscle—a short, strong muscle which extends from the lower end of the humerus to the olecranon process across the elbow joint.

Muscles activating the lower leg also pass through the forearm region. Included are the deep digital flexor, common digital extensor and the lateral digital extensor which attach at the upper ends of the radius and ulna.

In addition, the superficial digital flexor extends through the forearm. Closely associated is the superior check ligament which originates on the volar (back or bottom) surface near the middle of the radius and fuses with the superficial digital flexor near the knee.

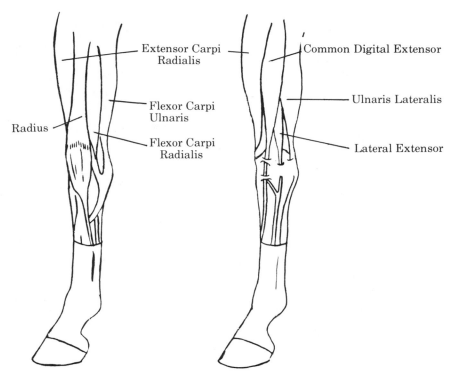

Fig. 7-3. Two medial views showing the muscles of the forearm.

What is good conformation of the forearm?

A forearm with good conformation is long, wide, thick and well directed. A well directed forearm is straight in line with the knee and cannon from all views. The forearm which is long, yet in proportion with the entire body, will provide the horse with more length of stride. The extension of the ulna (point of the elbow) determines the width of the forearm. Good forearm width (viewed from the side), when in balance with the horse's body, is desirable as major muscles for strength of propulsion are attached at this location.

Because very little body fat is deposited in this area, the amount of forearm muscling is a good indicator of the degree of muscling throughout the entire body of the horse. Forearm muscling is most concentrated at the top, becoming tendinous and slimmer at the bottom. The actual amount of muscling varies between breeds, but it should be smooth and lengthy rather than short and bunchy. Viewed from the front, the forearm should appear thick and strong due to the underlying muscles.

STRAIN OF THE SUPERIOR CARPAL CHECK LIGAMENT

What is the superior carpal check ligament?

As described under "Forearm Anatomy and Conformation," the superior carpal check ligament, along with the inferior carpal check ligament, assists the suspensory ligament in support of the fetlock. A strong fibrous band, the superior (or radial) check ligament is a branch of the superficial digital flexor that attaches to the distal end of the radius.

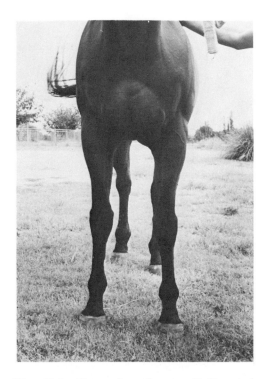

Fig. 7-4. Example of a well-directed forearm. Notice that the forearm is straight in line with the knee and cannon.

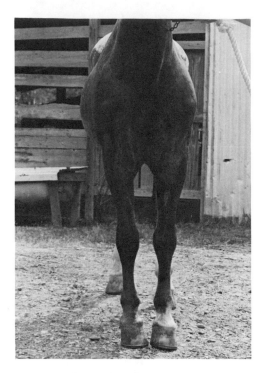

Fig. 7-5. Example of a poorly directed forearm.

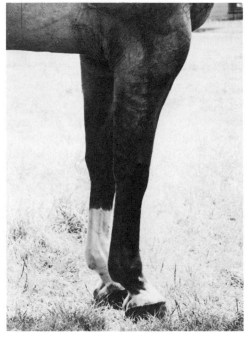

Fig. 7-6. Side view of a wide forearm, indicating greater strength and propulsion than a narrow forearm.

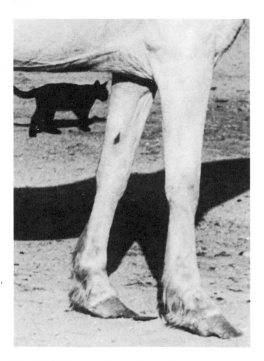

Fig. 7-7. View of a narrow forearm.

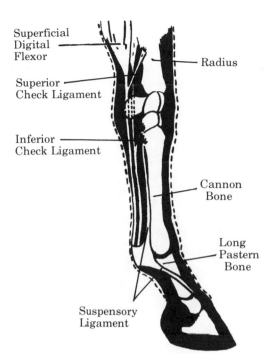

Superficial
Digital
Flexor

Radius

Superior
Check Ligament

Inferior
Check Ligament

Cannon
Bone

Long
Pastern
Bone

Suspensory
Ligament

Fig. 7-8. A side view of the foreleg, showing the locations of the check ligaments.

How can this ligament be injured?

The superior check ligament can be strained by a simultaneous dorsal (toward the front) flexion of the fetlock and overflexion of the knee. The result will be an acute or chronic lameness depending on the severity of the tendon tear. The superficial flexor tendon may be involved along with the superior carpal check ligament. Lameness will be more pronounced and the carpal sheath may be distended in the acute stage. Three to four weeks following the injury, X-ray examination will reveal the extent of injury and chances for recovery. If the case is chronic, X-rays of the ligament's attachment site may reveal periostitis.

What is the treatment for injury to the superior check ligament?

Corticosteroids to reduce the inflammation may be injected into the carpal sheath by the veterinarian in an acute case. This will be followed by a support bandage to be worn for two or three weeks and stall confinement for a month. Even light exercise should be discontinued for a three-month period following the injury.

RADIAL NERVE PARALYSIS

Where is the radial nerve?

The radial nerve is a major nerve in the forearm and shoulder that activates the extensor muscles of the elbow, knee and digit (fetlock, pastern and coffin joints) and the lateral flexor muscle of the knee. When the radial nerve function is impaired or destroyed, these muscles are partially or completely paralyzed.

What causes paralysis of the radial nerve?

The only cause is injury to the radial nerve. The injury can occur when a horse falls or is kicked on the lower shoulder, or it can even be brought about by lying on hard surfaces for extended periods of time. The radial nerve can be injured by being overstretched when the limb is hyperextended. Fractures in this area can also injure the nerve.

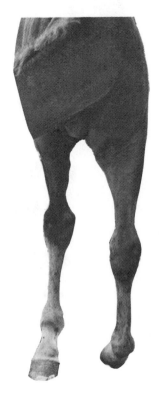

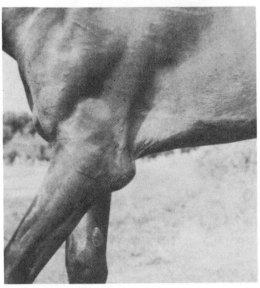

Courtesy of VETERINARY SURGERY, Edition VI, E. R. Frank, Burgess Publishing Co., Minneapolis, Minn.

Fig. 7-9. (Left) A front view showing radial nerve paralysis of a foal's left foreleg. Notice that the elbow is dropped, and the front of the hoof rests on the ground.

Fig. 7-10. (Above) Atrophy of the triceps muscle as a result of injury to the radial nerve.

What are the signs of radial nerve paralysis?

The signs vary depending upon the extent and degree of nerve damage. In mild cases the horse may move smoothly, but stumble when obstacles on the ground are encountered. In more severe cases the elbow will drop because the muscles are relaxed.

Complete paralysis of the radial nerve has distinctive signs. The horse is unable to move the leg forward to place weight on the foot. When he tries to do this, the leg is advanced to the normal position but the horse cannot extend the elbow joint and straighten the leg to a normal position for supporting weight. The knee and fetlock stay flexed. If the foot is manually placed under the horse in the proper position to bear weight, the limb can support weight.

When standing, only the toe of the affected leg rests on the ground because the muscles are relaxed. Since the shoulder and elbow are extended and the knee and digits flexed, the affected limb appears to be longer than the normal one. In severe cases the skin may be worn off the front of the fetlock and coronary band from being dragged over the ground. Also, the affected muscles will atrophy (waste away) within a few weeks.

Is there any treatment for radial nerve paralysis?

Most treatments are useless. If paralysis is complete, the horse should be kept in a stall to prevent additional injuries. Casts, leather boots, bandages, etc. can be used to protect the front of the fetlock. It is thought that regular manual massage of the inactive muscles might help somewhat.

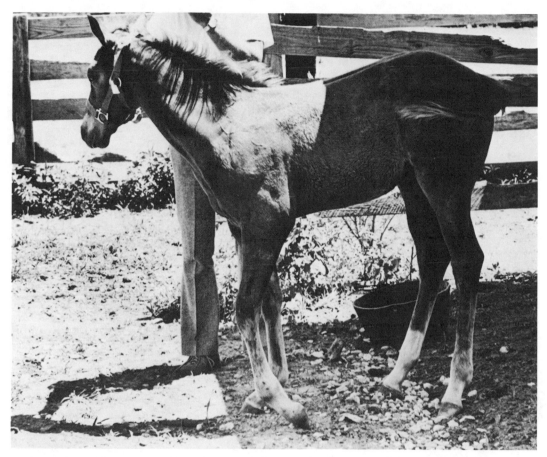

Fig. 7-11. A side view showing radial nerve paralysis of the left foreleg.

If there is not any specific treatment, does an animal recover from paralysis of the radial nerve?

The radial nerve has a limited ability to regenerate or heal. In cases of mild paralysis the prognosis is guarded, while for more severe paralysis the chance of recovery is extremely unfavorable.

FRACTURES OF THE FOREARM

What causes fractures of the forearm?

Of the two bones in the forearm, the ulna is more frequently broken. With either the ulna or the radius, the most common cause of fracture is slipping or falling.

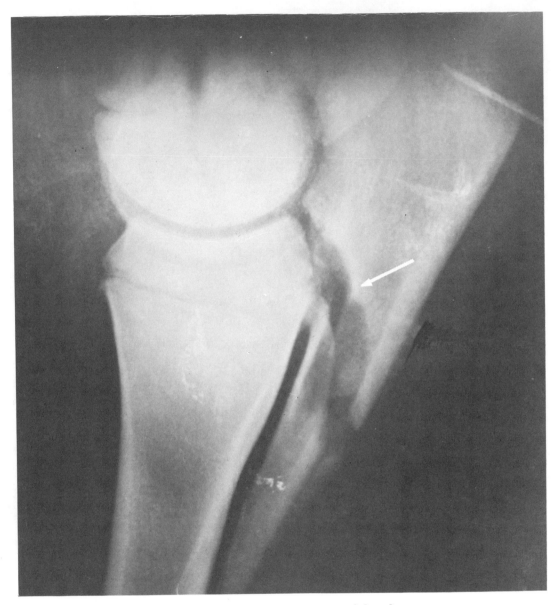

Fig. 7-12. X-ray showing a simple, oblique fracture of the ulna.

How is fracture of the forearm diagnosed?

In any case where fracture of the forearm is suspected, a veterinarian should be consulted to determine whether or not the fracture is treatable. The fracture will normally show considerable swelling, making palpation or crepitation (checking for clicking or grinding) difficult. Usually, accurate diagnosis must be obtained by X-ray.

How is fracture of the forearm treated?

A simple fracture of the radius may call for immobilization by a plaster cast strengthened by rods, and fixing the bone with transverse pins. This should be followed by confinement for six weeks. If the bone fragments override each other or either joint, or if the fracture is compound (fragments pierce the tissue), or comminuted (crushed), very little can be done.

The ulna is often fractured through the area where it joins the radius. This is particularly true with young colts, where ossification (growing together of the bones) is not complete.

Fig. 7-13. Side view showing fractures of the radius.

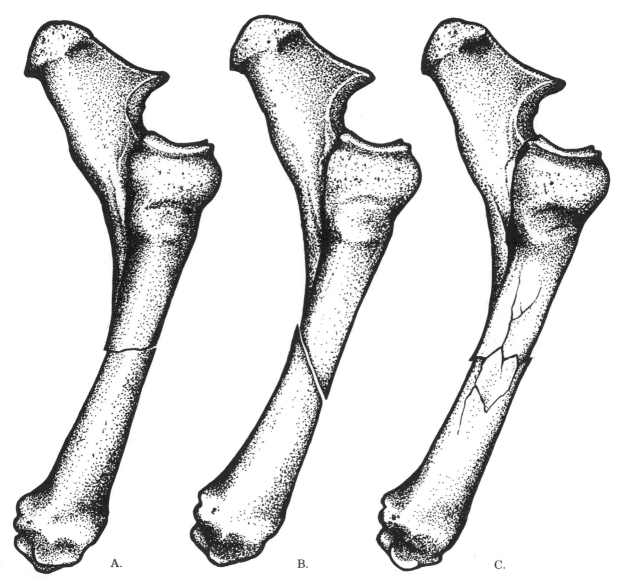

| A. Simple fracture. | B. Overriding fracture. | C. Comminuted fracture. |

Can a fracture of the ulna be expected to heal successfully?

Yes. If the ulna is fractured, it usually happens along the area adjacent to the radius. In these cases, if the veterinarian's X-ray examination shows that the

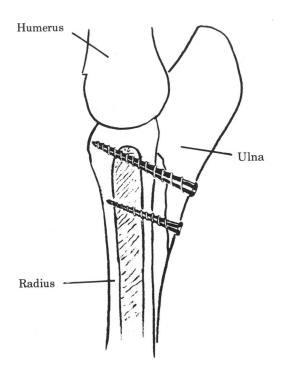

Fig. 7-14. A side view of transfixation screws, used to surgically repair fractures of the ulna.

interosseous ligament between the radius and ulna is fairly intact and displacement of the fractured parts of the bone is minimal, stall rest for about six weeks is all that will be necessary. If the displacement is severe enough, the veterinarian may surgically insert transfixation screws to reduce the fracture and hold it in place while it heals.

What if the radius is broken?

If the radius is broken, the outlook for recovery is not as good. This bone carries the full weight of the horse.

Can fractures of the radius be treated with any hope of success?

In some selected cases, especially in foals, there is reasonable hope for recovery. If the broken parts do not override or if the break is not completely across the bone, the veterinarian may suggest surgical treatment using a network of transverse pins through the fragments. These are bolted together with rods on the outside to hold the fragments in place. A cast will be applied over the leg from elbow to ground. In a few weeks, if X-rays show progress in healing, the cast can be removed and replaced with one that covers only the break area.

Are there any cases in which repair should not be attempted?

Fractures of the radius that override or are compound are not likely to be successfully treated. The mechanical forces required to reduce (put broken ends back together) and fix an overriding break are so great that damage to other structures of the leg is imminent. In a compound fracture the problem of bone infection is normally too great to cope with successfully.

Should overriding radial fractures ever be treated?

In the case of a very young foal the veterinarian might contemplate treatment, if an owner was insistent, but the prognosis would not be encouraging.

8

ELBOW

ANATOMY AND CONFORMATION

Where is the elbow of a horse located?

In the horse, the elbow is the uppermost joint of the front limb that is not within the shoulder girdle. It is the joint formed at the upper end of the foreleg, where the limb meets the body.

Which bones are involved in the elbow joint?

The elbow joint (humeroradial articulation) is formed by the junction of the condyles (paired, spool-like projections) on the lower end of the humerus, and the upper ends of the fused radius and ulna.

In the horse, the bones forming the elbow joint have specialized shapes to make up the joint surface. To provide a larger supporting surface for the humerus, the upper end of the radius is slightly dished and enlarged. In its surface, the ulna has a semilunar notch at the point where the ulna projects past the radius. The dished end of the radius and the semilunar notch of the ulna meet to form a smooth half-circle. The condyles of the humerus fit neatly into this half-circle forming the elbow joint.

It is important to remember, as explained in the "Anatomy and Conformation of the Forearm," that the ulna projects behind the elbow joint, making the point of the elbow and is called the olecranon process at this location. Although confusing, the following three terms are similar, but have distinct meanings: point of the elbow (olecranon process of the ulna); elbow joint (the actual joint located where the front leg joins the body); and elbow (the general area on the outside of the horse).

How does the elbow joint work?

The elbow joint is a true ginglymus (hinge) joint. Its only action consists of flexion and extension. Flexor muscles on the front of the joint and extensor muscles

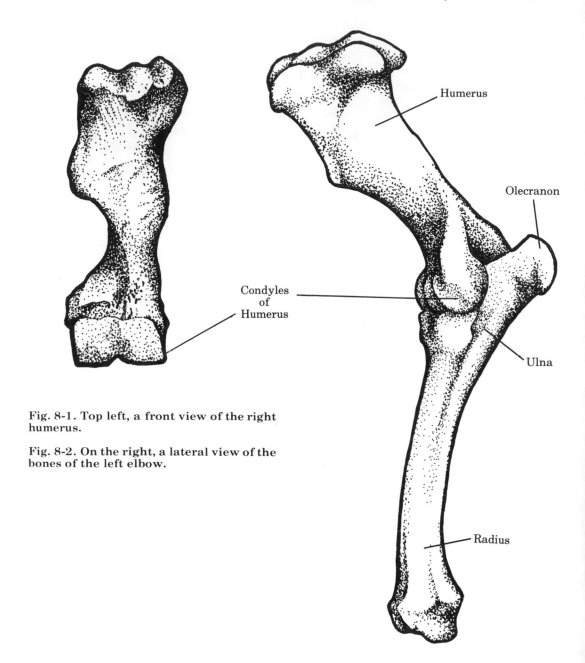

Fig. 8-1. Top left, a front view of the right humerus.

Fig. 8-2. On the right, a lateral view of the bones of the left elbow.

on the back provide power for this movement. As in all four-legged animals, the extensor muscles of this joint are stronger than the flexor muscles, since one of their purposes is to support the body weight, in addition to keeping the limb extended while the animal is standing.

Which muscles are extensors of the elbow joint?

The two extensor muscles of the elbow are the triceps and the anconeus. The triceps, as the name implies, has three separate heads or origins. One head originates at the back lower edge of the scapula (shoulder blade) and the other two originate on each side of the scapula. At their lower end, all three heads of the triceps attach to the olecranon process of the elbow (back of the elbow). The triceps is the longest extensor muscle of the elbow.

Underneath the triceps is the anconeus muscle. This small muscle covers and protects the back of the elbow joint capsule. The anconeus extends from the lower end of the humerus to the ulna, across the elbow joint, and aids in extending the elbow.

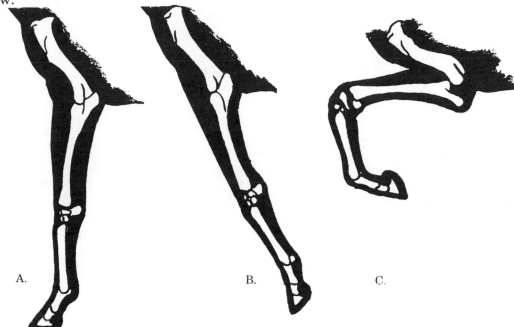

Fig. 8-3. Side view of the bones of the foreleg. A. Normal standing position. B. Extension of the elbow and knee joints. C. Flexion of the elbow and knee joints.

What are the flexors of the elbow joint?

The biceps brachii muscle and the brachialis muscle are the flexors of the elbow joint. The two heads of the biceps originate on the lower end of the scapula and attach at the front upper surface of the radius. The brachialis muscle originates near the top of the humerus and attaches on the front of the elbow joint below the biceps. The essential action of both of these muscles is to flex the elbow joint.

Are there any particular conformation characteristics to look for in a "good elbow"?

As in all joints, the elbow should have a clean appearance and be in balance with the entire body of the horse. The elbow should be neither out nor tied in, because both will restrict movement, to a certain degree.

Because the elbow is the uppermost joint of the front leg, improper positioning of the attachment of the leg at the elbow results in poor total leg conformation. Base wide and base narrow are both examples. From a front view, a base narrow horse has a greater distance between the front legs at the top of the legs than at the feet. In the opposite situation, base wide, the distance between the legs at the top is smaller than the distance between the legs at the feet.

"Pigeon-toed" and "splay-footed" are also conformation faults resulting from legs which are crooked at their origin. The feet of a pigeon-toed horse point in

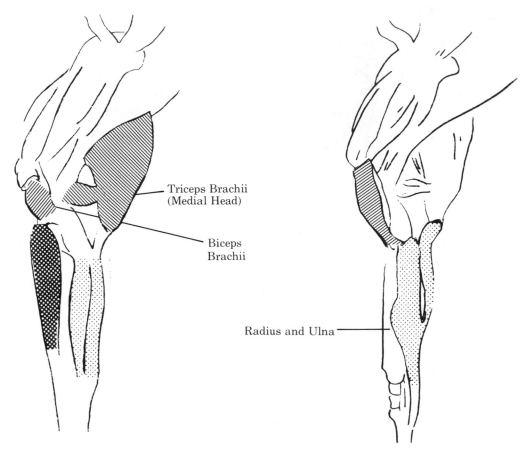

Fig. 8-4. Medial views of the right forearm. The diagram to the right displays a deeper dissection of the muscles.

Fig. 8-5. Two lateral views of the muscles of the right foreleg, with a deeper dissection to the right.

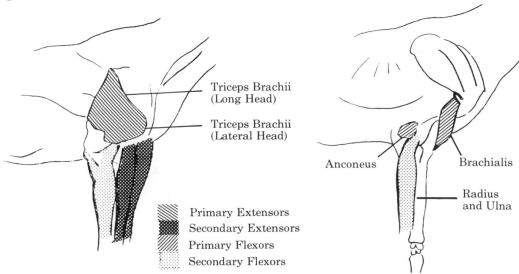

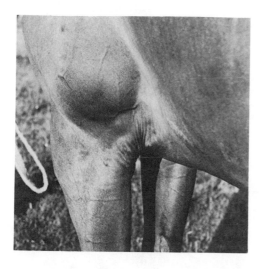 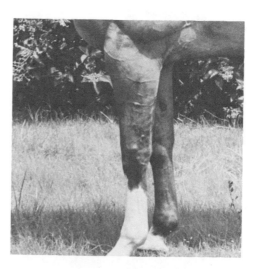

Fig. 8-6. A well-conformed elbow is in balance with the rest of the horse, and is directed neither in nor out. As a result, the horse naturally stands with the legs directed straight under the body.

Fig. 8-7. Front view of base narrow conformation caused by improper positioning of the attachment of the leg at the elbow. Notice that the distance between the feet is much less than the distance between the legs at the top. This horse also has osselets (large arrows) and periarticular high ringbone (small arrows).

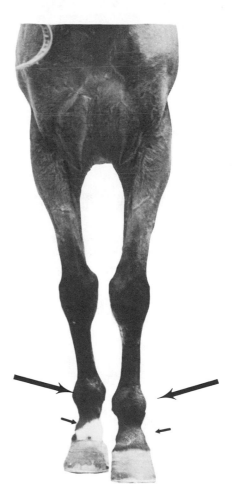

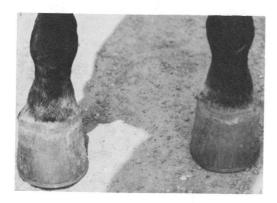

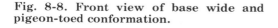

Fig. 8-8. Front view of base wide and pigeon-toed conformation.

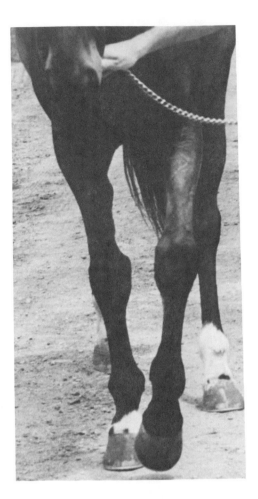
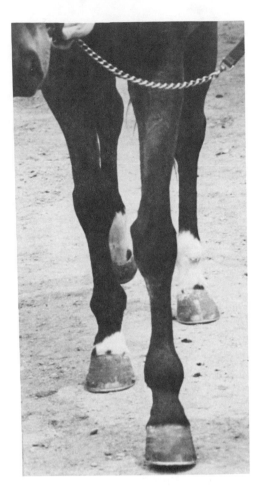

Fig. 8-9. Above, two front views of a horse with base narrow conformation. Notice the flight of the foot in this base narrow travel.

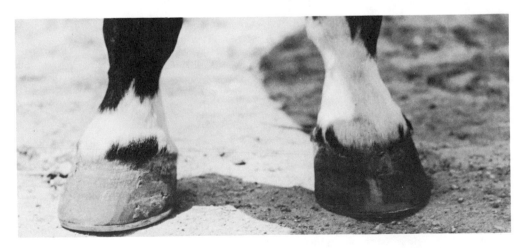

Fig. 8-10. A front view of base narrow and splay-footed conformation.

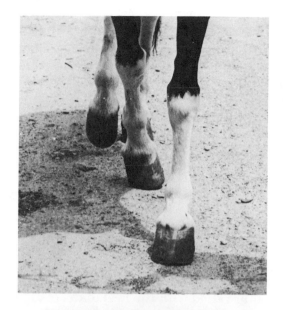

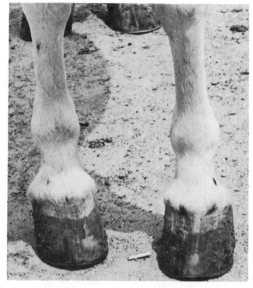

Fig. 8-11. A front view of severe pigeon toe.

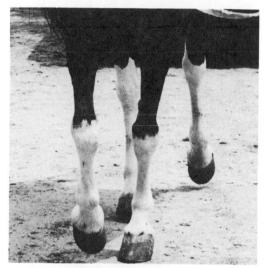

Fig. 8-12. On the left, top to bottom, front views of the travel of the pigeon-toed horse shown above. Notice the flight of the horse's right foot.

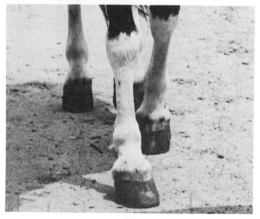

because the legs are turned inward from their origin down. The feet of a splay-footed horse turn out because the legs are turned outward through their entire length.

From a side view, "standing under" in front and "camped" in front are both results of legs improperly directed from their origin. Standing under in front means that the forelimbs do not extend straight down from the elbow, but angle under the body. With camped in front conformation, the forelimbs angle out away from the body.

CAPPED ELBOW

What is capped elbow?

Capped elbow or shoe boil, also known as olecranon bursitis, is a soft, flabby swelling over the point of the elbow due to trauma.

How is trauma incurred?

Trauma usually results from: (1) the shoe hitting against the elbow of the same limb while the horse is being exercised, (2) the horse hitting himself in stamping his foot while fighting flies, or (3) the horse being stabled with insufficient bedding. These conditions are common to horses that are shod with the heel of the hoof left too long and possibly shod with caulks or elevated and weighted shoes.

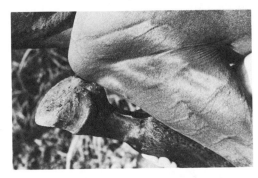

Fig. 8-13. View of the heel hitting the elbow region. This results in trauma to the elbow which can cause capped elbow.

Is the injury obvious?

The swelling over the point of the elbow sometimes develops rapidly and fluctuates in size. At other times, the swelling may not develop until after repeated trauma. When it does occur, it can be seen and palpated easily. The ailment is

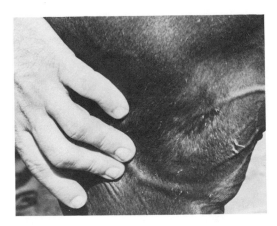

Fig. 8-14. A view of the elbow showing a skin inflammation which is precursory to capped elbow. Note the peeling fragments of skin tissue.

usually painless and does not cause lameness. If there is pain and heat, an infection is indicated, and lameness will be pronounced.

How is capped elbow treated?

First, the cause must be determined and removed. Then, if the injury is slight, daily applications of tincture of iodine or some other blistering method may be sufficient. When the condition has been allowed to become severe, the veterinarian may drain the lesion and administer corticosteroids. A longstanding injury composed mostly of fibrous tissue may require surgical removal.

Is there any other way to prevent or aid in the healing of this injury?

Applying a round "doughnut" roll below the fetlock to limit flexion or special shoeing will stop or ease the problem.

Does capped elbow heal easily?

If the cause is removed, a single injection of corticosteroid is often all that is necessary in acute cases. Persistent lesions will need to be surgically removed.

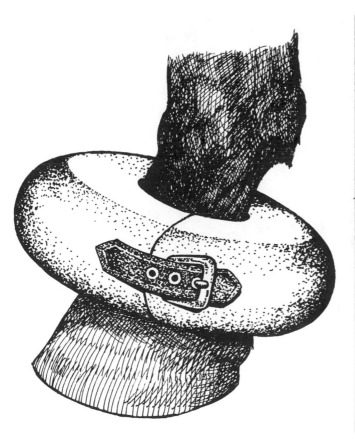

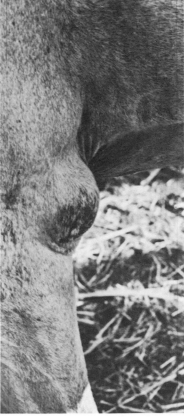

Fig. 8-15. A "doughnut" used in preventing capped elbow.

Fig. 8-16. View of capped elbow.

FRACTURE OF THE OLECRANON

What causes fracture of the elbow?

The olecranon (elbow) is a rough tuberosity (protuberance) at the proximal end of the ulna, and is the point of attachment for the triceps and several other muscles. It can usually only be fractured by a direct blow, such as the horse striking a solid object or being hit by an automobile. The most common cause is a kick over the elbow by another horse. These blows may cause a simultaneous fracture of the humerus or the radius, but they are fractured less often than the olecranon. (See humerus, page 181 and radius, page 181.) The olecranon has a bone growth center in young horses, which is relatively easily separated from the shaft of the ulna. In older horses the trauma may result in damage ranging from small bone chips to serious fractures.

How is fracture of the olecranon diagnosed?

The horse nearly always demonstrates some sign of radial paralysis or "dropped elbow." In this condition, the horse cannot bring the leg forward to bear body weight. There is usually pain. Bone crepitation may be difficult to detect because of

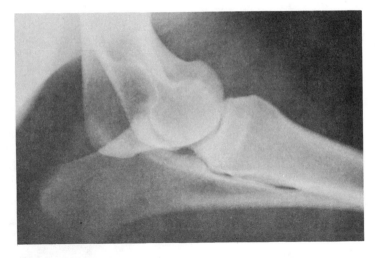

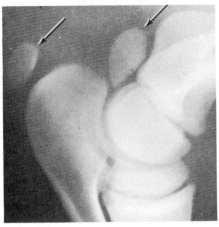

Fig. 8-17. Normal elbow of a mature horse.

Fig. 8-18. Elbow of a young foal. Notice the ossification centers (arrows).

Both photos courtesy of LAMENESS IN HORSES, Edition III, O. R. Adams, Lea and Febiger Publishing Co., Philadelphia, Pa.

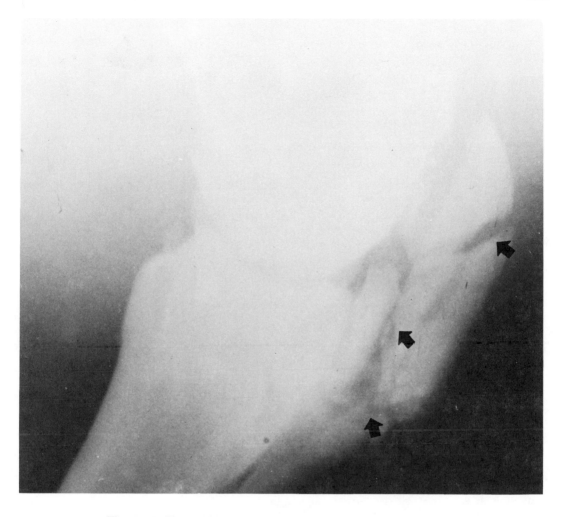

Fig. 8-19. X-ray showing a multiple fracture of the elbow.

swelling. X-rays are needed to determine the extent of the fracture, so a veterinarian should be called immediately.

How is fracture of the olecranon treated?

Bone chips are often removed successfully from the olecranon by surgery, and fractures with no separation of the bone sometimes heal properly with complete stall rest for six weeks. Other, more serious fractures are seldom treated successfully. This is so primarily because of the tremendous pressure put on the olecranon by the triceps muscle. It usually displaces most surgical pins, wire or bone screws.

Permanent lameness usually results. If a separated olecranon does heal, it generally overrides the shaft of the ulna. The outcome of comminuted (crushed) fractures or compound fractures (which pierce soft tissue) is generally bone necrosis (death) and the formation of sequestra (dead bone fragments). The prognosis is generally poor.

9

HOCK

ANATOMY AND CONFORMATION

What is the hock?

The hock is the joint between the cannon and the gaskin (thigh) in the hindleg of the horse. The hock joint is anatomically equivalent to the human ankle.

What is the structure of the hock?

The hock is a complex joint composed of small bones held together by numerous ligaments. However, they form only one major joint with a single joint capsule.

The fibular tarsal bone acts as a lever and projects upward and backward to form the point of the hock. This projection of the fibular tarsal bone is called the tuber calcis. Attached to the tuber calcis is the Achilles tendon, which works to extend and support the hock. If the Achilles tendon is cut, the hock would drop to the ground. The Achilles tendon is made up of the tendon of the gastrocnemius muscle and the superficial digital flexor which extends from the stifle to the coffin bone.

The tibial tarsal bone is anterior to (in front of) the fibular tarsal bone. The remaining bones of the hock are smaller than either the fibular tarsal bone or the tibial tarsal bone and are arranged between the distal (lower) end of the tibial tarsal bone and the proximal (upper) end of the cannon bone. These smaller tarsal (hock) bones are the central tarsal bone, first tarsal bone, second tarsal bone (the first and second tarsal bones are fused), third tarsal bone and the fourth tarsal bone.

All of the tarsal bones are bound together by short, strong ligaments. There is very little movement between them, consisting of only slight arthrodial (gliding) action.

The major joint of the hock is a ginglymus (hinge) joint formed between the distal (lower) end of the tibia and the tibial tarsal bone. The hock joint is partially flexed at all times, which helps to reduce concussion.

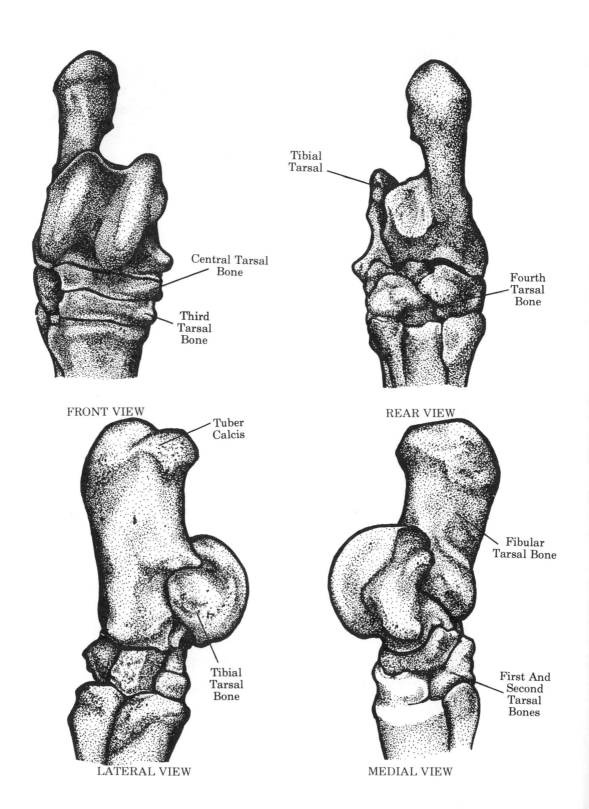

FRONT VIEW

REAR VIEW

LATERAL VIEW

MEDIAL VIEW

Central Tarsal Bone

Third Tarsal Bone

Tibial Tarsal

Fourth Tarsal Bone

Tuber Calcis

Tibial Tarsal Bone

Fibular Tarsal Bone

First And Second Tarsal Bones

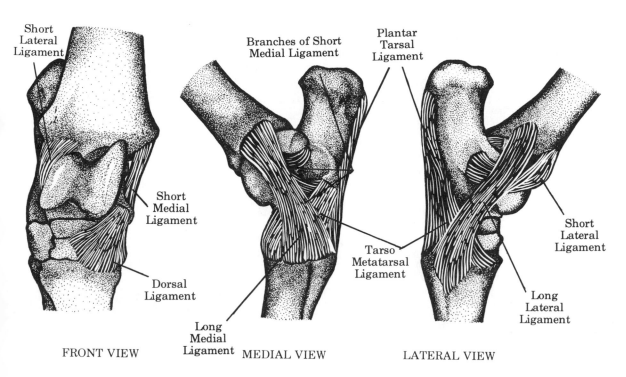

FRONT VIEW   MEDIAL VIEW   LATERAL VIEW

Fig. 9-2. Three separate views of the ligaments binding the tarsal bones together.

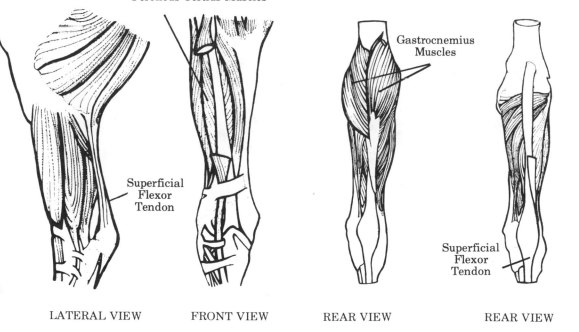

LATERAL VIEW   FRONT VIEW   REAR VIEW   REAR VIEW

Fig. 9-3. Four views of the muscles of the hock area.

The hock has reciprocal action with the stifle, meaning that the stifle joint cannot flex without flexing the hock joint. The structures responsible for this reciprocal movement are the superficial digital flexor and the gastrocnemius (on the back of the leg) and the peronius tertius muscle (on the front of the leg). The peronius tertius muscle extends from the upper end of the stifle joint to the hock region where it splits and attaches to both the hock and the top end of the cannon bone.

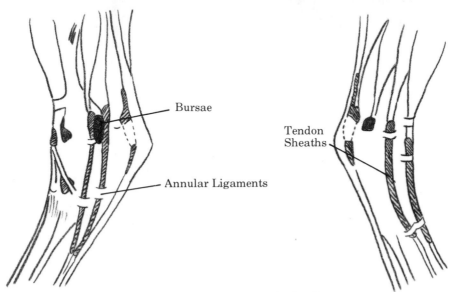

Fig. 9-4. Structures of the hock.

There are numerous other muscles, tendons and ligaments in the hindleg which aid in the complex movement and support of the hock and the entire limb.

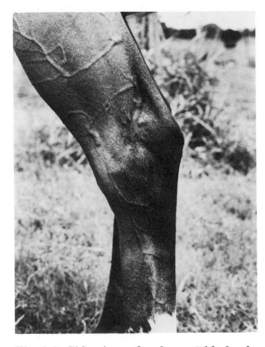

Fig. 9-5. Side view of a clean, wide hock.

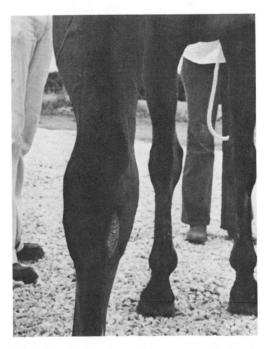

Fig. 9-6. Back view of a clean, wide hock.

What is considered good hock conformation?

The hock should be wide from front to back, giving width and strength to the gaskin. Ideally the point of the hock is long, so that the lever it forms is provided with increased length and power. The appearance of the hock should be clean cut, with no roundness or "meatiness." The joint should have a neat look with thin, supple skin covering it so that the bones stand out in clear relief.

Fig. 9-7. Side view of a "meaty" hock.

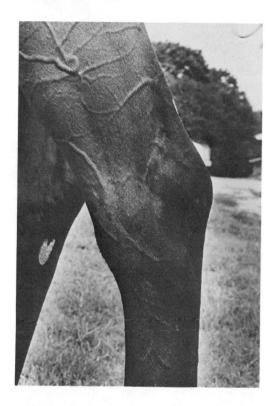

Good hock conformation is in proportion with the structure of the entire body of the horse—neither too fine nor too coarse, and the hock should be of ample size to bear the weight of the animal. For good conformation, hocks must be correctly set.

What does "correctly set" mean?

When viewed from the back, the leg should be straight with no deviation of the hock joint. From the side, the angles of the hock and stifle should appear neither too straight nor too angulated. A line dropped straight down from the point of the buttock should touch the point of the hock and the point of the fetlock.

What are the types of faulty hock conformation when the horse is viewed from the back?

"Cow hocks" and "bow legs" are both deviations of the hock joint, readily visible from the rear. With bow legs (or bandy legs), the hocks are set too far apart, frequently resulting in interference between the hindfeet as they pass one another in travel. In the case of cow hocks, the hocks are set too close together, causing excessive strain on the inside of the hock and predisposing the horse to bone spavin.

Another type of poor hock conformation is the narrow, thin hock. Usually this type of hock is weak and unable to adequately dissipate concussion.

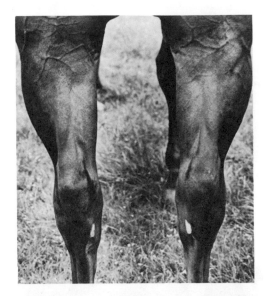

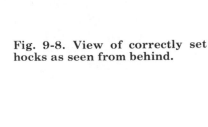

Fig. 9-8. View of correctly set hocks as seen from behind.

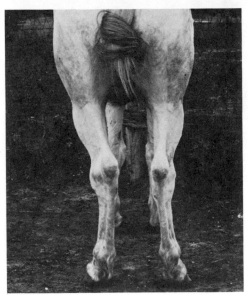

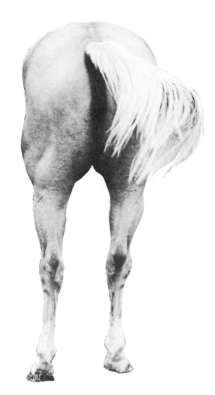

Fig. 9-9. An example of cow hocks as seen from behind.

Fig. 9-10. An example of bow legs. Notice that the heels are turned in, while the hocks are turned slightly outward.

What types of faulty conformation concern the angle of the hock?

Sickle hocks and straight hocks are deviations in the angle of the hock as seen from the side. A straight hock increases the tension on the front of the joint capsule of the hock. The "too straight" leg is easily injured by hard work. Bog spavin and upward fixation of the patella can be contributed to by a straight hock.

In the case of sickle hocks, the horse appears to be standing under from the hock down—the cannon slopes forward. This is due to the excessive angulation of the hock. Sickle hock conformation places increased strain on the back of the hock, predisposing a horse to curb, bone spavin and bog spavin.

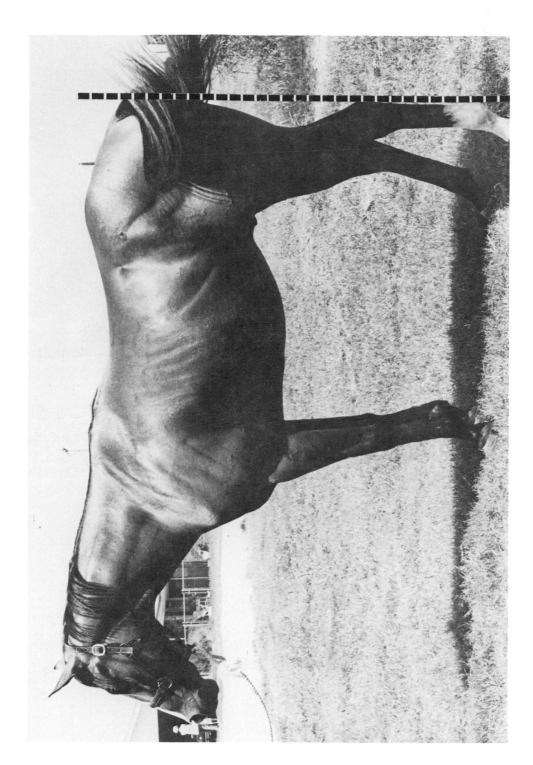

Fig. 9-11. Side view of a horse with correctly set hocks. Notice that a line dropped straight down from the point of the buttock will touch the point of the hock and the point of the fetlock.

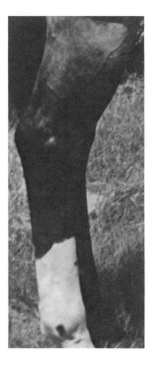 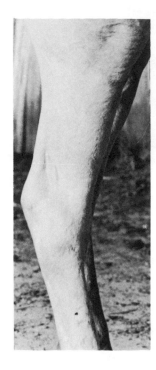 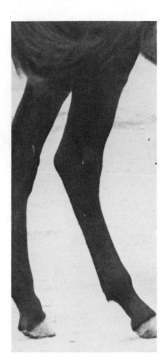

Fig. 9-12. Examples of faulty angle conformation of the hock. Normal hocks (left), too straight hocks (center), and sickle hocks (right).

CAPPED HOCK

What is capped hock?

Capped hock is an inflammation of the bursa over the point of the hock. As its names implies, a "cap" forms which may be soft and fluid filled when it is fresh. In time it will become a firm, fibrous enlargement of the bursa, especially if there has been recurrence of an old injury.

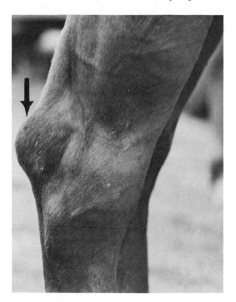

Fig. 9-13. Side view of capped hock.

What are the signs of capped hock?

At first the swelling of the bursa will be soft and varied in size but eventually it will harden. Lameness rarely occurs and almost never persists, and if it is present, it will be mild.

What are the causes of capped hock?

This condition is caused by trauma to the bursa over the point of the hock such as kicks, falls and bumps, or lying down for extended periods on a hard surface. Capped hock may be accompanied by a curb as the causes are essentially the same.

How is capped hock treated?

Acute, early cases may respond well to cold water treatments. Then the veterinarian may drain the synovial fluid and administer corticosteroid injections. Counterirritants may be used in cases where the initial inflammatory reaction has subsided and further reduction of the enlargement is desired.

Is the prognosis good in cases of capped hock?

If the injury is incurred several times and extensive fibrous tissue results, the prognosis is poor for cure of the blemish; but if the injury occurs only once and treatment is prompt, results are usually good. Some of the blemish is usually permanent. If the disfigurement is not acceptable to the owner, surgery can be performed to remove the bursa to try to improve the appearance of the hock. The chance of success for this procedure is fair.

STRINGHALT

What is stringhalt?

Stringhalt or springhalt is an involuntary, greater-than-normal flexion of the hock while the horse is in motion and may affect one or both hindlimbs.

How is this caused?

The true cause is unknown, but the condition is associated with nervous disorders, degeneration of the sciatic and peroneal nerves which supply the muscles of this area, and affectations of the spinal cord. At any rate, the condition is considered to involve some pathology of the lateral digital extensor muscle.

How does stringhalt affect the horse?

The effects are quite variable, but the disease is easy to diagnose from the signs. Because the syndrome is erratic, it is often not obvious during examination. Stringhalt is apparently not painful and does not cause lameness in the usual sense.

Some horses show a very mild hyperflexion of the hock during walking, while others jerk the leg up so violently that it strikes the abdomen and then pounds to the ground. Some horses show signs at each step, others only occasionally. In nearly all cases the signs are exaggerated when the horse is turning or backing. It usually is most noticeable after the horse has rested. The flexion may increase in cold weather and decrease or even disappear in warm weather. This syndrome is not characteristic of any particular breed or breeds of horses.

Does stringhalt prevent the horse from being usable?

Although regarded as a gross unsoundness, stringhalt may not materially hinder the horse's capacity for work, except in severe cases where the constant concussion gives rise to complications. The judgment of a veterinarian will be

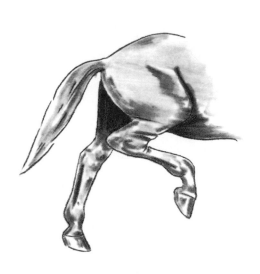

Fig. 9-14. Illustration of stringhalt. Notice the greater-than-normal flexion of the horses's right hock.

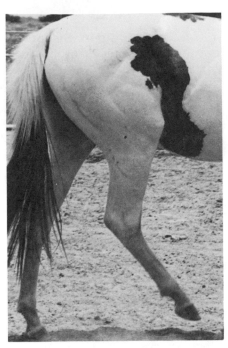

Fig. 9-15. Mild case of stringhalt.

valuable in deciding whether or not a horse may continue to compete in horse show performance classes. The veterinarian may or may not consider treatment of the syndrome necessary.

What is the treatment for stringhalt?

It is a surgical procedure to cut the tendon of the lateral digital extensor muscle. This may alleviate the condition and involves removing a section of the tendon and sometimes part of the muscle. The prognosis after surgery is guarded to favorable.

CURB

What is a curb?

A curb is a thickening of the plantar tarsal ligament. This is a short ligament which starts just below the point of the hock and runs down to the head of the cannon bone. Its purpose is to hold the point of the hock in position. When strained or injured, it ruptures along with the surrounding blood vessels. There may be a small amount of internal bleeding which causes swelling and filling in the area.

How does strain or injury occur?

The hocks are easily damaged by falling, slipping, or kicking stalls, trailers, etc. Strain can come from overexertion when jumping or pulling. Poor conformation such as cow hocks or sickle hocks is a primary predisposing factor in bilateral cases.

What are the effects of curb?

There is an enlargement below the point of the hock which is easily seen from the side. Acute curb is characterized by inflammation and lameness. The horse stands with the leg at rest and the heel elevated to reduce tension on the ligament. Swelling may increase rather than recede with exercise.

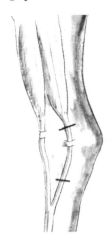

Fig. 9-16. Illustration showing the location for cutting the tendon of the lateral digital extensor in the surgical treatment of stringhalt.

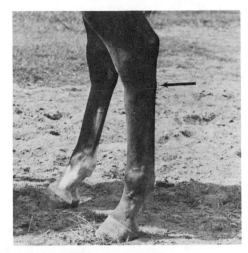

Fig. 9-17. Side view of curb (arrow).

In severe cases where trauma has been the cause, periostitis (see page 127) on the back surface of the fibular tarsal bone may result in new bone growth.

In chronic cases, the area often becomes infiltrated with scar tissue resulting in a permanent blemish, but usually no lameness results.

How is curb treated?

The inflammation requires cold packs and rest. The area over the enlarged ligament may be fired or blistered by the veterinarian, but this will be beneficial only if the inflammatory reaction has subsided. Otherwise, the condition will be aggravated and take longer to heal. Systemic corticoid treatment is of value in the acute phase of curb. Rest is essential for about 30 days.

Is the recovery rate good?

Yes, if the horse has good conformation and proper treatment. Poor conformation will tend to aggravate the situation which makes the prognosis less favorable and the required time for complete healing longer. In most cases there will be a permanent blemish, but this does not cause lameness.

THOROUGHPIN

What is thoroughpin?

Thoroughpin is a distension of the sheath of the deep flexor tendon resulting in swelling just above the point of the hock. It can vary from a quite small swelling up to about four inches in diameter, shaped much like a ball, that can be maneuvered from one side of the hock to the other by hand pressure.

How is thoroughpin caused?

Thoroughpin is usually due to trauma such as bumping, kicking, etc. Consequently, it is generally only on one leg. Other possible causes include tendon strain or pressure.

How is thoroughpin treated?

Since a distended tendon sheath will heal with time, rest is indicated. If the veterinarian sees the need to reduce pressure and swelling, the area can be drained and corticosteroids injected two to three times a week until the swelling does not recur. Results are generally good, although it is difficult to reduce the swelling permanently. Hock bandages are sometimes used. Firing and blistering will not help the condition.

What are the effects of thoroughpin?

Lameness will probably be present when the ailment first occurs. After the sheath heals the swelling may remain, but the lameness does not persist. Therefore, the usefulness of the horse is not affected but there will be a permanent blemish.

Thoroughpins that are set are not of much concern in working horses.

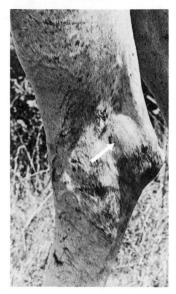

Fig. 9-18. Side view of thoroughpin. Notice the swelling above the point of the hock.

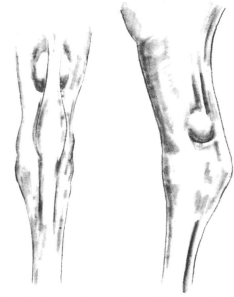

Fig. 9-19. An illustration of thoroughpin, as seen from behind (left) and from the side (right).

LUXATION OF THE SUPERFICIAL FLEXOR TENDON

Can the hock joint be dislocated?

Because it is composed of a number of small bones, the hock joint as a whole does not dislocate. However, the superficial digital flexor tendon, which serves to flex and support the hock, can dislocate either medially (inside) or laterally (outside) from the point of the hock (lateral luxation is more common).

What causes the superficial digital flexor tendon to luxate?

This tendon spreads as it passes over the point of the hock to cover the tuber calcis. At this point it splits so that two strong bands go off each side of the tendon to insert on the tuber calcis. The rest of the tendon continues down to the digit as a strong rounded tendon. An abnormal force or strain that tears or ruptures one of the side bands unbalances the network and allows the tendon to slip and dislocate.

What are the signs of a luxated superficial flexor tendon?

Lameness and swelling in the area of the injury will be evident immediately. Also the slipping of the tendon down the side of the tuber calcis (either side depending on the side of the injury) is visible from the side each time the horse takes a step. There will be no marked change in hock conformation although there may be excessive flexion with movement.

How is luxation of the superficial flexor tendon treated?

Attempts to manually hold the tendon in place or to correct the luxation with counterirritants to the area will be unsuccessful. Surgical repair by the veterinarian is required followed by immobilization of the hock in a cast for three to four weeks. The prognosis for successful treatment by this method is guarded.

Fig. 9-20. Illustration of the steps involved in repairing a luxated superficial flexor tendon, as seen from behind.

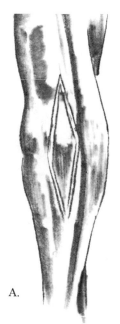 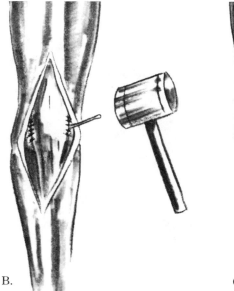 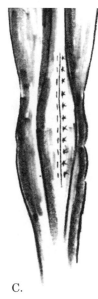

A.   B.   C.

A. An incision is made over the point of the hock. Notice that the tendon is displaced to the right.

B. The tendon is sutured into place and a Steinmann pin is inserted to prevent the tendon from luxating again.

C. The surgery is completed with skin sutures to close the incision.

Fig. 9-21. Two views of the hock joint as seen from behind. On the left, the normal position of the superficial flexor tendon on the point of the hock. On the right, luxation (dislocation) of the tendon.

Fig. 9-22. The hind leg is put in a cast to immobilize the hock after surgery to correct a luxated superficial flexor tendon.

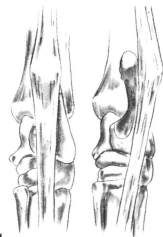 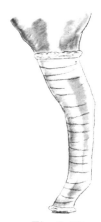

Fig. 9-21.   Fig. 9-22.

Occasionally the horse can become functionally sound again if the tendon establishes a new bed in its displaced position. However, if the tendon continues to slip off and on the tuber calcis, the horse will stay lame. Although it is a relatively new method for correcting luxation of the superficial flexor tendon, surgical repair appears to be a treatment with merit.

BOG SPAVIN

What is bog spavin?

Bog spavin is a chronic distension of the joint capsule of the hock with synovial fluid. The joint capsule is lined with synovial tissue which secretes synovia (synovial fluid) to lubricate the joint. Excessive production of synovial fluid causes overfilling of the hock joint.

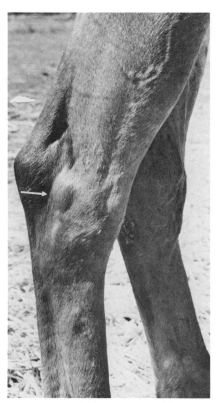

Fig. 9-23. Side view of bog spavin (arrow).

What causes bog spavin?

Faulty hock conformation (straight hocks, for example), places additional stress on the hock joint which tends to cause bog spavin. Hock injuries such as strains and sprains from quick stops or rapid turns also cause bog spavin.

Nutritional deficiencies or imbalances of calcium, phosphorus, vitamin A and vitamin D have also been cited as causes of bog spavin. Ordinarily this is a factor only with horses less than two years old because their bones are still immature and growing.

What are the actual signs of bog spavin?

The swellings of bog spavin are characteristic and appear in three specific places. Two small swellings appear on the inner and outer edges toward the back of

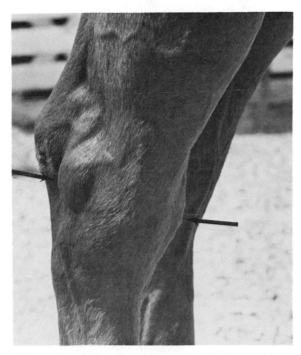

Fig. 9-24. Side view of bog spavin (arrows).

the hock, and a larger swelling appears on the inner aspect of the hock in front. When pressure is applied to one swelling, the fluid will be pushed toward the other swellings and they will enlarge.

Bog spavin rarely makes a horse lame. However, if the spavin was caused by a minor injury, the horse may be lame due to the injury. Bog spavin caused by an injury usually affects only one leg while conformationally and nutritionally caused bog spavins usually appear in both legs. Also, when due to the latter causes, the onset is gradual.

Bog spavin normally does not interfere with the usefulness of the horse, but does result in an ugly blemish. There is no bone involvement as there is in bone spavin.

Occasionally bog spavin spontaneously appears and disappears in young horses.

Is there any treatment for bog spavin?

Since it usually does not result in lameness, treatment is often not required or indicated for bog spavin. A veterinarian should be consulted though, so that the cause can be determined. If the bog is nutritional in origin, correcting the diet will normally cure it. A bog is sometimes a precursor to bone spavin and the veterinarian will consider this in determining how to treat or manage the bog to hedge against this possibility. Most treatments are limited to attempting to remove the blemish, and usually they are unsuccessful.

Removal of excess fluid, corticosteroid injections into the joint capsule, blisters, liniments and pressure bandages are examples of treatments which are tried. Massage several times daily is also used in an attempt to reduce the swelling. Even if treatment is successful, bog spavin swellings have a tendency to recur. This is especially true when faulty conformation is a factor since the cause is ever present. The blemish is permanent in most cases.

BONE SPAVIN

What is bone spavin?

Spavin is a general name for lamenesses originating in the hock. The bones of the lower, gliding articulations of the hock joint (page 193) are involved in bone spavin. There is either excessive new bone formation (exostosis) or bone destruction on the inner surface of the hock. Bone spavin begins with an erosion of the joint surfaces in the hock and is followed by new bone growth and ankylosis (fusing of the bones).

Are there other names for bone spavin?

Yes, the term "jack" spavin refers to an exceptionally large bone spavin. "Blind" spavin and "occult" spavin are terms for typical spavin lameness without external signs. The degenerative changes are present, but there is no exostosis visible externally.

What causes this disease?

Faulty conformation is a major cause of bone spavin. Cow hocks and sickle hocks both increase stress on the inside of the hocks, predisposing a horse to bone spavin. Narrow, thin hock conformation will also make a horse more susceptible to this disease.

Strains, sprains and direct injuries to the hocks which cause an inflammation of the surface of the bone resulting in new bone growth (bone spavin) are other common causes.

Mineral imbalances have also been blamed for some cases of bone spavin.

What are the signs of bone spavin?

The symptoms are not well defined. Even when a horse is lame and bony enlargements are apparent on a hock, the lameness may be due to another factor, so a veterinarian is needed to make a conclusive diagnosis. There may be an enlargement of variable size on the inner side of the hock except in the case of blind or occult spavin. There is no definite relationship between the size of the enlargement and the degree of lameness and usually no increase in heat over the area of the spavin. One or both hindlegs may be affected.

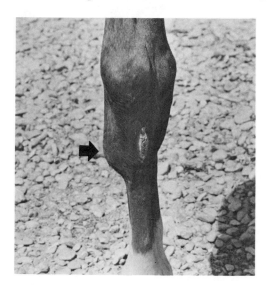

Fig. 9-25. Rear view of the hock area showing a bone spavin.

Bone spavin typically begins as a "cold" lameness, with lameness becoming constant as the disease progresses. This means that the horse will be lame but the lameness usually disappears with exercise and returns when the horse is rested.

The changes in the bones of the hock result in decreased flexion of this joint, forcing the animal to move with an exaggerated hip action. Instead of bending normally and moving smoothly, the lame leg is jerked upward and forward as the hip is raised and the toe generally drags on the ground. Therefore, when a horse has bone spavin, the hoof of the lame leg will show excessive toe wear along with slight heel wear. When the animal is at rest he generally stands on the toe of the hoof in an attempt to relieve pressure on the hock.

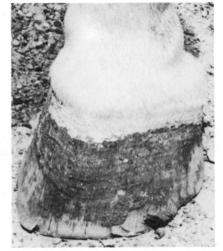

Fig. 9-26. View of a hind foot of a horse with bone spavin. Notice how the toe of the hoof is dubbed off as a result of the foot being dragged along the ground.

Positive reaction to a spavin test is not absolute, conclusive proof of bone spavin. The test is reliable in most cases, however, and is performed in the following manner: the affected leg is picked up and held acutely flexed for about two minutes, then it is released and the horse is immediately trotted. If lameness is markedly increased for the first few steps after the leg is released, the test is considered positive for bone spavin.

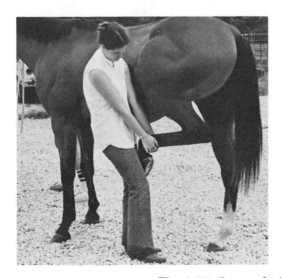 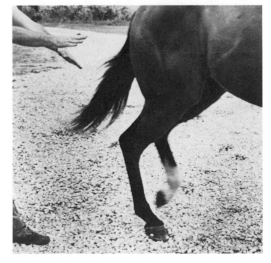

Fig. 9-27. Steps of a bone spavin test.

Generally, radiographic examination (X-ray) can be used to obtain a definite diagnosis of bone spavin. However, in a few instances spavin will not show up on X-ray, but evidence of degeneration will be found in necropsy (autopsy) when the joint is opened.

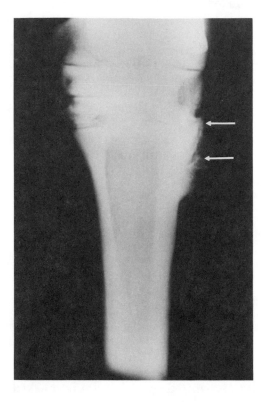

Fig. 9-28. X-ray of hock joint showing bone spavin. Arrows indicate areas of new bone growth (exostosis).

Is there any treatment for bone spavin?

Rest is ordinarily prescribed for this disease. Because the exostosis and erosion of the bone are irreversible, treatment is aimed toward making the horse sound enough to be used. This involves easing the pain by means of corrective shoeing or surgically ankylosing (fusing) the joint, depending upon the extent of the disease.

Corrective shoeing methods, including a shortened and rolled toe, plus a raised heel, will help the horse's way of going. In more extensive cases when the surfaces of

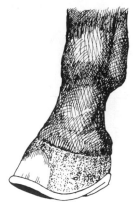

Fig. 9-29. Corrective shoeing to ease the pain involved in bone spavin.

the joint are extensively involved, corrective shoeing is used in conjunction with treatments to speed up the ankylosis of the joint. Point firing into the joint is one method that may be used by the veterinarian. A surgical procedure to drill out the

Fig. 9-30. Illustration of steps involved in surgically ankylosing the hock joint in the treatment of bone spavin.

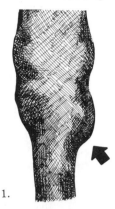

1.

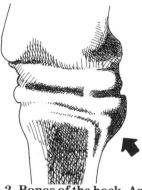

2.

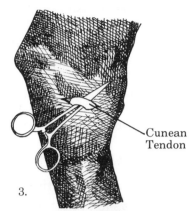

3.

1. Exterior view of hock with bone spavin (arrow).

2. Bones of the hock. Arrow indicates new bone growth on the third and central tarsal bones, causing the bulge seen in 1.

3. The cunean tendon, exposed through an incision over the hock joint.

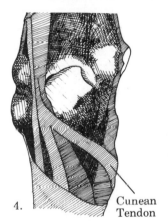

4. Cunean Tendon

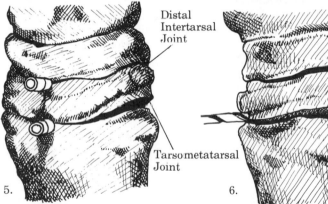

Distal Intertarsal Joint

Tarsometatarsal Joint

5.

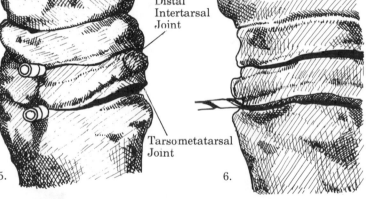

6.

4. View of the cunean tendon crossing the hock joint.

5. Needles inserted into the hock to identify the joints to be fused.

6. A drill bit in position at one distal intertarsal joint.

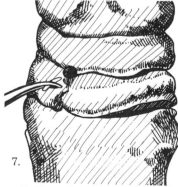

7.

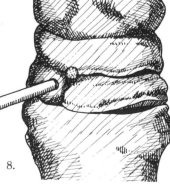

8.

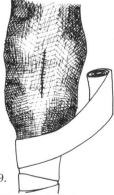

9.

7. Bone fragments from the tuber coxae being inserted into the drilled hole.

8. The bone fragments being firmly packed into the hole to contribute to the fusing of the joint.

9. The hock being wrapped after surgery has been completed.

joint space and destroy the cartilage may also be used to hasten the fusion of the bones.

In some cases of bone spavin the enlargement is under a tendon in the hock area. This is very painful to the horse because the tendon does not have a smooth surface to slide over. In this situation a portion of the tendon is often removed to alleviate the pain.

Does this mean that bone spavin cannot be cured?

This is true, but in many cases the horse can eventually become serviceably sound. By no means is this a complete recovery, but the horse can be used. Ordinarily the horse will be slightly lame until he is warmed up—especially in cold weather. However, when bone spavin has caused extensive changes on the joint surface of the hock, the outlook is not nearly as favorable.

BURSITIS OF THE CUNEAN TENDON

What is bursitis of the cunean tendon?

The bursae are small sacs of fluid in or near joints which serve as lubrication between layers of the body. Bursitis is the inflammation of one or more of these sacs. The cunean tendon is the medial (inside) tendon of the tibialis anterior muscle, and attaches to the hock joint. The bursa involved in bursitis of the cunean tendon is between the tendon itself and the ligaments overlying the tarsal bones. It is a common condition in harness racing horses.

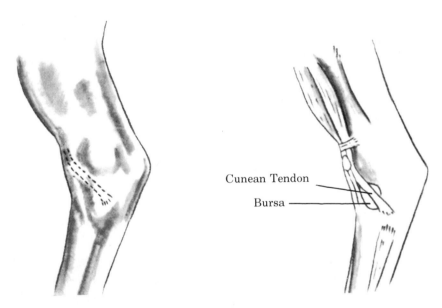

Cunean Tendon

Bursa

Fig. 9-31. Two medial views of the hock showing the location of the cunean tendon and bursa.

What causes bursitis of the cunean tendon?

Bursitis of the cunean tendon is thought to be caused by strain. It may be brought on by twisting or a jolt to the joint. Young trotters are commonly affected, probably because the joint is not at full strength. Horses with poor hock conformation are more likely to be affected.

How is bursitis of the cunean tendon diagnosed?

The horse will show signs typical of bone spavin. (See Bone Spavin, page 208.) Some of the signs are that the affected leg may remain partially flexed, or even be rested on the opposite hoof. When the lameness is first noticed, it may only occur before the horse has warmed up. As the inflammation gets worse, lameness may become constant. The horse will put as little weight as possible on the affected leg, move it in shorter steps, and carry it to the inside to relieve tension. Unlike bone spavin, pressure applied to the area will probably cause pain.

How is bursitis of the cunean tendon treated?

If bursitis of the cunean tendon is suspected, a veterinarian will be needed to confirm diagnosis and render appropriate treatment. Generally the injection of a corticosteroid is called for to temporarily relieve the pain. If this seems to bring favorable change, the veterinarian may prescribe rest to let healing take place or perform a tenotomy, cutting the cunean tendon where it crosses the bursa. Sometimes a tenectomy (complete removal of the tendon) is used. Both of these methods have been effective in restoring use of the limb. The prognosis is generally good.

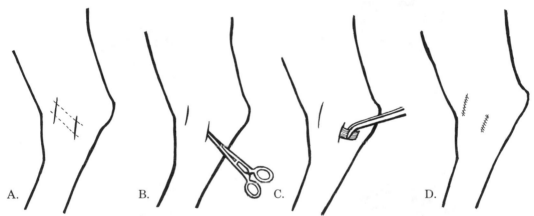

A. Two incisions made over the cunean tendon.

B. Cutting of the tendon through the incisions.

C. Removal of the cut section of tendon.

D. Sutured incisions after surgery.

FRACTURE OF THE HOCK JOINT

What causes fracture of the hock joint?

A hock joint fracture is usually caused by crushing or twisting or a direct blow to the joint. Any horse may incur a crush-type fracture, for instance, in a door or gate. The twisting injuries, though, are most common among barrel racers, horses shod with heel calks, or any animal exposed to a situation where the foot is held stable and the leg turns. The most frequent direct blow to the hock joint is a kick by another horse. Other direct blows causing fractures might include the horse striking a solid object, or being hit by an automobile.

The horse will probably show the same outward signs no matter what part of the hock joint is fractured. There is generally considerable swelling of the leg and pain is severe. The horse may refuse or be unable to stand. Many horses go into shock and die within two or three days. More specific diagnostic signs may vary with the area or areas injured. There are ten bones which articulate (form movable joints with each other) in the hock joint, but fractures may be dealt with in three basic groups.

The first group includes the tibia (main bone of the gaskin) and the second, third and fourth metatarsals (rear cannon bones). (See Cannon Area Fractures, page 140 and Gaskin Area Fractures, page 225.) Young animals are more likely to be injured in or near the articular surfaces due to the area of bone growth there, while mature animals are more likely to be injured in the shaft of the bone. Crepitation may be evident, but X-rays are necessary to determine the exact location of the damage.

The second group consists of five of the six tarsal bones, including the tibial tarsal bone, the central tarsal bone, the first and second tarsal bones (fused as one bone), the third tarsal bone and the fourth tarsal bone. These are the "internal" bones of the hock joint and all have articular surfaces. They are rarely fractured, but of this group the most likely to be fractured is the tibial tarsal bone. It is the most exposed and articulates with the tibia. Diagnosis may be made by crepitation, although X-ray is also necessary here to determine the exact location.

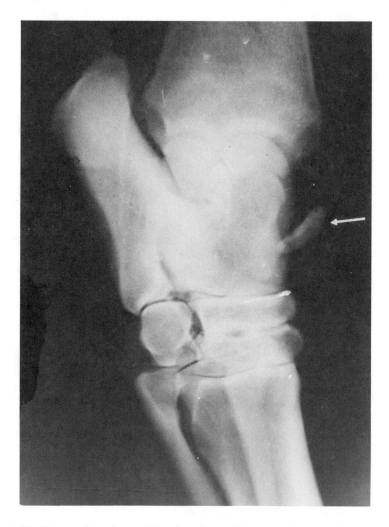

Fig. 9-33. X-ray showing a chip fracture of the tibial tarsal bone (arrow).

Finally, the fibular tarsal bone or point of hock should be considered by itself. Diagnosis is much the same as for other hock joint fractures, except that fracture here produces a peculiar wobbling of the Achilles tendon. The Achilles tendon is attached to a rough tuberosity on the fibular tarsal bone called the tuber calcis.

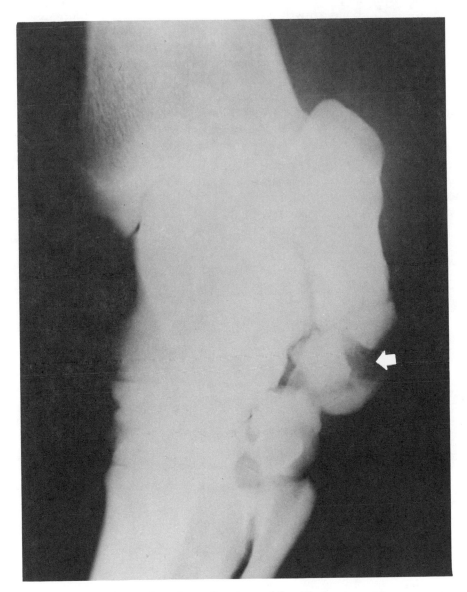

Fig. 9-34. X-ray showing a fracture of the fibular tarsal bone.

How is fracture of the hock joint treated?

Since the immediate symptoms of hock joint fracture may be easily confused with those of less serious disorders, a veterinarian should be consulted for the actual diagnosis.

A chip fracture to the tibial tarsal bone may sometimes be treated successfully. If the area of injury does not directly articulate with the tibia, surgical removal of the fragments or fixation by bone screws may be indicated. Some of these injuries may

216

be caused by osteochondritis dissecans, which causes lesions that break off in the joint. (See Osteochondritis Dissecans, page 235.) If the lesions are diagnosed by X-ray before avulsion (tearing) occurs, confinement for several months may help recovery. Otherwise, surgery is necessary.

In young animals, fracture of the tibia or the third metatarsal often results in breaking off at the bone growth center, with the shaft of the bone overriding the joint. Since treatment is difficult, the bone often heals in this position, creating a "false joint" and permanent lameness. A fracture of these major bones (or of the second or fourth metatarsals) nearly always results in ankylosis (immobility) if the break involves an articular surface.

A fracture of the point of the hock is sometimes healed successfully if the fracture is simple and the fragment is large enough to accommodate two or more bone screws. Generally, however, the force exerted by the biceps and other muscles continually displaces the bone and results in a "false joint" and lameness.

The majority of hock joint injuries that involve articulating surfaces result in permanent lameness. Bone necrosis (death), the formation of sequestra (fragments of dead bone), osteomyelitis (inflammation of the bone marrow) and other infections are commonplace. The prognosis is poor.

GASKIN

ANATOMY AND CONFORMATION

Which area of the horse is called the gaskin?

"Gaskin" refers to the area of the hindleg between the stifle and hock joints. The tibia and fibula are the bones of the gaskin.

How are the tibia and fibula shaped?

The wide top end of the tibia forms the bottom part of the stifle joint. The shaft of the tibia is slender and triangular in shape, and the lower end of the tibia forms the upper part of the hock joint. The head and shaft are present in the fibula, but it has no enlargement at the lower end.

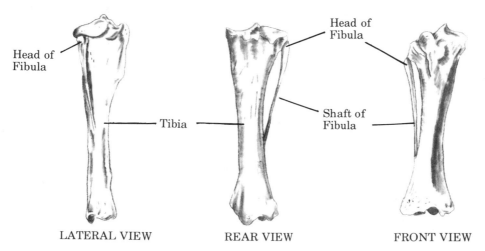

Head of Fibula

Head of Fibula

Shaft of Fibula

Tibia

LATERAL VIEW   REAR VIEW   FRONT VIEW

Fig. 10-1. Three separate views of the right tibia and fibula.

The tibia and fibula correspond to the radius and ulna in the forelimb. The tibia is the larger bone situated on the inside of the leg, while the fibula is much smaller and is found on the outside of the leg.

Which muscles and ligaments are involved in this area?

The muscles and ligaments found in the gaskin area are: (1) the long and lateral digital extensor muscles, (2) the tibialis cranius muscle, (3) the peroneus tertius (which is a powerful ligament connecting the stifle and hock so that they move together), (4) the proximal, middle and distal annular ligaments which encircle the hock to strengthen and protect the hock joint capsule and (5) the extensor digitalis brevis muscle which is vestigial in function.

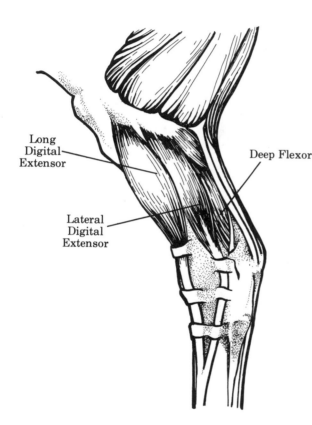

Long Digital Extensor

Lateral Digital Extensor

Deep Flexor

Fig. 10-2. Lateral view of the left hindleg, showing the muscles of the gaskin.

What is good conformation of the gaskin?

Although the muscling of the gaskin area varies according to breed, the muscles should be well developed because they give the horse power to pull, jump and run.

From a rear view, the medial outline of the gaskin may be slightly curved inward in some horses, like the Arabian, or almost vertical, as in the Quarter Horse.

The width of the gaskin, as judged from a side view, is dependent upon the position of the tuber calcis (point of the hock) and the Achilles tendon. The farther back these are, the better the leverage and the wider the gaskin, since the Achilles tendon forms the back line of the lower part of the gaskin.

The outer side of the tibia is heavily muscled while the inner part is directly under the skin. Since the muscles can be seen so clearly in this area, they can be used as an indicator of the condition of the entire animal.

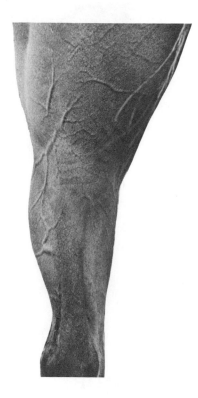

Fig. 10-3. Rear view of the gaskin area.

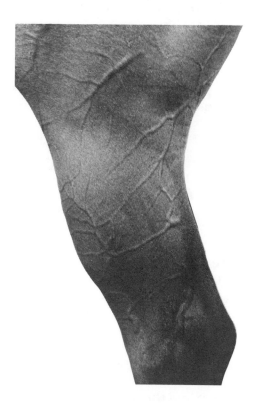

Fig. 10-4. Side view of the gaskin area.

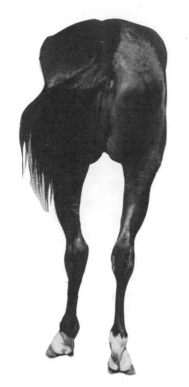 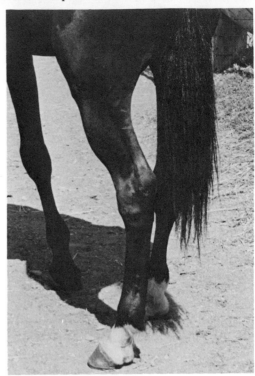

Fig. 10-5. Two views of a weak gaskin.

RUPTURE OF THE PERONEUS TERTIUS MUSCLE

What is the peroneus tertius muscle?

The peroneus muscle extends along the front of the gaskin from the stifle joint to the hock joint, and works to flex and extend both of these joints together. Rupture (forcible tearing of the tissues) of the peroneus tertius muscle is a serious condition in the horse.

What causes the peroneus tertius to rupture?

The peroneus tertius ruptures when the hock joint is overextended. This can happen when a horse kicks violently, falls with the rear leg extended, receives a deep cut on the front of the gaskin, overexerts during a fast start or struggles to free a caught hindleg. In the last instance, rupture occurs when the leg is pulled too far back while the horse is struggling. Severe trauma involving the front of the gaskin may also rupture the peroneus tertius.

What are the signs of a ruptured peroneus tertius?

Because the function of the peroneus tertius is lost, the signs of this disorder are very typical. The hock can be extended without extending the stifle, which a normal limb is not capable of doing. As the horse walks, the stifle flexes to advance the limb, but the hock is carried forward without flexing. In fact, the part of the leg below the hock hangs limp while the horse is in motion.

The limb will be able to support weight, causing little pain when the horse is standing. If the lower part of the limb is pulled backward, the hock will overextend. Also, the Achilles tendon will be relaxed, even to the extent that it dimples and folds.

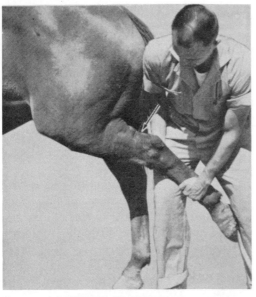

Fig. 10-6A. Rupture of the peroneus tertius. Arrow indicates dimpling of achilles tendon.

Courtesy of LAMENESS IN HORSES, Edition III, O. R. Adams, Lea and Febiger Publishing Co., Philadelphia, Pa.

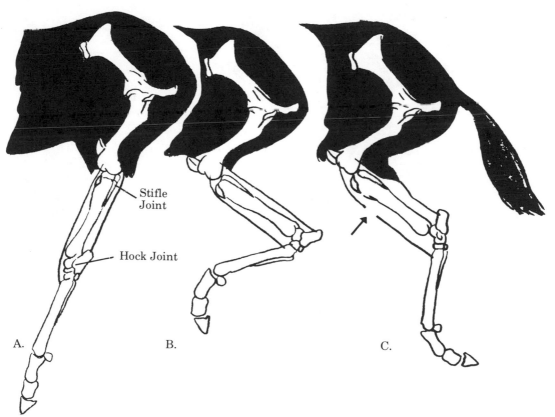

Stifle Joint

Hock Joint

A.   B.   C.

A. Extreme extension of a normal leg. Notice that both the hock joint and the stifle joint are extended.

B. Normal flexion. Notice that both the hock joint and the stifle joint are flexed.

C. Flexion with a ruptured peroneus tertius (arrow). Notice that the stifle joint is flexed but the hock joint is straight.

A veterinarian should be called to diagnose this condition since the signs could be mistaken for a fracture of the leg.

How is rupture of the peroneus tertius treated?

Veterinarians prescribe complete rest for treatment of this condition. Rest is essential for the muscle to heal properly. Casts and bandages are rarely used, but the horse should be kept as quiet as possible for one to two months, after which exercise can be initiated. Complete recovery usually requires two to three months.

If the horse is properly reconditioned, the limb will regain full normal action. Exercise that is excessive or premature may cause the peroneus tertius to heal longer than normal, resulting in impaired action.

RUPTURE OF THE GASTROCNEMIUS TENDON

What is a rupture of the gastrocnemius tendon?

Rupture of the gastrocnemius tendon may occur alone or in combination with the superficial flexor tendon, when it is considered to be a rupture of the Achilles tendon. Since the gastrocnemius ruptures before the superficial flexor tendon, this condition is more common than rupture of the Achilles tendon.

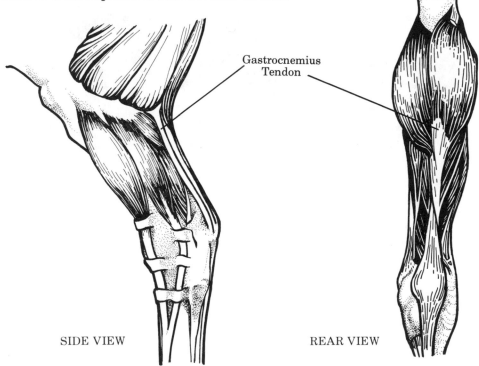

Gastrocnemius
Tendon

SIDE VIEW   REAR VIEW

Fig. 10-7. Side and rear views of the gaskin showing the location of the gastrocnemius tendon.

What causes the gastrocnemius to rupture?

Trauma is the cause of rupture; and in many cases it is the result of strenuous stops or starts. It is most vulnerable when great stress is being applied to the hock in an effort to extend the limb or to prevent its extension.

What are the signs of a rupture of the gastrocnemius tendon?

Rupture of the gastrocnemius tendon results in increased angulation of the hock joint, giving the impression that the horse is squatting, if both limbs are affected. The horse will be unable to straighten the affected limb, but he can walk without too much difficulty.

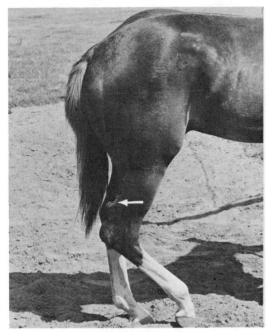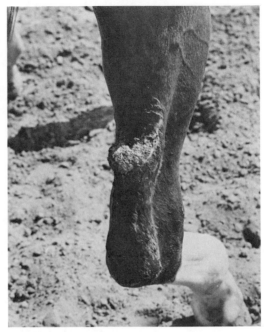

Fig. 10-8. Side and back views of the hindleg showing rupture of the gastrocnemius tendon. Notice that the horse is unable to straighten the leg.

What is the treatment for rupture of the gastrocnemius tendon?

Treatment of a rupture of the gastrocnemius tendon is the same as treatment of a ruptured Achilles tendon. Casting the whole leg and placing the horse in slings is an attempt to take pressure off the affected limb to allow the severed muscle ends to reunite. This procedure is difficult because many horses will not tolerate the restrictions of a leg cast and slings. If the horse does not cooperate with the required treatment methods, euthanasia may be required.

RUPTURE OF THE ACHILLES TENDON

What is the Achilles tendon?

The Achilles tendon is composed of the tendons of the gastrocnemius muscle and the superficial flexor in the hindlimb. These two in combination are called the Achilles tendon.

What is a rupture of the Achilles tendon?

Achilles tendon tearing is very unusual, but ruptures of both tendons involved is possible. Rupture of this tendon results in complete uselessness of the injured leg.

What causes rupture of the Achilles tendon?

Rupture of the Achilles tendon may be caused by trauma or lacerated wounds.

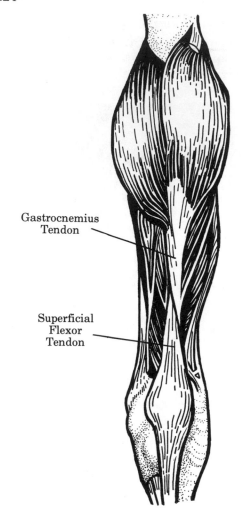

Gastrocnemius
Tendon

Superficial
Flexor
Tendon

Fig. 10-9. A rear view of the hindleg showing the two tendons that make up the Achilles tendon.

Severe stress may weaken the tendons, causing them to rupture when they are stressed again.

What are the signs of rupture of the Achilles tendon?

The signs of Achilles tendon rupture are easily identified. Without the support of the Achilles tendon, the hock may drop to the ground. The hock will be closer to the ground than it would be if only the gastrocnemius were ruptured. Severe angulation of the hock makes it almost impossible for the horse to move the affected limb forward. Because the limb cannot support weight, rupture of the Achilles tendon in both hindlegs makes a horse completely helpless.

What is the treatment for this condition?

If only one limb is involved, casting the whole leg (as high as possible) and placing the horse in a sling may be successful. Involvement of both hindlegs is more difficult because the horse does not cooperate with efforts to keep weight off his hindlegs. Many horses will not tolerate full leg casts and slings for the six to eight weeks necessary to accomplish healing of the ruptured tendons. In cases where the horse will not tolerate the required treatment, euthanasia is the alternative.

FRACTURE OF THE GASKIN AREA

What causes fracture of the gaskin area?

There are two bones in the gaskin area, the tibia and the fibula. The fibula is seldom broken, because it is a rather small bone which joins the proximal end of the tibia and lies on the lateral (outer) surface of the larger bone, where it is well protected by muscle.

Unlike the fibula, the tibia is a weight-bearing bone. It is most exposed to blows on the medial (inner) surface. The most common cause of fracture is a kick from another horse.

Can the gaskin area incur different kinds of fractures?

The tibia can be broken in the same manner as other large bones. That is, it can have simple fractures, in which there is little or no bone displacement, comminuted or "crushed" fractures, or compound fractures, in which bone pierces soft tissue. Another common tibial fracture is a chip fracture, in which small fragments of bone are dislodged. The tibia is usually fractured in this way at the malleoli, which are rounded processes near the hock joint that may be broken off. The tibia is also, however, the most common site of the deferred fracture. In this type of injury, bone displacement may not occur for as long as two or three weeks after the accident. The best explanation for this occurrence is that the tibia may be only fissured (cracked) and is held together by the deep fascia (fibrous tissue) surrounding the bone. Some time later, strain is placed on the limb and displacement occurs.

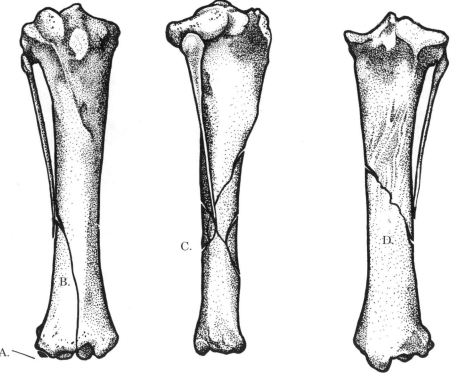

Fig. 10-10. Fractures of the tibia. A. Fracture of a malleolus. B. Fissured fracture. C. Multiple fracture. D. Simple oblique fracture.

How is fracture of the gaskin area diagnosed?

Fracture of the tibia where the bone is displaced is easily diagnosed. The horse will probably "swing" the leg, refusing to put weight on the injury. There is generally considerable swelling, which tends to bow the leg inward. Bone crepitation is usually evident. Fractures which were not originally compound usually become so after a few days, when the horse tries to bear weight on the limb. Bone fragments from complete fractures nearly always penetrate the medial skin surface, away from the muscles.

It is hard to diagnose a deferred fracture until actual displacement occurs. Until that point, the only dependable diagnosis is by X-ray.

Do fractures of the fibula occur?

Yes, but authorities disagree on the frequency of fracture of the fibula. Due to its location it is well protected by the peroneus muscle unless it receives a direct blow. What appears to be a "fracture" of the fibula in radiographs is said to be a normal fibrous junction in the upper and lower portions of the bone. Diagnosis of fracture of the fibula should be cautious if radiographs of the opposite limb show a similar "fracture."

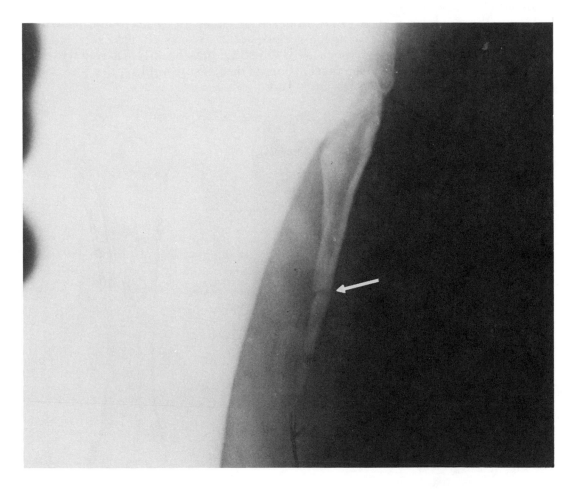

Fig. 10-11. X-ray of the tibia and fibula. Arrow indicates a normal fibrous junction which may be mistaken for a fracture of the fibula.

What is the treatment for fractures of the fibula?

No treatment is necessary since fracture of the fibula does not cause lameness. The tibia acts as a splint to prevent displacement of the fibula.

Fracture of the fibula has been treated by surgical removal of the bone fragment.

How is fracture of the gaskin area treated?

In all cases where fracture in the gaskin area is suspected, a veterinarian should be called to confirm the nature and extent of the injury before action is taken.

Bone fragments from a chip fracture are often successfully removed by surgery. For other types of tibia fractures, very little can be done. In the case of deferred fractures or simple fractures, plaster casts have been tried with limited success. It is common for necrosis (death of the bone) to follow, along with other disorders such as sequestra (dead bone fragments) and osteomyelitis (inflammation of the bone marrow). Prognosis is very poor.

STIFLE

ANATOMY AND CONFORMATION

What is the stifle joint?

The stifle joint is a hinge joint in the horse corresponding to the human knee. It is the largest joint in the body and is composed of two separate articulations, the femoro-patellar and the femoro-tibial. The stifle joint is in the forward part of the junction of the hindleg and the rest of the body. It is the extension of this joint in a forward angle by the large muscles of the hindleg which actually propels the horse forward and promotes speed.

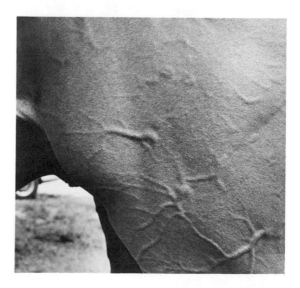

Fig. 11-1. View of the stifle.

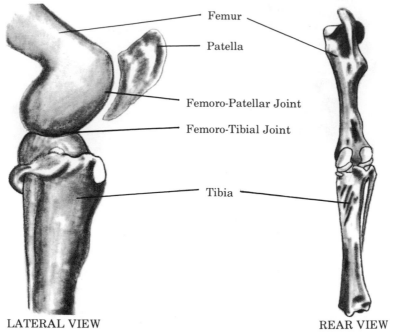

LATERAL VIEW   REAR VIEW

Fig. 11-2. Two separate views of the bones of the right stifle joint.

What is the structure of the stifle joint?

The stifle joint connects the lower end of the femur with the upper end of the tibia. There are two semilunar cartilages (menisci) which separate the ends of the femur and tibia and also help keep the joint in position and absorb shock.

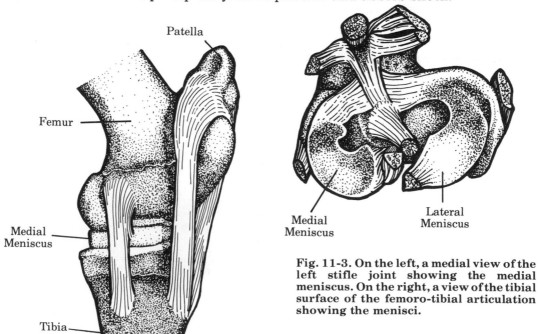

Fig. 11-3. On the left, a medial view of the left stifle joint showing the medial meniscus. On the right, a view of the tibial surface of the femoro-tibial articulation showing the menisci.

The patella (kneecap) rides on a "track-like" structure called the trochlea on the forward part of the large rounded lower end of the femur. It helps reduce friction and is involved in the transmission of extension power from the femur to the tibia.

How is the patella related to the femur and tibia?

The patella is connected to the femur by various ligaments and the quadriceps femoris. The quadriceps femoris is a large extensor muscle which runs along the front of the femur and is the major extensor of the stifle. The patella is connected to the tibia by the three patellar ligaments. The stifle is extended as the pull of the quadriceps reaches the patella, affecting the patellar ligaments and thus moving the tibia.

Are there any other ligaments involved in the stifle joint?

The stifle joint is held together by fourteen ligaments. Because of this, torn or strained ligaments are the chief cause of most stifle lamenesses. The stifle is surrounded, except in front, by heavy muscles. The efficiency of the joint is dependent on these muscles.

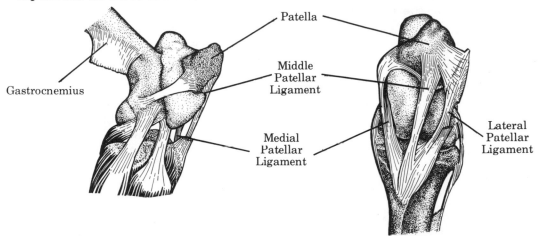

Fig. 11-4. Above, a lateral view of the right stifle joint showing the patellar ligaments.

Fig. 11-5. Front view of the patellar ligaments of the left stifle joint.

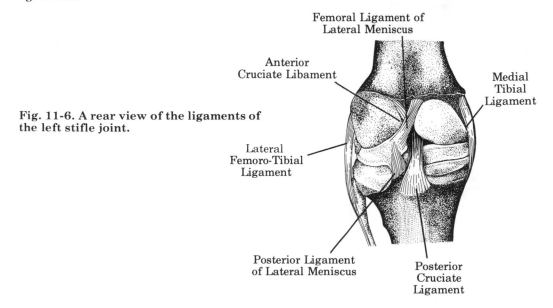

Fig. 11-6. A rear view of the ligaments of the left stifle joint.

Which are the flexors of the stifle joint?

The primary flexors of the stifle joint are the hamstring muscles which also extend the hip. They include the biceps femoris, the semitendinosus and the semimembranosus muscles. The gastrocnemius and the superficial digital flexor are muscles which originate on the back side of the lower femur and extend the hock and also help to flex the stifle. These two actions cannot happen simultaneously because of the dual action wherein the stifle joint and hock joint always move in unison, extending together and flexing together.

The popliteus is a small muscle behind the stifle which mainly helps flex but can also slightly rotate the tibia and fibula inward.

What is the function of the stifle joint?

The stifle joint is always in a semi-flexed position to aid in absorbing shock. This semi-flexed position can be seen from the outside as the patella points out against the skin. To make the limb rigid enough for standing, the muscles of the stifle joint which insert on the patella are the only ones that must contract. This is because of the dual action of the stifle and hock mentioned above.

As part of the overall movement of the limb, the stifle joint, as previously explained, always moves in conjunction with the hock joint. These two, however, are not directly related to the action of the fetlock and lower joints.

How should the stifle be positioned in the body?

The stifle should be in a well-forward position, giving a rectangular shape to the thigh from a side view. A stifle too far back is indicative of a short thigh and has a V-shape from a side view. Full muscling arching smoothly over the stifle area denotes strength and also gives a rectangular shape when viewed from the side or rear.

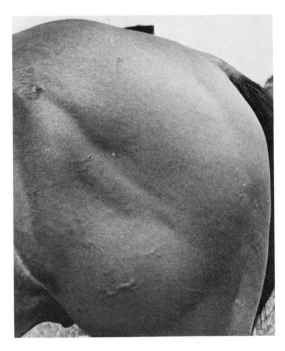

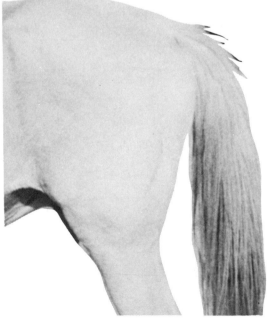

Fig. 11-7. A side view of the stifle in a well-forward position showing the rectangular shape of the thigh.

Fig. 11-8. A stifle that is too far back, showing a V-shaped thigh.

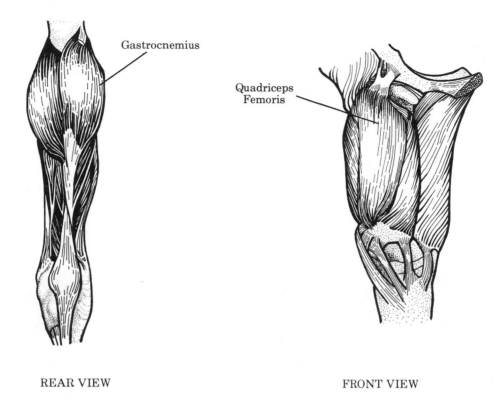

REAR VIEW   FRONT VIEW

Fig. 11-9A. Two views of the muscles of the stifle.

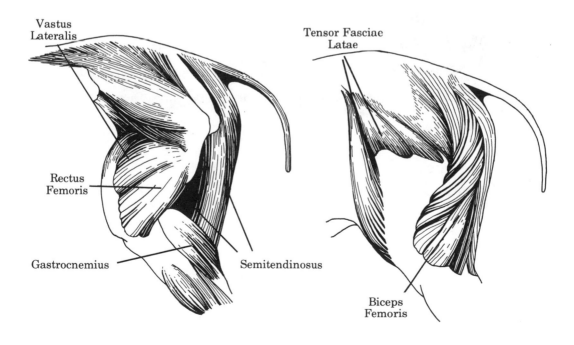

Fig. 11-9B. Two lateral views of the muscles of the hindquarters and stifle.

What are some conformation faults in the stifle area?

The term "straight behind" denotes excessively straight legs when viewed from the side. In this case there is very little angle between the tibia and femur. The hock joint and pastern are also straight. A horse with this defect is prone to bog spavin, upward fixation of the patella and is easily injured by heavy work.

"Standing under behind" describes a limb that is placed too far forward when viewed from the side. A plumb line from the hip joint would fall at the heel or behind the heel rather than halfway between the heel and the toe.

A limb that is placed too far back, when viewed from the side, is referred to as being "camped behind." A straight line drawn from the hip joint to the ground would hit at the toe or in front of it in this case.

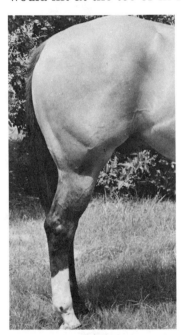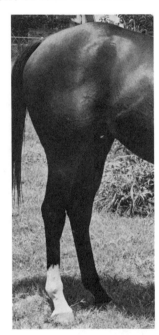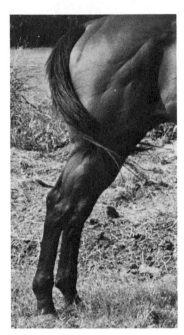

Fig. 11-10. Side views of conformation faults of the stifle area. A. "straight behind", B. "standing under behind", C. "camped behind".

GONITIS

What causes gonitis?

Gonitis is a very general term referring to inflammation of the stifle joint which may be acute or chronic. It is the result of a wide and complex range of causes that are frequently interrelated.

For instance, the most common cause of gonitis is chondromalacia of the patella (degeneration of the articular cartilage of the patella). (See Chondromalacia of the Patella, page 240.) This disorder results in gonitis as an inflammation of the synovial (lubricating) sac between the femur and the patella, called the femoropatellar pouch. Chondromalacia of the patella may be caused by trauma to the stifle joint, but is more often the result of pressure caused by upward fixation of the patella (kneecap). This may be accompanied by thickening of the synovium and roughening of the patella and medial trochlea (articulating surface) of the femur, which are other forms of gonitis.

Sprain or sprain fracture usually produces gonitis. The anterior cruciate ligament and the medial collateral ligament are most frequently damaged, and an injury to one of these often involves the other as well. The lateral collateral ligament and posterior cruciate ligament may also be damaged, but with less frequency. A complete rupture of the ligament generally causes complete osteoarthritis. Any degree of damage to the ligaments may be expected to cause damage to the menisci (cartilage of the stifle joint).

Inflammation of the menisci is yet another form of gonitis. It may result from damage to the ligaments, as mentioned, or it may be the result of osteochondritis dissecans. Most common in young horses (up to 3½ years), this ailment causes

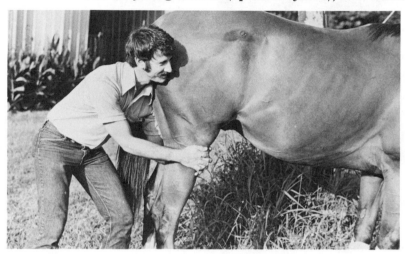

Fig. 11-11. Test for sprain of the anterior cruciate ligament. Hands and shoulder of veterinarian are placed as shown, then force is applied. Crepitation can be felt if the ligament is sprained.

lesions on the menisci, and small pieces of the menisci are torn off when the horse moves. Young horses, especially foals, are also susceptible to infectious arthritis resulting from septicemia. This in turn may bring on gonitis.

Rarely, the joint capsule may be injured and the fibrous portion partially torn from its attachment. This would also result in gonitis.

Finally, any type of fracture to the joint would cause gonitis, but this also is not a frequent occurrence. (See Fractures of the Stifle Joint, page 243.)

How is gonitis diagnosed?

Due to the complexity of gonitis, a thorough diagnosis should be made by a veterinarian.

The noticeable swelling in gonitis will cause the horse pain in movement, primarily in moving the limb forward. Consequently, the horse will normally not step fully forward with the affected limb. While standing, the stifle joint will be flexed either fully or partially, with the fetlock joint moved forward. The horse may swing the leg while standing or moving in order to keep from using the joint.

The affected joint is usually palpated to identify the area of involvement and checked for crepitation. If fracture is suspected, X-rays may be taken. If the condition is caused by arthritis, heat and temperature rise usually accompany the pain and swelling.

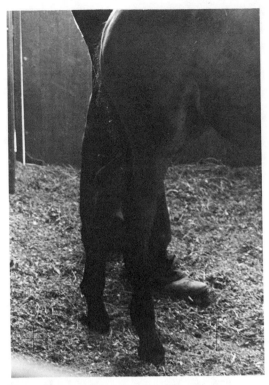

Fig. 11-12. Typical position of a horse with gonitis.

How is gonitis treated?

If the gonitis is due to chip fractures of the stifle, the chips may often be removed surgically with some degree of success. If a sprain to the joint capsule or ligaments is suspected, injection of the joint with a corticosteroid, followed by 30 days of stall rest may produce good results. In some cases, a sprain may be encouraged to heal by the application of a blister or by firing. This should never be done in conjunction with the injection of an anesthetic. If infection is involved, it may be necessary to administer antibiotics.

For any causes of gonitis other than chip fractures, the outcome is generally not favorable. Confinement and good nursing care may deter progression of the condition, but restoration of full use of the limb is unlikely. With osteoarthritis in particular, lameness may be predicted. The prognosis is poor.

UPWARD FIXATION OF THE PATELLA

What is upward fixation of the patella?

This condition is also called "stifling" and occurs when the stifle joint is fully extended. The patella becomes fixed on top of the medial ridge of the trochlea (track-like rounded projection on the lower end) of the femur and it is caught between the medial (inner) and middle patellar ligaments.

What causes the patella to become fixed in this position?

Trauma to the hindleg when the limb is overextended can cause upward fixation of the patella. Poor conformation, especially hindlegs that are too straight, is predisposing to this condition. Poor conditioning and loss of strength will also make a horse prone to upward fixation of the patella.

Once upward fixation of the patella has occurred, the ligaments are stretched and the horse will have a tendency toward recurrence of the problem.

What are the signs of upward fixation of the patella?

The stifle and hock joints will be locked in a fully extended position, unable to flex. The digital joints, however, will be able to flex, so the fetlock and front of the foot will rest on the ground. If the horse is forced to move forward, the front of the hoof will drag on the ground.

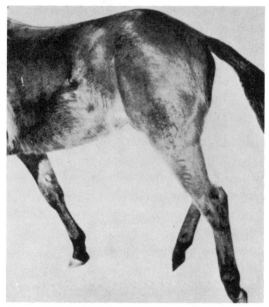

Fig. 11-13. Photograph of locked stifle. Notice that the stifle and hock joints are locked in a fully extended position.

Courtesy of LAMENESS IN HORSES, Edition III, O. R. Adams, Lea and Febiger Publishing Co., Philadelphia, Pa.

When the limb is locked in extension, palpation of the stifle by an experienced person will reveal that the patellar ligaments are tense, and the patella is locked above the medial ridge of the trochlea of the femur.

Upward fixation of the patella is somewhat erratic and may return to normal almost instantly or remain fixed for several hours or days. Sometimes there will be a momentary catching of the patella when the horse walks, which may be confused with stringhalt because there is a sudden upward jerking when the foot leaves the ground on its forward stride. This condition will be most noticeable when the horse is turned in a small circle or during the first few steps. Occasionally, the momentary catching is accompanied by a snapping sound each time the patella is released. To aid in diagnosis, the veterinarian may perform a test to determine if the horse is predisposed to upward fixation of the patella.

In some cases, upward fixation of the patella may occur simultaneously in both limbs. This is extremely painful for the horse and usually causes him to sweat and breathe rapidly because of the intense pain due to the weight on the affected legs. The horse will be unable to move.

How is upward fixation of the patella treated?

The treatment depends upon the severity and frequency of the occurrence of upward fixation of the patella. After considering the animal's history, the veterinarian will decide what type of treatment to use. An intimate knowledge of the anatomy of the stifle is needed to be able to correctly apply the mechanical forces necessary to remedy an upward fixation of the patella. The following practices should be employed by a veterinarian because he has the necessary familiarity with this joint for successful treatment.

The first time upward fixation of the patella occurs, the veterinarian may tranquilize the horse and attempt to replace the patella mechanically. He will fasten a rope below the fetlock and pull the leg forward. At the same time, pressure will be applied to the sides of the patella in an upward and outward direction to dislodge it. The stifle and hock joints will flex when the patella is returned to its normal position. In a small percentage of cases, forcing the horse to make a sudden movement, or back quickly, may force the patella to slip back into place.

In rare situations the horse may have to be given a general anesthetic to thoroughly relax the muscles and allow replacement of the patella.

The veterinarian will probably use a surgical procedure for repeated upward fixation of the patella. This operation is called a medial patellar desmotomy and means a "cutting of the medial patellar ligament." Since the medial patellar ligament is responsible for holding the patella in an upward position, severing the ligament will make the fixation mechanically impossible. It might seem that the severing of this ligament would impair normal function of the stifle, but horses do very well even in strenuous work after this type of surgery.

What is the prognosis for upward fixation of the patella?

The prognosis is good for this disorder since surgery can correct most cases. However, there is the possibility of arthritis of the stifle joint in longstanding cases which may result in persistent lameness, even after surgery.

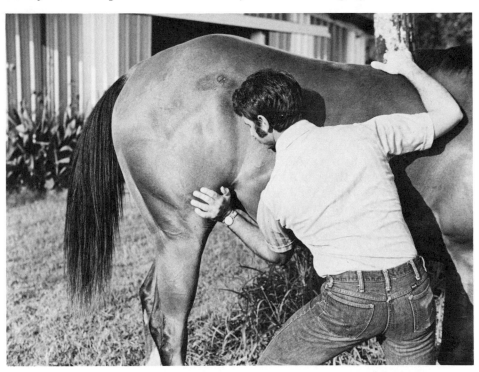

Fig. 11-14. The veterinarian attempting to free the patella.

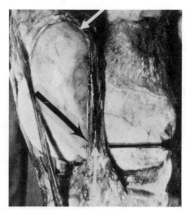

Fig. 11-15. Upward fixation of the patella. The lower arrow shows the approximate site for cutting the medial patellar ligament. The arrow above shows how the medial patellar ligament locks over the medial trochlea of the femur. The view is of the medial aspect of the left hind limb, and to reproduce locking, the patella must be pushed upward and laterally.

Courtesy of LAMENESS IN HORSES, Edition III, O. R. Adams, Lea and Febiger Publishing Co., Philadelphia, Pa.

LUXATION OF THE STIFLE JOINT

Can the stifle joint become dislocated?

Yes. A dislocation of the stifle joint is called a "luxation." This condition is rare because of the strong ligaments that support the stifle joint.

What happens to the joint when it becomes luxated?

Luxation of a joint means that it is out of normal position. This condition nearly always involves tearing or stretching of the ligaments. In severe cases, one of the bones forming the joint may push through the joint capsule. It comes to rest in the surrounding tissue where it is fixed by muscle spasm. The degree of dislocation and damage to the tissues depends on the severity of the injury. Severe violence to the joint may produce a compound dislocation in which the end of the bone may be forced through the skin. Exostosis (new bone growth on the affected surfaces) may result in many cases of luxation.

Is a luxation of the stifle joint easily detected?

The abnormal bone placement is obvious upon observation and examination. Not only the joint, but the whole limb, is deformed, resulting in lameness. The horse's gait may appear to improve during exercise, but will be much worse after "cooling down." Movement will probably be accompanied by crepitation, a dull clicking sound or grinding feeling noticed if the stifle is palpated as it moves.

What can result from a luxation of the stifle joint?

Since a dislocation may fix in a certain position, unlike a fracture, which would still allow free movement of the limb, a false joint may develop. A false joint is a joint out of place which becomes fairly functional due to the fibrous connective tissue which grows around the end of the bone and permits movement. No joint capsule or cartilage, however, will develop in a false joint as it will in a true joint There may be a shortening or lengthening of the limb.

How can luxation of the stifle joint be treated?

Treatment consists of putting the joint back into its normal position. Unless the horse is completely anesthetized by the veterinarian to relax all the muscles, replacement of the joint will be very difficult.

It is very important that the horse be treated as soon as the injury is discovered to prevent the joint capsule from filling with connective tissue.

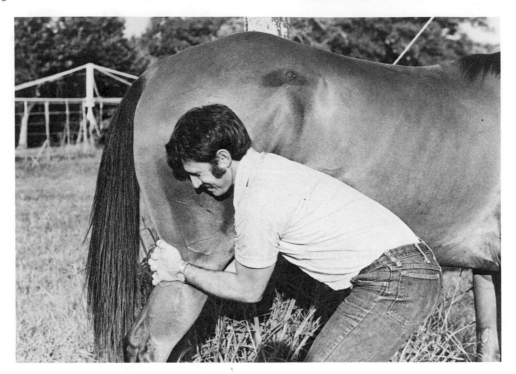

Fig. 11-16. Test for luxation of the stifle joint. Basically same procedure as test for anterior cruciate ligament rupture. (See Fig. 11-11, p. 235.)

What is the prognosis in the case of stifle joint luxation?

Recovery from luxation will not be complete or quick because of the extensive stretching and tearing of ligaments. The scar tissue which will form in the healing process would inhibit normal joint movement. However, if the horse is given sufficient rest, a return to near normal is possible.

CHONDROMALACIA OF THE PATELLA

What is chondromalacia of the patella?

Chondromalacia is a degeneration of the articular cartilage of the patella which may result from an inflammatory disease of the stifle joint. The condition may also be involved in inflammation and upward fixation of the patella.

What causes chondromalacia of the patella?

The most frequent cause of chondromalacia of the patella is the pressure produced between the patella and the medial trochlea of the femur. Caused by a partial fixation of the patella between the medial and middle patellar ligaments, the pressure results in erosions in the surface of the cartilage. Tears in the anterior cruciate or medial collateral ligaments of the joint can produce inflammation resulting in chondromalacia, in addition to inflammation from traumatic injuries to the joint.

What are the signs of chondromalacia?

The primary signs of chondromalacia are gonitis (inflammation of the stifle joint) and stifle lameness. Lameness is usually mild which may make it difficult to diagnose. Some horses will show a mild reaction to the spavin test because of the arthritis and may elevate the hip at the trot as in hock or stifle lameness. Most commonly, the flexion of stifle and hock will be reduced, the anterior (reaching-out) phase of the stride will be shortened, and the toe may be dragged as the horse moves. It is possible for chondromalacia to occur in both hindlimbs at once. When the patella is pressed upward and outward with the limb in an extended position, the joint may partially lock or there may be a soft tissue crepitation (crackling sound) between the patella and the medial femoral condyle. Crepitation is an indication of an inflammatory reaction and is considered to be a positive sign of chondromalacia.

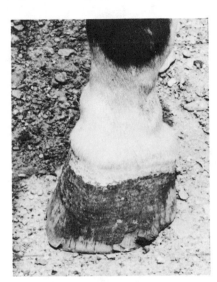

Fig. 11-17. View of the hind foot of a horse with chondromalacia of the patella. Notice how the toe of the hoof is dubbed off due to the foot being dragged as the horse moves.

How is this disorder treated?

Treatment of chondromalacia of the patella involves reducing the inflammation and removing its cause. Temporarily, injection of the femoropatellar pouch with corticosteroids will reduce the inflammation and prevent further deterioration. Pressure on the patella is relieved by severing the medial patellar ligament (as for upward fixation of the patella). At least six months are required for regeneration of the articular cartilage and relief of symptoms. If the degeneration of the articular cartilage is very advanced, regeneration may not occur and the horse may not return to soundness. However, if signs of chondromalacia are relieved within six months, the horse may remain sound.

OSTEOCHONDROSIS (BONE-CARTILAGE DISEASE) OF THE TIBIAL TUBEROSITY

What is osteochondrosis of the tibial tuberosity?

Osteochondrosis of the tibial tuberosity is a disease of the growth center (epiphysis) of the tibia. In true osteochondrosis, trauma causes death of tissue in the tibial crest followed by regeneration or recalcification of the tissue. This will make the epiphyseal line more irregular than normal, giving the appearance of great separation from the rest of the bone. The tibial crest is vulnerable to this type of injury until the young horse is three years old and the epiphyses have closed.

What causes osteochondrosis of the tibia?

The cause of osteochondrosis of the tibia is thought to be trauma to the tibial crest from tension on the patellar ligaments. If heavy training of the young horse

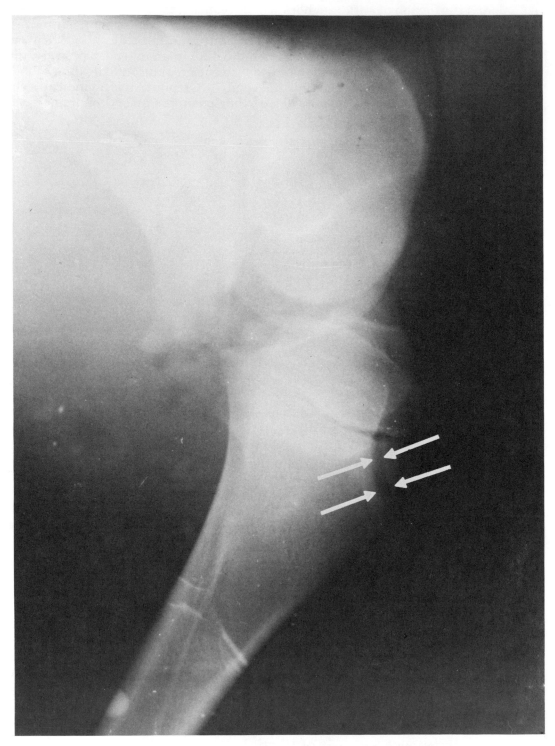

Fig. 11-18. X-ray of the stifle joint showing osteochondrosis of the tibial tuberosity. Arrows indicate the irregular epiphyseal line, causing a portion of the tibial crest to appear to be separated from the rest of the bone.

stresses these ligaments at their insertion on the tibial crest, disturbance of the epiphyses results. Partial upward fixation of the patella can cause similar signs which must be diagnosed by a veterinarian.

What are the signs of osteochondrosis?

The signs of osteochondrosis are not highly specific, which calls for careful diagnosis by the consulting veterinarian. In addition to pain, swelling and tenderness in the stifle region following exercise, the horse will trot with a short stride. The lesion may appear in both legs or only one limb may be involved. Lack of movement and a low arc of the foot in flight may cause the toe of an affected hoof to be rounded off by dragging or scuffing of the foot.

What is the treatment for osteochondrosis?

In any treatment chosen by the veterinarian for osteochondrosis, complete stall rest is essential. A minimum of three months is required and more may be prescribed if avulsion of the tibial crest appears possible. Corticoids and analgesics have not been effective in treating this condition. The most successful treatment is thought to be drilling of the tibial crest to produce inflammation (an effective treatment with humans). In some cases, subcutaneous injection of Lugol's iodine over the stifle area has seemed to hasten recovery.

FRACTURE OF THE STIFLE JOINT

What causes fractures of the stifle joint?

Different parts of the stifle joint are fractured in different ways. The patella, for instance, is mobile and cannot be fractured except by great force. Such injuries happen occasionally at racetracks where ordinary field-type rails are used, and the horse's leg hits the upright post at great speed. A kick from another horse may also cause this fracture. Whatever the cause, the damaging blow usually fractures the end of the femur as well.

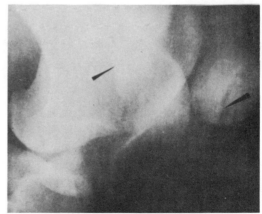

Fig. 11-19. Fracture of the patella. Severe trauma to the stifle joint accompanied by fractures can cause gonitis. In this case there was a fracture of the patella as shown by pointer and a fracture of one of the femoral trochlea indicated by the second pointer. Trauma to the anterior portion of the stifle causes this type of lesion.

Courtesy of LAMENESS IN HORSES, Edition III, O. R. Adams, Lea and Febiger Publishing Co., Philadelphia, Pa.

Fractures of one or both of the menisci (large halfmoon-shaped cartilages) are generally the result of crushing or twisting of the limb, and are usually accompanied by luxation (joint dislocation). Injuries to the articulating (joint surface) portions of the femur and tibia themselves are most frequent among colts. In fact, blows to these areas of the colt's body are more likely to fracture the joint than the shaft of the bone. Finally, the tibial spine, a small ridge on the end of the tibia and inside the stifle joint, may also be broken by crushing or twisting.

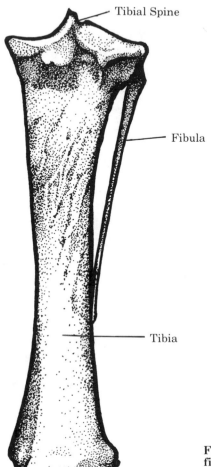

Tibial Spine

Fibula

Tibia

Fig. 11-20.

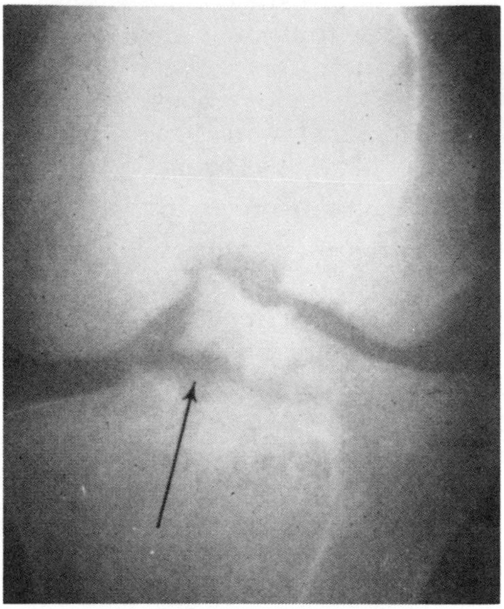

Courtesy of LAMENESS IN HORSES, Edition III, O. R. Adams, Lea and Febiger Publishing Co., Philadelphia, Pa.

Fig. 11-21. X-ray of fracture of the tibial spine.

Fig. 11-20. Rear view of the right tibia and fibula showing the location of the tibial spine.

How are stifle joint fractures diagnosed?

Attention may be first brought to a stifle joint fracture when the horse refuses to put weight on the leg, and shows evidence of pain. Swelling usually occurs shortly after the area is injured. An attempt to move the joint will probably produce crepitation (grinding sound). However, the exact location and extent of the fracture can only be determined by X-ray.

How are stifle joint fractures treated?

Treatment of stifle joint fracture is extremely difficult and generally meets with limited success. A fractured patella may sometimes be reunited with stainless steel screws or wire sutures, provided that it has fractured into only two or three pieces. Other stifle joint fractures have limited alternatives for treatment, and the horse is usually simply confined to prevent excess movement.

What are the effects of stifle joint fracture?

Stifle joint fractures of any nature frequently lead to other serious conditions, such as chondromalacia (cartilage degeneration), gonitis, immobility of the joints or atrophy (disuse degeneration) of the muscles. (See Chondromalacia, page 240, and Gonitis, page 234.)

When the tibia or femur is the site of the fracture, the bone often heals in a position overriding the joint, forming what is called a false joint. Even if the break was not originally compound, it may become so if the horse attempts to put weight on the leg.

12

SHOULDER

ANATOMY AND CONFORMATION

What is the structure of the shoulder joint?

The shoulder joint is an enarthrodial (ball and socket) joint. This type of joint allows movements in nearly all directions because a "ball-shaped" end of one bone fits into a round depression in another bone, forming a joint. A ball and socket joint is capable, to a limited degree, of the following movements: flexion; extension; rotation; abduction (move outward); adduction (move inward); and circumduction (move in a circle).

Which bones make up the shoulder joint?

Because it is formed by the scapula and the humerus, the shoulder joint is also called the scapulo-humeral joint. The humerus is the long bone in the upper forearm. Its lower end forms the elbow joint with the radius and ulna. The upper end of the humerus is spherical (the "ball" section of the joint) and forms the shoulder joint with the scapula. The protrusion produced by this upper end of the humerus is called the point of the shoulder. Also, the upper end of the humerus has many tuberosities (small, irregular protuberances) that serve as sites for the attachment of several strong muscles which function to move the front leg in locomotion.

The scapula (shoulder blade) is a flat, triangular-shaped bone. In its lower end is a cup-shaped hole (the glenoid cavity) into which the upper end of the humerus fits, forming the shoulder joint.

The lateral (outer) side of the scapula has a ridge, called the spine, extending from the top (vertebral border) to the lower edge of the bone, stopping short of the glenoid cavity. On each side of the spine is a fossa (hollow, depressed area). The upper front fossa is called the supraspinous fossa, and the lower rear is called the

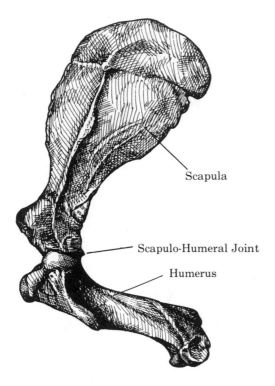

Scapula

Fig. 12-1. Lateral view of the bones of the shoulder joint.

Scapulo-Humeral Joint

Humerus

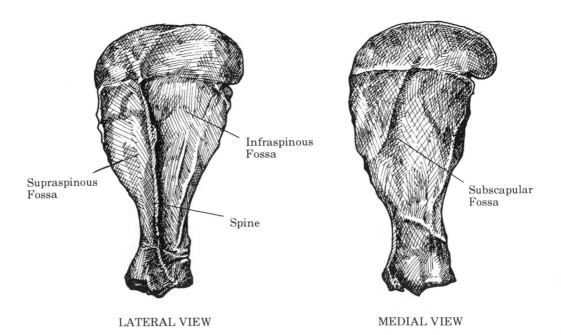

Supraspinous
Fossa

Infraspinous
Fossa

Spine

Subscapular
Fossa

LATERAL VIEW   MEDIAL VIEW

Fig. 12-2. Lateral and medial views of the scapula.

infraspinous fossa. There is also a large depression (subscapular fossa) on the medial (inner) side of the scapula. Most of the muscles which attach the front limb to the body attach to this underside of the scapula.

A large, extensive joint capsule encloses the shoulder joint. The ligaments which bind the joint together are weak and poorly developed, so some of the muscles surrounding the shoulder joint function as ligaments. Because muscles are more flexible than ligaments, this gives a greater range of movement to the joint. However, the heavy muscular arrangement in this particular area also partially limits joint action, making flexion and extension the chief movements of the shoulder joint.

Which muscles "work" the shoulder joint?

There are many strong muscles that function to move the shoulder joint. Each will be listed and explained separately.

Brachiocephalicus Muscle (brachio-arm/cephalicus-head)—This is a heavy, strong muscle which extends from the upper arm to the head. It begins at the point where the skull meets the spine and its lower end attaches to the lower front of the humerus. The brachiocephalicus muscle covers the front of the point of the shoulder and works to pull the shoulder forward and also raise the shoulder.

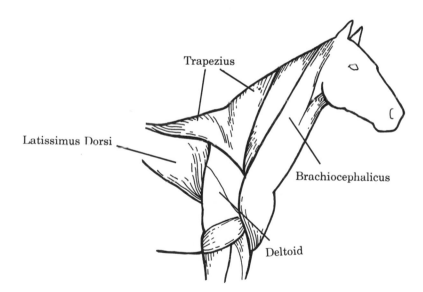

Fig. 12-3. Superficial muscles of the shoulder area.

Supraspinatus Muscle—This muscle works to extend the shoulder, but also functions as a ligament to strengthen and support the joint. This muscle attaches on the supraspinous fossa of the scapula and extends to the upper end of the humerus. The supraspinatus is one of the muscles that atrophies (shrinks) when a horse is afflicted with Sweeney (see page 253).

Infraspinatus Muscle—The infraspinatus muscle originates on the infraspinous fossa of the scapula and extends to the upper end of the humerus. It acts as a ligament of the shoulder and also works to abduct (move outward away from the center line) and flex the shoulder joint. (Sweeney also affects this muscle.)

Latissimus Dorsi—This is a strong, wide, triangular-shaped flexor muscle which works to pull the front limb backward (or the body forward if the foreleg is placed on the ground). The latissimus dorsi muscle is attached to that part of the spine which forms the back and loin by the lumbodorsal fascia (a wide aponeurosis, or band of tissue, that connects a muscle to a part it moves). The muscle narrows as it extends from this expansive attachment to the middle of the humerus, where it also attaches.

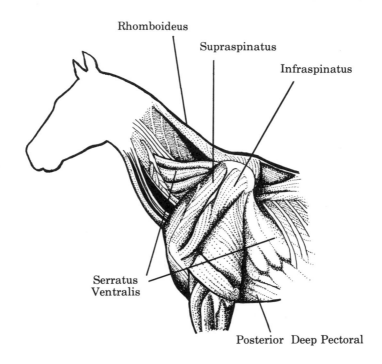

Fig. 12-4. Deeper muscles of the shoulder area.

Teres Major—This muscle is a flexor of the shoulder joint and extends from the lower edge of the scapula to the middle of the humerus on its inner surface.

Pectoral Muscles—These are large muscles that make up the substance of the chest, forming the inverted "V" of the breast. These extensive muscles attach along the length of the sternum (breastbone) and narrow as they attach to the upper part of the humerus. The function of the pectoral muscles is adduction (move inward toward the center line) of the forelimb. They also work to advance the body when the limb is placed on the ground. (These muscles are divided, named and identified separately in detailed anatomy studies as the superficial pectoral muscles and the deep pectoral muscles.)

Deltoid Muscle—This is a strong, important muscle which serves to flex and abduct the shoulder joint. It extends from the spine of the scapula to the deltoid tuberosity (projection on the outside of the shaft) of the humerus. As the name implies, the deltoid muscle is somewhat triangular in shape.

Coraco-Brachialis Muscle—The main function of this small muscle is to hold the joint together. The coraco-brachialis extends from the coracoid process (a small projection) on the lower end of the scapula to the inner side of the shaft of the humerus.

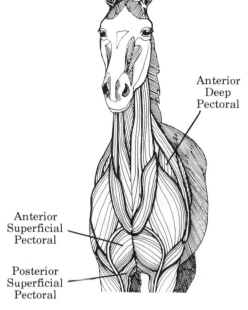

Fig. 12-5. Front view of the pectoral muscles.

Anterior Deep Pectoral

Anterior Superficial Pectoral

Posterior Superficial Pectoral

How is the shoulder attached to the body?

There is a group of large muscles which forms the shoulder (or pectoral) girdle. This group of muscles encircles the chest region to attach and support the front limbs.

In the horse there is no bony attachment (joint) of the scapula to the trunk of the body, so these muscles are extremely important and strong. Aside from holding the scapula in place, the muscles of the shoulder girdle also aid in its movement. They work together to move the scapula and hold it against the body.

The trapezius, rhomboideus and serratus ventralis muscles make up the shoulder girdle. All of these muscles are fan-shaped and layered, with the trapezius being outermost and the serratus ventralis being innermost.

The trapezius muscle attaches along the area of the spine from the head to just behind the withers. The muscle narrows as it extends to attach to the spine of the scapula. The trapezius is instrumental in holding the scapula in place against the body.

The rhomboideus muscle lies under the trapezius and attaches in the same region along the spine. From the spine, the rhomboideus extends to the inner side of the scapula.

The largest muscle in this group is the serratus ventralis. This muscle fans outward and downward from its attachment at the top underside of the scapula, ending in a curved line along the cervical vertebrae (neck) and ribs to behind the elbow. Together the serratus ventralis muscles on each side of the horse form a sling to support the trunk of the body between the front legs. They also work to swing the scapula forward and backward.

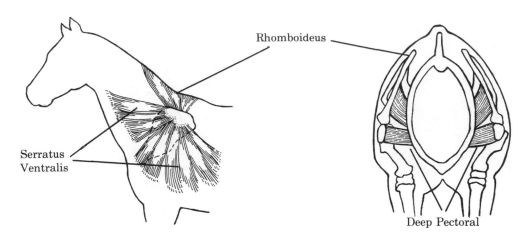

Fig. 12-6. Side view of the muscles attaching the shoulder to the body. The trapezius (not shown) lies on top of the rhomboideus.

Fig. 12-7. Front view of a cross-section of the chest showing how the shoulder is attached to the body.

What characteristics make up good conformation of the shoulder?

"Ideal" conformation for the shoulder varies to a large extent, depending upon the breed of the horse and what the horse is expected to do. However, there are certain characteristics desirable in all situations. Well developed, symmetrical muscling of the shoulder region, best fitting the purpose of the individual horse, is important.

The shoulder should be angled in relation to the front leg and entire body, although the exact degree of angulation varies. The angle of the shoulder is determined by the spine of the scapula—not a line between the point of the withers and the point of the shoulder.

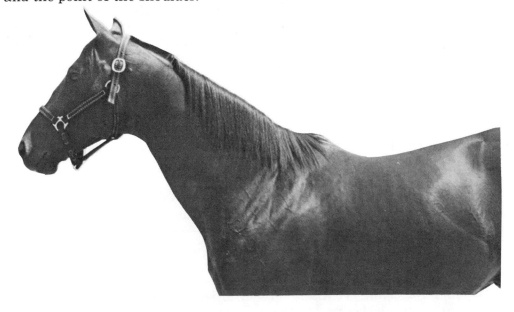

Fig. 12-8. Example of good shoulder muscling and a good shoulder angle.

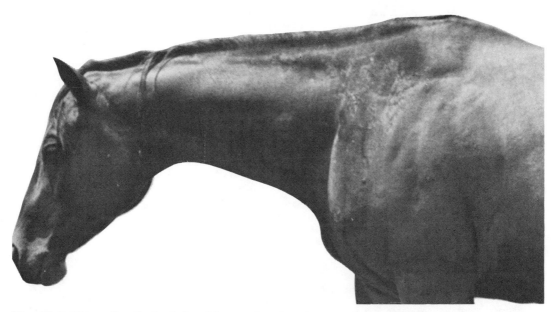

Fig. 12-9. Example of a bad shoulder angle, showing a straight shoulder.

Sloping shoulders (the angle between the scapula and the humerus) aids in decreasing concussion, supports weight and permits the foreleg to extend farther.

The scapula and humerus should be relatively long, yet in proportion with the entire body of the horse. Adequate length of the scapula provides room for the numerous attachments of large muscles at this location. The humerus is heavily muscled, and serves as a lever for the muscles attaching here. Because the humerus serves as a lever of attachment for these muscles, ample length will add power to the action of the muscles. A long humerus also increases the range of movement of the entire foreleg, but should be in balance with the scapula and entire body.

SWEENEY

What is sweeney?

Sweeney is an atrophy (shrinkage) of the supraspinatus and infraspinatus muscles in the shoulder of the horse. Other names for sweeney are slipped shoulder, shoulder atrophy and suprascapular nerve paralysis.

What causes these muscles to shrink?

The suprascapular nerve supplies the supraspinatus and infraspinatus muscles, and loss of nerve supply will cause these muscles to atrophy. Nerve supply to the muscles is lost when the suprascapular nerve is injured. Because of its location, this nerve is prone to injury. The suprascapular nerve runs around the front border of the scapula at the point of the shoulder.

Direct trauma to the point of the shoulder can easily injure the suprascapular nerve. Blows to the point of the shoulder, pressure from the harness collar used in draft horses, and extreme backward motion of the shoulder which stretches the nerve too much, are examples of trauma which can injure the suprascapular nerve. The severity of the nerve injury can vary from minor bruising of the nerve, resulting in temporary paralysis, to complete severing of the nerve.

Another cause of atrophy of the supraspinatus and infraspinatus muscles is disuse of the muscles. In this case there is no nerve injury, but there is usually a foot or leg lameness severe enough to cause the horse not to use the limb for an extended period of time. The muscles will atrophy if they are not used for a long period.

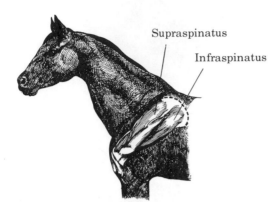

Supraspinatus

Infraspinatus

Fig. 12-10. Diagram showing the muscles involved in sweeney.

What are the signs of sweeney?

Sweeney may be difficult to detect in the early stages before atrophy progresses to a recognizable stage, especially if there is no sign of injury. The horse may have difficulty extending the affected shoulder. Also, the shoulder may suddenly move outward when weight is placed on the limb. In many cases, instead of using normal action the horse may swing the affected leg out and around when moving forward.

In more advanced cases, when the atrophy has begun, sweeney is easy to recognize. The shoulder joint will be more prominent and the shoulder area will appear flattened. In fact, there will be obvious hollow places on each side of the spine of the scapula, making the scapular spine prominent and readily noticeable.

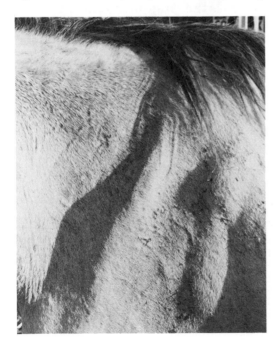

Fig. 12-11. View of a horse with sweeney.

The supraspinatus and infraspinatus muscles are responsible for most of the lateral support of the shoulder, so when the muscles atrophy, the joint becomes loose and wobbly. Occasionally there will be almost no change in action although the function of the muscles is lost.

A veterinarian should be consulted because even though advanced sweeney is easy to recognize, early sweeney is not and it may be difficult to determine whether the lameness is indeed sweeney or some other problem.

How is sweeney treated?

Before the veterinarian can treat this disorder, the cause must be determined. If the atrophy is the result of disuse of the muscles, the lesion causing failure to use the limb will have to be treated and removed.

For sweeney due to nerve injuries, treatment may be unrewarding because there is no known treatment for nerve injuries. Any apparent injury should be treated to reduce the inflammation. Liniments and massage are used frequently, but often there is no benefit. As a general rule the veterinarian will recommend that the horse be rested.

It is a common practice to inject counterirritants under the skin of the affected shoulder. This treatment produces scar tissue to fill out the shoulder and improve the appearance of the horse. This treatment is for cosmetic reasons only and will not aid in restoring the function of the muscles.

What is the prognosis for sweeney?

For cases of sweeney caused by failure to use the limb, the prognosis is entirely dependent upon the correction of the primary factor resulting in the disuse of the limb. The veterinarian will be able to advise in each individual case. If the sweeney is secondary, the muscles will regenerate to normal size after the horse begins to use them again.

When sweeney is the result of a suprascapular nerve injury, the prognosis depends upon the extent of the injury and the length of time that the paralysis has existed. For mild cases in which the nerve was merely bruised, the horse may recover in one to two months. However, the prognosis is guarded to unfavorable in most cases. If the suprascapular nerve has been completely severed, the injury will most likely be permanent, because the nerve has almost no ability to regenerate.

BICIPITAL BURSITIS

What is bicipital bursitis?

This is an inflammation of the bicipital bursa which lies under the biceps brachii muscle at the point of the shoulder. (See Flexors of the Elbow, page 183.) As previously explained, a bursa is a small sac of synovial fluid which acts as a "pad" between two structures that rub against each other during normal motion. The bicipital bursa is located in the groove at the upper end of the humerus and serves to cushion the sliding of the biceps brachii over the end of the bone.

As with any inflammation, bicipital bursitis can be either acute or chronic. Intertubercularis bursitis is another name for bicipital bursitis. This is the same type of bursitis that affects humans in the shoulder region.

What causes bicipital bursitis?

There are several factors which can cause the onset of bicipital bursitis. Severe trauma at the point of the shoulder, lacerations which pierce the bursa inviting infection, and strain of the biceps brachii can all cause bicipital bursitis. This condition has also been known to occur as a consequence of chronic navicular disease. General infections which may localize in joints (such as navel ill, influenza, respiratory infections, etc.) can be responsible for the development of bicipital bursitis. (The bursa becomes inflamed and sore due to an internal disease.)

What are the signs of bicipital bursitis?

When the inflammation is acute, direct pressure over the point of the shoulder will cause pain. The degree of the lameness varies greatly with the severity and extent of the inflammation. The "shoulder lameness" may consist of only slight stumbling, shortened stride, reluctance to bear weight on the leg and dragging the toe. In some cases, the horse may swing the leg out and around when in motion, instead of flexing the shoulder joint to advance the leg forward. Other cases may exhibit a more restricted movement of the shoulder joint when the horse is in motion.

Acute bicipital bursitis produces a more specific type of lameness. The main sign appears when the horse is moving forward. Instead of advancing the affected leg in a normal manner, the horse will carry it while making a short jump forward on the sound leg. However, the horse may use the leg almost normally when backing. The affected leg is usually positioned farther back than normal and rested on the toe when the horse is standing. Also it will be painful to the horse when the leg is pulled up and backward.

Bicipital bursitis occurring as a sequel to navicular disease will naturally exhibit signs very similar to navicular disease. (See Navicular Disease, page 69.) However, the horse will also be sensitive to pressure over the point of the shoulder; thus, anesthetizing the posterior digital nerves as a diagnostic aid will not result in a marked temporary reduction of lameness. The veterinarian may anesthetize the bicipital bursa to confirm his diagnosis.

Whatever the degree of inflammation, a veterinarian should be called to ascertain that the horse is suffering from bicipital bursitis. This is especially important because shoulder lamenesses are difficult to diagnose. Often a "shoulder lameness" is blamed when the seat of lameness is really somewhere else such as lower in the same leg or possibly in the opposite hind limb.

How is bicipital bursitis treated?

The veterinarian will select and administer treatment best fitting the individual case. For mild cases he may recommend cold water bandages for several weeks, followed by liniment and massage. It is a common practice to inject the inflamed area with corticosteroids. This treatment is often repeated at monthly intervals. Counterirritation, such as firing and blistering internally, is frequently used. In some cases, the veterinarian may use radiation therapy.

All situations require that the horse be rested until after all the signs of lameness have subsided. Longstanding cases, however, may not respond to treatment because of other complicating factors such as navicular disease, arthritis of the shoulder joint, etc.

What is the prognosis for bicipital bursitis?

Acute cases, especially when treated early, respond best to treatment. Bicipital bursitis, which is either chronic or secondary to another condition (disease, for example), has a guarded to unfavorable prognosis. Because permanent changes may have taken place, bicipital bursitis that was chronic before veterinary treatment was sought has a strictly unfavorable prognosis, due to the probability of development of permanent adhesions of scar tissue or pathological new bone growth.

ARTHRITIS OF THE SHOULDER JOINT

What is arthritis?

Arthritis is an inflammation of the structures of a joint. Any or all of the joint structures can be involved in the inflammatory process. This includes the bones, joint cartilage, joint capsule and associated ligaments. Therefore, arthritis may consist of changes in the joint capsule and bony changes of the joint surfaces.

Arthritis will be either an acute or chronic inflammation. Acute arthritis consists of a relatively new, severe inflammation in the joint, while chronic arthritis consists of a mild to severe inflammation in the joint lasting over a long period of time.

How is arthritis of the shoulder joint caused?

Trauma to the point of the shoulder is nearly always the cause of arthritis of the shoulder joint (omarthritis). Examples of trauma which may bring about this condition are falls, kicks, fractures and puncture wounds involving the point of the shoulder. Bacterial infections of the joint can also cause arthritis to develop.

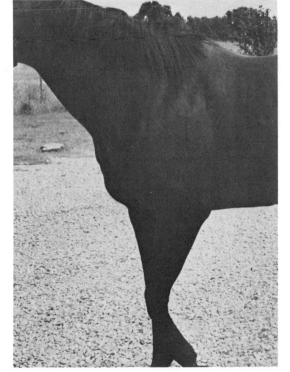

Fig. 12-12. Standing pose typical of lameness due to arthritis of the shoulder joint.

What are the signs of arthritis of the shoulder joint?

The signs can appear in a number of different forms and are not necessarily consistent. The services of a veterinarian are definitely needed to diagnose this disease. For example, lameness may be either severe or mild in either early or longstanding cases, depending upon the amount of pain the disease causes.

Ordinarily, when lameness is mild, the horse will swing the affected leg out and around when advancing it, instead of flexing the shoulder to move the leg normally. In more severe cases the horse will also exhibit a reluctance to bear weight on the leg when standing. In either case, the stride of the horse will probably be shortened. Forced extension of the foreleg, which pulls the shoulder forward, will frequently cause pain.

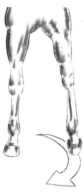

Fig. 12-13. Diagrammatic representation of the type of lameness associated with arthritis of the shoulder joint. The horse swings the leg out and around instead of flexing the shoulder as he moves.

The veterinarian may use nerve blocks and X-rays to aid in establishing a conclusive diagnosis.

How is arthritis of the shoulder joint treated?

There is no successful cure for arthritis of the shoulder joint. Treatment may be totally ineffective if joint damage has already taken place. However, veterinarians commonly treat omarthritis with intra-articular injections of corticosteroids and phenylbutazone to temporarily relieve the pain. Also, in acute cases, counter-irritants may be injected around the joint, but response to this therapy is erratic. If the X-rays reveal a chip fracture at the edge of the joint, surgical removal can meet with success in curing the shoulder lameness.

RUPTURE OF SERRATUS VENTRALIS MUSCLES

Because of the important demand made upon the serratus ventralis muscles, are they prone to rupture?

No. This condition is quite rare in horses, but it can occur. As explained in the "Anatomy and Conformation of the Shoulder" section, these paired, fan-shaped muscles are very extensive and are responsible for supporting the trunk of the body between the front legs. Together the serratus ventralis muscles on each side of the body form a sling for the trunk. (Refer to Anatomy of the Shoulder, page 251.)

What causes these muscles to rupture?

Extremely severe trauma to the area of attachment of these muscles (top underside of the scapula) is the only cause. An example is a heavy blow to the region of the neck and withers.

What are the signs of this rupture?

Because the serratus ventralis muscles support it, the trunk will sink between the shoulders following rupture of these muscles. In addition, the withers will be lower than the croup and the upper edges of the scapula will be above the vertebral column (backbone). This condition is extremely painful and a veterinarian should be called as soon as possible following the injury.

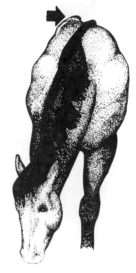

Fig. 12-14. Appearance of a horse with a rupture of a serratus ventralis muscle. Notice how the trunk sinks down between the shoulders, and the upper edge of the scapula (arrow) is above the backbone.

How is rupture of the serratus ventralis muscles treated?

For humanitarian as well as economic reasons, an initial decision should be made regarding whether or not to treat the horse at all.

If treatment is initiated, the veterinarian will immobilize the horse, using a sling to support the weight of the trunk of the body. Anti-inflammatory drugs may also be used. Because this type of injury is so extensive and severe, in most cases the horse never entirely recovers. Even after an extended rest period the withers will remain in a lower than normal position.

LUXATION OF THE SHOULDER JOINT

Can the shoulder joint be dislocated?

Yes, but it is quite uncommon in horses. The shoulder joint can be dislocated by a hard fall on the point of the shoulder area, trauma, or by excessive flexion of the shoulder and elbow joint which pushes the head of the humerus forward and upward out of the socket in the scapula (glenoid cavity).

How can a shoulder luxation be diagnosed?

The outward signs will be obvious in that the shoulder joint will be grossly misshapen and the horse will not try to support any weight at all on the affected leg. The veterinarian will probably X-ray the joint to be sure that no fracture is present.

If there is no fracture present, how will the dislocation be reduced (put back into place)?

Because of the large structures involved, the veterinarian will need to cast the horse and possibly use general anesthesia for muscle relaxation to effect reduction.

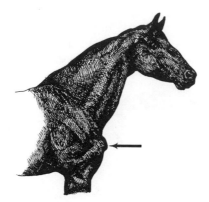

Fig. 12-15. Luxation of the shoulder joint. Arrow indicates the protruding head of the humerus.

What would the prognosis be for recovery from a shoulder luxation?

If it is properly diagnosed and promptly and correctly reduced, the chance of full recovery is good.

FRACTURE OF THE SCAPULA (SHOULDER BLADE)

What causes fracture of the scapula?

Only two areas of the scapula lack the protection of heavy muscle, and they usually receive the damaging blow. The first is the spine of the scapula, which is the prominent ridge dividing the lateral surface of the bone. The tuber spinae, where the trapezius muscle is attached, is the high point of the spine and very close to the surface of the skin. It may generally only be broken, though, by a direct blow. This usually results in a fracture of the scapular spine itself.

The second frequent site of injury is the coracoid process. This is the part of the bone which is farthest forward, located slightly back from the point of the shoulder. It is most frequently damaged when the horse is caught in a doorway or gateway. In a young horse, the resulting injury is usually fracture of the coracoid process itself. An older animal is more likely to fracture the neck, which is the narrowest portion of the body of the scapula.

How is fracture of the scapula diagnosed?

The most immediate signs of scapula fracture are refusal of the horse to bear weight on the limb, evidence of pain, and swelling in the area of the shoulder. These signs indicate the need to immediately consult a veterinarian in order to determine the extent of the injury.

A simple fracture of the spine of the scapula will yield very few signs other than those mentioned. Confinement to a stall for 30 days often produces good results. If, however, the spine is separated from the body of the scapula, this may cause necrosis (death of bone tissue), forming of sequestra (pockets of dead bone fragments) or atrophy (degeneration because of disuse) of the muscles. This often results in permanent lameness, and very little can be done beyond confining the horse.

Other fractures of the scapula may sometimes be diagnosed by crepitation, but the grinding may be so slight that it can only be heard with a stethoscope. It should

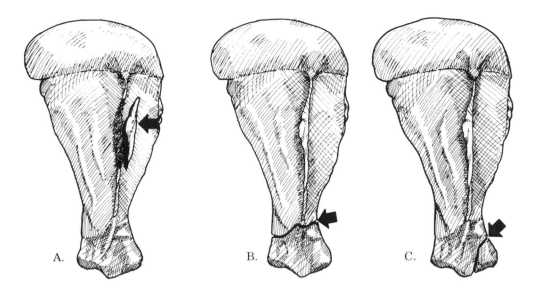

Fig. 12-16. Diagram showing types of fractures of the scapula. A. Fracture of the spine. B. Fracture of the neck. C. Fracture of the coracoid process.

be remembered that this causes great pain to the horse. It is generally not helpful to try X-rays in this region, due to the heavy muscles present and the awkward position of the injury.

Fracture of the coracoid process usually also involves the glenoid cavity, which is the point of articulation with the humerus. Ankylosis (immobility of the joint) can be expected, muscles will probably atrophy, necrosis and sequestra frequently occur, and the horse is generally permanently lame. Given the horse's lack of tolerance for devices such as slings, there is little hope of proper healing.

The neck of the scapula has a tendency, when fractured, to heal in a position overriding the joint. This creates a "false joint," and results in permanent lameness. Again, fractures of this nature are virtually impossible to treat, and recovery is rare.

WITHERS

ANATOMY AND CONFORMATION

What are the withers?

The prominent area that is the meeting point of the neck, the back and the peak of the shoulders is called the withers. Each of the structures that make up the withers is discussed in its respective anatomy and conformation section. Parts of the neck that are important components of the withers are the ligamentum nuchae and the various muscles illustrated and named in the accompanying drawing. These paired muscles act together to raise the head and neck, or act on one side only, to flex the neck to one side or the other.

What structures of the shoulder are involved?

The dorsal extremity of the scapula and the associated muscles, the trapezius, the latissimus dorsi, the suprasinatus, the infraspinatus and the serratus ventralis all contribute to the mass of the withers. The actions of these muscles are described in the section on Anatomy and Conformation of the Shoulder, page 247.

What about the back?

The spinous processes of the first ten or so thoracic (rib-bearing) vertebrae form the upper skeletal outline of the withers. Some of the muscles of the neck are also part of the back. Action of the muscles of the neck portion raises and laterally flexes the head and neck. Those muscles of the back that contribute to the mass of the withers are shown in the illustration. They flex the back a slight amount, dorsally and laterally, as in stretching.

What else goes into the makeup of the withers?

Several bursae are involved; the most important one is called the supraspinous bursa. It covers the tops of some of the first three to five thoracic spines, and lubricates the interfacing surfaces between the ligamentum nuchae and these

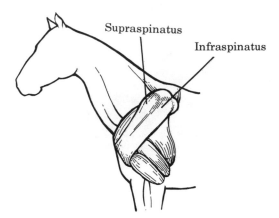

Fig. 13-1. Lateral view of the superficial muscles of the shoulder.

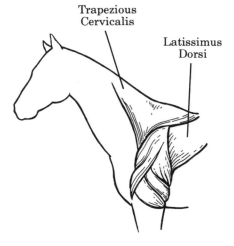

Fig. 13-2. Lateral view of the deeper muscles of the shoulder.

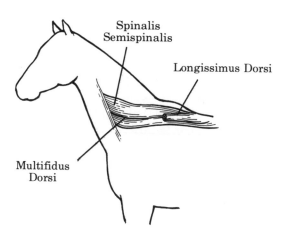

Fig. 13-3. Lateral view of the muscles passing over the withers.

spines. Inflammation of this large bursa leads to fistula of the withers. Each thoracic spinous process located behind the major bursa has a small bursa of its own that seems to have little practical value. Inflammation of any one of the small bursae may be caused by a poor fitting saddle, trauma resulting from rolling on a rock, a bite by another horse or a blow. This is a common problem in very high withered horses.

What conformation of the withers is good or bad?

Withers that are very low with little or no prominence are not desirable because a saddle depends on some prominence to help hold it in place laterally. Very high withers are also undesirable because they are too subject to injury by a saddle riding against the tops of the spines. Good withers fall about midway between these two extremes.

FISTULOUS WITHERS — POLL EVIL

What is the condition called fistulous withers?

Fistulous withers is an inflammatory disorder of horses which is identical to poll evil. Their only difference is that of location. Fistulous withers occurs in the supraspinous bursa area (withers); poll evil occurs in the supra-atlantal bursa area (poll).

In the early stage of the disease, bursitis is a more appropriate term for the condition, because a fistula (an abonormal passage leading from an internal organ to the body surface) is not present. When the inflamed bursal sac ruptures, or when continuous drainage and a secondary infection sets in after surgical intervention, then a true fistula occurs.

What is the cause of fistulous withers?

The actual cause of fistulous withers has not been determined, although numerous theories have been proposed. Mechanical injury may cause some cases, but the overriding opinion is that fistulous withers is usually infectious in origin. Tests indicate that the disease is frequently the result of a dual infection by the bacteria *Brucella abortus* and *Actinomyces bovis*. These are the causative organisms for the diseases of cattle called Bang's disease (Brucellosis) and lumpy jaw (Actinomycosis) respectively. (See Brucellosis, page 618.)

What is the appearance of fistulous withers?

The bursal sac becomes enlarged and its wall thickens because of the inflammation. Where the sac has little covering support, it may rupture to the outside and drain. In chronic cases of inflammation, the ligament and dorsal vertebral spines of the vertebrae are affected, and may even necrose (die).

In the early stage of the disease, the bursitis distends (fills) the bursa with a straw-colored fluid which contains bodies of fibrin that look much like grains of rice. The swelling, giving the withers its rounded look, may pouch out in several places, depending on the position of the bursal sacs and the direction they take between the tissue layers. The bursal sacs grow in loose tissue, developing to the point that they begin to open into other sacs through small openings among more dense tissues. Coagulated fibrin accumulates as it proceeds, but no running pus or secondary infection occurs until the bursal sac ruptures or opens to the outside. Once this has happened, other organisms enter the bursa, causing secondary infection which makes the discharge more pus-like in character.

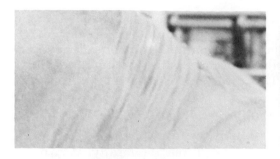

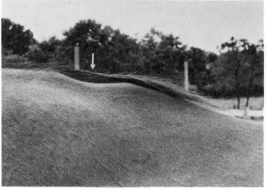

Fig. 13-4. Examples of conformation showing low, good and high withers. The horse with the good withers also has a vertebral spinous process missing (arrow).

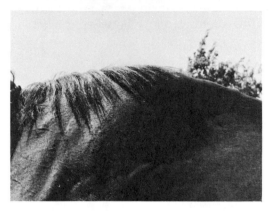

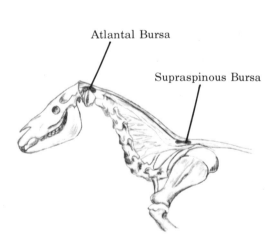

Atlantal Bursa

Supraspinous Bursa

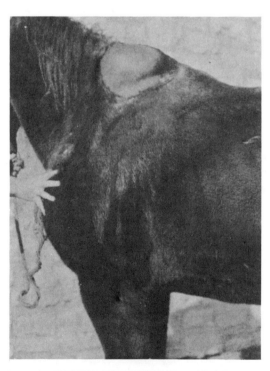

Courtesy of VETERINARY SURGERY, Edition VI, E. R. Frank, Burgess Publishing Co., Minneapolis, Minn.

Fig. 13-5. Diagram of the supraspinous bursa.

Fig. 13-6. Side view of withers showing bursitis in early stage of fistulous withers.

How is fistulous withers diagnosed?

Diagnostic signs vary according to the location and extent of the swelling, the potency of the bacteria and the resistance of the tissues.

The horse may evidence pain and stiffness before any swelling is obvious. There may or may not be heat in the local area. The bursa may even rupture before any swelling is evident because surrounding tissues prevent expansion of the sac. In this case, there will be one or more tracts leading out of the skin to discharge the straw-colored, "rice-body" material. If the bursa slips into underlying tissue, the swelling may show up in any of several locations in the area of the withers. In chronic cases, the draining tracts may heal and scar, only to reappear in another location.

Routine bacterial culturing and sensitivity testing of the bursal fluid are part of the diagnosis. X-rays are needed if bone involvement is suspected.

What is the treatment for fistulous withers?

Judgment on the manner of treatment must be left to the veterinarian since many diagnostic tests need to be done to determine the causative organisms. Many factors need to be considered based on these tests, such as whether or not the cause is known, whether the lesion is open and draining, the value of the animal, the extent of the lesion, and the danger of spread of the organisms to other animals and man. The earlier treatment is initiated, the better the chances of recovery. In longstanding cases, the treatment required may be quite extensive.

During treatment, the veterinarian will take extreme care to avoid spreading the bacteria that cause the disease because it is very dangerous to cattle and humans. It is highly important that only the veterinarian attempt treatment because of the required sanitary and safety measures. (For further information, refer to texts which include Malta disease and undulant fever of humans, and Brucellosis and lumpy jaw of cattle.)

According to the above-mentioned determining factors, the veterinarian may employ antibiotics, sulfonamides, anti-inflammatory agents, enforced rest, iodides, arsenicals, surgical drainage, or surgical removal of the bursal sac and necrotic material.

What is the prognosis for cases of fistulous withers?

Extensive necrosis of bone and cartilage is frequent with this type of infection, often involving degeneration of the bursal wall and ligamentum nuchae.

If the tissue damage is severe, surgical removal of the necrotic material to arrest further degeneration will be necessary. The primary aim in surgical intervention is the control of infection. When infection is controlled, the chances of recovery are fair. Treatment is usually long term and meticulous, often complicated by repeated relapses of the infection.

14

BACK AND BARREL

ANATOMY AND CONFORMATION

What regions of the horse are included in the back and barrel?

The back refers to the region between the point of the withers and the point of the croup. The barrel includes the thoracic (chest) cavity and the abdominal cavity.

How should the back and barrel be conformed?

A short back is usually considered a desirable feature. It should be in proportion to the withers, which are ideally of medium height and strong, and to the shoulders, which must not be "loaded" (thick). The best length of the back, however, is one that produces good balance in the individual horse. The back should be straight and level while the horse is standing, and allow for smooth, fluid movement.

A big barrel is an asset, since it provides space and protection for the heart, lungs, liver and stomach. If the barrel is too wide, though, the horse will be forced to swing the hindquarters around the barrel during normal movement, resulting in wasted motion.

The "ideal" barrel exhibits the greatest roundness behind the heart girth — the front is moderately slim, but there is a wide circumference over the back portion of the barrel. The ventral (lower) portion of the barrel is long in comparison to the back, and the ribs are well sprung (curved rather than slab-sided). The ribs should also be spaced widely, since this indicates strong respiratory muscles, greater flexibility of the thorax (chest) walls, and improved breathing capacity.

What are the basic mechanisms of the back and barrel?

The back and barrel are moved by a complex muscular-skeletal system. The bones primarily involved are the thoracic and lumbar vertebrae and the ribs.

Starting at the base of the horse's skull and moving toward the tail, the thoracic vertebrae are the second "set" of vertebrae. They immediately follow the cervical

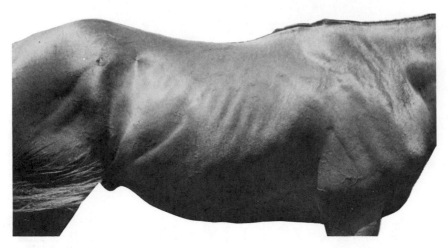

Fig. 14-1. Conformation of the back and barrel. This horse has well set-back withers and a long, Thoroughbred-type back which is balanced for his height and overall length.

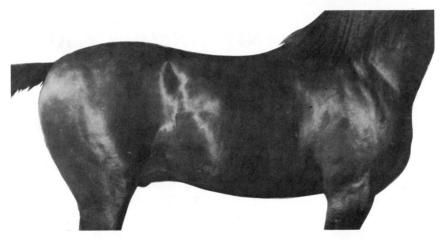

Fig. 14-2. Conformation of the Arab back and barrel. The back is shorter and the withers less prominent.

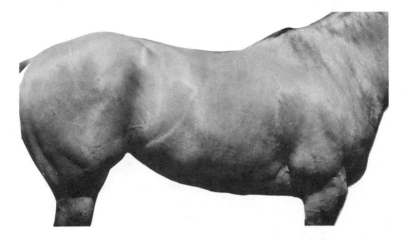

Fig. 14-3. Quarter horse back and barrel. Shortness is considered desirable, but withers and muscles are more pronounced than in Arabs.

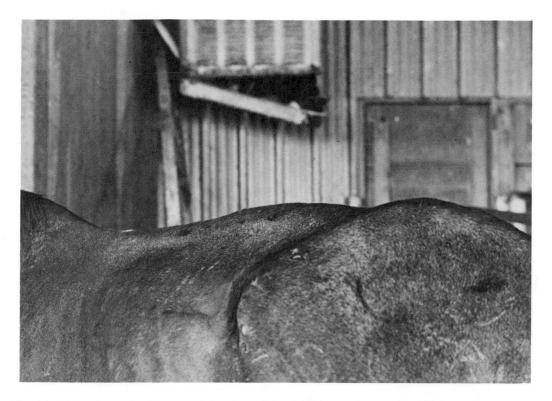

Fig. 14-4. Photograph of horse with a "roach back". Notice the rounded appearance over the loins.

(neck) vertebrae, and extend to the middle of the back. Usually they are eighteen in number. Horses have been known to have nineteen, however, and seventeen is not uncommon, particularly among Arabians. The thoracic and lumbar vertebrae have the same basic construction. That is, they are composed of a body or round mass of bone, an arch which forms the ring for the spinal cord, and several different processes (projections) which provide attachment and support for other bones, muscles, ligaments and nerves. There is generally a dorsal (upper) process, a ventral (lower) process, two transverse (lateral) processes and an articular process.

The thoracic vertebrae are unique, since they provide points of attachment for the ribs. Each thoracic vertebra (except the last one) has four costal facets (articulating surfaces) on the body of the vertebra, placed so that each one forms half a "socket." A facet on the adjoining vertebra forms the other half of the socket. The rib articulates with this socket and with similarly placed facets on the transverse processes of the vertebra.

The thoracic vertebrae also have rather tall dorsal processes. Those near the base of the neck are the largest and form the basis of the withers. Further toward the tail, these processes become shorter.

In both thoracic and lumbar vertebrae, the articular process, which articulates with the next distal vertebra, is rather small. The last three thoracic vertebrae are characterized by mamillary processes, which are between the dorsal and transverse processes. This characteristic continues in the lumbar vertebrae.

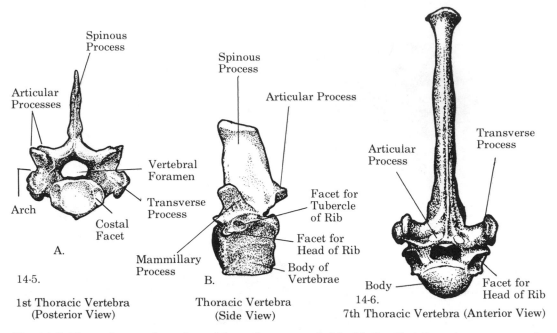

14-5.

1st Thoracic Vertebra
(Posterior View)

Thoracic Vertebra
(Side View)

14-6.

7th Thoracic Vertebra (Anterior View)

Fig. 14-5. Thoracic vertebra viewed from the rear and side. Notice that the spinous process is shorter on the thoracic vertbra (B.) that is closer to the lumbar vertebra.

Fig. 14-6. Seventh thoracic vertebra shows the basic construction of all vertebrae.

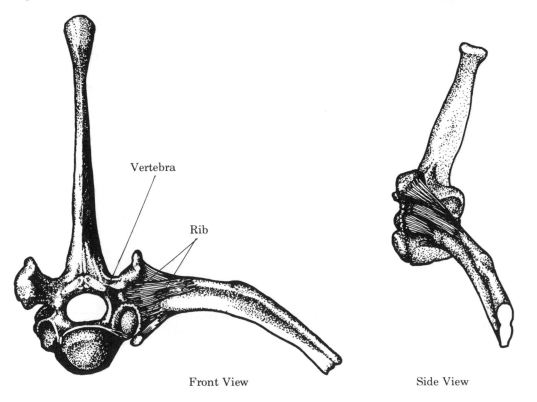

Front View

Side View

Fig. 14-7. Junction of the thoracic vertebra and the rib.

Fig. 14-8A. Illustration of first thoracic vertebra and rib. Notice the oval shape of the thoracic cavity.

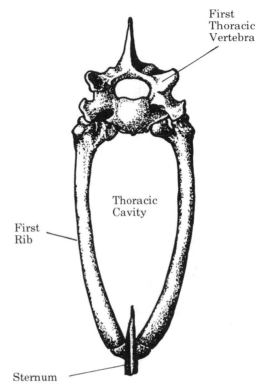

First Thoracic Vertebra

Thoracic Cavity

First Rib

Sternum

Fig. 14-8B. The bones of the back and barrel include 18 thoracic vertebrae and 6 lumbar vertebrae, in addition to the ribs of the thoracic vertebrae.

Thoracic Vertebrae　　Lumbar Vertebrae

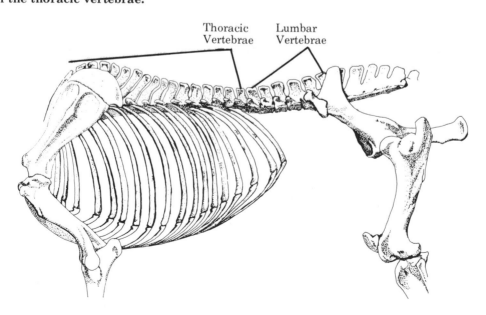

The lumbar vertebrae are usually six in number. Arabians in particular have been known to have five, and a horse with nineteen thoracic vertebrae may also have only five. These bones are distinguished from thoracic vertebrae in that they do not articulate with the ribs. The transverse process becomes progressively more prominent, being largest in the last lumbar vetebra.

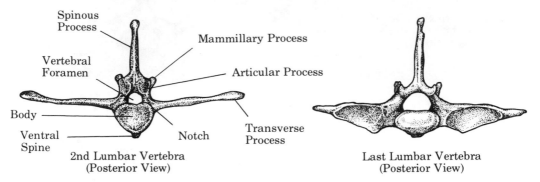

2nd Lumbar Vertebra
(Posterior View)

Last Lumbar Vertebra
(Posterior View)

Fig. 14-9. Lumbar vertebrae. Notice the longer spinous process on the last lumbar vertebra.

Although they vary in length and curvature, ribs consist of a curved shaft, two extremities, and are arranged in opposing pairs.

The first rib is directed slightly forward and down. The second is vertical and the remaining ribs are sloped backward and down. The intercostal spaces (gaps) between the ribs are well muscled. The vertebral extremity has a head, neck and tubercle by which it attaches to the vertebral column.

The head of the rib is a smooth, rounded articular surface connected to the shaft by a narrow neck. This is the portion of the rib that articulates with the sockets formed by the costal facets of the thoracic vertebrae. The tubercle is a small, knobby extension, slightly back from the neck of the rib, that articulates with the transverse process of the thoracic vertebrae.

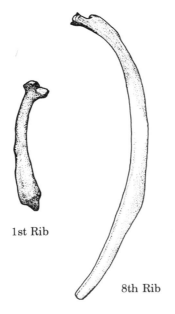

Fig. 14-10. Differences in shape of the ribs.

1st Rib

8th Rib

The first eight pairs of ribs are called the sternal or "true" ribs, because they are connected directly to the sternum (bony floor of the chest) by costal cartilage.

Asternal, or "false," ribs are not directly connected to the sternum. There are usually ten of these ribs, but eleven or nine are not infrequent. The number of ribs depends on the number of thoracic vertebrae present, because the ribs are attached to these vertebrae. The costal cartilages of most asternal ribs angle forward and fuse together, forming one common connection to the sternum. The last one or two pairs of asternal ribs are frequently called floating ribs because their sternal ends are often not attached to those of adjacent ribs.

What are the muscles of the back and barrel?

The longissimus dorsi is the longest and largest muscle in the body of the horse. It extends from the neck to the sacrum (peak of the croup), and is made up of many small bundles of muscle fibers. These connect one vertebra to the next, or overlap one or more vertebrae. The vertebrae are joined from the transverse process to the spinous process, from transverse process to transverse process, and from spinous process to spinous process. The longissimus dorsi has one-half of its mass on each side of the spine and is the most powerful extensor of the spinal column. It holds the spine rigid, allowing the horse to pick up the forequarters. Each half may act independently, flexing the spine laterally.

The abdominal muscles (four layers of specific muscles) are strong, extensive muscles which form most of the abdominal wall. These muscles support the digestive and reproductive organs (especially of the female during gestation). By compressing the abdomen, they aid in defecation, urination, expiration, coughing and sneezing, and parturition. They also arch the back, and can flex the trunk of the animal laterally by acting on one side only.

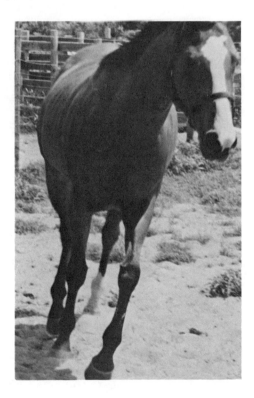

Fig. 14-11. Lateral flexion is accomplished by the muscles of the barrel. Notice the compression of the ribs on the left side and the expansion of the barrel on the right side.

The seven sets of muscles attached to the thoracic vertebrae, the ribs and their cartilages and the sternum are the muscles of respiration. They expand the thorax, causing inspiration (breathing in), and contract the thorax for expiration (breathing out). The most important of these are the external intercostal muscles, internal intercostal muscles and the diaphragm. (The diaphragm is presented in the "Respiratory System" chapter.)

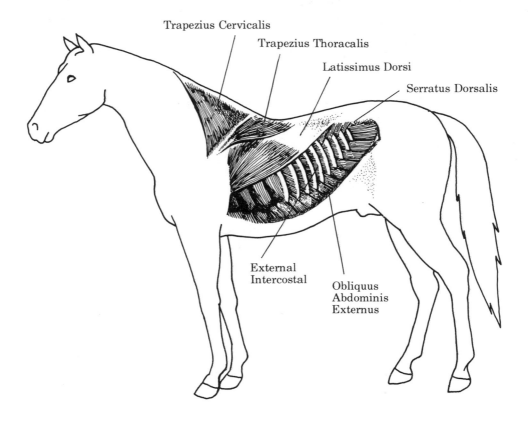

Fig. 14-12. Superficial muscles of the back and barrel.

The external intercostal muscles extend downward and backward from each rib to the next rib back. The action of the external intercostal muscles increases the size of the thorax by rotating the ribs upward and backward. Internal intercostals extend from each rib downward and forward to the next rib in front. These muscles are the next "layer" of muscle beneath the external intercostals. The internal intercostal muscles rotate the ribs backward, decreasing the size of the thorax.

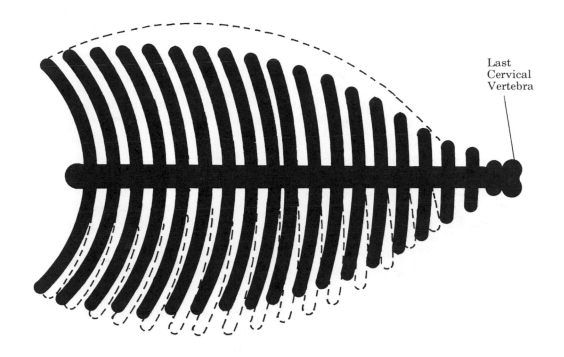

Last
Cervical
Vertebra

Fig. 14-13. Top view of the back and barrel, showing the ribs attached to the thoracic vertebrae. Dotted lines indicate expansion of the barrel and ribs.

UMBILICAL HERNIA

What is an umbilical hernia?

An umbilical hernia is the protrusion of contents of the abdomen through an opening in the muscles, forming a swelling or lump in the area of the navel. The external swelling contains the hernial sac. It is generally part of the peritoneum, which is the sac of tissue surrounding the internal organs. Sometimes, however, the hernial sac may be made up of, or include, part of the intestine. The part of the hernial sac lying within the ring (opening in the muscles) is called the hernial neck.

What causes an umbilical hernia?

Most cases of umbilical hernia are caused by a hereditary defect; the muscles around the navel simply did not close properly. Some cases though, may be caused by excessive traction on an oversized fetus, or by cutting the umbilical cord too close to the abdominal wall. Many umbilical hernias may not be evident at birth. Although they generally do not enlarge, an exceptional hernia may appear to be brought on by rearing, kicking, jumping, etc. These hernias are usually due to hereditary defects or some previous trauma, the effect of which was not evident at birth.

How is umbilical hernia diagnosed?

It may be assumed that a protrusion around the navel area of a young foal is a hernia. If there is reason to suspect a hernia, a veterinarian should be called immediately. Most hernias are not immediately dangerous, but a hernia may easily become strangulated and should be treated as a medical emergency unless it is very small. A strangulated hernia is one in which the hernial ring has narrowed, trapping a piece of the intestine. This affects circulation and may cause hemorrhage, peritonitis (inflammation of the peritoneum) and necrosis (death of the tissue). Death follows almost all cases of necrosis. Strangulation of the hernia has probably occurred if the swelling becomes painful and warm to the touch and the horse begins to act colicky.

Most umbilical hernias are the "reducible" type, meaning that the contents of the hernia may be moved back into the abdominal cavity. The tissue is not inflamed or painful and it is soft and elastic. It will return into the body when pushed, or when the horse is lying down. In any hernia, vibrations will be felt in the swelling if coughing is induced, and the hernial ring should be detectable with a finger.

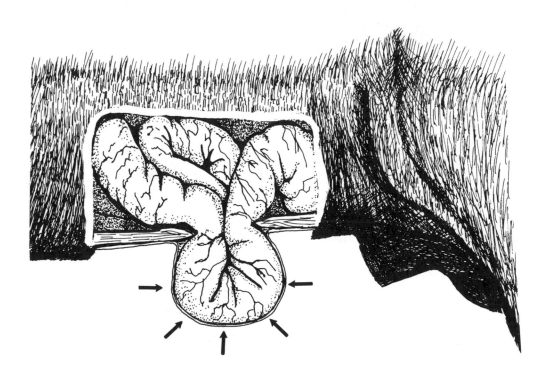

Fig. 14-14. Irreducible hernia. This hernia can only be corrected by surgery because adhesions have formed (arrows).

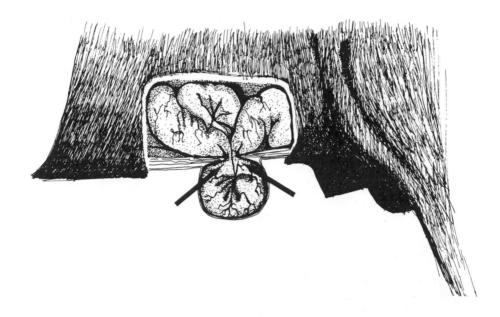

Fig. 14-15. Strangulated hernia. The hernial ring has closed in (arrows) around the escaped intestines, making it impossible for them to return to the abdominal cavity. This causes necrosis and gangrene in the herniated tissues.

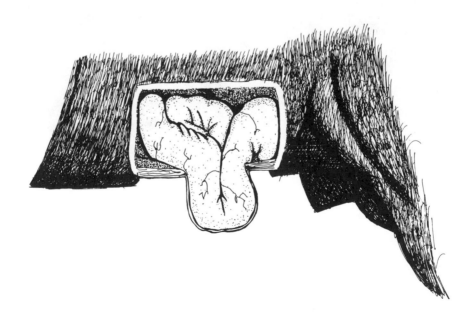

Fig. 14-16. Reducible hernia. The intestines can easily be pushed back into the abdominal cavity.

How is umbilical hernia treated?

Many cases of umbilical hernia need no treatment at all. They do not enlarge as the foal grows and may be invisible within twelve months. If a hernia is not strangulated, it may be reduced in size by the application of a mild blister, repeated in four to six weeks.

One method, no longer in popular use, consists of laying the foal on its side, pushing the internal contents of the hernia back into the body, and applying a clamp. The clamp shuts off circulation to the tissue, which drops off in about ten days. The disadvantages of having the foal wear a clamp for this period of time are obvious.

Some large reducible hernias may be corrected by surgery, and it is the only known method of treatment for irreducible or strangulated hernias. The procedure involves pushing the contents of the hernia up into the abdominal cavity while the foal is lying down. An incision is made into the swelling, the hernial ring is sewn shut, and the excess skin is removed before the incision is closed.

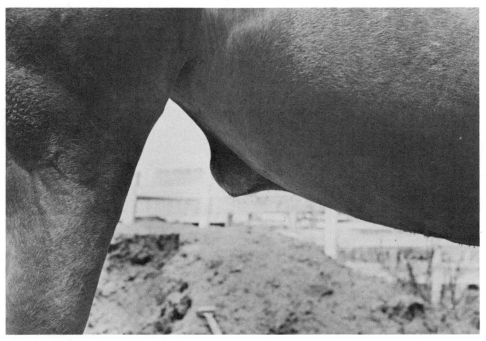

Fig. 14-17. Photograph of an irreducible umbilical hernia. The intestines cannot be pushed back into the abdominal cavity due to the formation of adhesions.

MYOSITIS OF THE PSOAS AND LONGISSIMUS DORSI MUSCLES

What is myositis of the psoas and longissimus dorsi muscles?

Myositis is an inflammation of the muscles, in this case, the longissimus dorsi and psoas muscles. The longissimus dorsi extends from the sacrum and ilium to the neck, making it the largest and longest muscle in the body of the horse. There are two psoas muscles, the psoas major and the psoas minor, that are subject to inflammation from stress.

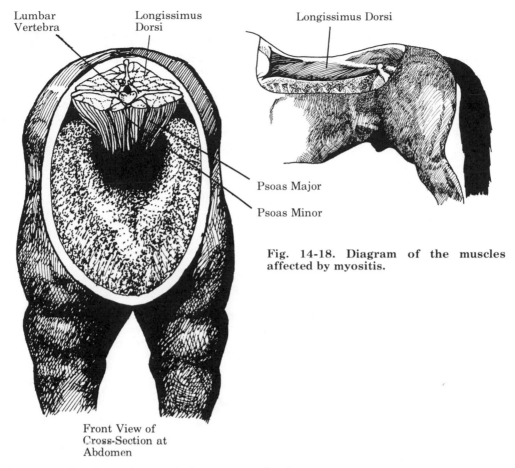

Fig. 14-18. Diagram of the muscles affected by myositis.

What are the functions of these muscles?

The longissimus dorsi is the most powerful extensor of the back and loins. It flexes the spine laterally and assists in extending the neck.

There are different functions for each psoas muscle. The psoas major flexes the hip joint and rotates the thigh outward, while the psoas minor flexes the pelvis on the loins and inclines it laterally.

What causes myositis in these muscles?

Inflammation of the longissimus dorsi and psoas muscles is usually due to strain of these muscles in racing or fast starts. In some cases, myositis is secondary to active degeneration of bones or joints in the back or hindlegs. Lesions of the tarsus and stifle frequently cause signs of myositis. Azoturia and tying-up (see Azoturia, page 626) can also cause inflammation of these back muscles.

What are the signs of myositis of the psoas and longissimus dorsi muscles?

The signs of myositis must be carefully differentiated by a veterinarian from the signs of sacroiliac subluxations and overlapping of the thoracic or lumbar dorsal spinous processes. Indications of strain in these muscles may cause the horse to act as if he had kidney trouble. Stiffness causes the hind limbs to be carried up under the body and the back will be arched. Some horses may seem tucked up in the abdomen and move with a very short stride. Pressure over the loins is very painful and causes the horse to drop his back.

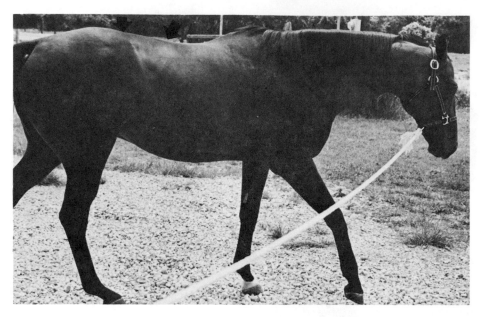

Fig. 14-19. Stiff, rounded back which is typical of soreness. The head will be raised and the stride even shorter when weight is placed on the back.

How is myositis treated?

Rest is the most important treatment if the myositis is primary. If the inflammation is caused by or accompanies some other disease process, anti-inflammatory drugs (corticosteroids or phenylbutazone) may help alleviate the inflammation and relieve the pain. The horse should not be returned to work until all signs of pain have been absent for at least three weeks. Vitamin E and selenium have proved helpful in treating and preventing some muscle disorders, and may be prescribed by the consulting veterinarian.

SUBLUXATION OF THE SACROILIAC JOINT

What is a subluxation of the sacroiliac joint?

A subluxation is a partial displacement of a joint. The sacroiliac joint is composed of the sacrum and the ilium. These two structures are joined together by strong ligaments which are designed to prevent movement in this joint. Any movement in the sacroiliac is due to partial dislocation of this fused joint.

What causes a subluxation of the sacroiliac?

Partial dislocations of this joint may be caused by falls, slipping, or any other trauma that twists or stresses the sacroiliac joint.

What are the signs of a displacement of the sacroiliac joint?

The most common signs of a displacement of the sacroiliac joint are pain and stiffness in the hindquarters. Pain is usually caused by reflex muscle spasms which attempt to maintain the immobility of the sacroiliac joint. Prominence of the tuber sacrale (hunter's bumps) may develop if one or both sacroiliac joints are displaced. When the horse is walked, one or both tuber sacrale may be seen to move. Old (chronic) displacements will show prominence of the tuber sacrale.

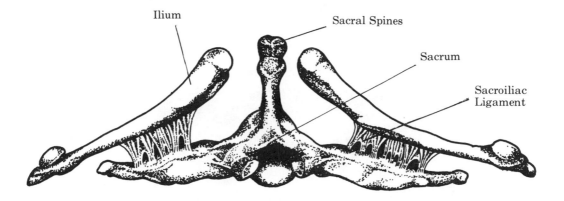

Fig. 14-20. Illustration of the sacroiliac junction.

How are subluxations of the sacroiliac joint treated?

Treatment of partial displacement of the sacroiliac joint begins with complete rest and confinement for at least 30 days. Irritants may be injected locally to stimulate formation of scar tissue which will help to immobilize the joint. Lameness must be treated by limitation of movement in the sacroiliac joint. All treatment should be carefully supervised by a veterinarian since errors in diagnosis and treatment could lead to infection and cause chronic lameness. Injuries of this type which eventually heal are relatively susceptible to re-injury.

OVERLAPPING OF THE THORACIC AND/OR LUMBAR DORSAL SPINOUS PROCESSES

What are the thoracic and lumbar dorsal spinous processes?

The spinous process is the "ridge" on the dorsal side of the vertebrae. There are usually eighteen thoracic vertebrae, beginning just behind the cervical (neck) vertebrae, and extending to the middle of the back. Working toward the tail, the next are the lumbar vertebrae, usually six in number, which extend to the peak of the rump.

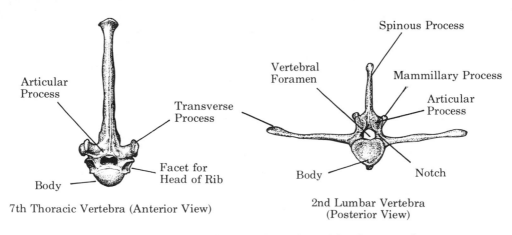

7th Thoracic Vertebra (Anterior View)

2nd Lumbar Vertebra (Posterior View)

Fig. 14-21. Diagram comparing the thoracic and lumbar vertebrae.

What causes overlapping of the spinous processes?

Usually the horse has suffered an injury from a trauma such as going over backwards, falling, or has struggled in a casting harness. After the injury, the ends of the spinous processes enlarge due to exostosis (abnormal new bone growth), causing the overlapping and consequent pain.

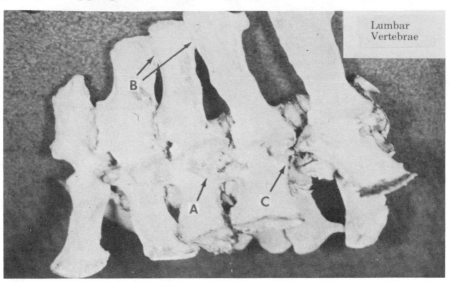

Courtesy of THE HORSE, by Peter D. Rossdale, M.A., F.R.C.V.S., published by The California Thoroughbred Breeders Association. Photo by Peter Rossdale.

Fig. 14-22. Overlapping spinous processes (B.) following an injury that resulted in inflammation and the formation of exostoses. Inflammatory lesions between the joints are seen at (A.). (C.) is a normal joint.

How is overlapping of the spinous processes diagnosed?

A horse affected with overlapping of the spinous processes will generally show a change in behavior and temperament. It may resent grooming and saddling, sometimes bucking or lying down after saddling. It may groan and show other signs of discomfort as the cinch is tightened. Pressure along the back may cause pain. Hunters and jumpers, which are most commonly affected, will often refuse to jump.

The location of the injury may often be revealed by palpation. The examination should begin at the withers and work backward, looking for irregularities in the size of the summits of the spinous processes.

It is also helpful to test the spine for flexibility. In a normal horse, pushing down in the middle of the back should make the spine dip, while pressure at the base of the tail produces arching. Overlapping of the spinous processes will reduce this movement to little or none.

Finally, an X-ray examination may be needed to determine the extent of the problem.

How is overlapping of the spinous processes treated?

Surgery will generally relieve overlapping, but it is rather extensive. Basically, the procedure involves removing the summit of the affected process.

After surgery at least two months' stall rest and one month of exercise in hand are required before healing is complete enough to allow riding. It sometimes takes several months for good results to show. The prognosis is guarded.

RIB FRACTURES

What causes rib fractures?

Rib fractures may be caused by blows, kicks, falling or accidents in transport, among others.

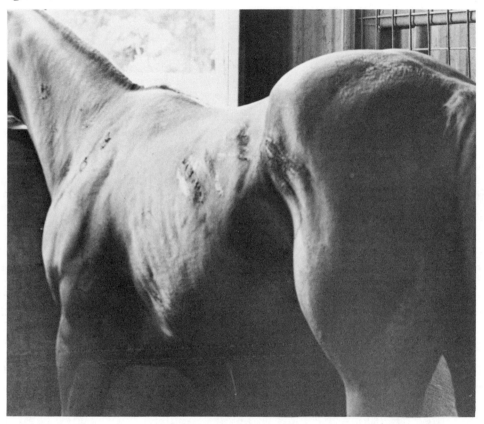

Fig. 14-23. Wounds over the shoulder do not usually injure the ribs, but kicks on the rest of the thoracic ribs often cause simple fractures.

How serious are rib fractures?

Many rib fractures which are "simple" (have no protruding or crushed bones), are never detected, never treated and cause no problems. Others can be painful, harmful and in some cases, fatal.

Fracture of the first rib, for instance, often produces radial paralysis or "dropped elbow," because the break interferes with the functioning of the radial nerve. In this case the horse cannot advance the affected front leg to bear the weight of the body. If the leg is advanced for the horse, however, bearing the weight is not difficult.

The second to the sixth ribs are seldom broken, since they are well protected by the shoulder blade and the muscle and bone of the forearm.

Compound fractures in which a bone or bone fragment pierces tissue can cause serious, sometimes fatal, difficulties. A broken rib that punctures the pleura (tissue lining the thoracic cavity), or the lung itself is not uncommon. Puncture of the pleura can result in pleuritis or pneumothorax, either of which may be fatal (see Pleuritis, page 429, and Pneumothorax, page 421).

Fractures of the last four or five ribs may pierce the peritoneum, or tissue surrounding the organs. This may result in serious infection.

Comminuted fractures are those in which the bone is crushed, rather than broken sharply. Both comminuted and compound fractures can result in necrosis, or death of the bone tissue, sequestra (dead bone fragments) or inflammation of the bone marrow (osteomyelitis).

A sequestrum will be treated by the body as foreign matter. It will be attacked by white blood cells as if it were an infection, pus will form, and the result may be a constantly draining abcess called a fistula. Abscessing may also result if the broken bone in a compound fracture is exposed and infected.

How are rib fractures detected?

Unless there is considerable swelling of the soft tissue, fractures can generally be found by feeling with the hand. If a horse shows signs of pleuritis, such as hurried breathing, frequent coughing, reluctance to move and discomfort, rib fracture may be suspected. A lung puncture usually results in frothy blood coming from the nostrils. In any case involving rib fracture, a veterinarian should be consulted immediately.

How is rib fracture treated?

Simple fractures are frequently not treated. Compound or comminuted fractures may call for removal of bone fragments, broken bone, and sometimes nearby healthy bone to avoid infection. Any opening into the body is closed, and antibiotics may be given to combat infection.

SADDLE SORES (SADDLE GALLS)

What causes saddle sores?

Saddle sores are caused primarily by friction between the horse and the saddle or harness. In some cases, the friction is the result of faulty conformation of the horse. If the withers are too low, for instance, the saddle may sit too far forward. If they are too high, the withers may be compressed by the saddle. A narrow chest can make it difficult to cinch the saddle tightly. A thin horse has poor padding between itself and the saddle, making it a likely candidate for saddle sores.

More often, working conditions are the cause. A poorly made or poorly adjusted saddle, a rider or load sitting in an unbalanced position, excessive uphill and downhill riding, or wet skin caused by rain or sweat are the primary offenders. A combination of any of these factors greatly increases the chances of saddle sores.

How are saddle sores diagnosed?

Saddle sores are usually quite evident when present. The most common type of saddle sore is a simple inflammation of the hair follicles. This causes heat and is painful to the animal when touched. Left untreated, the area may swell, blister and develop pus. The final stage of this development is necrosis (death of the tissue). The necrosed skin is commonly called "sitfast," which must be removed before healing by granulation can take place.

The withers are more likely than the back to develop chronic saddle sores, because they are the most prominent point on which a saddle sits. A chronic saddle sore is generally recognized by the total absence of hair and the presence of calluses, caused by damage or destruction of the hair follicles in the area. If the follicles are

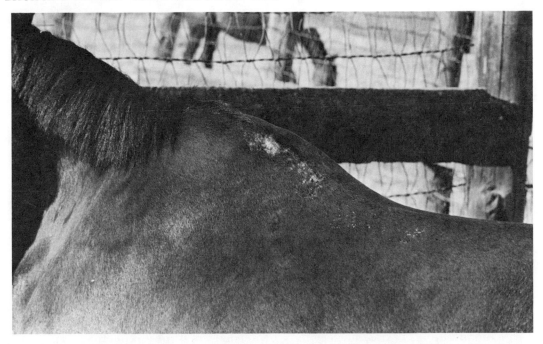

Fig. 14-24. Saddles that are improperly fitted can cause calluses on the withers. These sores will eventually heal in with white hair, leaving a permanent blemish on the horse.

not destroyed completely and sufficient rest is given to allow the hair to grow back, it is generally white in color. These saddle sores may be further characterized by folliculitis (hard nodules around the base of the hair). Any saddle sore on the withers may lead to inflammation of the bursae (small, fluid lubricating sacs) in the area or further complication of the saddle sore due to the swelling of bursitis.

Saddle sores of an equally serious nature may result when the skin itself is injured rather than just the hair, by a split, tear or cut. This may occur, for instance, when a saddle or harness sticks to the skin and then is suddenly moved. This normally results in extremely painful swelling of the deep layers of skin, sometimes accompanied by rupture when the saddle or harness is removed. These injuries are known as galls, and are most painful when located on the withers.

Fig. 14-25. This is an example of a girth sore caused when the cinch or girth pinches the folds of skin behind the foreleg.

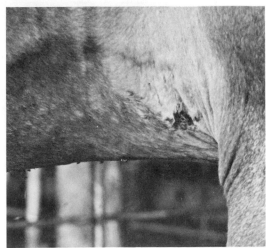

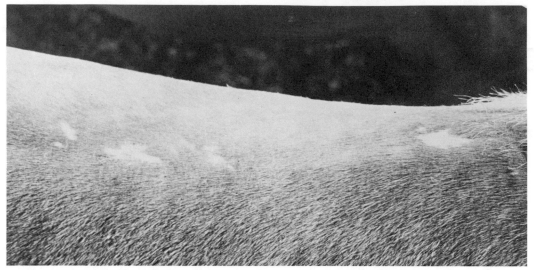

Fig. 14-26. Growth of white hair which characterizes an old saddle sore.

How are saddle sores treated?

Particularly with open sores, a veterinarian should be consulted. If hematomas (large blood blisters) exist, surgery may be needed, as it may if necrosis is present. Antibiotics may be given to combat infection, and antiseptics applied to open wounds.

A saddle sore on the withers must have immediate attention, since it is an indication that pressure is being applied to the spinous processes (bony ridge in the withers). Continued work under the conditions which caused the sore can lead to bursitis, or even damage the bone itself. Bursitis is generally treated by draining the excess synovial (lubricating) fluid from the bursa and the injection of corticosteroids in the hope that the swelling will not return. If it does so, surgical removal of the bursa may be necessary. Bone damage of this sort can contribute to overlapping of the spinous processes (individual "projections" that make up the bony ridge), resulting in lameness. (See Overlapping of the Thoracic and/or Lumbar Dorsal Spinous Process, page 283.)

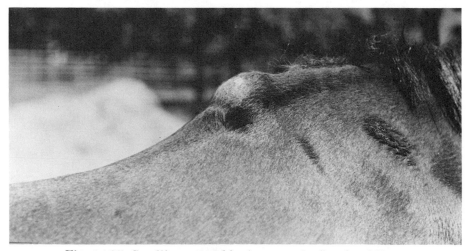

Fig. 14.27. Swelling caused by improperly fitted saddle.

In all cases, total rest from any work which would involve the affected area is necessary. For sores that are not advanced, astringent packs and massage with stimulating ointments is useful. Provided that treatment is given before the condition becomes advanced, the prognosis is good.

15

HINDQUARTERS

ANATOMY AND CONFORMATION

How should the hindquarters be conformed?

The correct conformation of the hindquarters is different for various kinds of horses, and is a direct function of the kind of work the horse is called upon to do. In judging the hindquarter conformation of any horse, it should be kept in mind that the hindquarters supply much more power toward locomotion than do the forequarters. Their connection to the spine is more direct, giving them a solid base for propulsion, and their muscles are larger and more powerful.

A horse that is asked to run must have considerable freedom of movement. This means that the hindquarters must straighten out as far as possible, to allow the greatest amount of "ground gain" with each stride. The successful racer usually has a straight and level croup, and the angles formed by the hip joint and stifle are as straight or "open" as possible.

If a horse must push or jump, however, the hindquarters must be constructed in a way to supply greater leverage or "push" than is needed to run. The croup should have a slightly more downward angle, so that the horse can get the hind feet "under" itself. A little more "closed" angle of the hip and stifle joint is also an aid in pushing.

The key to judging the appearance of the hindquarter muscles is usually the squareness or rectangularity of their shape. A posterior view of the hindquarters should produce a "square" look, with the croup rounded. The notable exception to this is the Quarter horse, in which a pear-shape is considered more desirable. The inside of the thigh and the outside of the stifle should be well developed, and should produce a "square" or rectangular look when viewed from the side, or when the leg is viewed as an individual limb from the rear. Again, well developed muscles here and in the buttocks are normally standard for the Quarter horse.

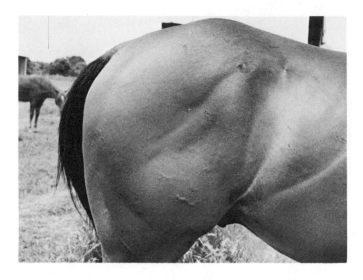

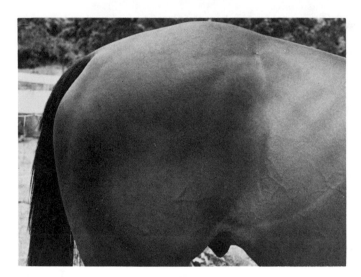

Fig. 15-1. The croup on the top is comparatively level, and would be desirable in a race horse. The croup on the bottom shows the rounder conformation needed for jumping.

What is the bone structure of the hindquarters?

The pelvic girdle is the structural basis for the entire hindquarters region. Its major bone is the os coxae, or hip bone, which is flat and has three parts. The largest of the three parts is the ilium, which is actually two separate halves. Each half is roughly triangular, giving the appearance of a wing on either side of the pelvis. The floor of the pelvis is formed by the pubis, the smallest of the three bones, and the ischium, which is roughly square with the sides curved inward. Again, these bones are actually right and left halves. The ilium forms the upper arch of a large, roughly elliptical opening, and the bottom arch is formed by the pubis and ischium. A gap at the top of the opening serves to hold the sacrum, a triangular portion of the spinal column that is actually five fused vertebrae.

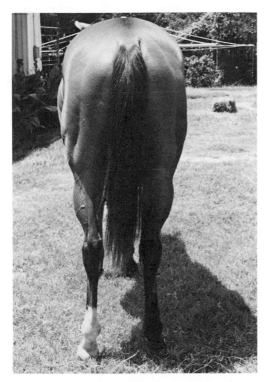

Fig. 15-2. Well-conformed Thoroughbred hindquarters, showing a generally "square" look with a rounded croup.

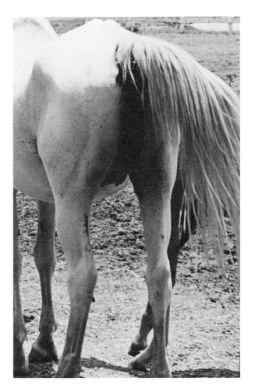

Fig. 15-3. A defect in hindquarters conformation, commonly known as "hunter's bumps."

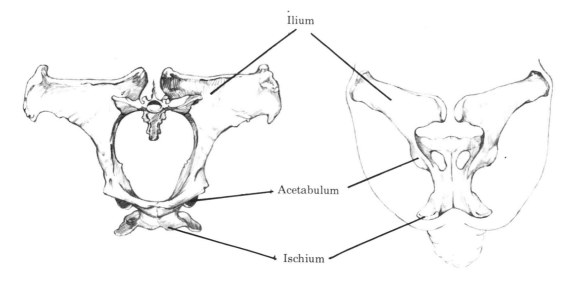

Fig. 15-4. A diagram of the pelvis bones of a mare, as seen from the front (left), and from the top.

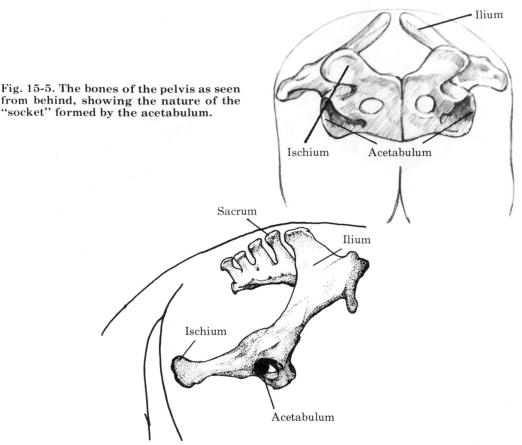

Fig. 15-5. The bones of the pelvis as seen from behind, showing the nature of the "socket" formed by the acetabulum.

Fig. 15-6. Bones of the pelvis region, side view. The processes (bony projections) on the sacrum show that it is part of the spinal column.

The three parts of each side of the pelvis meet at the acetabulum, which is on the ventral side of the bones. This is the surface where the femur articulates.

The femur is the largest of the long bones. The proximal (upper) end of the femur articulates with the acetabulum, the head of the femur being ball-shaped for this purpose. The shaft of the bone has several prominences for the attachment of muscles, and the distal (lower) end terminates in two other articular surfaces. One surface is the trochlea, which has two extensive track-like ridges that articulate with the patella (kneecap). The second surface is the lateral and medial condyles, which articulate with the stifle joint.

What muscles move the hindquarters?

The muscles of the hindquarter may be considered in groups, according to their location. There are usually five muscles counted in the sublumbar group. As a group, their general effect is to flex the hip joint, and rotate the thigh outward. The largest muscles doing this work are the psoas major and the iliacus, sometimes considered as a single muscle called the ilio-psoas.

The lateral muscles of the hip and thigh lie on the outer surface of those regions, and form their posterior contour. The muscle farthest forward is the tensor fasciae latae, which acts to flex the hip joint and extend the stifle. The gluteus medius is a large, powerful muscle that figures strongly in kicking, rearing and forward motion.

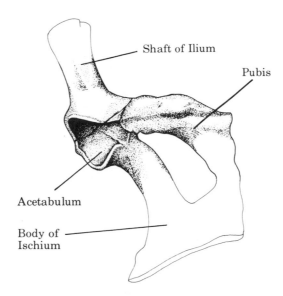

Fig. 15-7. Ventral view of a portion of the hip bone, showing the inside of the acetabulum.

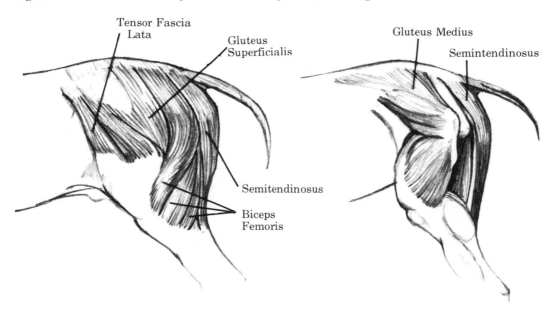

Fig. 15-8. These views illustrate the powerful muscles of the hindquarters. The gluteus superficialis lies over the powerful gluteus medius muscle.

It acts in conjunction with the biceps femoris, which is large and complex, and performs other functions as well.

The medial (inside) muscles of the thigh act to flex the hip joint, adduct the limb (draw it toward the body), and to rotate the thigh.

There are three anterior muscles of the thigh, the largest of which is the quadriceps femoris. It covers the front and sides of the femur, and has four different parts which act to extend the stifle and flex the hip.

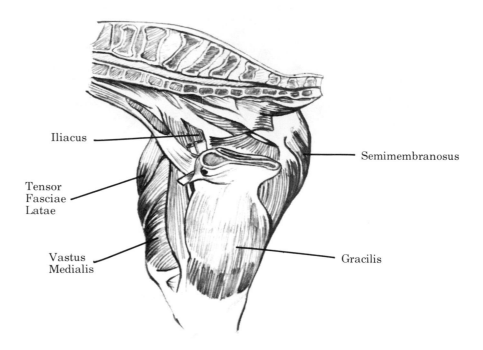

Iliacus

Tensor
Fasciae
Latae

Vastus
Medialis

Semimembranosus

Gracilis

Fig. 15-9. The outermost layer of muscles on the medial (inner) side of the thigh. These muscles flex the hip, rotate the thigh and draw it toward the body.

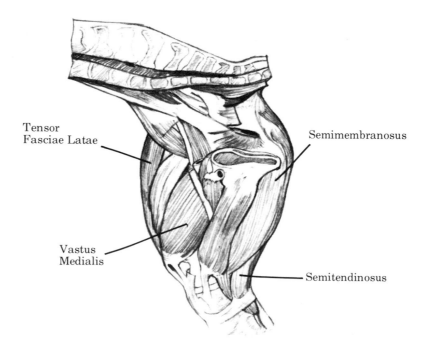

Tensor
Fasciae Latae

Vastus
Medialis

Semimembranosus

Semitendinosus

Fig. 15-10. Deeper layer of muscle on the inside of the thigh. The semitendinosus (also seen in illustration 15-9) is to the lower right.

COXITIS (INFLAMMATION OF THE COXOFEMORAL JOINT)

What causes coxitis?

Coxitis may often be traced to a violent action which affects the joint. Improper restraint of the rear leg, excessive strain on the joint or indirect blows due to slipping or falling may be suspected. This is particularly true if damage has been done to the acetabulum (hip socket), the rim of the acetabulum, or if a tear or fracture involves the articular surface in this area. Coxitis often develops in a younger animal as the result of an infection that settles in the joint.

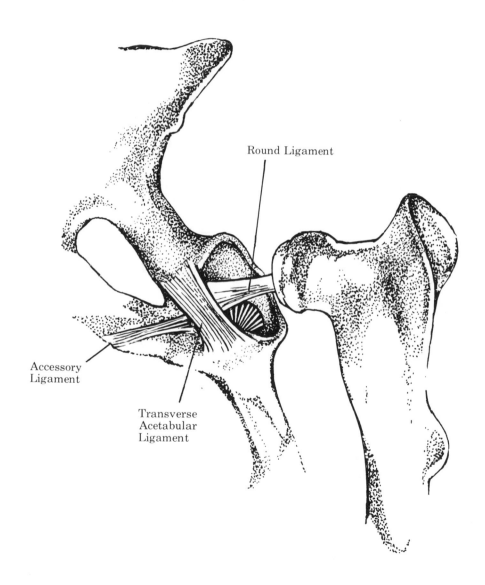

Fig. 15-11. Diagram showing the ligaments which help hold the femur (thighbone) to the hip, forming the coxofemoral joint.

How is coxitis diagnosed?

An animal affected with coxitis will develop a distinctive gait and stance. In severe cases, the leg will be carried. In less severe cases, the horse will avoid bearing weight on the leg while standing, and may move the foot forward in front of the opposite leg. Walking, the hindquarter will be elevated, making for a rolling gait. The leg will move in a semi-circular motion, stifle out, hock in. The leg is not moved fully forward in the stride, and the toe may be worn from dragging. The gluteal muscles eventually atrophy, but bone crepitation (clicking or grinding) is usually not noticeable. If these signs are in evidence, a veterinarian should be consulted to confirm the diagnosis. Further examination by the veterinarian may include palpation of the joint through the rectum, which sometimes shows enlargement of the acetabulum. X-ray examination is very difficult due to the heavy muscles surrounding the area, and requires special equipment. If done, the radiographs may reveal further irregularities.

The veterinarian may also draw fluid from the joint. If it shows the presence of excess or discolored synovial (lubricating) fluid, small pieces of cartilage or fibrin (evidence of blood clotting), joint damage and infection are probable.

How is coxitis treated?

A local anesthetic injected into the joint often produces temporary relief. However, no hope of permanent recovery may be offered. Rest may encourage some healing, but permanent lameness should be expected. The prognosis is poor.

RUPTURE OF THE ROUND LIGAMENT OF THE COXOFEMORAL JOINT

What is a rupture of the round ligament of the coxofemoral joint?

Rupture of the round ligament of the coxofemoral (hip) joint is a tearing of the strongest ligament in the hip joint which often accompanies dislocation of the hip. This rupture allows the head of the femur greater than normal motion and may lead to osteoarthritis in the joint.

What causes this rupture?

Direct injury or stress may cause the round ligament to rupture. Although rupture of the round ligament always occurs when the hip is dislocated, this ligament may be torn without displacement of the hip. This injury is not frequent, but can result from a foot caught in a rope or a sideline, if the horse struggles violently.

What are the signs of round ligament rupture?

When the round ligament is ruptured, the affected limb assumes a toe-out, stifle-out and hock-in appearance. There will be no shortening of the limb, however, as when the hip is dislocated. The veterinarian may wish to obtain a radiograph to rule out the possibility of a dislocated hip, especially if the injury is not recent. A crackling sound (crepitation) may be heard when the joint is moved because of degeneration, looseness and poor fit in the joint causing increased friction.

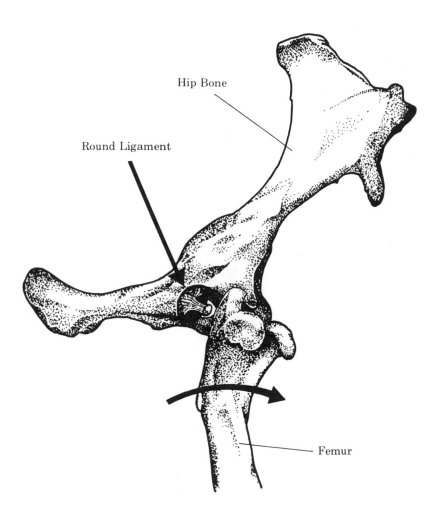

Hip Bone

Round Ligament

Femur

Fig. 15-12. Diagram of a rupture of the round ligament of the coxofemoral joint. Curved arrow indicates direction of movement of the femur to reveal the round ligament.

What is the treatment for rupture of the round ligament?

Stabilization of the joint with a toggle pin may make the animal sound for breeding purposes, but treatment does not usually prevent osteoarthritic degeneration in the joint. Immobilization of the joint is very difficult in the horse and rarely permits the horse sufficient healing for soundness. The joint will never be sound enough to permit galloping or strenuous work.

LUXATION OF THE COXOFEMORAL JOINT — DISLOCATION OF THE HIP JOINT

What is luxation of the coxofemoral joint?

The luxation (dislocation) of the coxofemoral (hip) joint is uncommon in horses. It can only happen if the round ligament of the hip is ruptured.

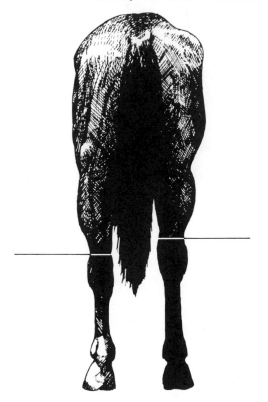

Fig. 15-13. Rear view of luxation of the hip. The trochanter of the femur protrudes upward causing a shortening of the right hind leg, as shown by the point of the right hock being higher than the left.

What causes dislocation of the hip?

It is rather difficult to dislocate the hip since the ilium tends to fracture before this occurs. However, this can happen if the horse catches a hindfoot in a rope and struggles violently. Major trauma is required for dislocation of this well-protected joint.

What are the signs of a dislocated hip?

If the hip is dislocated, there will be a marked shortening of the forward part of the stride due to a physical shortening of the limb. The limb is shortened because the femur is above its normal placement which may cause it to rub against the shaft of the ilium. Swelling of the injured tissues may make it difficult to detect any prominence at the point of the hip. As with a simple rupture of the round ligament, the injured limb will assume a toe-out, hock-in, stifle-out position and may appear to dangle.

How is a dislocated hip treated?

Treatment of a dislocated hip should only be attempted by a veterinarian because it requires general anesthesia and surgery. The veterinarian should be called promptly if dislocation is suspected; delay will allow contraction of the muscles and make reduction impossible. If the head of the femur can be relocated and it remains in place for three months, the muscles will usually keep it in place. Toggle pins may be used to try to keep the hip in place, but they do not hold up well under stress.

Recovery is usually limited to breeding soundness, but some horses may become completely sound. The veterinarian usually recommends treatment for valuable breeding animals only, due to the poor chances of complete recovery.

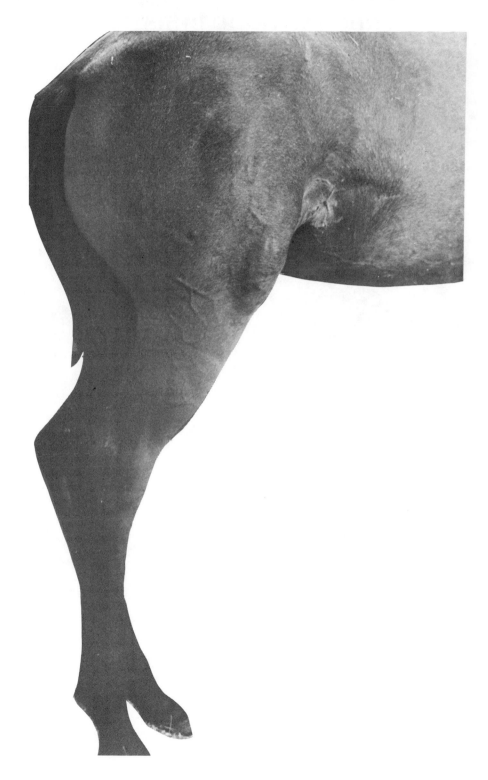

Fig. 15-14. This stance is typical of luxation of the hip, and several other hip injuries. Note that the hock is carried in, stifle out.

TROCHANTERIC BURSITIS

What is trochanteric bursitis?

Trochanteric bursitis is an inflammation of the bursa of the trochanter. This bursa lies between the tendon of the middle gluteus muscle and the great trochanter of the femur. In trochanteric bursitis, the tendon of the middle gluteus muscle may also be inflamed.

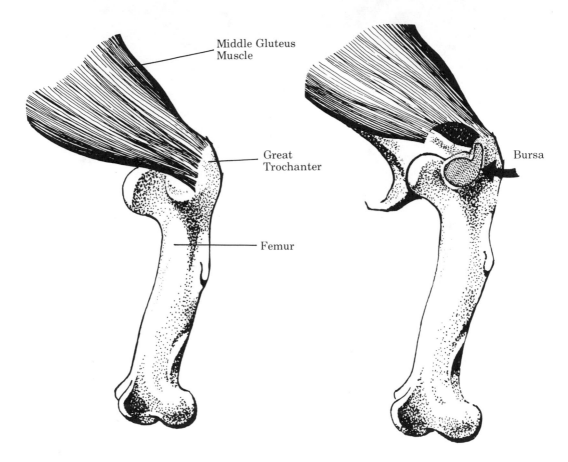

Fig. 15-15. Diagram showing the location of the bursa of the trochanter.

What causes trochanteric bursitis?

This condition may be caused by a direct blow to the trochanter, or strain on the middle gluteus tendon due to excessive circling or running on non-adhesive surfaces. It may also follow distemper, bone spavin and myositis.

What are the signs of trochanteric bursitis?

Trochanteric bursitis may cause signs of lameness and pain in the affected limb. If only one limb is involved, the horse may travel "sideways behind" in an attempt to move away from the painful side. The shoe will be worn more on the inside of an affected limb and the horse may stand with all the joints of that limb flexed. If the bursitis is caused by a direct kick, radiographs may disclose fracture of the cartilage or bone of the trochanter. Pressure over the affected hip joint may cause the horse to shy from pain, although many sound horses shy from pressure on this region.

How is trochanteric bursitis treated?

If the inflammation is acute, rest, heat and massage of the involved muscles may be prescribed. The veterinarian may also inject the area with corticosteroids or with a counterirritant. Counterirritants are more useful in chronic cases, however, where corticosteroids are ineffective. Some success has been achieved with ultrasonic treatments in cases of chronic bursitis. Surgery may be required if the cartilage or bone has been damaged. Treatment may result in recovery in four to six weeks, or the condition may become chronic, leaving the horse persistently lame or liable to a breakdown when he returns to training.

THROMBOSIS OF POSTERIOR AORTA OR ILIAC ARTERIES

What is thrombosis of the posterior aorta or iliac arteries?

Thrombosis is a blood clot that forms where a vessel has been damaged. If the clot becomes large enough, it will partially or may even completely occlude (block) an artery, cutting off the flow of blood to the organ or area supplied by the artery. The posterior aorta and iliac arteries are the major suppliers of blood to the hind limbs. When this blood supply is diminished by thrombosis, severe lameness may occur.

What causes a thrombus?

Damage to the intima (smooth inner lining) of the arteries allows the formation of a thrombus (blood clot). Many things may damage the delicate inner lining of a blood vessel, but the most common cause of this type of injury is the attachment of migrating larval forms of *Strongyles* (bloodworms). These larvae use the blood vessels to travel through the circulatory system before they mature. After this migration they return to the stomach, liver and intestines, depending on their species. Severe damage can cause the posterior aorta or iliac arteries to become completely blocked, resulting in muscle pain and lameness in the hind limbs.

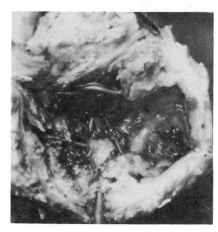

Photo Courtesy of THE HORSE, by Peter Rossdale, M.A., F.R.C.V.S., Published by The California Thoroughbred Breeders Association. Photo by Peter Rossdale.

Fig. 15-16A. The photograph shows the larvae of *S. vulgaris* in the intima of an artery.

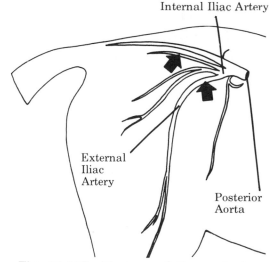

Fig. 15-16B. Diagram of the posterior aorta and iliac arteries. The arrows indicate the sites where a blood clot (thrombus) most commonly forms.

What are the signs of thrombosis of the posterior aorta or iliac arteries?

The signs and the time of their appearance vary with the size of the blood clot and the amount of blockage it causes. If the thrombus is small and there is minimal blockage of the vessel, the horse may be able to perform vigorous exercise before he becomes lame. In most cases, however, very little exercise is required to cause lameness. A veterinarian is usually required to diagnose the cause of lameness since the signs are very similar to azoturia (see Azoturia, page 626). Some blockages are severe enough to cause extreme lameness even when the horse is walking.

At the time the horse becomes lame, profuse sweating, pain and anxiety may be observed, especially if the horse is forced to continue the exercise. Due to the poor circulation in the affected limb, the femoral pulse will be weak and the limb will feel cooler to the touch than an unaffected limb. The most outstanding characteristic of this condition is the rapid appearance and disappearance of the signs. After the animal has rested, he may trot soundly again until the poor circulation causes a shortage of oxygen in the muscles supplied by the blocked vessel. If the thrombus blocks the aorta where it divides, both hindlegs may be affected, making it difficult for the horse to support his hindquarters.

What is the treatment for this condition?

The most effective treatment for thrombosis is prevention of *Strongylus* infestation by good sanitation and a regular, effective worming program. The veterinarian is the best source of reliable information on the subject of worm control. When the condition seems to be getting progressively worse, destruction is often necessary. Drugs to safely dissolve blood clots in horses have not yet been developed, so the veterinarian will probably rely on worming the horse with thiabendazole once a week for three weeks. If further damage can be prevented and rest is provided, collateral (alternate) circulation will sometimes develop sufficiently to allow the horse to function in a normal fashion.

FIBROTIC AND OSSIFYING MYOPATHY

What is a myopathy?

Myopathy is a term used to describe disease of a muscle. Fibrotic myopathy is a disease in which damaged muscles heal, forming connective tissue fibers (fibrotic) instead of normal muscle tissue. Ossifying myopathy means that the healing tissue is composed of bone cells, usually fibers that have become abnormal as they matured.

Where do fibrotic and ossifying myopathy occur?

Fibrotic and ossifying myopathy are most frequently found in the hindquarters where they affect the semitendinosus muscle. The semimembranosus and biceps femoris muscles are involved as the fibers spread and develop from the semitendinosus muscle. (See Anatomy of Hindquarters, page 295.)

What causes myopathy?

The cause of fibrotic myopathy and ossifying myopathy is thought to be trauma (injury) to the muscles. Muscles involved in myopathy are most commonly injured when the horse performs sliding stops, resists a sideline or hangs a foot up in a halter. These movements place a limb in a position that causes the thigh muscles to contract in a jerking manner. When this causes partial rupture or tearing of the semitendinosus muscle, the torn muscle fibers may heal abnormally, forming adhesions which restrict the full movement of the thigh muscles. If these fibrotic lesions turn to bone, similar restriction of movement results.

What are the signs of myopathy?

The signs of myopathy are due to the adhesions formed between the muscles when they do not heal normally. Frequently present in one hindleg, the lesions may

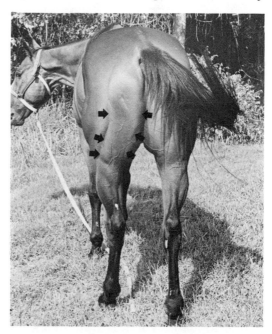

Fig. 15-17. Well-defined musculature in this horse's hindquarters shows the semitendinosus (arrows) very plainly, which is the first muscle affected by myopathy.

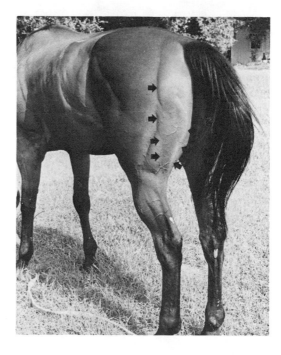

develop in both legs, or in a foreleg. Characteristically there is an abnormality of gait in which the horse does not reach forward normally. Just before the affected hindleg hits the ground, it is jerked back three to five inches. Most noticeable at the walk, this lameness is present in both fibrotic and ossifying myopathy. Firmness can be felt in the affected muscles just above the stifle joint.

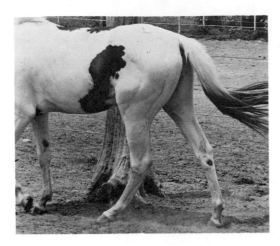 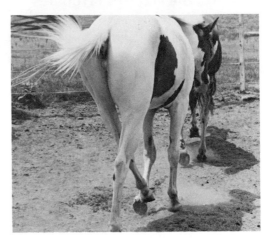

Fig. 15-18. The "goose-stepping" gait shown here is typical of a horse affected by myopathy.

What is the treatment for fibrotic and ossifying myopathy?

The most effective treatment in cases of myopathy is surgical removal of the affected tissue. A veterinarian must remove the affected tendon and part of the muscle after the diagnosis is confirmed. Since the surgery is complicated, it will not be described here. Before performing surgery, however, the veterinarian will be sure to distinguish myopathy from stringhalt by the direction in which the foot is jerked.

If surgery is performed to remove adhesions, the horse should be rested for the first seven to ten days. Then light exercise may gradually be increased to prevent new adhesions as the tissue heals. Most cases show some relief a few days following surgery although complete recovery does not always occur.

MYOTONIA

What is myotonia?

Myotonia is a condition of the muscles which causes them to contract rigidly after movement of any sort.

What causes myotonia?

There have been so few reported cases of myotonia that causes have not yet been firmly established. It is known that the condition is congenital, and that it is apparently a condition of the muscle rather than the nerve.

How is myotonia diagnosed?

The most obvious symptom of myotonia is over-development of the muscles in the hindquarter. The afflicted horse is unable to walk smoothly after a period of rest, but this condition improves temporarily with exercise. Laboratory examination has shown that the electrical current in affected muscles is different from that in normal muscles, and that the muscle fiber itself is larger than normal.

How is myotonia treated?

The rarity with which myotonia occurs has not allowed for the establishment of standard treatment. The condition has been treated with some success in humans through the use of quinine and related drugs. Since myotonia in horses seems to closely resemble the same ailment in humans, a veterinarian may decide, under specific circumstances, to try the same drugs already used on people. It should be kept in mind, however, that no data is available on the success or failure of this method.

Cases of myotonia have been known to improve with the passing of time, even to the point that gait appears to be normal.

NEURAL PARALYSES OF THE HINDQUARTERS

What is neural paralysis?

Neural paralysis is an inability to use certain muscles, due to damage to, or pressure upon, a nerve.

What causes neural paralysis?

There are several different kinds of neural paralysis, each resulting from damage to a different nerve. Exceptions exist with respect to specific disorders, but the general causes are: fractures in which a bone crushes a nerve, abscesses or tumors along the nerve, callus formation following fractures, overstretching of a limb, or infection of various types.

What are the types of neural paralysis?

Some forms of neural paralysis are observed frequently. Others are rare, or limited to certain geographic areas. Perhaps the best known is equine ataxia or wobbles. (See Wobbles, page 562.) Other common paralyses include femoral nerve paralysis, gluteal nerve paralysis, sciatic nerve paralysis and peroneal nerve paralysis.

Femoral nerve paralysis is caused by injury to the femoral nerve, which acts upon the quadriceps femoris muscle. (See Anatomy of the Hindquarters, page 295.) This affliction is unique, in that it is often caused by azoturia. (See Azoturia, page 626.) The femoral nerve passes between two muscles that are often affected in azoturia, and may be acted upon by the lactic acid present during this condition. Femoral paralysis prevents the horse from extending the stifle joint. When an attempt is made to put weight on the limb, the stifle and hock flex suddenly and the stifle drops. The quadriceps muscle will atrophy.

Peroneal paralysis usually results from the general causes already mentioned. The peroneal nerve moves the lateral and long extensors of the foot and the tibialis anterior muscle. The condition is recognized when the horse extends the leg back, but contacts the ground with the anterior (front) part of the hoof when it is brought forward. Recovery may be expected in 24 to 48 hours if the paralysis is due to being restrained with the legs flexed, or being laid out on his side with a casting harness.

Gluteal paralysis affects the gluteal muscle group and other muscles important in pushing with the rear limb. The gluteal nerve is seldom injured, but may be affected by abscesses, tumors or difficult delivery of a foal.

The sciatic nerve activates a group of large muscles in the thigh, including the biceps femoris, semitendinosus and semimembranosus muscles. Sciatic paralysis causes the limb to hang loosely, relaxation of the Achilles tendon, and inability to flex the hip, hock or stifle. The horse can support body weight while standing, but forced movement forward causes the leg to jerk upward and the flexed foot will be dragged on the ground.

Forms of neural paralysis encountered less frequently include obturator paralysis, pudic nerve paralysis, cauda equina paralysis, and "pseudo-amyloid" multiradicular degeneration of spinal nerve roots.

Obturator paralysis affects four of the muscles that pull the leg in sideways toward the body. It is a common condition in cattle, rarely affecting horses. It may be the result of tumors or abscesses, but occasionally happens after foaling.

Pudic nerve paralysis causes inability to retract the penis, which hangs limply. Cauda equina paralysis prevents voluntary movement of the tail. Both of these problems may result from the common causes previously mentioned.

"Pseudo-amyloid" degeneration has been reported only among Shetland pony foals. It is a congenital defect in the spinal nerve roots, and causes symptoms resembling wobbles.

How is neural paralysis diagnosed?

If neural paralysis is suspected, a veterinarian should be consulted to confirm the diagnosis. While the gait caused by a neural paralysis is generally distinctive, it could easily be confused with another disorder that calls for different treatment. Other than the change in gait, the primary indicator of neural paralysis is atrophy of the afflicted muscles.

How is neural paralysis treated?

If a neural paralysis is caused by pressure exerted on the nerve by a tumor or abcess, surgical removal of the source of pressure often restores use of the affected part. Spontaneous recovery is possible, but little hope can be offered in cases where the nerve itself has been damaged. Complete rest and good nursing care may provide some relief, but the prognosis is generally fair to poor.

LATHYRISM

What is lathyrism?

Lathyrism is an illness or set of symptoms brought about by eating toxic plants of the genus Lathyrus. The plant usually responsible for the poisoning is Lathyrus sativus, also called Indian pea, dogtooth pea, flat pea and Singletary pea. It is grown in Africa, Canada and mountainous regions of the United States. The common sweet pea, which is grown in flower gardens, is closely related but does not cause this syndrome.

How is lathyrism diagnosed?

The single most obvious symptom of lathyrism is gradual, progressive paralysis of the hindlimbs. The affected horse moves the hindlimbs stiffly at first, transferring weight to the forelimbs. As the condition becomes worse, the entire body weight may be carried on the forelimbs, the hindlimbs merely "treading". This seems to be the result of lesions of the spinal cord.

Pulse, respiration and temperature may at first be normal, but will probably be affected if the condition reaches the vagus nerve. Pulse usually becomes rapid and weak, and death may be caused by respiratory paralysis.

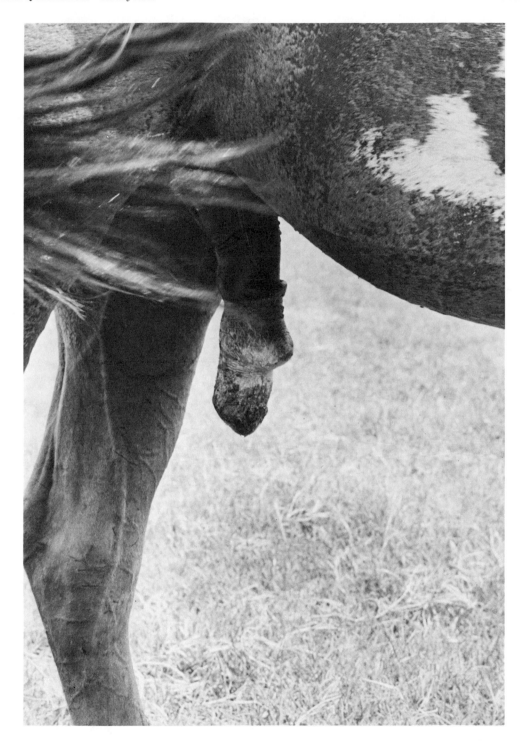

Fig. 15-19. Inability to retract the penis (paraphimosis) may be the result of damage to the pudic nerve, but is more often caused by swelling of the prepuce, penis, or inguinal region. This not only exposes the penis to injury, but also invites infection. Little can be done to correct paralysis of the pudic nerve, but other forms of paraphimosis should receive veterinary attention.

Other systemic changes may include chronic enteritis, fatal hemorrhages in the heart area, and congestion of the lungs.

How is lathyrism treated?

Since the signs of lathyrism may easily be confused with those of other disorders, a veterinarian should be consulted. Feed should be examined, since only large amounts of lathyrus seeds, fed continuously, will bring on the condition. A veterinarian may treat specific symptoms to give relief, but unless it is in advanced stages, horses frequently make full spontaneous recovery from lathyrism when the lathyrus plant is removed from the feed.

FRACTURE OF THE PELVIS

What is a fracture of the pelvis?

The pelvis may fracture in more than one region, but most common is a fracture in the shaft of the ilium. It is the shaft of the ilium and the tuber coxae that usually fracture before the hip is dislocated. Fractures of the pelvis can also occur in the symphysis pubis and the obturator foramen.

What causes fractures of the pelvis?

Fractures of the pelvis are frequently the result of a fall. Whether due to a slip, a struggle while being cast, or to fighting a sideline, fractures usually occur before dislocation of the well-protected hip joint. The ilium often fractures when the horse falls hard on its side.

What are the signs of a pelvic fracture?

Since there are many sites of fracture in the pelvis, the signs may vary. Fractures of the tuber coxae, commonly called dropped or knocked down hip, cause very little lameness. They are recognized by the flat appearance of the fractured hip when viewed from behind. If the skin is broken, the fractured ilium may protrude through the skin where the tuber coxae is broken off. Surgical removal of loose pieces of bone may be necessary and must be done by a veterinarian.

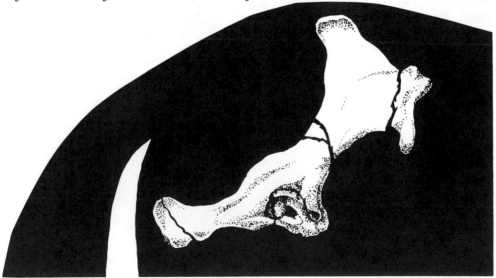

Fig. 15-20. This diagram shows fractures of the pelvis in the sites where they most commonly occur.

The shaft of the ilium may fracture in front of, behind or through the acetabulum. Severe lameness accompanies fractures of these areas, which may cause the affected limb to appear shorter if the ends of the fractured bone overlap. Pressure placed upon the affected limb will cause extreme pain and the horse will shorten the anterior (forward-reaching) part of his stride.

Fractures of the symphysis pubis or through the obturator foramen cause the horse to appear lame in both hind limbs. If these areas are affected, the horse will move with a short, mincing gait behind.

What treatment is recommended for fractures of the pelvis?

There are no surgical corrections for fractures of the pelvis. Treatment consists of confining the horse to a box stall and limiting his movements. Slings may aid healing if the horse can be kept in them for six to eight weeks. Complete healing of the pelvis takes at least a year and the horse must be closely confined during this period. Movement must be limited to prevent movement of the bone ends which might sever the iliac artery. At least the first three months must be spent in a box stall, depending on the location and severity of the fracture. In some cases, if the horse is suffering great pain, euthanasia may be recommended because of the long, slow healing process.

16

HEAD AND NECK

ANATOMY AND CONFORMATION

How should the head and neck be conformed?

The head of the horse is generally considered to reveal the intelligence, character, condition and breeding of the individual animal. As a result, it is given a great deal of attention, and characteristics that set a breed apart are often supposed to be most evident in the head. Some features, however, are universal standards.

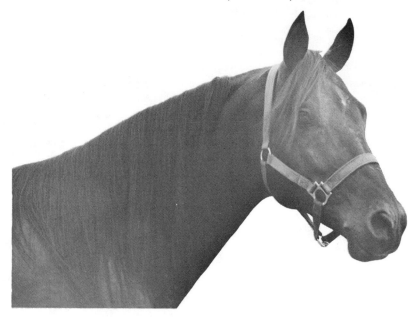

Fig. 16-1. View showing good conformation of the head.

For instance, it is important in every breed that the size of the head be compatible with the size of the body. Also, the features should be chiseled: that is, the bones, muscles and blood vessels well defined. Ears need to be refined (rather than thick), active enough to display alertness, and placed close together over a wide forehead.

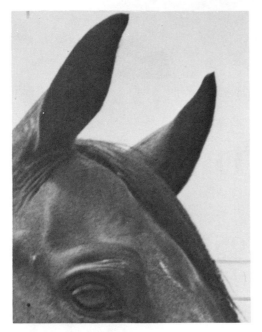

Fig. 16-2. Refined ears.

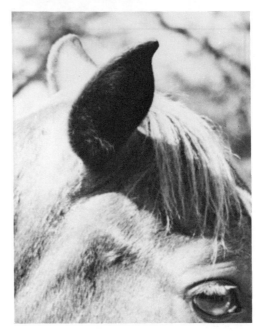

Fig. 16-3. Thick ears.

Eyes that are widely spaced, dark and uniform in color, and large, round and "intelligent looking" are considered of value. Large, thin-walled nostrils combined with wide jowls indicate that the horse can withstand the heavy breathing associated with hard work. A narrow muzzle is preferable, and when open, the mouth should reveal sound lips and sound teeth which mesh firmly together.

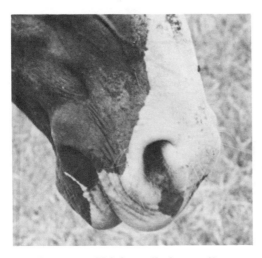

Fig. 16-4. Thick-walled nostrils.

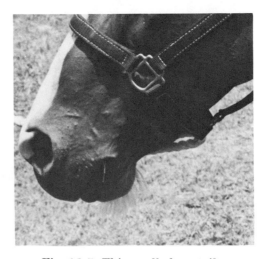

Fig. 16-5. Thin-walled nostrils.

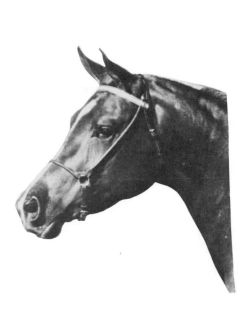

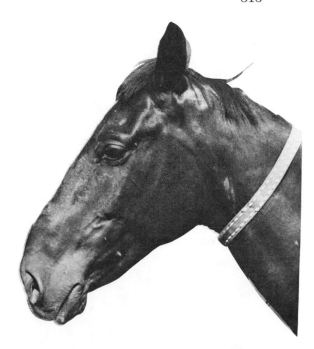

Fig. 16-6. Good conformation of the head, showing a refined muzzle.

Fig. 16-7. Poor conformation of the head, showing a coarse muzzle and a Roman nose.

Further refinements are usually based on the standards of appearance for the Thoroughbred, the Arabian or the Quarter Horse. The Thoroughbred standard demands that the profile of the head show a straight line from ears to muzzle, and prefers a head that is long. Arabians value an undulating profile, or one which demonstrates a bulging forehead and a "dish" below the eyes. Both the Arabian and the Quarter Horse should have short heads, and the Quarter Horse should have large jowls as well. Although it is not always achieved, small, "fox-like" ears are sought in the Quarter Horse.

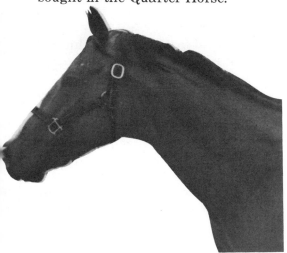

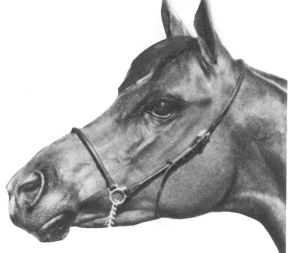

Fig. 16-8. Example of a Thoroughbred head. Notice the long head and the straight line from ears to muzzle.

Fig. 16-9. Example of an Arab head. Notice the short head and the undulating profile.

It is generally agreed that the neck must be in proportion to the head and body, and that the bottom line of the shoulder (from point of shoulder to throatlatch) should be straight. All standards call for a throatlatch small enough for easy breathing, and all accept some degree of arch to the top line of the neck. The Arabian standard is unique in requiring a considerable arch to the neck.

What are some of the common deviations from standards of conformation?

A horse's head may have any number of undesirable conformational traits, but some occur frequently enough to have characteristic names. Ears placed too far apart, for instance, are considered "lopped." "Mule" ears are too long. Too small an eye is called a "pig-eye."

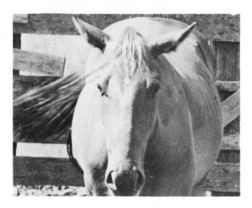

Fig. 16-10. Lopped ears, which are ears placed too far apart.

Even an Arabian may have too much "dish" to its face, or have the dish in the wrong place. A "parrot" mouth is the equivalent of bucked teeth in a human.

The neck is likewise subject to frequently encountered faults. Probably the most common of these is the "ewe" neck. This term indicates that the upper and lower sides of the neck are arched — down. A "swan" neck is properly arched, but is too thin, and sometimes too long. A "close-coupled" neck may indicate jowls that are too large, or a throatlatch that is too thick, either of which prevents the neck from arching properly.

What is the basic bone structure of the head and neck?

The entire complex of bones within the head is referred to as the skull, which is shaped roughly like a four-sided pyramid. Three divisions of the skull, grouped together by function, are commonly made for ease in description.

The function of the cranial bones (or cranium) is to enclose the brain and to form part of the cavities for the eyes and the nasal passages. The spinal cord enters the base of the skull through an opening in the occipital bone, which has an irregular, vaguely triangular shape. The peak of the occipital bone is the nuchal crest, which forms the poll. With the exception of one small bone known as the sutural bone, the roof of the cranium is formed by flat pairs of bones. The largest of these is the parietal bone. The forehead is the widest part of the surface, and is formed by the frontal bone. This bone forms the process (or ridge) immediately over the eye, and this process arches away from the face, joining the cranium at the temporal bones. The "bar" this forms is called the zygomatic arch.

The temporal bone, in addition to forming the zygomatic arch, provides the "canal" or opening into the skull which leads to the middle and inner ear. It also forms the glenoid cavity, which articulates with the mandible (jaw).

The face of the horse includes the lower part of the frontal bones. Other major bones include the nasal bones and the maxilla. The maxilla, premaxilla and palantine bones form the hard palate (roof of the mouth), which contains the upper teeth. This area of the skull houses the nasal cavities, and supports the pharynx and larynx.

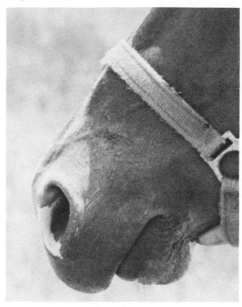

Fig. 16-11. Parrot mouth, similar to bucked teeth in a human.

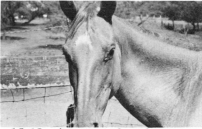

Fig. 16-12. An example of ewe neck, showing the downward arch of the upper and lower sides of the neck.

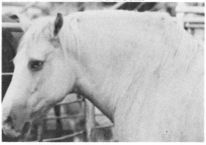

Fig. 16-13. Example of a short, thick, close-coupled neck.

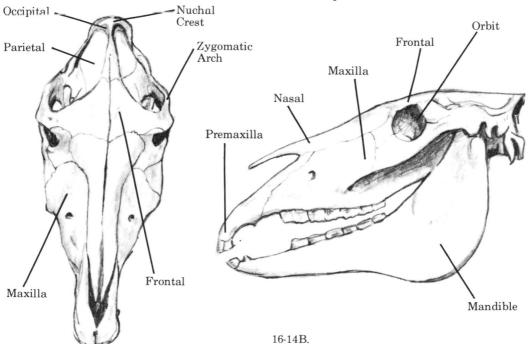

16-14A.

16-14B.

Fig. 16-14. Bones of the skull. A. Top view. B. Side view.

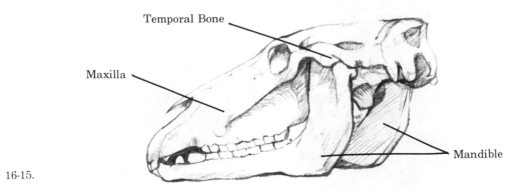

16-15.

Fig. 16-15. View of the bones of the skull, seen from the side and slightly from behind, showing how the mandible hinges on the temporal bone at each side.

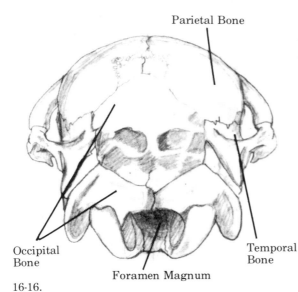

Fig. 16-16. View of the cranium of a newborn foal as seen from behind. The spinal cord enters the cranium through the opening in the occipital bone known as the foramen magnum.

16-16.

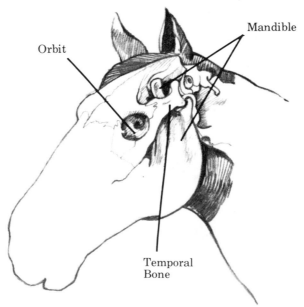

16-17.   Fig. 16-17. A view of the head exposing the ear area of the skull.

The mandible (lower jar bone) of the horse is the largest bone in the face. When seen from the side, it is shaped like a boomerang, one end at the mouth, the other in the area of the cranium. Here it articulates with the temporal bone, at a joint formed by the temporal fossa and the coranoid process. It is actually composed of right and left halves, which are ossified (fused together) in the area of the mouth before birth. The area of fusion forms a flat, horizontal surface, the front of which contains the incisor and canine teeth. The jowls are formed by the rami, which contain the cheek teeth.

With the exception of an occasional extra cheek tooth (premolar) in the upper set, the number of teeth in the lower set is normally the same as in the upper set. The lower jaw of the horse normally contains six permanent incisors, but the two canine teeth may be noticeable only in a male. They have usually all "erupted" into the mouth, replacing deciduous (baby) teeth by the time the horse is five years old. At this age the lower jaw usually has all six premolars and all six molars.

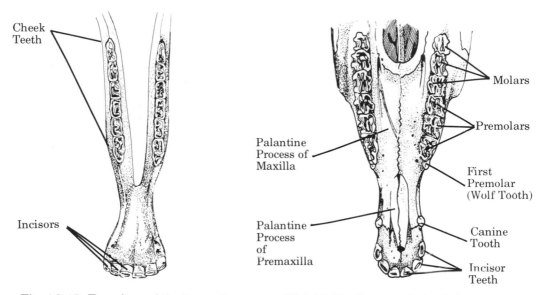

Cheek Teeth

Incisors

Palantine Process of Maxilla

Palantine Process of Premaxilla

Molars

Premolars

First Premolar (Wolf Tooth)

Canine Tooth

Incisor Teeth

Fig. 16-18. Top view of the lower jaw.　　**Fig. 16-19. Bottom view of the upper jaw.**

The cheek teeth of the horse may require dental work, due to the way they mesh. That is, the lower arcades (rows) are closer to each other than are the upper arcades, so that the outside edge of the upper teeth and the inside edge of the lower teeth do not mesh with anything. In addition, the crowns of these teeth are not level, but meet on a line that points upward and inward, toward the roof of the mouth. This conformation predisposes the horse to chew on only one side of the mouth at a time, and to apply pressure to the jaw only when it is moving on the path of least resistance; upward and inward. As a result, the outside edge of the upper teeth and the inside edge of the lower teeth are not worn away by chewing, but become sharp ridges. This can result in cuts inside the mouth or incomplete chewing of feed, either of which can lead to further complications.

The hyoid bone looks much like a smaller jawbone, and it is situated between the two rami of the mandible. Its upper end also attaches to the temporal bone, its lower end to the thyroid cartilage of the larynx. Jutting out of the lower end is a bony spine called the lingual process, which inbeds in and supports the root of the tongue.

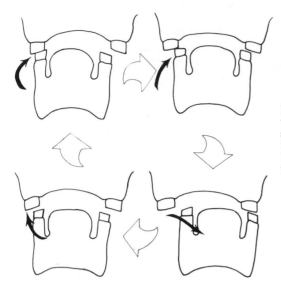

Fig. 16-20. View of the teeth showing the way they mesh, as the horse chews on one side of the mouth at a time. Dark arrows indicate the direction of movement of the lower jawbone as it moves in a circular path.

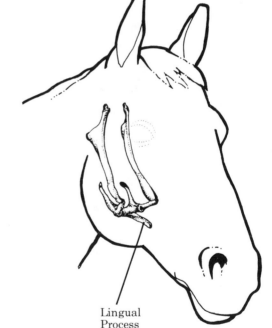

Lingual Process

Fig. 16-21. A view of the head showing the location of the hyoid bone. The lingual process supports the root of the tongue.

What are the bones of the neck?

There are seven bones of the neck, known as cervical vertebrae. For purposes of description they may be divided into three functional groups. The first group consists of the first and second vertebrae, known as the atlas and the axis. The atlas articulates with the occipital bone of the skull, which projects two hook-like bones, called occipital processes, for that purpose. Two deep, oval pockets, the anterior articular cavities, receive the occipital processes. The location of the cavities on the ventral (bottom) side of the atlas forms the joint in a way that allows the head to move up and down independently. The atlas is wide and short, and the dorsal (upper) surface of its ventral arch forms the fovea dentis, a wide, slightly concave articular surface. On this surface rests the odontoid process (dens) of the axis.

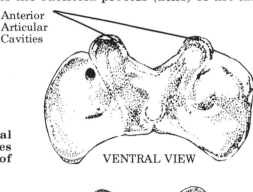

Anterior
Articular
Cavities

VENTRAL VIEW

Fig. 16-22. Atlas or first cervical vertebra. The anterior articular cavities articulate with the occipital processes of the skull.

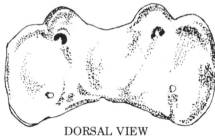

DORSAL VIEW

The axis is the second cervical vertebra. It is the longest of the vertebrae, and is characterized by the presence of the dens, a process that has a profile resembling a thumb. The joint formed by the fovea dentis and the dens allows the head to move independently from side to side. Saddle-shaped anterior articular surfaces are situated on either side of the dens.

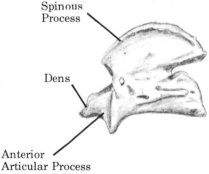

Spinous
Process

Dens

Fig. 16-23. Axis or second cervical vertebra.

Anterior
Articular Process

The third, fourth and fifth cervical vertebrae are very similar to each other in design and function. Each is large compared to other vertebrae, and each has a foramen (opening) for the spinal cord. The ventral portion of the foramen is formed by the body, the upper side by the arch. There are four transverse processes, two to a side, located ventro-laterally from the foramen, and two articular processes, one to a side, dorso-laterally, above and to each side, of the foramen. The spinous process is on the upper surface, the ventral spine on the lower surface. The articular processes of each vertebra slope backward, and articulate with the articular process of the vertebra immediately following. Each vertebra also has an articular surface immediately below the vertebral foramen, front and back.

The sixth vertebra is much like the others in formation. The most notable difference is it is shorter and wider than the preceding vertebrae and the spinous process is larger. The seventh is again shorter and wider, and has a spinous process about twice as high as that of the sixth vertebra. Unlike any other cervical vertebrae, it has two facets on the posterior of the body, which articulate with the first rib.

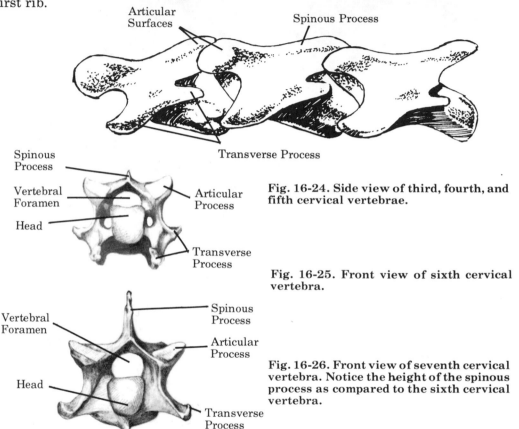

Fig. 16-24. Side view of third, fourth, and fifth cervical vertebrae.

Fig. 16-25. Front view of sixth cervical vertebra.

Fig. 16-26. Front view of seventh cervical vertebra. Notice the height of the spinous process as compared to the sixth cervical vertebra.

What are the basic muscles of the head?

The muscles of the head comprise four different groups. The first group is the superficial (close to the surface) muscles, including those of the lips, cheeks, nostrils, eyelids and external ear. Muscles of the eye are considered as a separate group, as are the jaw muscles and hyoid muscles.

The lips are directly acted upon by at least seven separate muscles. They are closed by, among others, the orbicularis oris, which acts like a sphincter. Often a muscle in this area will act in several ways. For instance, a single muscle may serve both to evelate the lip and dilate the nostril. Each ear is moved by seventeen muscles, in a complex fashion that resembles ball-and-socket joint movement.

Each set of eyelids is acted upon by four muscles. The orbicularis oculi closes the eye, and its opening is assisted by the levator palpebrae superioris.

The lower jaw is moved by six muscles. The largest and strongest of these is the masseter, which covers the jowls and serves to bring the jaws together. The hyoid bone is acted upon by eight muscles, some of which also move the tongue. The genio-hyoideus muscle, for instance, draws both the hyoid bone and the tongue forward.

The neck is directly acted upon by twenty-four pairs of muscles. They are usually considered in two divisions, the ventral cervical muscles, and the lateral cervical muscles. Of the twelve pairs of ventral cervical muscles, three act to flex the head. The remaining ventral cervical muscles act largely to flex the neck.

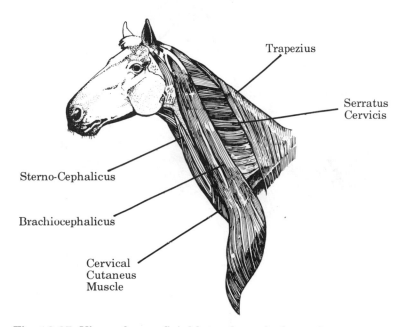

Fig. 16-27. View of superficial lateral cervical muscles.

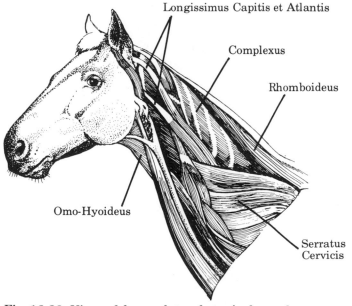

Fig. 16-28. View of deeper lateral cervical muscles.

Fig. 16-29. Muscles Of The Head.

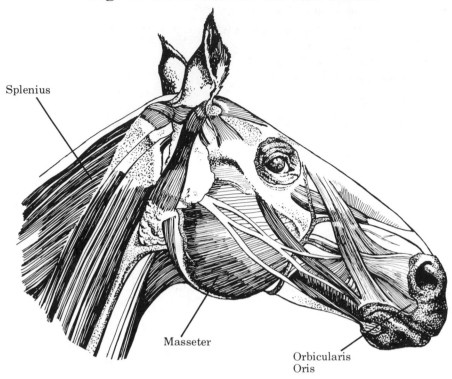

Splenius

Masseter

Orbicularis
Oris

A.

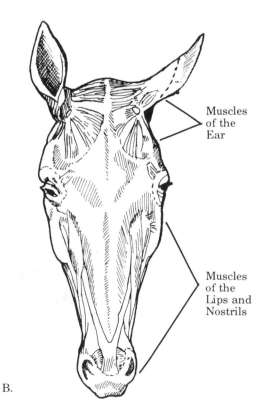

Muscles
of the
Ear

Muscles
of the
Lips and
Nostrils

B.

Fig. 16-30. Muscles Of The External Ear.

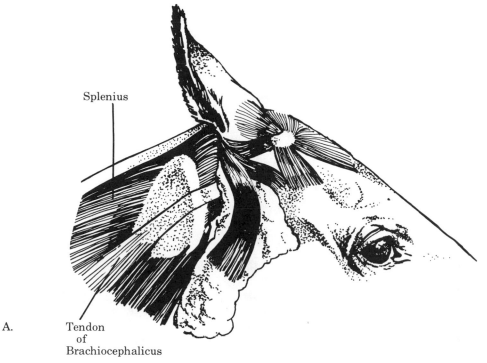

Splenius

Tendon
of
Brachiocephalicus

A.

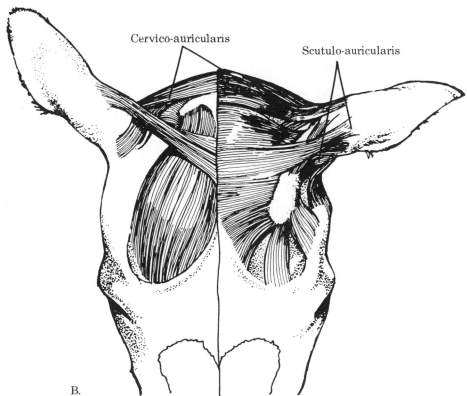

Cervico-auricularis

Scutulo-auricularis

B.

The lateral cervical muscles are arranged in four layers, eight of them being in the fourth (deep) layer. This entire group acts to extend, rotate, flex, incline and elevate the head, and to extend, flex and rotate the neck. In many cases, one muscle can perform several functions. The splenius muscle in the third layer, for instance, can elevate the head and neck, or incline it to one side or the other.

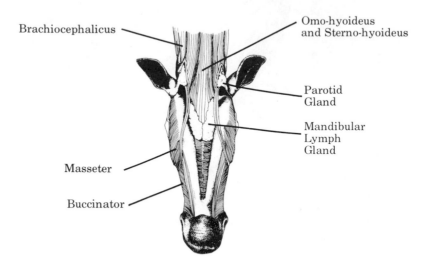

Fig. 16-31. The muscles of the head and neck, as seen from beneath the jaw.

In addition to the musculature, the head is "held up" by a strong, elastic ligament called the ligamentum nuchae. The ligament has two parts, which differ strikingly from each other. The funicular section resembles a cord, and is strung between the nuchal crest (poll) and the peak of the withers. The cord is heavy, flat and thick where it is attached to the skull, but becomes smaller in diameter (about one-half inch) on the back of the neck. Where the cord rubs against the atlas, friction is reduced by the presence of the atlantal bursa (lubricating sac). At the withers the cord flattens and becomes five to six inches wide. The supraspinous bursa lies between it and the bones of the withers, protecting the ligament from rubbing.

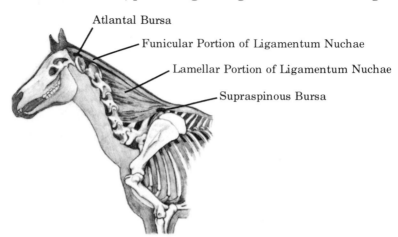

Fig. 16-32. Side view showing the position of the ligamentum nuchae and the atlantal and supraspinous bursae.

The second identifiable part of the ligament is the lamellar part. It consists of two layers of slender fibers. They are strung loosely, attaching to the cervical vertebrae at the upper end, and to the thoracic spines and funicular part of the ligament at the lower end.

THE SENSE OF SMELL

How does the sense of smell work?

Each nostril contains three delicate bones called turbinates. They are covered by a thick, soft, mucous membrane, which is yellow-brown in color.

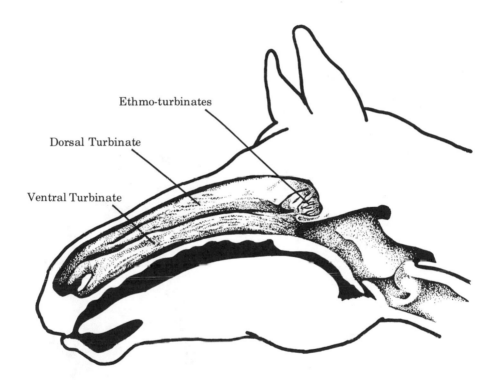

Ethmo-turbinates

Dorsal Turbinate

Ventral Turbinate

Fig. 16-33. Internal view of the head, showing the location of the turbinates.

The dorsal (upper) and ventral (lower) turbinates are long, rolled into the shape of a scroll, and penetrated by many holes, like a sieve. Together with the membranous covering, this contributes to the accuracy of the horse's sense of smell by providing a broad surface for warming and filtering the air.

The ethmo-turbinate is a group of plate-like projections into the back portion of the nasal cavity, originating at the ethmoid bone. The surface of the mucous membrane which covers this structure is penetrated by long, narrow rods which are olfactory nerves. The nerve cells lie just beneath the surface of the membrane, and they project tufts of fine, hair-like cilia into the nasal cavity. It is through these cilia that a chemical interaction is performed with the environment, and a bio-electric impulse is sent along the nerve to the olfactory bulb of the brain.

Each side of the nasal cavity is connected, directly or indirectly, to four air-sinuses. These pockets in the bone lie immediately beneath most of the surface

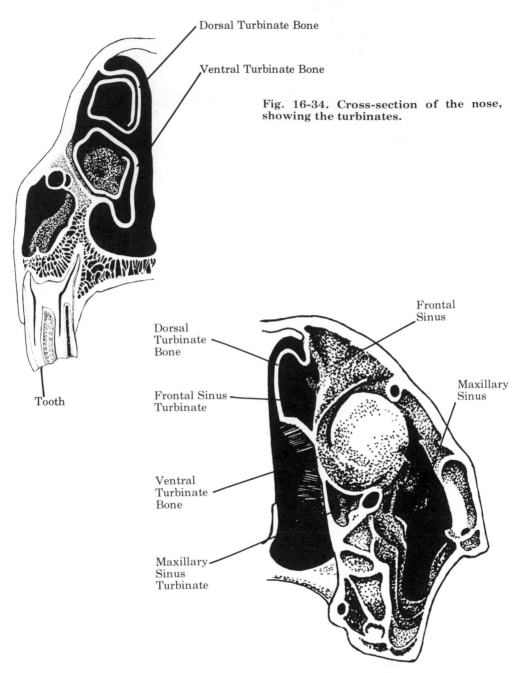

Dorsal Turbinate Bone

Ventral Turbinate Bone

Fig. 16-34. Cross-section of the nose, showing the turbinates.

Tooth

Dorsal Turbinate Bone

Frontal Sinus Turbinate

Ventral Turbinate Bone

Maxillary Sinus Turbinate

Frontal Sinus

Maxillary Sinus

bones of the forehead and occupy some space under the facial bones, immediately beneath the eyes. Lining the interior walls of the sinuses is a thin epithelium (tissue), which may become inflamed in a condition called sinusitis. Sinuses serve no evident purpose beyond rounding out the facial areas of the skull, giving them a smoother appearance.

The nasal cavity itself is quite sensitive, and may be easily damaged. One source of injury is a stomach tube directed through the nasal cavities. Handled too roughly, it can cause pain and prolific bleeding.

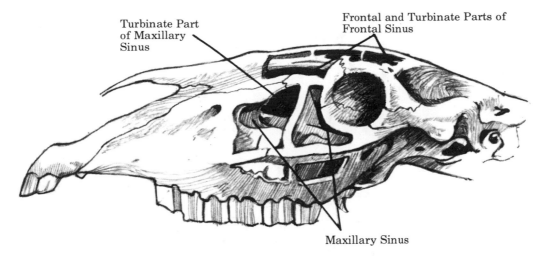

Turbinate Part
of Maxillary
Sinus

Frontal and Turbinate Parts of
Frontal Sinus

Maxillary Sinus

Fig. 16-35. View of the skull, showing the sinuses.

THE SENSE OF SIGHT

What is the basic mechanism of the eye?

The eye of the horse, seen from the outside, has several distinguishing characteristics. The most obvious is the presence of the third eyelid, or nictitating membrane. It consists of a curved plate of cartilage, roughly triangular in shape, that is surrounded by mucous membrane. The third eyelid is positioned at the inside corner of the eye where it serves to "wipe" foreign objects from the eye, in the same manner as a windshield wiper.

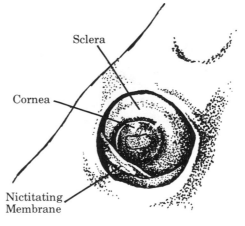

Sclera

Cornea

Nictitating
Membrane

Fig. 16-36. The third eyelid, or nictitating membrane, at the inside corner of the eye.

The eye is lubricated by lacrimal fluid, as is the human eye, which emanates from the lacrimal gland. A further similarity to the human eye is the presence of the lacrimal caruncle, which is the pea-sized prominence at the inside corner of the eyelid. There are two tiny holes near the caruncle. They come together to form a tear duct about 12 inches long that opens into the nasal cavity just above the nostril. This is called the naso lacrimal duct. It carries tears from the eye down into the nose. Clear, watery fluid found in the nostril is lacrimal fluid from the eye above it. If tears from the eye pour out onto the horse's face, there is a good possibility that the naso lacrimal duct is plugged with dirt or other debris.

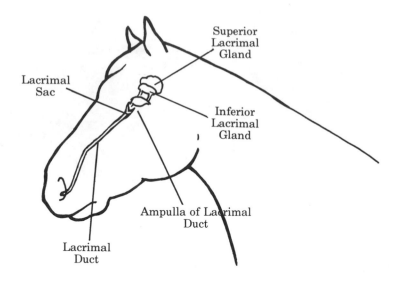

Fig. 16-37. View of the eye and lacrimal apparatus.

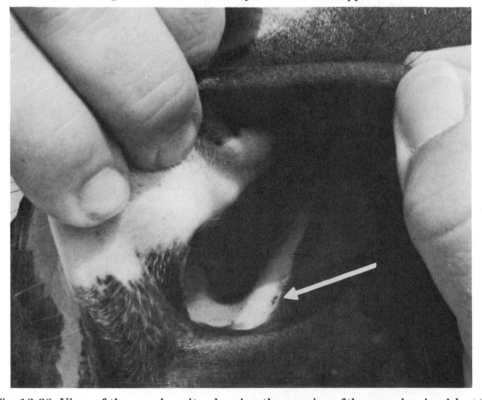

Fig. 16-38. View of the nasal cavity showing the opening of the naso-lacrimal duct (arrow).

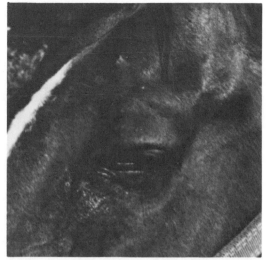

Fig. 16-39. Tears from the eye, caused by blockage of the naso-lacrimal duct.

The eyeball itself is completely surrounded by muscle, fat and tissue, and is directly exposed only at the cornea. The cornea is transparent, colorless, and composed of five layers of tissue. The inside surface of the cornea forms the front wall for a "pocket" called the anterior chamber. Light passes through the anterior chamber to its back wall, where the iris acts as a "valve" to govern the amount of light that continues through. The iris is a muscular diaphragm, the internal edges of which form an opening called the pupil. The edges of the iris directly touch the lens, but the rest of the iris tissue is separated from the lens by another, smaller "pocket" called the posterior chamber. The pupil closes more tightly when the amount of light entering the cornea is greater than the sensitive inner eyeball can withstand. The opening widens when the light is insufficient to permit adequate vision.

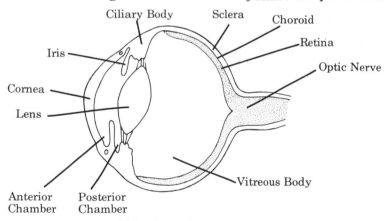

Fig. 16-40. Side view of the structures of the eye.

The pupil opens directly onto the lens, which is convex on both sides. Light admitted through the lens travels through the inner eyeball and strikes the tissue on its back wall, called the retina. This highly sensitive covering picks up the images focused by the lens, which are transmitted to the brain by the optic nerve.

The chambers in front of the lens are filled with a fluid called the aqueous humor. It circulates through the chambers, aiding in nutrition and in the visual process. It passes out of these areas through tissue at the angle created by the cornea and the iris. Blockage of this flow is the cause of several eye disorders, including glaucoma.

The area behind the lens is filled with a clear, gelatinous substance called the vitreous humor, which also serves in the visual process.

How is the eyeball moved?

The eyeball is rotated in the socket by seven muscles. Four straight muscles, called the recti, move the front of the eye up and down, or from side to side. The two oblique muscles draw the eye up and down at an angle, and the retractor muscle pulls the eye back into the head.

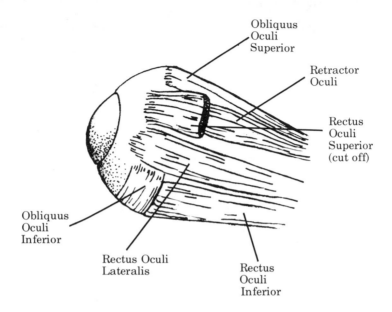

Fig. 16-41. A deep dissection of the eye, showing the muscles which move the eyeball.

THE SENSE OF HEARING

How does the sense of hearing work?

Sound must pass through three different areas in order to reach the auditory nerve, which transmits to the brain.

First, of course, the sound is "collected" by the auricle (external ear). Cartilage forms the basis of the ear, which is funnel-shaped, and in its natural position faces outward and slightly back. This cartilage also forms the upper end of the external auditory canal, while the lower end is composed of an extension of the temporal bone, called the external acoustic process.

The second area is a sound "chamber" called the tympanic cavity or middle ear. It is separated from the external auditory canal by the eardrum. Within the chamber are three small bones that transmit vibrations to the inner ear. The hammer, which is the first bone in the "chain" formed by the three, is moved by the vibration of the eardrum. Its movement in turn disturbs the anvil, or second bone, which articulates with the third bone, the stirrup. Although described separately, these bones actually move as one unit, transferring sound vibrations that occur from the external eardrum to the inner ear.

As in other animals, the horse has a eustachian tube which connects the pharynx to the middle ear. The pharynx is a muscular mechanism in the throat, which is involved in both breathing and swallowing. The eustachian tube is normally closed, except when the horse swallows. At this time, the passage opens into the pharynx, and the resulting flow of air into the middle ear assures that air pressure is equal on both sides (internal and external) of the eardrum. Unlike other domestic animals, the horse has an additional mechanism of the eustachian tube known as the guttural pouch. Air moves in and out of the pouch during respiration, but its purpose is not known.

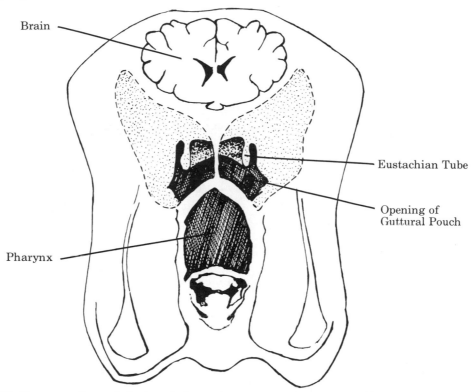

Fig. 16-42. Cross-section of the head through the base of the external ear, showing the location of the eustachian tube and guttural pouch, which is indicated by the dotted line.

The internal ear contains the receptors of the auditory nerve. There are many theories concerning the functioning of the internal ear, but none is completely satisfactory. It is known that the stirrup of the middle ear rests on the oval window of the inner ear, vibrating the perilymph (fluid) it contains. This in turn vibrates a second membrane and the vibrations are finally picked up by the cilia (hairs) of the auditory nerve cells. These are located in a structure called the cochlea, which lies inside the inner ear.

THE SENSE OF TASTE

How does the sense of taste work?

As in man, the taste buds of horses are essentially chemical receptors. They may activate the glosso-pharyngeal nerve, or the trigeminus nerve. Ovoid in shape, the majority of them are on the base of the tongue, or on the soft palate (also on the "floor" of the mouth). Unlike man, the horse also has taste buds on the epiglottis, which is a flap of skin that covers the opening into the windpipe during swallowing. There are normally no taste buds, however, on the tip of the tongue.

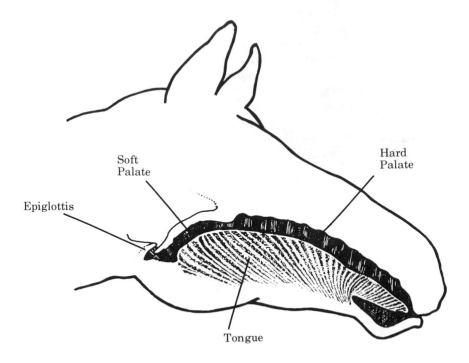

Fig. 16-43. Side view of the head, showing the area of the tongue. The horse has taste buds on the base of the tongue, the soft palate, and the epiglottis.

TORTICOLLIS (DROPPED NECK) (BENT NECK)

What is torticollis?

Torticollis is a condition characterized by a twisted or distorted neck. Many variations are seen, but most commonly the head is lowered and twisted to one side.

What causes torticollis?

Most frequently, torticollis is caused by a fall or severe trauma that bends the neck. The horse may fall over on his side, pinning his neck and head under his body while he is in a stall or in a pasture. Horses often fall when they step on a lead rope that is attached to their halter. This type of injury may also occur if the horse is tied to an object at a point lower than his head and gets a leg over the rope. In the resulting struggle, he may injure his neck muscles, causing a kink or twist. Twisting of the head and neck may be due to spasm or paralysis of the neck muscles, a dislocation of some of the neck vertebrae, or it may be caused by tearing or rupture of one or more muscles in the neck.

What are the signs of this disorder?

This disorder may be so mild that it is difficult to recognize, or it may be so severe that it is obvious. Obvious torticollis is evident if the horse carries his head and neck lowered and to one side. Swelling may be present on the prominent (bulging) side or there may be dips or depressions, if the muscles are torn. The horse will show signs of severe pain, especially if attempts are made to straighten the neck. Some horses with bent neck may be unable to rise when they are first discovered lying down after a fall. Such cases often do not recover much usefulness.

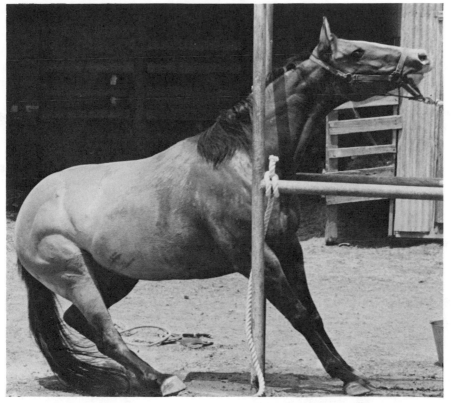

Fig. 16-44. Straining against a rope tied to a pole can injure the neck muscles, resulting in bent neck.

Fig. 16-45. Horse with bent neck. Notice that the head is lowered and twisted to one side.

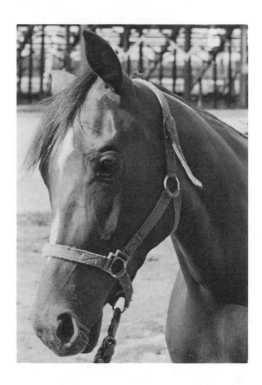

What is the treatment for torticollis?

One of the best treatments for any disorder is prevention. Young horses are especially prone to neck injury when they are tied, so care must be taken to make sure they are tied high enough to be safe. In addition to the danger of getting a foot over the rope, tying a horse lower than his head can cause damage to neck muscles because of the angle of pull. Allowing horses to run free with ropes attached to halters is a common cause of falls and neck injuries, in addition to the equipment breakage it can cause.

If horses are injured, the best immediate treatment is gentle massage of the affected area. The horse may be gently encouraged to straighten his neck as it is rubbed. After the pain has lessened, the veterinarian may suggest a rope with a weight be run through a pulley to the halter to help straighten the neck. In most cases, the veterinarian may want to take X-rays to be sure that the vertebrae are not dislocated or broken. If they are injured, splints may be applied to keep the bones in place while they heal.

GOITER

What is goiter?

Goiter is the term used to describe a swelling of the thyroid gland due to increased stimulation by hormones.

What causes goiter?

The presence of goiter indicates that something is wrong with the mechanism that produces thyroxin, which is a hormone produced by the thyroid that directly affects growth and development. Goiter is usually the result of hypothyroidism, which is insufficient thyroxin in the system. Generally this has a dietary cause, but occasionally animals are born with some physical defect that prevents the circulation of thyroxin through the system.

Hyperthyroidism (excess thyroxin) could also bring about goiter. However, it occurs so rarely in animals that it is thought not to occur naturally.

Hypothyroidism is frequently brought about by a lack of iodine in the diet, which appears to be a critical element in the formation of thyroxin. This hormone is produced by the thyroid gland after stimulation by a hormone from the pituitary gland. In turn, the presence of thyroxin in the system "turns off" the stimulating hormone, and the two maintain a balance. When the lack of iodine prevents the formation of thyroxin, the thyroid continues to be stimulated and its cells multiply in an effort to "catch up" in thyroxin production. The presence of these additional cells results in swelling of the gland called hyperplastic (meaning increased growth in numbers of cells) goiter.

Goiter may also be brought on if the diet of the horse includes goitrogenic (goiter causing) substances, eaten in large amounts. Goitrogens are contained, for instance, in linseed and soybeans, and to a lesser extent in cabbage and its near relatives. Although its presence is required in the body to manufacture thyroxin, excessive amounts of iodine may have the same net effect as a goitrogen. Its excess presence in the system apparently prevents the production of thyroxin.

Are there things other than lack of iodine that can cause goiter?

Mild goitrogens may bring on goiter of a different sort. Colloid goiter occurs when the acini (small, membranous sacs) of the thyroid gland are enlarged, and contain excessive amounts of their natural fluid, colloid. This type of goiter is diagnosed more frequently than hyperplastic goiter. Evidence suggests that this is because a hyperplastic goiter may become a colloid goiter as it degenerates.

Either type of goiter may become a nodular goiter, which means that the swelling of the thyroid localizes into small lumps.

How is goiter diagnosed?

Normally, the presence of large lumps immediately beneath the throatlatch indicates the presence of goiter. In cases of goiter caused by hypothroidism, the signs of that disorder will be present as well. The affected horse will avoid strenuous activity, may put on weight, and demonstrate mental as well as physical laziness. The condition rarely occurs, however, in mature animals. When hypothyroidism is congenital, the result may be stillborn or weak foals, foals with long hair, contracted tendons or poor muscle development. Their weakness leaves them susceptible to infection, and leg fracture is more frequent due to incomplete bone growth. In more advanced stages, cretinism (from the French *cretin,* meaning idiot) results. Cretinism impedes growth in stature and sexual development, and is thought to cause the same mental retardation in animals that it does in humans.

How is goiter treated?

Since the swelling of the thyroid may occasionally indicate an infection rather than a hormonal disorder, a veterinarian should be consulted for further diagnosis. Insofar as hypothyroid-caused goiter is concerned, the best measure to be taken against it is the proverbial "ounce of prevention." This is usually accomplished by making certain that iodine intake is balanced, and that goitrogenic substances are not fed excessively. When goiter is already present, it may be treated with programmed, regular doses of iodine. The prognosis for mature animals is generally good, but is poor for animals severely affected at birth.

GUTTURAL POUCH DISORDERS

What is a guttural pouch?

The guttural pouches are large mucous sacs opening off of the eustachian, or auditory, tube. They are located above the pharynx, below and between the base of the skull and first cervical vertebra.

What type of disorders affect the guttural pouches?

Since the eustachian tube connects with the pharynx, infection and pus formation in the guttural pouches can occur as an extension of pharyngitis (inflammation of the pharynx, see page 427). The infection may spread to the eustachian tube and extend to the lining of one or both guttural pouches. Infection can occur secondary to other respiratory diseases such as "strangles," a bacterial infection.

The formation of pus in the guttural pouches during an infection can lead to another condition involving the presence of chondroids. Chondroids are cheese-like or solid masses formed by mucus and pus which thicken and dry out within the guttural pouch.

A condition which may be a congenital defect of the eustachian tube or a result of inflammation involves an accumulation of air within the guttural pouch known as tympany. A fold of mucous membrane at the mouth of the pouch acts as a valve in

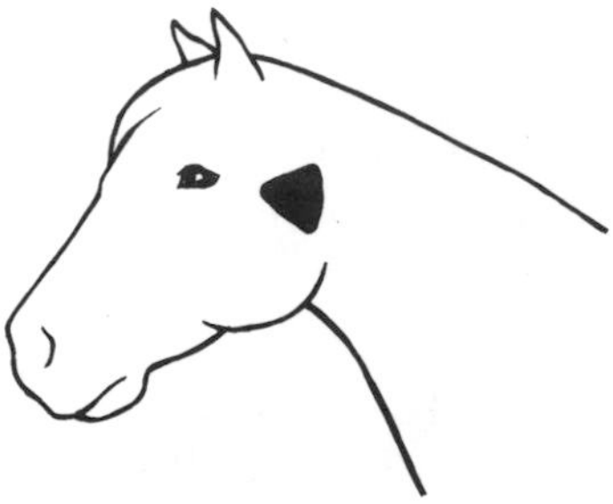

Fig. 16-46. View of the head showing the location of the guttural pouch below the ear.

Fig. 16-47. Internal view of the head showing the location of the guttural pouch.

16-46.

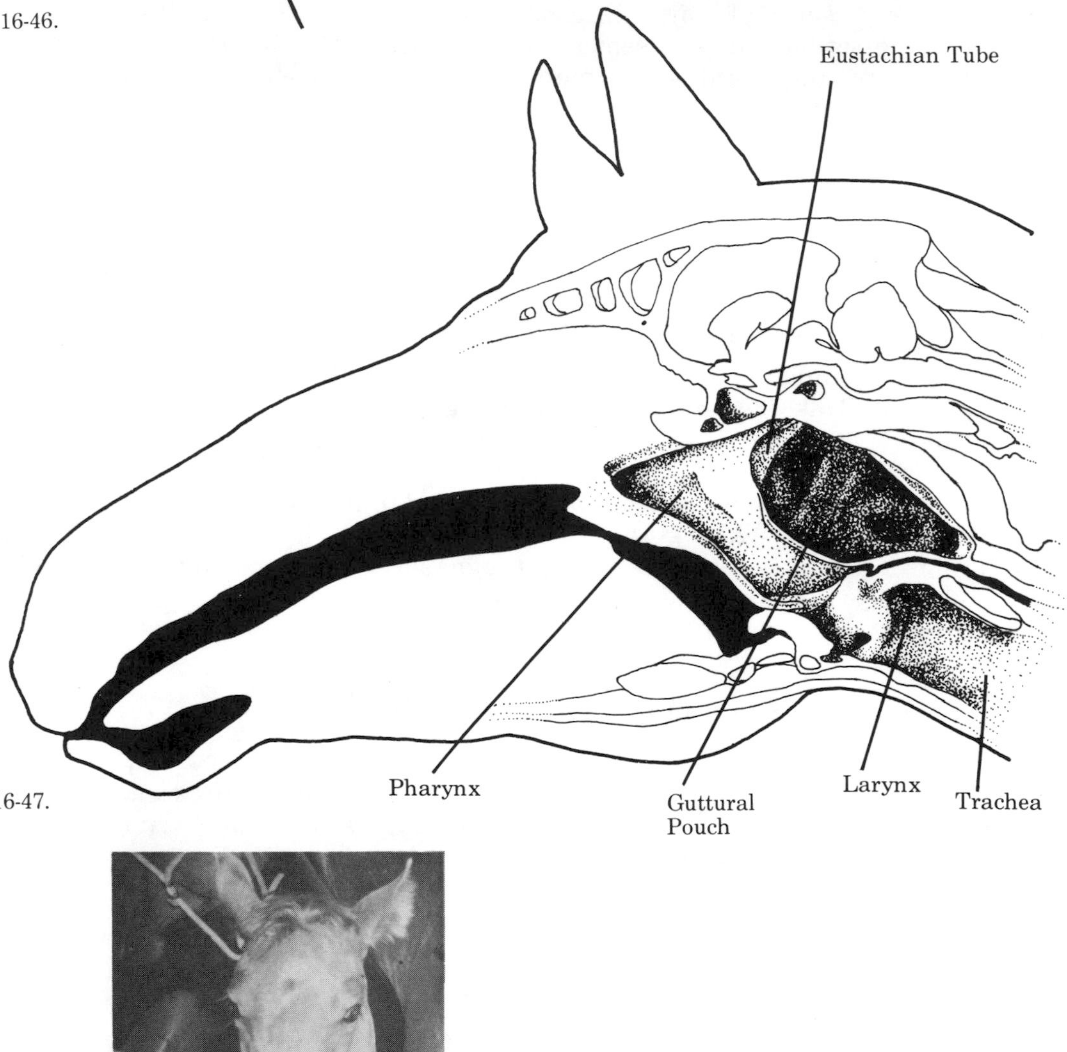

Eustachian Tube

Pharynx

Guttural
Pouch

Larynx

Trachea

16-47.

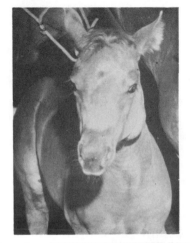

16-48.

Fig. 16-48. A foal with tympany of the left guttural pouch, which is distended with air.

*Photo courtesy of VETERINARY SURGERY, Edition VII,
E. R. Frank. Burgess Publishing Co., Minneapolis Minn.*

tympany and prevents air from leaving the pouch after it has entered the pouch during breathing.

What are the signs of an abnormal condition of the guttural pouch?

When there is pus, whether or not it is in the form of chondroids, present in the guttural pouch, some of the material will be discharged from one and occasionally both nostrils. Blood may be present with the pus; nosebleed can sometimes be due to a fungal infection of the guttural pouch. The nasal discharge is increased when the head is lowered or shaken and the horse may seem to have difficulty swallowing. There may be a painless swelling of the parotid gland located below the ear and behind the jaw, which when compressed results in an increased nasal discharge.

Tympany is characterized by a large painless swelling in the same area, the region of the parotid salivary gland. The horse often has difficulty breathing and may stand with the head and neck extended. Eating may result in coughing and a discharge of food particles through the nostrils. If the swelling is aspirated (sucked out, usually with a syringe and needle) by a veterinarian during diagnosis, air may escape from the pouch with considerable force. This would indicate a large amount of pressure on the area of the eustachian tube and pharynx and would explain a difficulty in breathing and swallowing.

How are these conditions treated?

Conditions involving the guttural pouch usually involve surgery by the veterinarian. The carotid artery (main artery of the neck) and several cranial nerves are adjacent to the guttural pouches and may be easily injured, hence the procedure is more involved than the lancing of a superficial abscess. Infections of the guttural pouch may not always require surgery, but if not, the pouch still must be repeatedly catheterized and flushed with sterile saline solution and antibiotics. Attention must also be given to the treatment of any underlying infections.

Chondroids and tympany usually require surgery to open and examine the guttural pouch. Chondroid masses are removed, along with any fluid present, and the pouch is allowed to drain. The guttural pouch is then flushed daily with an antibiotic solution until healing is completed in two to four weeks. Surgical treatment of tympany may not be successful and the air will continue to accumulate in the pouch. In some cases, surgical removal of the membranous flap is successful and air will then pass freely between the guttural pouch and eustachian tube.

LAMPAS

What is lampas?

Lampas is not a disease. It is a swelling or filling of the mucosa and mucosal tissue that covers the roof of the mouth just behind the front teeth.

What causes lampas?

Most frequently, the swelling occurs when the permanent incisor teeth erupt, usually at the ages of 2½ to 4 years. Older animals may develop swelling in this area if they are fed ear corn, grazed on coarse pasture, or are affected with inflammations of the mouth and gums.

What are the signs of lampas?

The swelling behind the front teeth forms a ridge that projects below the level of the upper teeth, causing severe irritation. This irritation may make it very difficult for the horse to eat, causing him to seem disinterested in food. If this region is examined, it may be hard and swollen. Drooling may occur and the horse may smack his lips frequently.

How is lampas treated?

Feeding should be made easier for the horse with mashes and rolled grains which require less chewing. Good quality hay should be fed from a manger or rack, to avoid excessive contamination with gravel or sand. No specific medical treatment is usually required, unless lampas accompanies other inflammations or infections of the mouth. Harsh treatments (lancing, rubbing salt in the wounds) are ineffectual and should not be used.

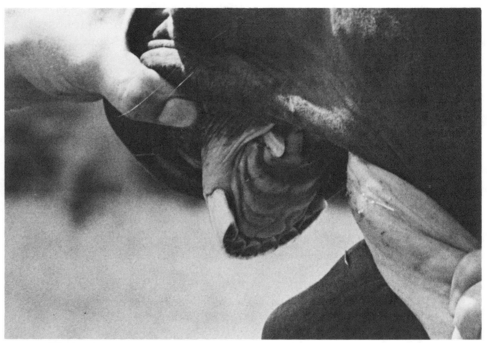

Fig. 16-49. View of horse's mouth showing lampas. Notice the swelling of the hard palate behind the front teeth.

DENTISTRY

What regular dental care does a horse require?

Horses, more than any other large domestic animal, have difficulties with their teeth. In light of this fact, veterinarians generally examine teeth at birth, and at about two years of age the horse is put on a regular dental program. Not every point of the program is covered in each examination, but teeth should be examined every six months. In younger horses, the program should include removal of wolf teeth, which hamper movement of the bit, and removal of parts of deciduous (first set) teeth that do not fall out naturally. Teeth of older horses must sometimes be corrected for "waving" or uneven wear. In all cases, it is necessary to check for and correct damaging sharp edges on the cheek teeth.

What are the signs that a horse needs dental attention?

The most obvious sign of dental trouble is a change in chewing habits. For instance, the horse might pause for short periods while chewing or hold its head to one side. The horse might be observed in a habit called "quidding," in which food is rolled into balls rather than chewed and then dropped on the ground. Rather than chew on a painful tooth, a horse may swallow before chewing is complete. This can cause colic and indigestion. Other signs include the presence of excess saliva, blood in the saliva, halitosis, swelling of the face or jaw, refusal to eat hard grain and loss of condition.

Occasionally a problem with dental origins will show up in a place other than the mouth. An ear fistula (seeping lesion) called a dentigerous cyst, for instance, is a tumor that involves dental material, but drains to the outside of the face near the ear. However, this is an exceptional problem.

What dental problems can a horse have at birth?

Some congenital (inborn) problems include teeth which do not mesh properly for chewing, the presence of extra teeth, or individual teeth that are improperly placed. Imperfectly meshed teeth (such as parrot mouth, similar to bucked teeth in humans), can only be filed periodically to prevent worsening of the condition. Individual teeth need not be pulled unless they interfere with eating or working. Deciduous teeth that do not "shed" properly are easily removed with forceps.

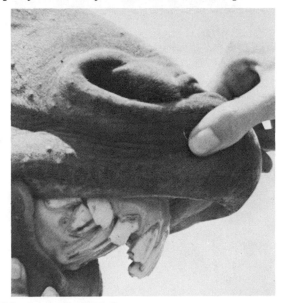

Fig. 16-50. View of parrot mouth, a congenital defect.

What commonly causes dental trouble in later life?

Mature horses can generally expect their dental problems from irregular wear, disease or injury. Irregular wear is not at all uncommon, and treatment usually consists of filing the teeth to conform more closely to normal wear. In very old horses or in severe cases, this may not be successful.

There is some question as to whether or not horses form dental cavities. The usual source of tissue degeneration is the gums. One common problem of this sort is alveolar periostitis, in which an infection of the gum results in the growth of an infected tumor on a tooth. An involved tooth must be removed, since further infection or the formation of fistulae may follow.

The most frequently fractured tooth is the fourth molar, which may be broken when a rock or other hard objects are picked up in feeding. Incisors may be damaged in accidents or by a direct blow.

Fractures of the teeth are usually treated by removal of the fragment, or of the entire tooth if the root has been injured.

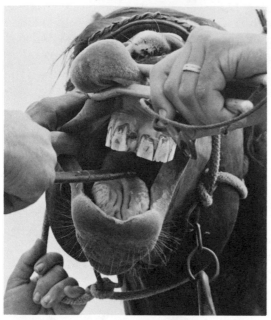

Fig. 16-51. Filing the teeth, a common practice referred to as floating the teeth.

How is extraction of teeth accomplished?

For any dental extraction, the horse is normally given a general anesthetic. While incisors may be removed with forceps, long roots make this an unsatisfactory procedure for cheek teeth. Molars are generally removed by drilling into the jaw above (below, for the lower jaw) the affected tooth, and tapping it out with a mallet and dental punch. This should only be attempted by a veterinarian, since it entails the risk of injury to other teeth, the jaw and facial nerves.

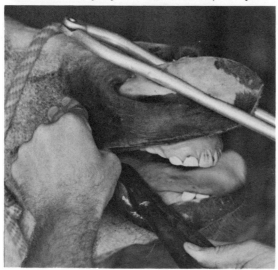

Fig. 16-52. Removing the first premolar tooth (wolf tooth).

DENTIGEROUS CYST

What is a dentigerous cyst?

A dentigerous cyst is a type of tumor which contains different kinds of tissue, including hair, teeth and sebaceous material, a thick oily substance of fat and epithelial cells. The cyst is also known as an ear fistula or conchal sinus.

What does a dentigerous cyst look like?

The cyst appears as a swelling at the base of the ear, arising from the temporal bone at the side of the skull. A discharge of sebaceous material and fluid continually drains from the lesion and sinus underneath, causing a loss of hair around the area of the ear.

A dentigerous cyst is usually seen in young horses, and may exist before birth. Its growth can be slow or rapid at the time it is first seen, but in most cases growth is very gradual over a long period of time before the cyst becomes evident.

How is the cyst treated?

The veterinarian will surgically remove the cyst by careful dissection, detaching it from the temporal bone where it is often attached by small dental fragments. The contents of the cyst are removed after surgery and the cavity will be packed to control hemorrhage. The packing will be removed on the second day after surgery, and the cavity flushed with a saline solution and an antibiotic. The lesion will usually heal in about ten days.

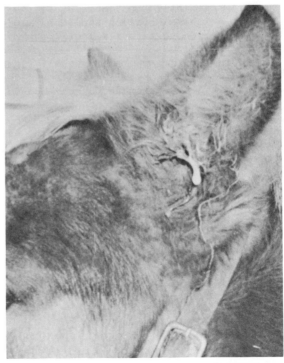

Fig. 16-53. Dentigerous cyst. Notice the discharge at the base of the ear.

Photo courtesy of VETERINARY SURGERY, Edition VI,
E. R. Frank, Burgess Publishing Co., Minneapolis, Minn.

MECHANICALLY INJURIOUS PLANTS

What are mechanically injurious plants?

Mechanically injurious plants are those which cause injury to the sensitive tissue in the mouth of the horse. They may cause injury by scraping or scratching the mucous membranes or gums, or they may lodge between the teeth and in the tissues of the mouth.

What are some of the plants that cause mechanical injury?

Very dry hay may cause damage in the mouth, along with the various types of thistles, cacti, foxtails, thorny shrubs, stickers and bristles that are available to horses. Frequently, injurious material is baled in the hay. In particular, yellow bristle grass is known to cause acute irritation to the gums, tongue and lips. When material lodges in the mouth, ulcers may develop and infection can spread rapidly.

What are the signs of this type of injury?

Affected horses may have a great deal of difficulty eating if lodged material prevents movement of the tongue and lips. Visible signs may include swelling of the nose and lips, swelling and irritation of the tongue, drooling or the discharge of pus from the mouth. The breath may have a terrible odor if the membranes have become infected or if food material is decomposing in the mouth.

How are plant injuries of the mouth treated?

Most injuries of the mouth heal very rapidly if the foreign material is removed. The veterinarian may have to tranquilize the horse, or deaden areas of the mouth, in order to remove lodged thistles and thorns. Prevention of injury includes the removal of possibly injurious plants from pastures and hay. Frequent examination of the mouth, in most cases, can prevent the development of ulcers and infection.

VESICULAR STOMATITIS

What is vesicular stomatitis?

Stomatitis is an inflammation of the soft tissues of the mouth. When the lesion is a vesicle, or blister, and is localized, the condition is referred to as vesicular stomatitis. It is an infectious disease characterized by the development of vesicles in the mucous membranes of the mouth or on the skin of the foot.

How does the horse contract the disease?

The disease is caused by a virus which may be transmitted by biting insects such as mosquitoes, stable flies and horseflies. Insect bites or skin abrasions appear to be necessary for infection to occur, but contagion can be caused by consuming feed or water that has been contaminated by saliva and vesicular fluid from an infected animal. Transmission was once believed to occur by contact between animals or with contaminated objects such as common feed troughs, but it is often impossible to explain the spread of the disease by contact. The method of transmission is still not completely clear. Insects appear to play a large part in the spread of the disease both locally and from infected to clean areas since the incidence of vesicular stomatitis is high during hot weather and in low lying areas. Few cases are seen during cold weather, with about 90% of the cases occurring in August and September.

What are the signs of vesicular stomatitis?

Excessive salivation is usually the first sign of the disease; saliva dribbles from the lips and drops on the food. Vesicles varying in diameter from a few millimeters to three centimeters (about ¼ to 1¼ inches) may be seen on the mucous membranes of the lips and tongue, but they usually rupture so rapidly that they may not be observed. They can last up to 24 hours, and vesicles on the tongue usually grow together and cover half of the tongue's surface before rupturing. The lesion becomes deep, raw and bleeding, with shreds of dead skin at the margin. This irritation causes the profuse salivation and the horse eats very little at this time because chewing is so painful.

Will the horse have lesions only in the mouth?

The horse may sometimes have secondary lesions on the feet, with lesions appearing on the coronary band. Pressure on the hoof is painful and causes the animal to limp. Separation of the hoof wall from its underlying structure can occur, in rare instances, causing a loss of the entire hoof. Vesicular stomatitis is similar to foot-and-mouth disease in other species, but the horse is not susceptible to the foot-and-mouth disease virus.

Is diagnosis of vesicular stomatitis difficult?

Diagnosis is not difficult since other viral or bacterial infections in horses do not produce a similar set of signs and lesions. It is similar to horse pox but can be differentiated by the absence of pustules in vesicular stomatitis. A diagnosis can be confirmed by a veterinarian by isolating the virus from a sample of skin tissue, saliva or vesicular fluid.

What is the treatment for vesicular stomatitis?

The animal should be made as comfortable as possible and provided with plenty of water and soft feed. Treatment is seldom undertaken but mild antiseptic mouth washes may contribute to the horse's comfort and recovery. If there is evidence of a complicating infection, a veterinarian should provide the proper symptomatic treatment. Ordinarily, recovery is prompt and complete in about two weeks.

Can the disease recur after recovery?

Within ten days to two weeks after development of the infection, antibodies to the virus can be detected in the blood. These give the horse a fairly firm immunity, of at least a few month's duration, to reinfection by the same type of virus. Vesicular stomatitis can be caused by two similar but distinct viruses, and there is no cross-immunity between the two viruses. Neither killed nor live virus vaccines have been used to immunize horses.

How can the disease be prevented?

Prevention has been based primarily on management. An animal which is kept stabled and protected from insects apparently has little chance of becoming infected, even in an area where the disease is being transmitted. Hygienic and quarantine precautions will help keep infection from spreading to nearby animals, and the disease will usually die out of its own accord.

HORSE POX

What is horse pox?

Horse pox is a contagious disease characterized by ulcers and pustules on the mucous membranes of the mouth, the skin of the lips and the skin in the pastern-fetlock region. In general, it is not a serious disease, but badly infected horses become weak and occasionally young animals will die. Horse pox occurs in Europe only rarely and no cases have been reported in the United States.

What causes the disease?

Horse pox is caused by a virus which is identical with the virus of true cow pox. Individual outbreaks stem from a previous case of horse pox, and possibly from a case of cow pox or a human being recently vaccinated against small pox.

How is the disease spread?

The infective material is contained in the vesicles, or blisters, and pustules, and is spread by contact with brushes, combs, saddles and other contaminated equipment. The virus can also be spread by handling, as in shoeing.

What are the symptoms of horse pox?

In the leg form, the first noticeable sign is heat, tenderness and swelling of the back of the pastern, causing pain and lameness. In about four days the area begins to exude drops of slightly yellowish fluid, which later forms a crust on the surface of the skin as a yellow mass matting the hairs together. After about ten days, with treatment, the inflammation subsides and healing begins.

When the disease is located at the lips and nostrils and mucous membranes of the mouth, various stages can be seen. First nodules form, which develop into vesicles with clear, straw-colored contents, then into pustules about the size of a pea, and finally into scabs. These lesions in the mouth will cause salivation and a lack of appetite. Recovery occurs in about 15 to 20 days, after which the horse will have a solid immunity to the virus.

How should horse pox be treated?

The affected parts should be treated with ordinary astringent and antiseptic dressings. The infected horse should be isolated and anything which may have become contaminated should be disinfected. This would include feed troughs, bits, grooming tools, and even hands and clothing of attendants. The virus is easily destroyed by ordinary antiseptics.

RHINOSPORIDIOSIS

What is rhinosporidiosis?

Rhinosporidiosis is a nonfatal fungal infection which is characterized by growths on the mucous membrane of the nasal cavity.

What do the growths look like?

The growths, in one or both nostrils, vary in size from ½ to 1¼ inches (about 1 to 3 cm) in diameter. They are attached to the mucous membrane and protrude into the nasal cavity, sometimes blocking the passage enough to make breathing difficult. The growths are soft, mottled pink in color, and covered with a thin glistening membrane. They are well supplied with blood vessels and will bleed easily.

Do these growths appear only in the nostrils?

The infection only affects the nostrils and will not spread to other parts of the body.

Are there other signs of the infection?

There may be nasal discharge of mucus and pus, sometimes mixed with blood, from the lesions. The horse will have difficulty in breathing, caused by large growths blocking the air passage in the nostrils, and will make loud snoring noises.

What causes rhinosporidiosis?

The infection is caused by a fungus but its source is not yet known. It has been suggested that the natural habitat of the fungus is in water, since infected animals have often used stock tanks or ponds, streams and rivers as sources of drinking water. The infection is not contagious.

How is rhinosporidiosis treated?

A veterinarian must make a microscopic examination of the nasal discharge or the contents of a lesion to make a definite diagnosis and to differentiate the infection from similar fungal infections such as cryptococcosis (see Cryptococcosis, page 437). The lesions can be surgically removed, but they may return if the entire mass is not removed. Healing is usually complete within a few weeks.

NEOPLASMS

What are neoplasms?

Neoplasms are new, abnormal growths of cells commonly referred to as tumors. They resemble the healthy cells they arise from but they do not have a useful function. Their cause is not yet clearly understood, but possible explanations include viruses, parasites, chemicals, irradiation and injury.

Are neoplasms harmful?

The cells multiply rapidly without control, and it is this uncontrolled growth that makes neoplasms so destructive. They may be classified as either malignant or benign, depending on the type of growth and its effects. In a malignant tumor, cells invade and destroy surrounding cells, and by a process known as metastasis, can spread the disease to other parts of the body by being carried away in the bloodstream or lymph. Without treatment, these tumors may cause enough damage to the body that the animal eventually dies. Benign tumors are much less dangerous and can usually be successfully treated so that the animal fully recovers from the effects of the growth. Benign neoplasms do not recur but malignant ones may reappear even after treatment.

How are neoplasms treated?

Surgical removal is the preferred treatment for all tumors, although radiation therapy is useful in some cases. Medication may be completely successful in treating neoplasms, but the tumor will often recur in six months to two years.

What type of tumors commonly affect the horse's head?

The most common tumor in horses is the cutaneous sarcoid which usually appears around the head but may be transferred to other sites (see page 403). These tumors appear as soft, fleshy nodules on the skin (cutaneous) with a consistency of hardened cottage cheese. They have not been known to spread to internal organs of the body, and the only problem seems to be that they detract from the horse's appearance. Cutaneous sarcoids may be surgically removed, but they usually reappear at the same site. Their precise cause is unknown, but sarcoids and papillomas (warts) are probably caused by viruses.

Can warts on the surface of the head spread to the mouth?

Cutaneous warts on the face and lips sometimes spread to the mucous membranes of the mouth. Warts that occur only in the mouth probably are caused

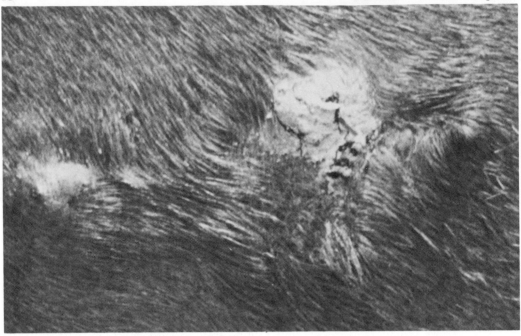

Fig. 16-54. An area of the skin showing a cutaneous sarcoid which has been surgically removed but is regrowing.

Fig. 16-55. Cutaneous warts on the muzzle, which is a common site for warts.

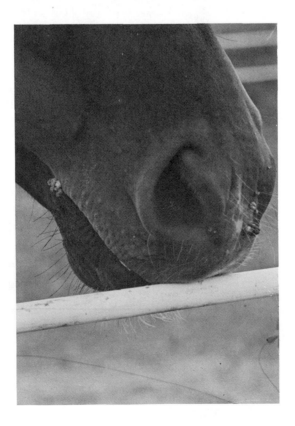

by a different virus from the one that causes warts on the skin. (For more information on Warts, see page 401.)

What other types of tumors may appear in the mouth?

Squamous-cell carcinoma is a common type of neoplasm affecting the mouth and pharynx of the horse. This tumor is a malignant growth of one type of epithelial cell. Some growths on the horse's gums may not be actual tumors but merely abnormally large masses of tissue caused by injuries or dental abnormalities.

Are the teeth ever affected by neoplasms?

Dental tumors have been found in horses, especially in young animals. One type of dental tumor, seen in newborn foals, is usually fatal because it causes an abnormal distortion of the face and prevents the foal from nursing. It may be the result of hemorrhage within the developing tooth.

Most dental tumors are benign, but their surgical removal is usually impossible because of their size and the amount of facial or jaw distortion that they cause.

Do neoplasms ever appear in the nose and throat?

Tumors of the sinuses and the nose are rare in horses. When they do occur, they may involve the structures of the tear ducts, causing an excessive overflow of tears. Tumors in the throat region may cause swallowing difficulty if allowed to grow. These tumors can usually be seen and felt on the lower neck region.

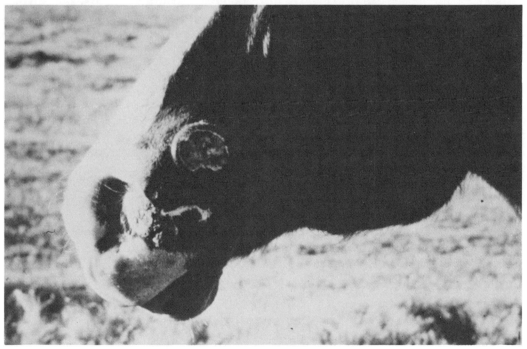

Fig. 16-56. Neoplasm involving the nose.

Do tumors within the eye commonly occur?

Various types of tumors may occur within the eye, but are not as common as those involving the eyelids. Tumors of the orbit surrounding the eye are rare and are usually an extension of a tumor from the nictitating membrane (third eyelid). Signs of orbital tumors include exopthalmos (protrusion of the eyeball), squinting and limited movement of the eyeball.

Are there such obvious signs when other tumors of the eye occur?

Other tumors may occasionally involve the deeper structures of the eye but are not as noticeable as those of the eyelids and orbit. Corneal neoplasms are rare but may arise from the membrane covering the eyeball. They can usually be treated by surgically removing the outer layer of the cornea, or by radiation treatment. The eyeball can then be saved but the horse will usually be blind in the affected eye. Treatment of a corneal dermoid, a congenital tumor (see page 361), is usually more successful and the horse's vision is limited only by the presence of scars on the cornea.

What type of tumor may involve the eyelid?

The most common type of neoplasms affecting the eyelids are sarcoids and squamous-cell carcinomas, which involve the upper and lower lids, the lid margins, and the conjunctiva lining the lids. Sarcoids of the eye are flesh-like nodules which contain connective tissue cells. They are seen more often in young animals than in old ones. Squamous-cell carcinomas are malignant new growths of one type of epithelial cells.

How do these neoplasms affect the eye?

Both types of neoplasms are malignant and will invade and destroy the surrounding areas, seriously damaging the rest of the eye. The cells can later transfer by metastasis to other parts of the body, spreading the disease further. Metastasis is when cells break off the tumor and are carried by the blood vessels until they lodge up in a small artery (embolism) and grow at this new site. Sarcoids and squamous-cell carcinomas will often recur after treatment.

How are tumors of the eyelids treated?

Radiation therapy is usually effective for squamous-cell carcinomas, but is not very successful in the treatment of sarcoids. In most horses, these tumors can be surgically removed, restoring normal vision and normal use of the eyelids. Recent developments in plastic surgery of the eyelids may also help the horse regain normal function of the eyelid. Full recovery of the use of the eye depends on the size and position of the tumor and how long it has been there.

STRANGLES

What is strangles?

Also known as distemper, strangles is a contagious pus-forming abscess of the lymph nodes in the upper respiratory and cheek mucosae.

What causes strangles?

Strangles is caused by infection with *Streptococcus equi* which only infects horses. The infection begins in the pharyngeal and nasal mucous membranes, then drainage carries the infection to the lymph nodes. Severe infection, in rare cases, may spread to other organs, causing suppurative (pus-forming) processes in the kidney, liver, brain, spleen, tendon sheaths and joints. Young horses are most susceptible, but strangles may occur in animals of any age. Infection is passed among horses by contamination from nasal discharges which may be ingested or inhaled in droplets. Water troughs, pastures or feed may be contaminated and remain sources of infection, even if horses are not present, for almost a month. Horses can spread the infection for at least four weeks after a clinical attack of strangles.

What are the signs of strangles?

Following an incubation period of three to eight days, the first sign of strangles is reluctance to eat or drink. Proper diagnosis at an early stage can greatly reduce the extent and spread of the disease, which may be destructive if a veterinarian is not called. Fever (103°— 106°F) and violent inflammation of the pharyngeal and laryngeal mucous membranes are accompanied by a thick, mucus nasal discharge which quickly becomes heavy and full of yellow pus. Pain from the seeping abcesses may cause the animal to stand with the neck stiffly extended. A moist, painful cough is usually present, and the animal is reluctant to swallow. Development of swelling and abscesses in lymph nodes of the throat (usually the sublingual node) may take three or four days. This is the stage in which most glands discharge pus and may rupture. Strangles usually begins to subside after the tenth day of infection, particularly if it is treated effectively. Death from strangles is rare and is usually due to general poor condition and inability to withstand the infection.

What is the treatment for strangles?

Infected animals should be isolated immediately and treatment begun with penicillin. Other drugs may be used, such as chlortetracycline or tetracycline if the disease is rather advanced when diagnosis is made. Treatment usually prevents systemic involvement, but abscessed lymph nodes may continue to enlarge and eventually rupture. Abscesses are usually not opened surgically unless it is for diagnostic purposes. Pure cultures of S. equi for diagnosis are difficult to obtain any other way because contaminants, especially S. zooepidemicus, invade abscesses very rapidly after they begin to drain. Applications of warm compresses to abscessing nodes will encourage them to break open and drain. Penicillin should be continued for at least a week after the abscesses drain and the temperature returns to normal.

How can strangles be prevented?

Vaccination is the best general preventative for strangles. Isolation of infected animals can prevent epidemics of strangles and is recommended for new additions to a herd or group. In some horses, purpura hemorrhagica may follow vaccination, though this is relatively rare. Previously unvaccinated horses should receive the S. equi bacterin in three 10 ml. doses at weekly intervals. The vaccine is not given to newborn foals, and is reduced to one "booster" shot for horses that are known to have had strangles. Vaccination on a yearly basis involves a single "booster" dose.

STREPTOCOCCUS ZOOEPIDEMICUS

Is there another respiratory disease similar to strangles?

A bacterial infection by Streptococcus zooepidemicus will produce signs similar to those of strangles. Differences between the two infections involve the presence of fever and the rapid development of abscesses in strangles, and the two species of bacteria responsible for the diseases can be easily distinguished from one another.

Does S. zooepidemicus always cause infection?

The bacterium does not always cause infection since it may be normally present in the skin and mucous membranes of healthy horses. It usually cannot produce disease unless those areas of the body have already been affected by viral respiratory infections or wounds. S. zooepidemicus is a common cause of wound infections and will often attack the upper respiratory tissues after they have been damaged by an upper respiratory virus.

What are the signs of *S. zooepidemicus* infection?

The horse will usually have a nasal discharge of mucus and pus. Many small abscesses will form in the region of the pharynx above the soft palate and in the lymph nodes draining that area. The infection usually spreads to other nearby lymph nodes, but abscesses do not form as rapidly as in strangles. Infection may involve other parts of the upper respiratory tract, including the sinuses and tear ducts.

Can the infection be fatal?

Streptococcal pneumonia almost always occurs after influenza in foals, and is the usual cause of death from influenza in young horses. Pneumonia caused by *S. zooepidemicus* can occur immediately after influenza or some other viral infection in horses of any age. The streptococcal infection may result in chronic pleuritis, an inflammation of the membrane surrounding the lungs. This causes the horse to cough and have difficulty breathing, which after a few months destroys the horse's usefulness.

Does the infection only involve the respiratory tract?

S. zooepidemicus can also infect the mare's reproductive organs. A healthy mare will usually not be infected unless she is injured while giving birth or becomes infected with other bacteria. *S. zooepidemicus* can affect various parts of the reproductive tract, causing inflammation of the cervix and lining of the uterus. Infection in a pregnant mare often results in abortion.

Can the foal of an infected mare become infected?

Foals may become infected in the uterus or during birth. Inflammation of the umbilical stump will then be observed during the first two weeks after birth, and the foal may have a mild fever. The infection can rapidly lead to septicemia (blood poisoning) or severe arthritis, with fatal or crippling effects.

How can the infection be treated?

Diagnosis and treatment should be undertaken by a veterinarian, since the infection may resemble other conditions which would require a different regimen of treatment. Penicillin, administered to the mare and newborn foal, is effective in killing *S. zooepidemicus*.

Can this bacterial infection be prevented?

Hygienic breeding procedures and treatment of genital diseases before breeding help prevent bacterial infections which may cause abortion in the mare. *S. zooepidemicus* is easily killed by the ordinary chemicals used in disinfection. Infection in the respiratory system is much more difficult to prevent since it occurs with influenza and other viral infections. There is no useful vaccination available yet to immunize horses against *S. zooepidemicus*.

Can a horse have a natural immunity after the infection?

Horses recovering from strangles develop some immunity to it that is of variable duration, but horses recovering from *S. zooepidemicus* infection do not. They may be infected repeatedly, but the infection may be from different strains of the bacteria. So far, 15 types of *S. zooepidemicus* have been found and there may be more, but no one type has been identified yet with a specific effect of the infection.

SINUSITIS

What is sinusitis?

Sinusitis is any inflammation or infection of the nasal sinuses, the air cavities within the head.

What causes sinusitis?

Infection of the sinuses can be secondary to respiratory diseases such as strangles (see page 350) and other infections of the nasal passages, or from diseases of the molar teeth. The anterior maxillary sinuses on each side of the cheek and the posterior maxillary sinuses just below each eye contain the roots of the upper molars. These sinuses may become infected when the involved teeth are diseased. In chronic sinus infections, the septum, a thin wall of bone and cartilage dividing the sinuses, may erode. Infection can spread from the nasal passages to the maxillary sinuses by direct extension through the small openings which connect them to one another. These sinuses are also common sites for tumors which often become infected with streptococcal bacteria.

What are the signs of sinusitis?

There will be a continual discharge of pus from one nostril and occasionally from both. Tapping with one knuckle on the bone just below the eye will cause pain to the horse, indicating an accumulation of pus in the posterior maxillary sinus. A veterinarian should be consulted since a nasal discharge of pus is a common symptom of many diseases. There may also be other infections present related to sinusitis that will need to be diagnosed and treated by the veterinarian.

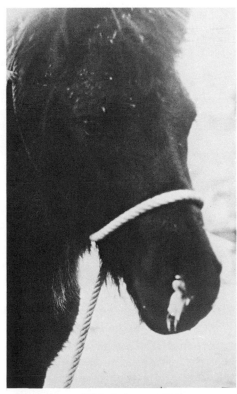

Fig. 16-57. A pony with a nasal discharge, which may be a sign of sinusitis.

Photo courtesy of W. L. Anderson, D.V.M.

How is sinusitis treated?

The infected sinus is usually trephined, a process of removing a small circular disk of bone from the area of the sinus, leaving an opening into the cavity. The pus in the cavity is aspirated and any dead membrane and bone removed. The trephine hole is then plugged with cotton or gauze.

The cotton plug is removed daily and the sinus is flushed with warm saline solution or warm water and antibiotics. The plug is replaced and the horse is exercised so the fluid can drain through the sinuses and nasal passages out through the nostril. This treatment is continued for several days until pus no longer drains from the nostril. The trephine hole is kept plugged to prevent it from healing over before treatment of the sinus has been completed.

Is a trephine hole always necessary to treat sinusitis?

When there is not a heavy accumulation of pus in the sinus, trephination may be unnecessary if the infection responds to medication. In the case of a sinus infection caused by a diseased tooth, removal of the tooth will allow for drainage and the sinusitis will respond well to post-operative treatment with antibiotics. Trephination of a sinus may eventually be necessary to clear up a persistent nasal discharge.

LACERATIONS OF THE EYELID

What causes lacerations of the eyelid?

A horse's eyelid can be lacerated or torn by such objects as barbed wire, nails, thorns, etc. The eyelid can be bruised or scraped from an external injury such as a blow or fall.

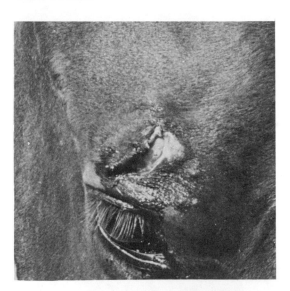

Fig. 16-58. A laceration above the eye. The torn edges will be sutured together to close the wound.

How should a lacerated eyelid be treated?

When an eyelid is torn, never remove the hanging portions, since all of the fragments still attached will be needed for healing. If too much of the eyelid is removed, the scar tissue that forms after healing may contract and pull the eyelid out of shape. Have a veterinarian examine the horse immediately, since injuries to the eyelids are difficult to handle unless treated early. Although eyelids are often torn, they are rarely completely removed. Most lacerations can be repaired by a veterinarian by suturing the torn edges of the lid. An antibiotic and a corticosteroid, if there is a lot of swelling, may be applied to the eyelid after it is repaired. The horse should be cross-tied or wear a neck cradle to prevent it from rubbing the eye until the lid is healed.

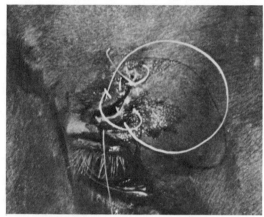

Fig. 16-59. Suturing the edges of the skin lacerations seen in 16-58.

TRAUMA TO ORBIT

What is trauma to the orbit?

Any injury to the bony cavity containing the eyeball is a trauma to the orbit.

What causes a trauma to the orbit?

The orbit can be damaged in trailer accidents, horse fights, blows inflicted by the handler and contact with foreign objects. Simple to compound fractures may occur in the supraorbital process of the frontal bone or the zygomatic arch. In these cases, the amount of damage to the eyeball depends on the extent and displacement of bone fragments.

How should this injury be treated?

A veterinarian should examine the eye and check for a bone fracture. Fractures with a minimal displacement of bone fragments usually do not require surgery. Repair of compound fractures with several fragments and extensive displacement involves cleaning the wound, removing the small bone fragments and immobilizing the larger ones. Treatment for the eyeball usually involves application of antibiotics and other medication.

Is recovery from the injury complete?

A simple orbital fracture should heal without problems, but compound fractures with a lot of trauma to the orbit may create further problems because of possible damage to the eyeball and possible infection of orbital tissues.

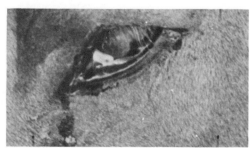

Fig. 16-60. An atrophied, dysfunctional eye caused by trauma to the orbit and damage to the eyeball.

ORBITAL CELLULITIS

What is orbital cellulitis?

Orbital cellulitis is an inflammation of the tissues surrounding the eyeball.

What causes the condition?

The condition occurs in injuries and as an extension of bacterial infections of the sinuses, salivary glands, teeth and other organs in close proximity to the eye.

What are the signs of orbital cellulitis?

Signs usually develop within 24 to 48 hours and are normally in only one orbit (the bony cavity around the eye). The eyelid and tissues around the orbit are swollen and red, with the swelling causing the eyeball to protrude. Any eye movement is painful to the horse, and there may be a discharge of mucus and pus from the corners of the eye. The horse usually has a fever and lacks appetite.

How is orbital cellulitis treated?

The horse should be examined by a veterinarian since most diseases of the orbit require early diagnosis and treatment to prevent irreversible damage to the eye. The horse should be kept in a darkened stall, with warm compresses frequently applied to the eye. The veterinarian may sedate the animal to relieve pain, and will administer antibiotics until the inflammation and swelling have subsided. If abscesses form in the orbit, they should be surgically drained. The eye should be covered with a protective bandage if the eyelid cannot cover the protruded cornea.

Will the horse fully recover from orbital cellulitis?

Recovery depends on how soon the diagnosis is made and how soon the condition responds to treatment. The more rapidly the infection responds to treatment, the better the chance of normal vision being restored. If inflammation of the orbit continues over a long period of time, the muscles around the eye may be damaged. The fat surrounding and cushioning the eye may be reabsorbed, and the optic nerve may eventually be damaged. A horse that has one eye set normally and one eye set deeply in its orbit has probably suffered orbital cellulitis in the past. An eye so affected probably has lost most, if not all, of its vision.

CONJUNCTIVITIS

What is conjunctivitis?

Conjunctivitis is an inflammation of the conjunctiva. It is one of the most frequent ocular diseases in the horse. The inflammation can be acute or chronic, and primary or secondary. Conjunctivitis may be unilateral or bilateral.

What causes conjunctivitis?

Foreign objects such as a seed hull or any of a number of bacterial or viral infectious agents that get into the conjunctival sack can cause primary conjunctivitis. One bacterial agent that has been identified in primary conjunctivitis is *Moraxella*. *Thelazia* is a small nematode (unsegmented worm) that can live in the conjunctival sack, causing conjunctivitis. Irritation caused by flies getting around the eyes and feeding on the secretions of the eye are a frequent cause of conjunctivitis. This usually becomes secondarily infected if effective fly control measures are not quickly put into practice.

Secondary conjunctivitis is a sequel to other ocular and systemic diseases. Many viral and bacterial infections may be accompanied by conjunctivitis, such as influenza, rhinopneumonitis, equine viral arteritis and strangles.

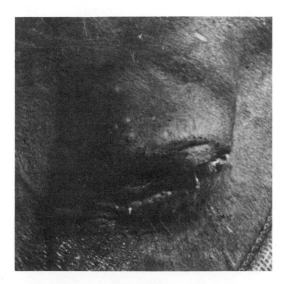

Fig. 16-61. Conjunctivitis. Notice that the eyelids are swollen and there are tears on the face.

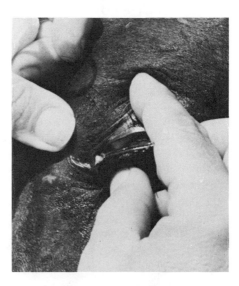

Fig. 16-62. Conjunctivitis, showing the exudate at the corner of the eye.

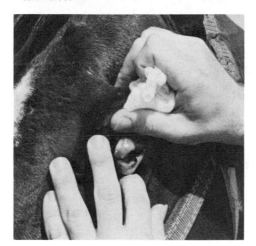

Fig. 16-63. Conjunctivitis. The membranes lining the eyelids are exposed to show the inflammation.

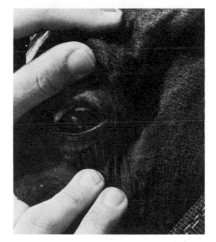

Fig. 16-64. A normal, healthy eye.

Chemical agents such as soaps, tick dips, or a foreign object of any type or size may initiate acute conjunctivitis. Often dust, mud, pollen, sprays, smoke, grain husks or grit are the causes.

What are the signs of conjunctivitis?

With conjunctivitis there is evidence of inflammation of the conjunctiva (membrane that lines the eyelid), swelling of the eyelids, and exudation which may be serous, mucous or purulent in nature. Erosion of the lid margins is common in cases that have been established for several days or more. *Thelazia* cases can be chronic with numerous enlarged lymph follicles and a discharge that is part serous and part mucoid.

If a foreign body becomes embedded in the conjunctiva, there will be muscle spasms which nearly close the eylid, moderate pain and excessive lacrimation (tear secretions) in nature's attempt to wash out the object. Due to the pain, the horse will be reluctant to allow the eye to be examined. At first the discharge will be watery, but will become thicker and stickier with time (mucopurulent exudate).

How is conjunctivitis treated?

Antibiotics are applied topically to treat primary conjunctivitis caused by a *Moraxella* infection. A *Thelazia* infection will require the veterinarian for treatment. He will administer a local anesthetic to locate and remove the white nematodes with forceps. Use of a topical organic phosphate miotic (drug which constricts the pupils) will help locate the nematodes since it induces their rapid movement.

Of course, any foreign bodies embedded in the conjunctiva must be removed. Treatment of acute conjunctivitis involves the use of antibiotics and corticosteroids about four times daily for 7 to 10 days. Chronic cases may take four to six weeks of treatment. Laboratory culture and sensitivity tests to determine the causative agent will help in selection of an effective antibiotic.

As a first aid measure, the affected eye can be washed with a lukewarm saline solution. Allergic reactions will need cold packs and corticosteroid ophthalmic ointments. Affected horses should be kept in a darkened stall as bright light seems to add to their discomfort.

INJURIES TO THE CORNEA

How do eye injuries affect the cornea?

Damage to the cornea, the thick, tough clear covering of the front of the eyeball, may take the form of erosions of the corneal surface (known as ulcers), lacerations and penetrations. Any of these injuries can be caused by sharp objects such as thorns and branches or by the lash of a whip.

What effects do ulcers of the cornea have on vision?

Corneal ulcers, lacerations and penetrations of the cornea may all leave scars after healing. These scars are opaque areas which will partially block the horse's vision. A scar's effect on vision depends on its position on the cornea, its thickness, and its size. A large, thick scar in the center of the cornea will drastically decrease the field of vision in the affected eye. Most superficial scars can be surgically removed to reduce their size by 80 to 90%, improving vision and the appearance of the eye.

What are the signs of a corneal ulcer?

An ulcerated cornea will usually be cloudy, and the site of the erosion can often be clearly seen. The conjunctiva, the delicate membrane lining the eyelids and covering the front of the eyeball, will be swollen and congested. The horse will avoid light and there may be a serous discharge from the eye at first, often becoming a discharge of pus at later stages.

How are corneal ulcers treated?

With most corneal injuries, the animal should be kept in a darkened stall and warm compresses may sometimes be applied to the eye. Minor shallow abrasions that involve only the outermost layer of the cornea may heal spontaneously in 24 to 36 hours, with little or no scarring. An antibiotic should be applied to the area to prevent infection.

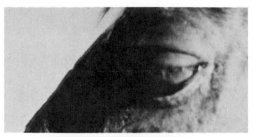

Photo courtesy of W. L. Anderson, D.V.M

Fig. 16-65. Ulceration of the cornea. Notice that the cornea is cloudy and the eyelids are swollen.

Fig. 16-66. Severe ulceration of the cornea.

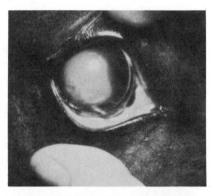

Photo courtesy of EQUINE MEDICINE AND SURGERY, Edition II, American Veterinary Publications, Inc., Wheaton, Ill.

Deep ulcers should also be treated with topical application of antibiotics and checked daily for the formation of blood vessels in the cornea. This vascularization may occur after any injury to the cornea, especially one resulting in an ulcer. Starting at the edge of the cornea, branching blood vessels grow across the cornea within a few days. The horse's vision is then limited since light must pass through the blood vessels in the cornea, which is normally clear, before reaching the retina. Some deep ulcers will heal of their own accord within 10 to 14 days, and the blood vessels will disappear spontaneously. Chronic ulcers that do not heal may need to be cauterized by a veterinarian with heat or special chemical preparations to stop the growth of blood vessels on the cornea. If vascularization of the cornea is not controlled, many layers of epithelial cells may develop over the blood vessels, making areas of the cornea thick and opaque.

If spontaneous healing of a corneal ulcer can occur, is treatment necessary?

If a corneal ulcer or other injury is not treated surgically or with a specific antibiotic, secondary bacterial infection may set in and cause inflammation of the eye. The eye may be bandaged to protect the cornea until the ulcer has healed. If a bandage is not used, the lids may be sutured together to protect the cornea, or a flap from the conjunctiva may be used to cover the cornea and provide support. Inflammation will almost always leave noticeable scars on the cornea, resulting in partial blindness. If the entire eye becomes severely inflamed and does not respond to treatment, the eye may have to be removed.

What are the signs of a lacerated cornea?

After an injury by a sharp object, a tear (laceration) may be seen in the cornea. The tear may be partial or complete, cutting through all the layers of the cornea. In full-thickness lacerations, the aqueous humor (the fluid in the anterior chamber behind the cornea), will escape through the tear and the eyeball will collapse as it loses fluid. The iris may prolapse and protrude through the tear in the cornea. When this happens, a gelatinous coat around the iris usually forms a plug, stopping the leakage of the aqueous humor and securing the iris within the cut edges of the cornea. With a prolapse of the iris, a dislocation, or luxation, of the lens (see page 366) may occasionally occur.

How are lacerations of the cornea treated?

A partial-thickness laceration, which can weaken the cornea, is sutured and an antibiotic is applied to the area at least five times daily for two to three weeks. Antibiotics may also be given systemically.

In full-thickness lacerations with a recently prolapsed iris, the iris should be replaced in the eyeball. If the prolapse has existed for a while, the protruding portion of the iris should be surgically removed. The cornea will then be sutured and air injected into the anterior chamber to rebuild the pressure within the eye, bringing it back to its normal shape. This will prevent the iris from adhering to the cornea during healing as it would if the eyeball were allowed to remain collapsed. The injected air in the chamber will soon be replaced with aqueous humor. The cornea should be protected while healing by suturing the lids together or suturing a conjunctiva flap or nictitating membrane (third eyelid) flap over the cornea.

What are the chances of the horse recovering its vision?

If the laceration is deep and the entire eye is affected, the eye may eventually have to be removed. If the entire thickness of the cornea has not been cut and the laceration is treated soon after it occurs, the horse will probably regain most of the sight in that eye. Otherwise, the chances of recovery of full vision are slight, especially when other structures of the eye are affected and possibly lost, and when there are post-operative complications such as infection in the eye.

How does penetration of the cornea affect the eye?

Penetration of the cornea by a sharp object such as a thorn or splinter can often cause inflammation which may leave opacities in the cornea, partially blocking normal vision. A penetrating object which causes a large tear in the cornea may cause problems similar to a full-thickness laceration, including collapse of the eyeball and prolapse of the iris. Complete perforation of the cornea can lead to loss of sight in the eye, but if there is no secondary infection, most of the sight can be restored. Vision would then only be limited by the position and size of the scar or opacity in the cornea.

How are penetrations of the cornea treated?

A thorn or splinter still in the cornea should be removed by a veterinarian after the horse has been tranquilized and the eye has been locally anesthetized. The puncture wound may need to be sutured. An antibiotic is administered topically and systemically until the cornea has healed. If the puncture wound is so deep that the iris, lens and vitreous humor (the fluid between the lens and retina) are involved, the eye may need to be removed immediately.

CORNEAL DYSTROPHY

Are there any defects of the cornea not caused by injury?

There are several types of corneal disorders or deformities that are medically defined as dystrophies. Some of these have been occasionally observed in horses. Dense white deposits, which are possibly fat deposits, may form at the edges of the cornea. Blood vessels may also form across the surface of the cornea, limiting the horse's vision. This superficial vascularization may occur in diseased corneas and in corneas that are apparently normal.

A corneal disease involving the appearance of small, irregular lesions throughout the cornea occurs occasionally in the horse. The lesions may represent areas of tissue degeneration, local inflammation, or the presence of Onchocerca larvae, minute worm larvae.

Irregularities in the cornea, especially the lower half, are apparently due to an uneven thickness of the front portion of the cornea. They may cause astigmatism, a condition in which the horse's vision is blurred since the uneven surface of the cornea prevents light from being sharply focused on the retina.

Opaque areas in the cornea may be associated with a high tension within the eye (glaucoma, see page 367), or a low tension. With a low tension within the eye, the cornea is swollen and covered with superficial blood vessels. It contains irregular lines which are folds in the membrane at the back of the cornea. There is no satisfactory treatment for corneal changes associated with this reduced tension within the eye.

CONGENITAL ANOMALIES OF THE CORNEA

Are there any congenital defects of the cornea?

A few congenital defects or anomalies of the cornea have been observed in horses. Melanosis and dermoids can be surgically corrected, but microcornea is a condition that cannot be treated.

What is microcornea?

Microcornea is the condition of an abnormally small cornea. It usually occurs with microphthalmia (abnormally small eyeball), although it has been seen in foals with normal-sized eyeballs. The cornea may measure less than 10 mm. in diameter, and the horse's field of vision will be much less than normal.

What is melanosis?

Congenital melanosis in the eye is an increase in pigmentation of some of the structures of the eye. It rarely affects the horse's cornea, but when it does, the pigmentation is usually located in the center of the outer layers of the cornea. Blood vessels are usually present in the pigmented areas. The areas present at birth usually do not become larger and are sometimes surgically removed if they are large enough to obstruct vision.

What are dermoids?

Corneal dermoids are benign tumors which can be successfully treated and will not recur.

What do these tumors look like?

The lesions are small, flat, skin-like growths located at the lower edges of the cornea in one or both eyes. Long hairs usually grow from the surface of the growth, adding to the irritation of the eye. The eye will have a serous discharge and a corneal ulcer (see page 358) may occasionally occur as a result of a dermoid. Dermoids in horses are often pigmented and may be mistaken for malignant melanomas, a more serious type of tumor.

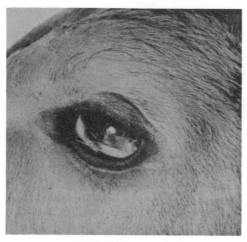

Fig. 16-67. Corneal dermoid. Notice the long hairs growing from the surface of the growth.

Photo courtesy of VETERINARY SURGERY, Edition VI, E. R. Frank, Burgess Publishing Co., Minneapolis, Minn.

Can dermoids be treated?

Dermoids can be treated by surgically removing the outer layers of the cornea. Perfect vision will not be restored, though, since there will be some scarring of the cornea after surgery. When dermoids are observed in the foal, some veterinarians recommend removing the growth at an early age (four to six weeks) to avoid complications.

DISORDERS OF THE IRIS

What type of disorders may affect the iris?

The iris is a muscular sheet containing a central opening, the pupil. The muscles of the iris increase and decrease the size of the pupil to adjust the amount of light entering the eye. Conditions affecting the iris include cysts of the iris and congenital anomalies.

What do cysts of the iris look like?

Cysts of the iris are bulging, fluid-filled sacs which may appear as dark areas above the pupil.

How do cysts of the iris affect the eye?

Cysts may occur in one or both eyes, in the iris and in the corpora nigra. Corpora nigra are small black structures at the edges of the iris which act as shades, absorbing excess light after the pupil has fully contracted in bright sunlight. The cysts may then interfere with the normal function of the pupil in dilating and contracting, which is regulated by the iris and corpora nigra. They can accompany atrophy of the iris, and can also be congenital.

How are cysts of the iris treated?

The front wall of the cyst is usually surgically removed, reducing the size of the cyst enough to allow the pupil to function normally. If an iris cyst is not serious enough to interfere with vision, it may not need to be treated. Iris cysts may rupture with intensive use of a mydriatic, a medication causing the pupil to dilate.

What are congenital anomalies of the iris?

Congential anomalies are abnormalities present at, and usually before, birth. They may or may not be hereditary; some defects may actually be hereditary but have not yet been proven to be inherited. Congenital anomalies of the iris include pigmentation, hyperplasia of the corpora nigra and aniridia.

What are pigmentation abnormalities of the iris?

The iris of the horse is usually dark brown. Congenital anomalies in pigmentation, or coloration, involve differences in color in the two irides, or in different areas of the same iris. These differences in color (heterochromia) are not common in horses and no diseases have been associated with them. The colors involved are usually combinations of brown, white and blue. Heterochromia in part or all of the iris is referred to as wall eye, or partial albinism in the affected eye. Glass eye, or total albinism in the eye, refers to an eye with an iris that is nearly white with pigmentation only in the corpora nigra. A glass eye is sometimes seen in a white or palomino horse or a horse (of any color) which has a blaze surrounding the eye. The eye not covered by the blaze may be partially albinistic, although this will probably not occur in horses with black skin, such as bays and browns.

What is hyperplasia of the corpora nigra?

Hyperplasia is greater than normal growth and development of the corpora nigra. The corpora nigra, located at the edges of the iris, may become so large that they block the horse's vision, especially when the horse is in bright sunlight. The horse may show signs of poor vision and tend to shy from objects more than normal. The condition can be corrected by surgical removal of the enlarged corpora nigra.

What is aniridia?

Aniridia is the absence of an iris. Hereditary aniridia in both eyes occurs occasionally in Belgian horses, but has not been reported in any other breeds. The vision of affected horses is poor or absent, with the iris nearly totally absent. Various types of cataracts are usually present, along with the aniridia.

CATARACTS

What are cataracts?

Cataracts are opacities that affect the lens of the eye. A cataract may be congenital, i.e., present at birth, and may continue to grow. The condition may also be acquired sometime in life because of an eye injury or infection. Although cataracts affect only the lens of the eye, they can affect either the lens substance or its capsule.

Are all cataracts alike?

No. There are many variations of cataracts. These variations are classified according to cause, maturity, age and position in the lens. Cataracts classified by cause are listed as congenital, primary or secondary.

Maturity classification progresses through incipient (beginning) to immature to mature to hypermature. Age classification concerns itself with the time of life in which the horse is stricken, i.e., congenital, juvenile and senile. A broader means of classification of cataracts lists them as developmental or degenerative.

Congenital cataracts can affect any part of the lens but are generally found in the central, posterior cortical area. Congenital cataracts may be associated with abnormally small eyes and are usually bilateral. If a horse has a cataract in only one eye, it is usually the result of trauma or disease and, consequently, there is a better chance of clearing up the problem.

Developmental cataracts are those which arise during growth because of hereditary, nutritional or inflammatory changes and alter the normal development of the lens fibers and epithelium. This grouping includes the various congenital cataracts.

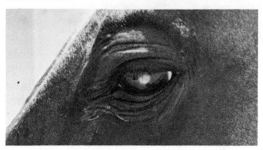 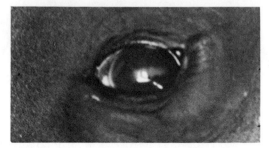

Fig. 16-68. A cataract. A portion of the opacity is clearly visible to the left of the square area of reflected light in the center of the eye.

Fig. 16-69. A cataract. Notice the round opaque area in the center of the eye.

Degenerative cataracts are those which arise, after normal development, from various causes such as trauma, diabetes, etc. and include senile nuclear and cortical cataracts.

The position of the cataract may determine whether the opacity will progress, regress or remain stationary; e.g., nuclear cataracts often remain stationary and may reduce in size as the lens ages, while equatorial cataracts are generally progressive.

What causes cataracts?

As stated before, a cataract can be present at birth, or it can be the result of some injury or disease later in life. Related diseases could be any systemic disease, inflammations of the eye parts, glaucoma, luxation, etc.

Changes in the layers which make up the lens sometimes result in cataracts, but most often the development involves some slight excess of fluid between the layers of the lens.

What are the effects of cataracts?

The effect of cataracts on vision is dependent on the size, density, shape and position of the cataract. Congenital cataracts will often be extensive enough to cause blindness in the foal.

How is a cataract diagnosed?

Unless a cataract is very extensive and mature, the use of an ophthalmoscope is the only way for the veterinarian to make a definite diagnosis. This instrument can help determine the presence and position of a cataract. Knowing the precise location of the opacity may indicate the possible cause and future progression of the cataract.

How is a cataract treated?

Treatment of cataracts is still in the experimental stage for horses. All attempts at treatment involve surgery or aspiration of excess fluid from the cortex of the involved lens.

DISORDERS OF THE INNER EYE

Is vision ever affected by eye disorders that are not obvious?

A horse's vision can be affected by defects and disorders in the deep structures of the eye, which may only be observed during a veterinarian's ophthalmologic examination. Some of these disorders may show no outward signs other that a change in behavior due to a partial loss of vision. The horse may shy, stumble or react to changes in light differently than usual.

The causes, effects and treatments of some disorders of the deep structures of the eye are not yet fully understood since equine ophthalmology is still a new field. Techniques of small animal medicine are often applied to the horse. Some of the conditions to be discussed will be merely observations of changes in the eye, since their specific effects on vision have not been explained.

Eye disorders that may not be easily observable include various disorders of the retina, the vitreous humor between the retina and lens, the iris, the aqueous humor between the iris and cornea, and the cornea.

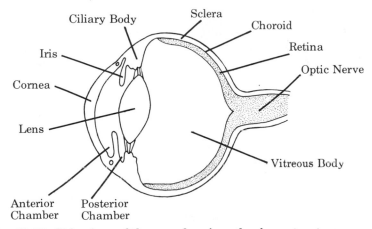

Fig. 16-70. Side view of the eye showing the deep structures.

What are some disorders of the retina?

Disorders of the retina include papilledema, optic nerve hypoplasia and atrophy, retinal detachment and chorioretinitis. They may develop as an aftereffect of systemic disease, ocular disease, a congenital defect or a hereditary condition. All diseases affecting the retina affect the horse's vision, to some degree.

What is papilledema?

Papilledema is an edema or swelling of the optic disk, the portion of the optic nerve formed by fibers converging from the retina, and appearing as a pink to white disk on examination with an ophthalmoscope. The blood vessels of the retina are congested, and small hemorrhages may be seen in the area of the retina around the optic disk. This condition may be a complication of advanced chorioretinitis, tumors of the optic nerve, or increased pressure within the cranial cavity (brain case) caused by abscesses or some other condition. It occurs in 80% of brain tumors. Treatment of papilledema would involve relieving any underlying disorder that caused it.

What is optic nerve hypoplasia and atrophy?

Hypoplasia, or incomplete development, of the optic nerve connecting the retina and the brain has been reported in foals. The blindness may not be noticed until weaning time, since the foal usually follows the mare closely for the first six months after birth. Optic nerve hypoplasia has been reported in the horse with other eye disorders, including cataracts, retinal detachment, and abnormally small eyes (micropthalmia). The pupil will respond to changes in light by contracting or dilating only slightly or not at all. When an affected animal is tested in an obstacle course, it usually collides with most of the obstacles.

Atrophy, or a decrease in size, of the optic nerve and disk occurs most commonly following periodic ophthalmia, an inflammatory disease of the eye (see page 368). The pupil usually does not respond to light and vision is partially or totally lost in the affected eye.

What is retinal detachment?

Detachment of the retina from the underlying layers is usually associated with periodic ophthalmia (see page 368) or injuries that may affect the eye. Retinal detachment in one eye may cause blindness in that eye, but it may not be detected unless the functional eye is covered while testing for vision.

What is chorioretinitis?

Chorioretinitis is an inflammation of the retina and the choroid, a thin, pigmented layer supplied with blood vessels lying between the retina and optic nerve. It is the major abnormality of the retinal area in periodic opthalmia, and can be associated with severe blood loss after surgery or injury. It may also be associated with certain fungus infections. Chorioretinitis may result in partial or complete blindness.

What type of disorder affects the vitreous humor?

The vitreous humor is a transparent, jelly-like material between the retina and the lens. It helps to support the lens from behind and also holds the retina in place against the back of the eyeball. Disorders of the vitreous humor include a persistent hyaloid vessel and luxation of the lens.

What is a persistent hyaloid vessel?

The hyaloid vessel is an artery present in the eye of the fetus, which comes forward from the central retinal artery through the vitreous body to supply the lens. The hyaloid artery is commonly present at birth, but usually degenerates during the first two weeks of life. Occasionally, it will persist in the horse, and remnants of the hyaloid vessel may be mistaken for a type of cataract.

What is luxation of the lens?

Luxation of the lens is a dislocation of the lens from its normal position, where it is held in place by ligaments attached to the ciliary body next to the iris.

What causes luxation of the lens?

A severe blow to the eyeball may damage these ligaments and dislocate the lens. Luxation can also occur in glaucoma, periodic ophthalmia, congenital defects and old age.

Can the condition be treated?

Some loss of vision is inevitable with luxation of the lens, but surgical removal of the luxated lens will prevent the horse from becoming totally blind.

What kind of disorder can affect the aqueous humor?

The aqueous humor, a fluid contained in the anterior chamber directly behind the cornea, is normally clear. Its clarity may change if there is inflammation in, or injury to some part of the eye, usually the iris, such as in hyphema and hypopyon.

What is hyphema?

Hyphema is a hemorrhage into the anterior chamber, usually after an injury to the head and eye. The horse may then show such signs as continual contraction of the pupil, eyelid irritation or an avoidance of light.

How is hyphema treated?

The veterinarian will administer a mydriatic, to dilate the pupil and constrict the internal blood vessels of the eye, to help stop the hemorrhage within the eye. Corticosteroids should be used to prevent blood clots from forming too rapidly, which could cause further injury to parts of the eye.

Will the horse's vision be affected by hyphema?

The hemorrhage often requires four to six weeks to be reabsorbed, but the horse may not always fully recover from the effects of the hemorrhage. Aftereffects of hyphema can include cataracts, shrinkage of the eyeball, and the formation of fibrous bands extending from the iris to the cornea. These bands may cross the pupil and interfere with vision, in which case they should be surgically removed.

What is hypopyon?

Hypopyon is the presence of pus in the anterior chamber behind the cornea, causing the normally clear fluid in the chamber to become an opaque yellow or white. The condition is a symptom of inflammation of the iris, as in periodic ophthalmia (see page 368).

How is hypopyon treated?

Treatment by a veterinarian involves controlling the underlying inflammation of the iris. Medications, such as corticosteroids, are applied to the eye to reduce the release of pus from the iris into the anterior chamber. Puncturing the eyeball to remove the pus is not recommended, since it could result in the formation of a clot in the aqueous humor that would be more extensive than the original hypopyon.

GLAUCOMA

What is glaucoma?

Glaucoma, an increased intraocular pressure, is rare in horses. This increased pressure results from impairment or complete stoppage of the normal drainage system of the aqueous humour. (See page 331.) As a result, the function and health of the structures within the eye in front of the lens are impaired.

Glaucoma comes from trauma or congenital abnormalities and is classified as primary or secondary. Secondary glaucoma is preceded by a recognizable, previous pathological condition within the eyeball. It is possible for secondary glaucoma to result from lens luxation. Rarely, recurrent uveitis (inflammation of the iris) occurs, leading to glaucoma in the horse. Primary glaucoma has no apparent pathological condition of the eye as a cause.

Another term used to classify glaucoma is "absolute." This is the terminal stage of primary or secondary glaucoma, by which time the parts of the eye have been damaged to the extent that the horse is blind.

What are the signs of glaucoma?

Enlargement and distension of the fibrous coats of the eye do not occur as obviously in horses with glaucoma as with other animals, therefore it is hard to detect. Enlargement of the globe, a relatively easy sign to see, is more noticeable in foals, where the eye is not so deeply set in its bony orbit.

Signs usually displayed in horses with glaucoma are extreme dilation of the pupil, edema of the cornea, congestion of the covering of the white coat of the eye, mild muscle spasms of the eyelid, and a pale, slightly cupped optic disc. The pupil responds poorly or not at all to light and the whole eyeball feels hard. The affected horse will be quiet, depressed and irritable. Corneal edema will make the eye look hazy, and possibly even opaque, when the pressure within the eyeball is very high.

How is glaucoma treated?

Although treatment of primary glaucoma in the horse has not been researched extensively, it has been found that long-acting organic phosphate miotics are effective. (Miotics are agents which cause the pupils to contract.) Use of these miotics aids in a reduction in intraocular pressure by forcing open the aqueous drainage network. A return of transparency to the cornea can be expected after the pressure is relieved.

If a luxated lens is involved, surgical removal of the lens may result in relief of glaucoma and prevent complete loss of vision. Secondary glaucoma resulting from uveitis, complicated hypermature cataracts, and wounds also require surgical treatment.

In cases of absolute glaucoma, the veterinarian may inject alcohol (an "alcohol block" of the nerve of the eye) behind the eyeball to relieve the pain, or he may remove the eyeball.

PERIODIC OPHTHALMIA

What is periodic ophthalmia?

Periodic ophthalmia is an inflammatory disease of the eye and is the most common cause of blindness in horses. It is characterized by the sudden onset in one or both eyes of acute clinical signs which gradually subside in a week or more, but recur after quiescent periods varying from a few days to several months. Each recurrent attack adds to the damage to the eye, usually ending in complete blindness in the affected eye. Periodic opthalmia is often referred to as "moon blindness," since the periodic outbreaks were once thought to be affected by the lunar cycle. The disease is seen more frequently in mature horses, four years and older, and both eyes are eventually involved.

What are the symptoms of periodic ophthalmia?

Acute signs of an attack appear suddenly and include severe photophobia, or dislike of light, and excessive lacrimation. Because the eye is extremely sensitive to light, the eyelid is held closed and sticky tears accummulate on the lower lid and cheek. The pupil is tightly contracted and fails to dilate in darkness. The cornea is intensely inflamed and the blood vessels in the sclera surrounding the cornea are so congested as to be clearly visible. After one or two days, the cornea is cloudy and yellowish at its margins. In two or three days, the lower half of the pupil becomes built up with a cheese-like exudate which partially blocks the passage of light into the eye. After about ten days the symptoms subside, and in another week the eye may seem nearly normal again. Following several relapses, the eyeball becomes atrophied and the sclera thickened, eventually resulting in complete blindness.

What causes periodic ophthalmia?

The cause of the disease is still unknown. There may be more than one cause, including riboflavin deficiency, *Onchocerca cervicalis* microfilariae (minute worm larvae), leptospirosis (see Leptospirosis, page 618), and hypersensitivity or allergic reaction. Nutrition studies indicate that there is an inverse relationship between the incidence of the disease and the level of riboflavin in the diet. Infection by *Onchocerca cervicalis* microfilariae (which die in the eye) produces symptoms of periodic ophthalmia. Affected horses often have a high level of antibodies to *Leptospira pomona* in their blood serum, but the nature of the relationship of leptospirosis to periodic ophthalmia is unclear. The ocular inflammation may also be a localized hypersensitivity or allergic reaction after a secondary infection or toxemia. The disease is neither inheritable nor congenital.

What is the treatment for periodic ophthalmia?

After diagnosis of the disease, treatment by the veterinarian involves reducing the inflammation by means of corticosteroids given topically or systemically and dilating the pupil by topical administration of mydriatics. The horse should be kept in a dark stall to decrease its discomfort during the period of photophobia and to help keep the pupil dilated. Adding riboflavin to the diet and administering antihistamines appears to be ineffective.

The prognosis for the disease is poor, depending upon the severity of the inflammation and the presence of ocular damage from previous attacks. Long-term application of topical corticosteroids may be helpful, treatment which involves much time and effort.

SKIN AND HAIR

ANATOMY

What is the nature and purpose of the skin and hair?

Considered as a unit, the skin, hair and hoofs of the horse are called the common integument (covering). It acts as the largest single organ of the body, and is remarkably well adapted to perform a variety of functions.

The most obvious function of the organ is to provide protection from external, violent damage. It performs this task by providing more protection to parts that are most subject to damage. The "covering" also keeps at a minimum the penetration of toxic substances and sunlight.

Another observable function of the skin is that it possesses the sense of touch. Heat, cold, pressure and pain are all observed through the medium of the skin. Linked directly to the sensing function, is the fact that skin participates in regulating the temperature control of the body.

Finally, the skin is the site in the body where vitamin D is manufactured from simpler elements.

What mechanisms does the "covering" provide for protection?

The hair is the body's first line of defense. It considerably reduces the danger of cuts, abrasions, extremes of temperature and chemical irritation. It allows very few things to actually touch the skin. The visible portion of the hair is called the shaft, the root being lodged into the skin in a depression called the hair follicle. The root extends to the second layer of skin, where an enlargement called the bulb holds it in place.

The skin itself provides an outer layer of tissue called the epidermis. The surface is actually composed of dead cells, which are acted upon by the glandular emissions of the skin to form keratin. This substance forms a dry, horny, protective layer

Fig. 17-1. Diagram of a hair follicle, including the sebaceous gland and pilo-erector muscle.

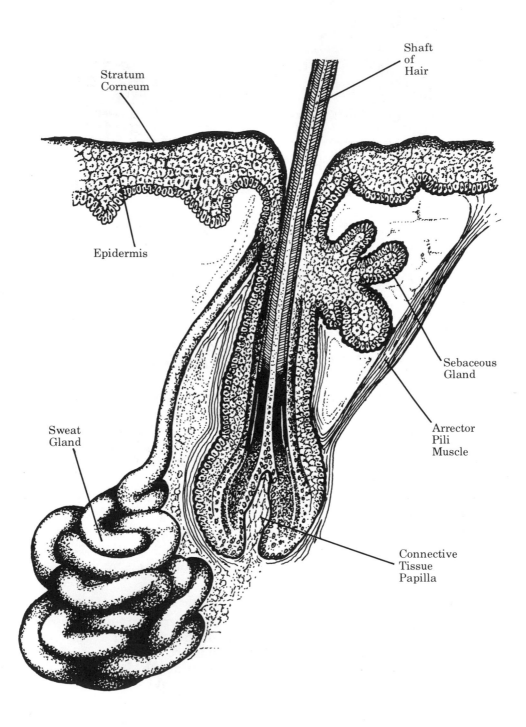

Shaft
of
Hair

Stratum
Corneum

Epidermis

Sebaceous
Gland

Sweat
Gland

Arrector
Pili
Muscle

Connective
Tissue
Papilla

called the stratum corneum. Hard portions of the hoof are simply accumulated layers of this growth that have evolved to protect the softer parts (see Anatomy and Physiology of the Hoof, page 34). Cells of the stratum corneum eventually fall away and are replaced by the constant growth of new keratin-forming cells from the second epidermal layer. In addition to keratinizing cells, this layer of skin further protects the animal with melanin. Melanin is simply skin pigment that acts as a filter for ultraviolet light, which is potentially harmful. This layer adheres to the second layer of skin through small indentations which receive small corresponding "nubs" of the dermis (second layer) called papillae.

The dermis itself is made largely of collagen, a protein substance that provides nourishment to the epidermis. It also contains the nerve endings, blood vessels and glands of the skin.

The skin of the horse is connected, in some regions, to muscles which lie in the fatty subcutaneous (under the skin) tissue. The twitching of the skin produced by these muscles may be seen as further external defense in that it shakes off dirt, flies and foreign objects.

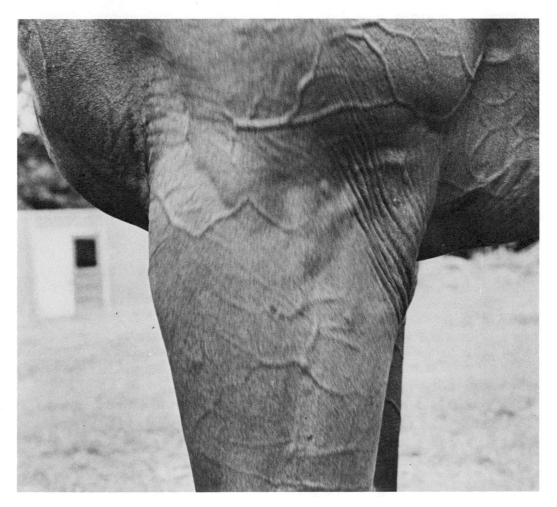

Fig. 17-2. Muscular skin twitching, often used by horses to "fend off" flies and foreign objects.

Finally, the sebaceous glands of the horse provide defense from penetration. The sebaceous glands are usually attached to hair follicles. Through these channels, they emit to the surface a fatty substance known as sebum. Sebum lying on the surface of the skin inhibits, to some extent, the penetration of toxic substances.

How does the sense of touch work?

The papillae of the dermis contain not only capillaries, but in many locations, small nerve endings. This means that the receptors are extremely close to the surface. When stimulated, they convey bio-electric impulses through major nerves to the central nervous system (see Nervous System, page 551).

How does the skin react to temperature change?

In extreme heat, it is well known that the horse sweats. This serves to maintain a lower body temperature, using the same logic as a car radiator, which exposes water to blowing air in order to cool it down. Sweat glands in the horse are of two different types with very similar composition. The gland itself is located in the dermis, and resembles a wound-up ball of tubing. The duct of the gland is the part of the tubing that carries the sweat up to the surface of the skin.

Apocrine sweat glands produce a sweat with more odor, because it includes some of the cell matter of the gland. They are usually activated by the "fight or flight" mechanism of the autonomic nervous system, or some emotional stimulus. Eccrine sweat glands emit mostly water, and are activated by heat.

In either extreme heat or extreme cold, the hair of the horse may appear to stand on end. This response creates additional insulation against temperature extremes, by creating air "pockets" next to the skin.

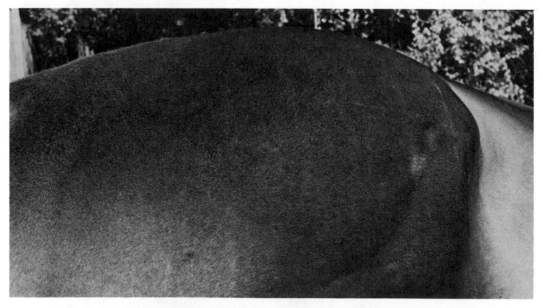

Fig. 17-3. The "fuzzy" appearence of this horse's hindquarters is caused by the action of the pilo-erector muscles, which raise the hairs on end to insulate against extremes of temperature.

How is vitamin D formed in the skin?

The fact that vitamin D is manufactured in the skin is well established. It is understood that it does so through a bio-chemical process using ultraviolet rays and simple elements already present in the skin. The exact means for accomplishing this end are not so well established. The presence of vitamin D allows the body to absorb calcium and phosphate. Both these elements are critical to normal bone growth.

PIGMENTARY DISORDERS

What is a pigmentary disorder?

Skin pigment (coloration) is largely due to the presence of a substance called melanin, which is manufactured by cells known as melanocytes. An excess of melanin (hyperpigmentation) is rarely a problem in horses. Melanin deficiency (hypopigmentation) is seen much more frequently.

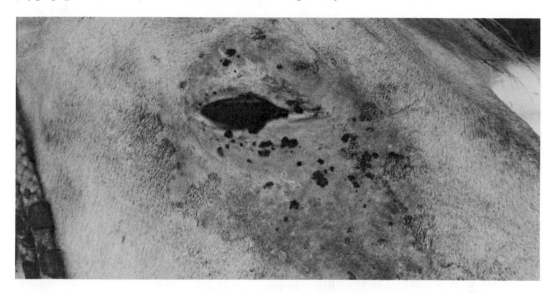

Fig. 17-4. Spotted skin pigmentation around the eye is evidence of "sun allergy," which is common in horses with hypopigmentation.

What causes pigmentary disorders?

Albinism, or total absence of pigmentation, is an inherited defect. The existence of a true albino horse is seriously questioned, since the vast majority of those reported have pigment in the iris of the eye.

Leukoderma is a loss of pigmentation which occurs following some other disorder. Wounds or lesions which are repeatedly irritated, for instance, may result in permanent color loss. A good example of this is the saddle sore. Repeated contact with rubber, such as a rubber bit, has also been known to destroy pigment. Certain kinds of inflammation may result in color loss, but this is mostly temporary.

Vitiligo is a color loss in later life, but the tendency toward it may be inherited. It also occurs in man, and is thought to have its origins in the autonomic nervous system.

How are pigmentary disorders treated?

At present, there is no satisfactory treatment for any pigmentary disorder. Lack of melanin poses relatively little danger in itself, but it does increase the danger from other problems, such as photosensitization (see Photosensitization, page 386).

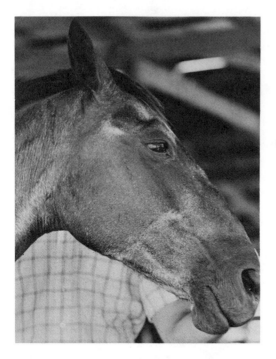

Fig. 17-5. This change in coloration is the "graying" that accompanies old age.

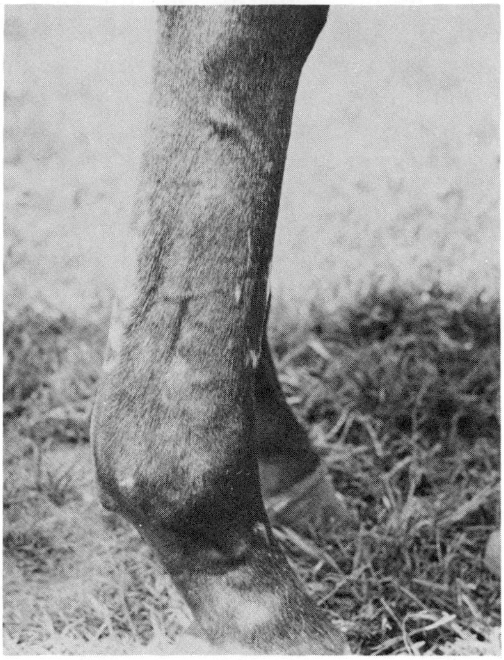

Fig. 17-6. Loss of pigment in the hair is caused by a scar from an old injury.

ANHIDROSIS

What is anhidrosis?

Anhidrosis is the loss of the ability to sweat. It is also known as "dry-coat" and is found in hot, humid areas when horses are brought in from temperate regions.

What causes anhidrosis?

Sweating serves to cool the body, and it is probable that heat regulating centers in the hypothalamus are not capable of adjusting to the higher temperatures. Other proposed explanations of anhidrosis question involvement of low blood chloride and sodium levels in affected horses and the lack of reaction of the sweat glands to epinephrine, which causes normal horses to sweat profusely. Horses raised in humid areas rarely develop anhidrosis.

What are the signs of anhidrosis?

Within a year of the horse's arrival in the hot, humid region, the horse will sweat and "blow" excessively after exercise or when standing in the stable. The nostrils may be constantly dilated and pulse rate elevated. Some horses will show these beginning signs and then begin to sweat normally, while others will go on to develop dry-coat, retaining the ability to sweat only under the mane, in some cases. Very advanced cases have poor condition, scurfy skin and dull, patchy hair. Temperatures of anhidrotic horses may reach 105°-108°F if worked. Polyuria (excessively large amounts of urine) compensates for the lack of sweating in elimination of body fluids. Horses showing the signs of anhidrosis should not be worked due to the possibility of collapse and cardiac failure.

What is the treatment for dry-coat?

Since the exact causes of anhidrosis are not understood, treatment is best kept simple. The preferred treatment (100% cures) is removal of the horse to a cooler climate. If this is not possible, air conditioning, sprinkling with cold water after work, and treatment with alpha tocopherol (vitamin E, as found in wheat germ oil), 1,000-3,000 units daily, for one month has been effective. Iodinated casein (Protamane) and intravenous administration of physiologic saline solution have also been used to treat anhidrosis. Treatment, especially with alpha tocopherol, seems to be effective only when some of the stress is taken off the horse's cooling system, so air conditioning and fans should not be overlooked in attempting to treat this condition.

What is the response to treatment?

If the horse is going to respond to treatment, the first signs will be the absence of labored breathing and dilated nostrils. Gradual replacement of the dry, broken hair with a healthy, shiny coat and smooth, elastic skin will be noted when the first sweating returns. Areas first to recover are around the anus and on the neck, followed by the regions between the hindlegs and in the flank and girth. Normal sweating patterns are usually restored within several weeks.

Can anhidrosis be prevented?

The only way to prevent susceptible horses from developing anhidrosis is to avoid hot, humid areas with horses that have been raised in temperate areas. Maintenance of adequate sodium and chloride levels may help (keep salt available), and is a good precaution in warm weather with any horse. Prompt recognition of the signs and proper treatment can prevent collapse or death.

ALOPECIA

What is alopecia?

Alopecia is a local or general loss of hair and is usually associated with some type of inflammatory skin disease. Most skin conditions that cause itching will result in some degree of hair loss as the horse rubs and bites at the skin in attempts to relieve the itching.

What are some of the conditions that can cause alopecia?

Alopecia can occur in infectious fungal diseases affecting the skin and hair, such as ringworm (see page 408), and in generalized diseases involving a fever in the horse. Loss of hair can result from the presence of certain poisonous compounds in the body; it is a symptom of selenium toxicity which occurs when the horse is grazed on a pasture that contains a poisonous mineral, selenium, in the soil. Injuries to the hair fibers caused by the horse continually rubbing or biting the areas of the body is a common cause of partial hair loss. Alopecia which occurs in connection with these infectious diseases, toxicities, and self-inflicted injuries is usually temporary, with a regrowth of hair in the affected areas.

When is alopecia permanent?

A loss of hair is permanent when the hair follicle (the skin tissue surrounding the hair) is destroyed and scar tissue is formed. Permanent alopecia may occur as a result of certain skin wounds, severe burns, excessive radiation and exposure to caustic chemicals. Alopecia associated with a hormone imbalance often occurs in

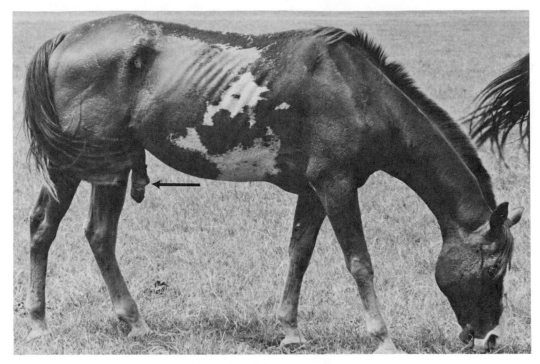

Fig. 17-7. An infection that becomes systemic (see arrow) can cause this general hair loss.

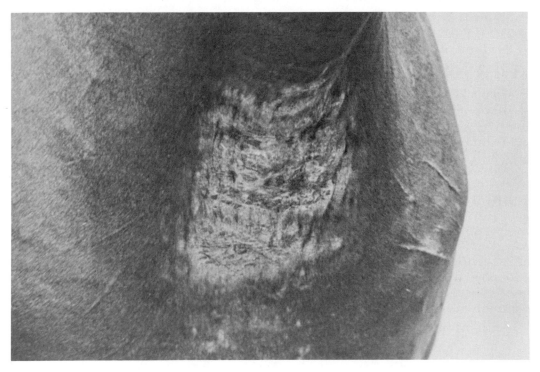

Fig. 17-8. Hair fibers in this area have been seriously damaged by rubbing, but can probably regenerate.

other animals but rarely in the horse. A hormone imbalance caused by a pituitary gland tumor in the horse often causes an abundant growth of hair, rather than a loss of hair. One type of permanent alopecia is congenital, in which there is a partial or complete lack of hair growth at birth that is permanent.

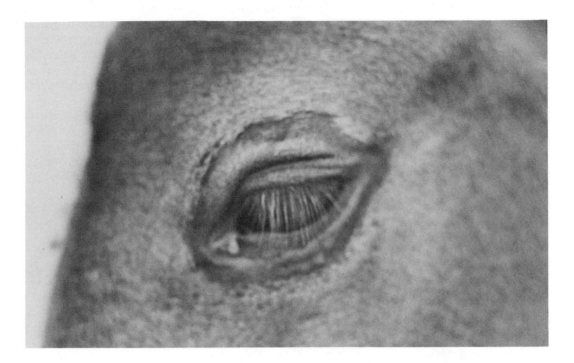

Fig. 17-9. Loss of a foal's fine "baby hair" is a good example of normal hair loss.

When is a loss of hair normal?

Normal shedding of hair is a constant process and occurs most rapidly in the spring when there is a change in temperature. The long winter coat is shed in response to warmer spring temperatures and increased hours of sunlight. Some horses tend to shed their winter coats unevenly, resulting in patchy haircoats and varying degrees of alopecia. This uneven hair loss is only temporary and is a variation of normal shedding rather than a disease.

The horse's haircoat normally grows in again as the weather becomes colder in the autumn. Horses with alopecia are then more susceptible to sudden changes in environmental temperature since they lack a protective haircoat.

A temporary loss of hair is also normal in the mare during advanced pregnancy and while she is nursing a foal.

How is alopecia treated?

Treatment involves diagnosis by a veterinarian to determine the cause of the hair loss. There is no specific therapy for alopecia, but the underlying cause, such as a skin infection, should be determined and treated. Regrowth of the haircoat then depends on how long the condition of alopecia has been present and the amount of damage to the hair follicles.

HIRSUTISM (LONG HAIR SYNDROME)

What is hirsutism?

Hirsutism is a condition in which the horse has an excessive growth of hair, resulting in a long wavy haircoat. The hair is often four to five inches in length, and may remain long throughout the year. The horse may fail to shed in the spring, or it may shed its coat normally and then have an abnormally abundant regrowth of hair. The skin may be dry and scaly, or slightly greasy. The horse is occasionally drenched in sweat and often shows signs of excessive thirst or excessive urination. Hirsutism is usually caused by a tumor of the pituitary gland, which regulates the level of hormones.

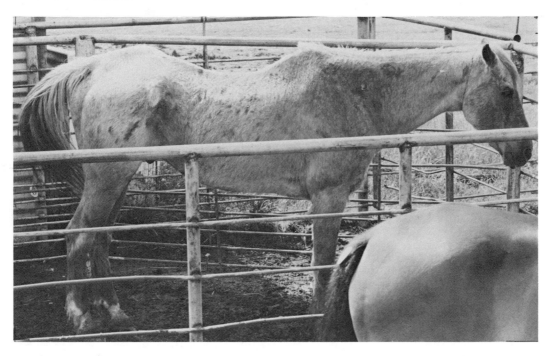

Fig. 17-10. This emaciated horse shows a moderate amount of excessive hair growth, known as hirsutism. Notice the slick coat of the horse in the foreground.

AURAL PLAQUES

What are aural plaques?

Aural plaques are white or grey spots that occur on the inner surface of the pinna (external ear).

What causes aural plaques?

Although the bites of flies are suspected to cause aural plaques, there is no real evidence that indicates any cause.

How are aural plaques diagnosed?

If white or gray spots in the ear are aural plaques, they may be painlessly "peeled" away. The skin under the plaques is generally pink, and does not appear to be harmed. Where there is one plaque, there are usually several, all measuring less than one-fourth inch in diameter.

How are aural plaques treated?

Many treatments have been tried for aural plaques, all without favorable results. However, since they do no apparent harm, this is of no great consequence.

SEBORRHEA

What is seborrhea?

Seborrhea is a dermatological (skin) disease that had been thought to be the result of an overproduction of sebum (secretion of the sebaceous glands). However, in the light of more recent studies, it is more probable that seborrhea is an abnormal keratinization rather than overproduction of sebum. The cause of this syndrome is unknown. It has been found that stimulation of sebum production occurs with increased blood supply to the skin and increased hair growth.

Seborrhea is generally a secondary disease in horses following dermatitis or eczema; rarely is it a primary condition in horses.

How is seborrhea classified?

Seborrhea can be classified into three types (1) seborrhea sicca—dry scales; (2) seborrhea oleosa—greasy scales and crusts, often with a foul smell; (3) seborrhea dermatitis—inflammation and irritation also present.

It is thought that greasy heel is a type of secondary seborrhea (see page 89). If so, it is the most commonly encountered type of seborrhea in horses.

What is the diagnostic procedure for seborrhea?

Diagnosis will concern itself with determining the primary cause which may be either parasitic or bacterial. Any irritant or systemic disease that might cause scaling should be considered first. It must be noted that greasy heel in its early stages may be mistaken for chorioptic mange, as the lesions are similar. Irritation is greater in mange, though, which causes the horse to stamp his feet as he would in attempting to knock off flies that are bothering him. Demonstration of the mange mites in skin scrapings would be diagnostic.

What is the treatment for seborrhea?

Seborrhea is a chronic disease. Therefore, treatment must be continuous since a cure cannot be expected, unless it is secondary, in which case correction of the inciting factor should lead to spontaneous remission of the seborrheic syndrome. Special shampoos designed for cases of seborrhea, used frequently, will remove the oily crusts and help maintain good condition. Good nutrition and proper management will also aid in controlling seborrhea.

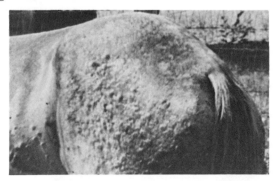

Fig. 17-11. This type of secondary skin irritation is often diagnosed as seborrhea.

VENTRAL MIDLINE DERMATITIS

What is ventral midline dermatitis?

This is a skin condition affecting the ventral midline, the area along the middle of the chest and abdomen. This type of dermatitis, which is a general term referring to an inflammation of the skin, produces itching and occurs in the warmer spring and summer months, later regressing in the fall. The disease is more common in horses over four years of age.

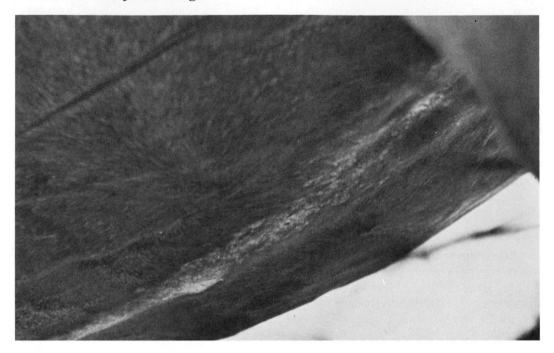

Fig. 17-12. Ventral midline dermatitis.

What causes this dermatitis?

Ventral midline dermatitis can be caused by Onchocerca microfilariae (parasitic worm larvae) but they are not the sole cause. Horn flies often attack in the area of the ventral midline and may be responsible for the condition. Ventral midline dermatitis occurs in the spring and summer when horn flies and other biting insects are prevalent, which suggests that it may be caused by the bites of horn flies alone or in connection with the bites of flies that carry Onchocerca microfilariae.

How does ventral midline dermatitis affect the horse's skin?

Lesions will appear on the horse's chest and abdomen as areas of thickened skin varying in size from less than one inch to ten inches in diameter. The skin is scaly and there is a loss of hair in the area of the lesions. Surface lesions may erode, forming ulcers which later develop a crust. The skin usually becomes depigmented, causing the area of the lesions to appear white.

How is the condition diagnosed?

Examination by a veterinarian is necessary to differentiate the disease from infection by Onchocerca microfilariae, known as cutaneous onchocerciasis. If the

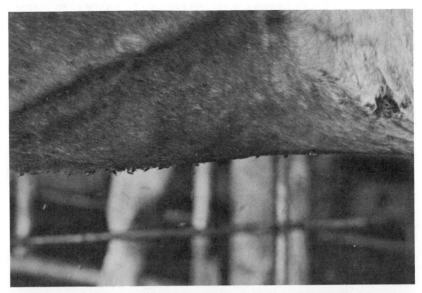

Fig. 17-13. This kind of hornfly activity is thought to cause or contribute to ventral midline dermatitis.

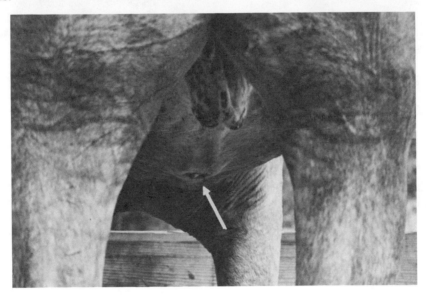

Fig. 17-14. As dermatitis advances, it can cause lesions of the type seen here (arrow).

horse has skin lesions on the face or signs of eye disease, and the dermatitis persists through the winter, the condition may be diagnosed as cutaneous onchocerciasis. Ventral midline dermatitis is seen only during the warmer months of the year and the lesions are much smaller and more sharply defined than those of cutaneous onchocerciasis.

How is the dermatitis treated?

After the type of dermatitis has been diagnosed by a veterinarian, the skin is cleansed with a mild soap and any crusts present are removed. A corticosteroid-antibiotic ointment is applied for several days until the lesions have healed, after which a fly repellent should be used to prevent re-infection.

ALLERGIC DERMATITIS (SUMMER ITCH) (SPANISH ITCH) (MEXICAN ITCH)

What is summer eczema?

Summer eczema is a common condition involving an inflammation of the skin which causes an intense itching. It occurs in the late spring, summer and early fall. Most cases of summer eczema seem to be allergic reactions to insect bites and are referred to as examples of allergic dermatitis.

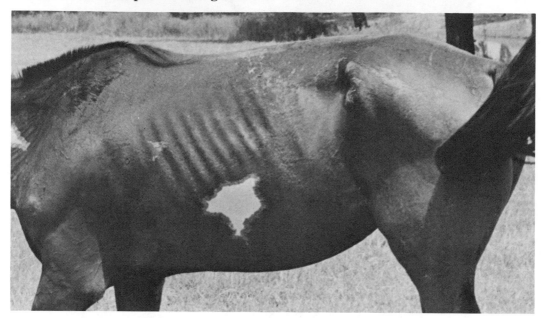

Fig. 17-15. The coarse, uneven, unthrifty coat of this horse is characteristic of summer itch.

What are the signs of allergic dermatitis?

Allergic dermatitis develops from a sensitivity of the outer layer of skin, the epidermis, to insect saliva. Eczema is the first sign, characterized by a redness, scaliness and itchiness of the epidermis. An inflammation of the deeper layers of the skin (dermatitis) soon develops. Other symptoms will be discussed in connection with Queensland Itch, an allergic dermatitis in Australia which is similar, if not identical, to allergic dermatitis in the United States, France, India and elsewhere.

What causes allergic dermatitis?

Allergic dermatitis has been shown to be caused by saliva from bites of specific species of mosquitoes and flies. The condition can also be caused by the microfilariae of *Onchocerca cervicalis,* a type of minute parasitic worm larvae. (See *Onchocerca cervicalis,* page 408.)

Whether allergic skin responses in the horse may possibly be due to other substances which are eaten, injected or inhaled is unknown. Inhaled allergens do not appear to cause allergic dermatitis in horses, and the only definite cause of the condition seems to be insect bites.

Are all horses, exposed to the same mosquitoes or flies, susceptible to allergic dermatitis?

Insect bites of the particular species of mosquitoes and flies may be harmless to

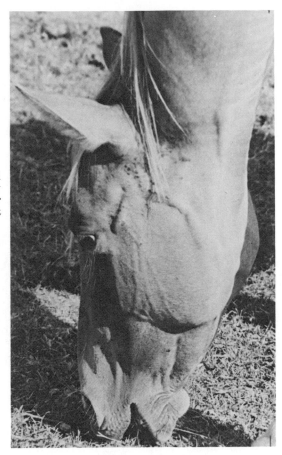

Fig. 17-16. Red, irritated bumps around this horse's ears are probably caused by insect bites, and can lead to further dermatitis if the irritation is not eliminated.

some horses and cause allergic skin reactions in others. Many horses confined with affected animals on the same pasture never show signs of the condition.

Does allergic dermatitis occur only in the summer?

Allergic dermatitis due to insect bites is first noticed in late spring or early summer, when many biting insects are present. Most cases occur in the hot, humid months of the summer and disappear in cooler weather; the skin of affected horses often returns to normal during winter months. Horses kept in wooded areas with slow running streams or ponds often show signs of allergic dermatitis since these areas are ideal breeding sites for several species of biting flies and mosquitoes. The insects responsible for allergic dermatitis, including Queensland Itch, are most active in the late afternoons and evenings.

How is a diagnosis of allergic dermatitis made?

A veterinarian will need to examine the horse and make a microscopic examination of several deep layers of skin to eliminate the possibility of external parasites on the skin. He may also stable the horse in an area free of biting insects to see if the skin lesions regress. If the lesions reappear when the horse is re-exposed to insects, the dermatitis is probably an allergic reaction to the insect bites. Another method of diagnosis involves a skin test with an injection of an extract of the insect that may be responsible for the dermatitis. A swelling will arise at the site of the injection within 24 hours if the horse is susceptible to allergic dermatitis. The use of these skin tests in horses is still limited.

How is allergic dermatitis treated?

Treatment and prevention of any allergic reaction involves removing its cause. In the case of allergic dermatitis, the horse should be moved to an area free of insects, or kept in a stall or screened shelter during the late afternoon and evening when the biting insects are active. Insecticides and repellents applied to the skin may be useful but they must be applied often and will irritate the skin of some horses. Fogging the insect breeding grounds in the horse's pasture is usually costly and may not be effective.

When the horse is protected in some way from biting insects, the skin may return to normal in three to four weeks, and further treatment may not be necessary. Corticosteroids administered by a veterinarian will relieve the itching for the first four to six days, but repeated injections become less effective. Antihistamines may also relieve the irritation but are very costly.

QUEENSLAND ITCH

What are the signs of Queensland Itch?

This allergic dermatitis, caused by a species of sandfly, is characterized by skin lesions on the base of the tail and ears. In older animals that have been exposed continually to the fly, lesions may also be seen over the withers and rump. Only in severe cases do the lesions occur on the sides of the body, neck, face and legs. The most obvious sign is a continuous effort to relieve itching, particularly at night when the horse will rub for hours against branches, fences, and other objects.

What do the lesions look like?

In the early stages there are small swellings of skin, with the hair standing erect. The skin is scaly, and there is a loss of hair on the ears and base of the tail caused by the horse's constant scratching. This scaliness and loss of hair are the most noticeable lesions and may be the only ones observed in mildly affected animals. The hair may become brittle and crinkled, with a ragged appearance of the tail and a further shedding of hair over the rump, withers and mane. When the dermatitis recurs each summer for several years, the skin becomes thickened, dry, rough and hairless in spots.

The general condition of the horse is unaffected, with a loss of condition only in severe cases. The appetite and body temperature are normal except when occasional secondary bacterial infection occurs.

How is Queensland Itch treated?

The treatment of Queensland Itch is similar to that of allergic dermatitis in general. When the horse is protected against sandfly bites by being stabled in an insect-free stall or sprayed with insecticides, the lesions often disappear within three weeks.

PHOTOSENSITIZATION

What is photosensitization?

Photosensitization is an abnormal reaction of the skin to sunlight. Sensitizing agents in the skin are affected in hairless or unpigmented areas, causing sharp lines of demarcation between the reacting area and normal skin.

What causes photosensitization?

The presence of a sensitizing agent in the skin is the cause of photosensitization. It occurs only if the horse is exposed to sunlight and affects relatively unprotected areas of the body. Sensitizing agents may be ingested by the horse if he grazes heavily on St. John's wort, Klamath weed, or buckwheat. Some horses also react to phenothiazine by developing this light hyper-sensitivity. Most commonly, the sensitizing agent is present in the skin because the liver has failed to remove the substance. The sensitizing agent is an end product of chlorophyll digestion, which is normally removed by the liver. If the liver is not functioning properly, this substance collects in the tissues, making the animal photosensitive. Some evidence indicates that the photosensitive reaction may occur in areas following skin contact with certain plants.

What are the signs of photosensitization?

The prinicipal signs of this disorder are skin lesions that are carefully limited to unpigmented areas of the body that have been exposed to sunlight. They occur mainly on the muzzle, nostrils (blue nose), eyelids and face but follow the white hair pattern on painted or spotted horses. These lesions are characterized by redness, swelling and a great deal of itching. Infections may occur, followed by necrosis and sloughing of considerable areas of skin.

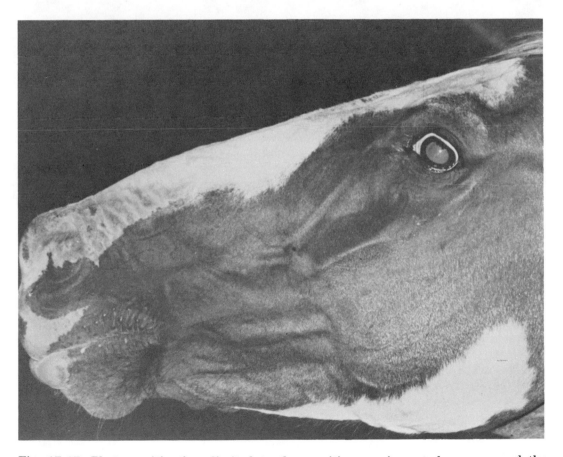

Fig. 17-17. Photosensitization, limited to the sensitive, unpigmented area around the nostrils.

How is photosensitization treated?

Affected animals should be protected from the sun and placed in a darkened box stall. The skin lesions should be carefully cleaned and dressed with protective ointments, mild astringents, antiseptics or corticosteroids, according to the directions of a veterinarian. Corticosteroids are usually administered to reduce the systemic inflammation and itching with an antibiotic to control infection. Prevention consists of removing the cause of the irritation from the pasture and limiting exposure to sunlight until the liver regains enough function to remove the sensitizing agent.

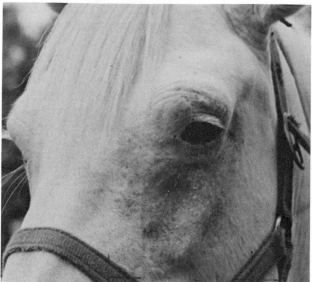 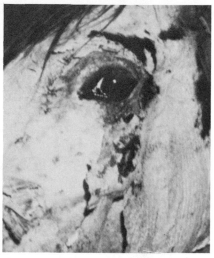

Courtesy of EQUINE MEDICINE AND SURGERY, Edition II, American Veterinary Publications, Inc., Wheaton, Ill.

Fig. 17-18. Photosensitization of the skin around the eyes.

Fig. 17-19. A severe case of photosensitization in which large portions of the skin were sloughed.

CONTACT DERMATITIS

What causes dermatitis?

Contact dermatitis is an inflammation of the skin usually caused by direct contact with an irritating substance. Irritants may include certain medications and strong compounds such as acids; application of an undiluted dip can result in inflammation. Continued exposure to feces, urine, or a wound secretion such as pus or other fluid may also be irritating to the skin. Contact dermatitis is sometimes caused by an allergic reaction of the skin to contact with certain chemicals. These chemical allergens may be preservatives or dyes used in the leather of bridles and saddles. Other allergens can be present in soaps, insect repellents, topical medications and some pasture plants. Most horses do not show allergic reactions to these substances, but once a hypersensitivity to a substance has developed, it tends to persist indefinitely, and any further contact with the allergen will result in dermatitis within one to three days.

What are the signs of contact dermatitis?

Redness of the skin appears on areas of the body which may have come into contact with an irritant or allergen. The head, legs, and abdomen are most commonly affected. The reddened areas of skin will form small swellings which ooze fluid and later develop crusts. There is a loss of hair from the affected areas which is increased as the horses bites at the skin to relieve the itching caused by the lesions.

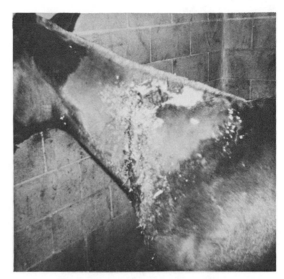

Fig. 17-20. Redness of the skin and small swellings are typical of contact dermatitis.

Photo courtesy of W. L. Anderson. D.V.M.

How is contact dermatitis diagnosed?

A veterinarian can usually make a tentative diagnosis of contact dermatitis based on the location and appearance of the lesions, but the cause must be identified. Irritants which the horse may have come into contact with are often easily determined, but specific allergens may be more difficult to identify. Factors to consider in diagnosing allergic reactions include how often the horse is washed and the type of soap used, insect repellents, and medications such as ointments or creams which may cause a skin hypersensitivity.

How is contact dermatitis treated?

The affected areas should be washed with a mild soap and further contact with the irritant or allergen should be avoided. Application of an antibiotic ointment may be effective for small isolated lesions. In severe cases, a systemic corticosteroid may be necessary and an antibiotic may be administered to control secondary bacterial infection.

URTICARIA (HIVES)

What is urticaria?

Urticaria is an allergic condition characterized by the appearance of wheals on the skin surface. They may accompany either a local or a systemic allergic reaction.

What are the signs of urticaria?

Urticarial lesions involve only the skin and appear as round, steep-sided elevations which vary in size. Located on the back, flanks, neck, eyelids and legs, the tops of the lesions are flat, tense to the touch and are without exudation or weeping. Unless they are due to plant or insect stings, there is no itching. When urticaria accompanies a systemic reaction, other signs may appear. Restlessness, anxiety, rearing, kicking at the abdomen, colic, sweating, diarrhea and fever might be signs of severe systemic allergic reactions.

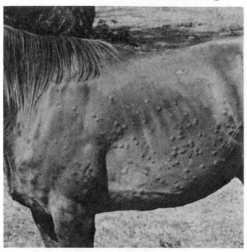

Fig. 17-21. These large, round bumps have an appearance characteristic of urticarial lesions.

What causes urticaria?

Various causes have been found for urticarial lesions. Basically, primary dilation of the capillaries causes reddening of the skin from congestion. Seepage from the damaged capillary walls results in local edema (fluid swelling) of the skin, with swelling and pallor due to compression of the capillaries. These skin lesions may be caused by contact with stinging nettles, various infections, insect bites, ingestion of unusual or high protein feeds, inhaled pollen or by contact with chemicals such as carbolic acid, turpentine, carbon disulfide or crude oil. Some highly sensitive horses may develop urticaria-like lesions (dermographism) from rubbing or whipping.

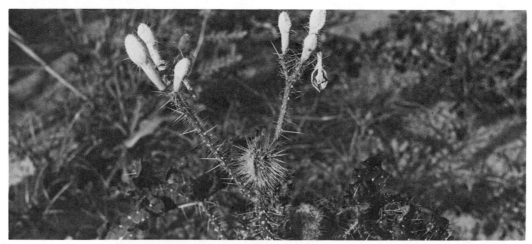

Fig. 17-22. Stinging nettles of this sort cause urticaria, often enough that it is sometimes called "nettle rash."

What is the treatment for urticaria?

The best treatment is removal of the irritating substance, if it can be determined. Most urticarial lesions disappear within a few hours without treatment. If the allergic reaction is systemic, the irritant injection should be discontinued immediately. Antihistamines, adrenalin, and corticosteroids are used when treatment is required. One treatment is usually sufficient.

Can urticaria be prevented?

When the allergen is known, it should not be administered or contact with it should be prevented. Caution should be exercised whenever a drug is given repeatedly or intravenously. Rations that are extremely high in protein should be closely supervised, since it is the protein content in most allergens that causes the allergic reaction.

FLYING INSECTS

What are the effects of flying insects on horses?

Flies, mosquitoes and gnats cause irritation and injury by their blood-sucking and egg-laying activities. Through their contact with the blood, they may spread anthrax, equine infectious anemia, tularemia, equine encephalomyelitis, surra and nagana. By causing openings in the skin, they also permit screwworms and blowflies to infect wounds.

Injury may also be caused if the horse attempts to escape flying insects by standing in water or running away. The intense annoyance may cause a horse to lose 15 to 20 percent of his body weight due to fly irritation while he is attempting to eat. Grazing horses are particularly affected by flies and other insects.

What are some of the characteristics of blood-sucking insects?

The best known blood-sucking insects are the stable fly, mosquito, horse fly, buffalo (or horn) fly, horse louse fly and black fly. These insects can inflict very painful bites that bleed and attract more flies. Stable flies are known for their rapid reproduction rate (30-60 day life cycle) and their preference for breeding in manure or urine-soaked bedding. Black flies characteristically raise wheals when they bite

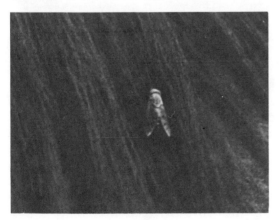 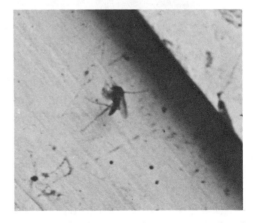

Fig. 17-23, 24. Both horseflies and mosquitoes can carry diseases, and are a source of physical and psychological irritation.

due to a toxin that they inject. These flies prefer to bite the legs, belly or head of the horse and may cause severe injury if they attack in large numbers. Horse flies are the large blood-suckers that attack the legs and belly of horses in summer. They are most frequently found near water because they prefer to lay their eggs on bushes near the water's edge. Although buffalo (horn) flies are principally pests of cattle, horses that are pastured with or near cattle are subject to the bites of these flies.

Buffalo flies are found on the shoulders, flanks and eyes of horses. Mosquitoes can be very annoying to horses, but they are more important as pests because of their ability to carry disease. Almost all biting flies are capable of mechanically transmitting disease when they bite, but the bodies of some species of mosquitoes serve as important incubators of viruses or bacterial infections such as VEE (see Encephalomyelitis, page 571). These mosquitoes lay eggs on the ground where they are hatched by rains or irrigation. This repeated dampness is the reason that some summers have several "cycles" of mosquitoes.

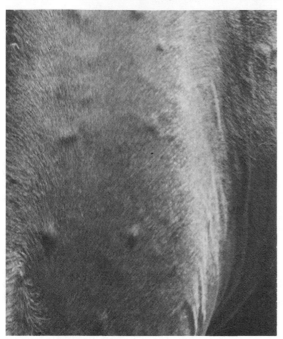 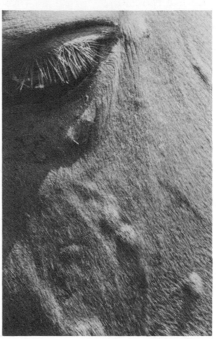

Fig. 17-25, 26. Insect bites of this sort can often be found on these areas of the body, because the horse cannot reach the insects here to brush them away.

What is important about insects that don't bite?

Pests of the horse that don't cause injury or annoyance by biting can still be a disturbance to the horse. House flies are especially bad as numerous pests whose sheer numbers (life cycle 12-14 days) cause great aggravation to horses and horsemen. In addition to numbers, the house fly feeds on manure that may contain eggs of the stomach worm (*Habronema*) (see Summer Sores, page 406). This can be a means of wound contamination or infesting the horse with worm larvae. Face flies cause great annoyance to the horse and they may also carry various infections that cause the eyes to weep and swell. "Blown-up" fly eyes are frequently seen on horses at pasture or where fly control is inadequate. These flies are frequently found sitting on vegetation around pastures where they lay their eggs on the leaves over manure. At this time, screwworm flies are primarily pests of the regions bordering Mexico. Due to the release of sterile male flies, this insect has disappeared from most other parts of the country. They lay eggs in shingled batches around the edges of wounds and the larvae burrow in the wound when they hatch (in 6 to 21 hours). During the 5 to 8 days that they feed in the wound tissues, screwworm larvae cause irritation and a peculiar-smelling bloody discharge. Fly-infected wounds heal slowly, if at all, and may be the source of systemic infections during fly season.

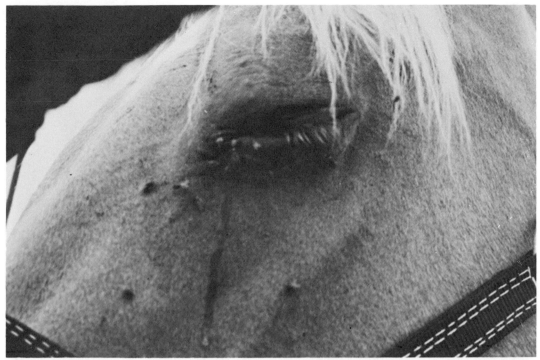

Fig. 17-27A. Where fly control is not practised, fly "clusters" commonly gather around the horse's eyes.

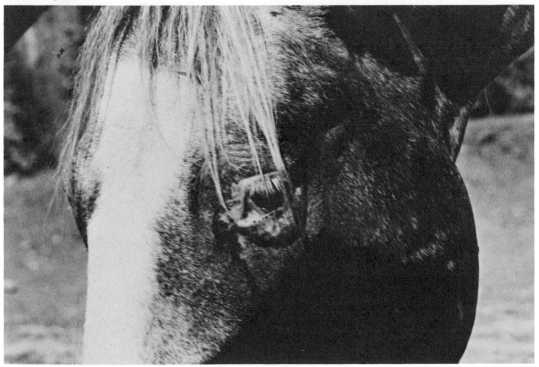

Fig. 17-27B. One of the painful results is severe swelling of the conjunctiva (lining of the eyelids).

FLY CONTROL

Insecticide	Concentration	Methods of Application	Cautions
Carbaryl (Sevin)	0.5% suspension	8 lb. 50% Carbaryl wettable powder/100 gal. water; spray	Do not use on lactating mares
Ciodrin	1.0% oil solution 3.2 lb. ciodrin per gal. emulsifiable sol.	Mix 3.2 lb. sol. with 100 gal. water; spray	Do not use more than once/week
Coumaphos (Co-Ral)	0.125% suspension	4 lb. 25% coumaphos wettable powder per 100 gal. water	Do not use on lactating mares
Dioxathion (Delnav)	0.15-0.6% oil solution	2 qt. 30% dioxathion oil solution/100 gal. water; spray	Do not use on lactating mares
Dichlorvos (Vapona)	1.0% oil base spray	1 part dichlorvos/99 parts spray base oil and inerts; area spray or mix with sugar for use as a bait	
Dimethoate (Cygon)	1% emulsion	2 gal. 25% dimethoate sol. per 100 gal. water	Do not use on animals; do not contaminate feeders or mangers or water; have animals out of barn during spraying
Malathion	0.5% suspension or emulsion	16 lb. 25% wettable powder or 0.8 gal. 57% emulsifiable solution/100 gal. water; spray or used with sugar for bait	Do not use on lactating mares

FLY CONTROL

Insecticide	Concentration	Methods of Application	Cautions
Methoxychlor	0.5% suspension or emulsion	8 lb. wettable powder or 2 gal. emulsion/100 gal. water	Premise spray only
Ronnel	0.25% suspension	8 lb. 25% wettable powder/ 100 gal. water; residual spray for premise spraying only	Do not use on animals, feed troughs or waterers
Ruelene	0.5% emulsion	½ gal. 25% emulsion concentrate/25 gal. water	
Toxaphene	0.5% suspension or emulsion	10 lb. 40% wettable powder or 2/3 gal. 60% solution per 100 gal. water	Do not allow any exposure of dogs or cats to toxaphene
Pyrethrins + synergist	(0.05-1.0% + 0.5-1.0%	Sprays	

Data for this table derived from Prescription section of *The Merck Veterinary Manual*, MERCK & CO., Inc., Rahway, N.J., 3rd ed., 1967.

How may flying insects be controlled?

Various insects have different breeding habits, but the best control can be achieved by proper manure disposal and stable hygiene. Low pastures with standing water are favorite breeding sites for mosquitoes, but this can be corrected by landfill and drainage. Around stables, containers with standing water should be eliminated or regularly cleaned. Good drainage is essential within barns and stables and manure should not be allowed to accumulate in nearby pens and corrals. If manure is broken up and spread thinly in pastures, worm fly larvae cannot survive. This breaks up the reproductive cycle and can bring immediate improvement in the numbers of insects around barns. The veterinarian can recommend sprays for stables and wipe-on spray repellents for application to horses. Area fly and mosquito control should be attempted with the help of local agencies and officials due to the possible danger of insecticide residuals and food and water contamination.

FLEAS, TICKS AND LICE

How does a horse become infected with fleas, ticks or lice?

Fleas are most likely to be picked up in an infested barn or stable. This is because of their preference for cracks, crevices or bedding as a place to lay eggs. A tick larva hatches on the ground and waits on plants for a likely host to pass by. The usual source of infection by lice is direct contact with an animal that is already infested, since lice usually spend their entire lives on the host. Lice separated from a host can, however, survive for nearly a week, so the surroundings of an affected animal are another potential source of infestation.

What are the signs of flea, tick or louse infestation?

Excessive biting or rubbing of the skin, accompanied by nervousness, loss of appetite and irritability are signs which may indicate the presence of these parasites. Unusual sensitivity around the ears, shying from a bridle or halter or shaking the head frequently and holding it in odd positions are common indicators pointing to ear ticks, of which there are several species.

If large numbers of any of these parasites are present, they may be seen by parting the hair. The eggs of lice may be evident close to the body, where they are "cemented" on short, fine hairs in areas that the horse cannot reach with its mouth.

What are the dangers from these infestations?

The most immediate danger to the horse is caused by the irritation of the presence of parasites. Since fleas, ticks, and lice are parasites, they live on the blood of their host. In order to get blood, they must bite or pierce the skin, which is painful in itself. In addition, the constant movement, typical of all but blood-sucking lice (as opposed to biting lice) can cause tremendous nervousness and aggravation. The horse's natural response to this is to bite, kick, rub or scratch at the area. This often brings secondary infections, which pose a further danger.

A large number of blood-sucking lice or ticks can bring about anemia. Whether as a direct result of the bites, or as a result of the severe irritation, a gross infestation may cause loss of appetite, weight and condition. Ticks in particular are responsible for transmitting diseases that may be fatal to horses, such as equine encephalomyelitis and equine babesiosis (see Encephalomyelitis, page 571, Babesiosis, page 478).

How are infestations of fleas, ticks and lice treated?

Dusting, spraying or dipping in insecticides are all acceptable methods of reducing the parasites. Among others, malathion has been successful in eliminating all three kinds of pests. With fleas and lice, it is usually necessary to discard old bedding and spray with insecticide in the horse's living quarters. Ear ticks can usually be routed by the direct application of small amounts of oil. Covering the tick's body with oil prevents it from breathing, and it leaves very quickly to avoid suffocating. A tick-infested area presents more of a problem, since it is likely to be widespread, and the ticks tend to develop resistance to many insecticides. Horses kept in areas where ticks are a problem must be sprayed or dipped regularly.

MANGE

What is mange?

Mange is a very contagious disease caused by any of several species of mites. The different types of mange occurring in horses are sarcoptic (the most serious), psoroptic, chorioptic and demodectic.

What are the signs of mange?

Sarcoptic mites are most commonly found on the head, neck and shoulders. They prefer areas where the hair is thin. Small papules (solid, round elevations of the skin) which are due to females burrowing beneath the skin to lay eggs cause intense itching and are the first signs of this form of mange. Dry crusts form, and the encrusted patches enlarge as the skin thickens. Folds form in the neck region and very extensive cases may spread to the entire body.

Psoroptic mange affects primarily the sheltered body parts covered with long hair—beneath the forelock and mane, and at the base of the tail. The lesions are similar to the sarcoptic type, except the scabs are moist and the mites remain on the surface of the skin. This type of mange is more contagious than sarcoptic mange.

The chorioptic mites prefer the leg regions of the horse, especially those horses which have heavy "feathering" on the backs of the cannons and fetlocks. Secondary infection is frequent with chorioptic mange, and "grease" development is common. Hair is removed by licking and rubbing and the skin becomes thickened and hardened. Horses frequently stamp their feet due to the irritation when infected with chorioptic mites.

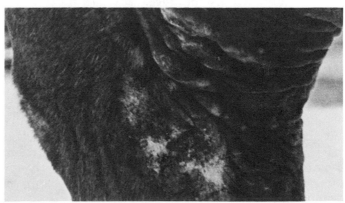

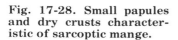
Fig. 17-28. Small papules and dry crusts characteristic of sarcoptic mange.

Demodectic mites live in hair follicles and sebaceous glands, causing tissue damage by the toxins they produce. They frequent areas around the eyes and on the forehead, sometimes spreading to the shoulder region and the entire body. The skin becomes covered with scales but does not itch. This does not occur frequently in horses.

Are mites contagious?

Yes. They are quite contagious. They have the ability to live for long periods away from a host if conditions are moist and cool. They may be transferred by blankets, pads, saddles, bridles and grooming equipment. Bedding is not usually a source of contamination, though it can harbor mites. Direct contact with an infected animal is an excellent means of spreading infection.

How can mange be controlled?

Dipping infected animals in a lindane solution is most effective. All animals kept together must be treated at the same time and dipped or sprayed thoroughly. The treatment should be repeated in 10-14 days to kill parasites that survived the first application.

Can mange be prevented?

Proper supervision of pastured animals, frequent grooming and good health are the best preventative measures. Mange is more prevalent in horses in poor condition.

STAPHYLOCOCCAL INFECTIONS

What are staphylococcal infections?

These are infections by a type of bacteria which normally resides on the skin and mucous membranes. The two species of staphylococcus, *Staph aureus* and *Staph epidermidis,* are parasites of animals, but *Staph aureus* is the only species known to be involved in disease processes. It is capable of infecting and producing disease, with the formation of pus, in nearly all animals and in almost all organs and tissues.

How does the bacteria enter the body to cause disease?

Since the staphylococcus organisms are often present on normal skin, they commonly infect wounds and can be found in abscesses and boils of the skin. *Staph aureus* alone rarely produces disease, but it occurs with other bacteria in contaminated wounds such as castration wounds, deep skin abrasions or compound fractures. It may also enter through fly bite lesions commonly seen on horse's necks, chests, and shoulders during the summer.

What is the disease process caused by the bacteria?

Once in the body, *Staph aureus* produces various substances which can cause such toxic events as coagulation of the fluid portion of the blood and damage to the blood cells. These toxic substances and enzymes contribute to the disease process but are not the only method of producing disease. The complete role of *Staph aureus* infection in the body is not yet understood. Infection can spread to other tissues in the area of a skin wound, but *Staph aureus* rarely spreads to the internal organs of the horse. *Staph epidermidis* is not thought to be capable of producing toxins or causing disease.

What are the signs of staphylococcal infections?

When pus is present in any wound or skin lesion, the veterinarian should be consulted to ensure that a more virulent pathogen than staphylococcus is not involved. If *Staph aureus* is responsible for or involved in the condition, it can be identified by culture of a sample of pus or blood. *Staph aureus* can sometimes cause a specific type of acne in horses known as pyoderma. This disease involves the formation of lesions on the horse's back similar to saddle sores, and may occur as a secondary bacterial infection of saddle sores which are already present. The staph organisms enter through the breaks in the skin on the horse's back, causing the area to become swollen and sensitive. Pustules develop and rupture, forming crusts on the skin. There is often a loss of hair from the lesions.

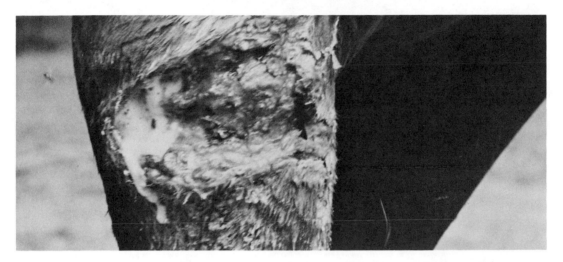

Fig. 17-29. The pus present in this wound indicates a possible staphylococcus infection.

How are staph infections treated?

After the condition has been diagnosed, the skin should be cleaned and the lesions drained of pus. A disinfectant should be applied to the area to control the infection. An antibiotic may be administered if the infection is more extensive than the area of the wound or skin lesions. The condition may sometimes disappear spontaneously within several weeks.

Can the horse be re-infected with staphylococci?

The horse does not become immune to staphylococci and may be re-infected. Prevention involves good sanitation and proper care of skin wounds.

CONTAGIOUS ACNE AND RELATED DISORDERS

What causes contagious acne and its related disorders?

Three different diseases, including contagious acne, have been directly linked to *Corynebacterium pseudotuberculosis* (hereafter called *C. Pseudotuberculosis*), a small, intra-cellular parasite. One disease, ulcerative lymphangitis, was widespread during the last century, but is now reported only sporadically. Abscesses, one of the other forms, occurs more frequently, but seems limited to California and surrounding states. Contagious acne itself is not often reported.

What are the signs of *C. pseudotuberculosis* infection?

All forms of the infection are normally accompanied by lesions on the skin, which vary in size according to the particular disease affecting the horse. They usually become quite painful to the touch, and emit a creamy, greenish pus.

Ulcerative lymphangitis most frequently affects the lymph vessels of the hindquarters, particularly in the region of the fetlock. The lesions begin as an inflammation or nodule and reach a diameter of about one inch. Infrequently, infection may extend to the lymph nodes and lesions spread throughout the body, resulting in death.

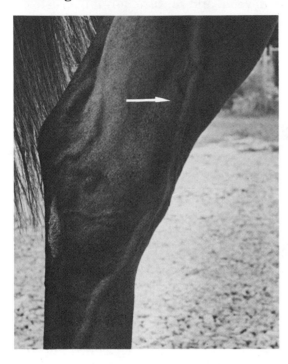

Fig. 17-30. The exaggerated lymph duct on this horse's leg is probably normal. Infected by lymphangitis, the duct would become larger and develop nodules.

Abscesses, also known as false distemper, are first noticed in the pectoral region, and in the majority of cases remain there. More advanced cases involve the lower half of the body, although some lesions have reportedly erupted near the ears. The lesions themselves may range in size from one-half inch to three inches in diameter, and may rupture spontaneously within ten days to two weeks.

Contagious acne is generally limited to areas that come into contact with the harness or tack. It is thought to develop most easily in areas already affected by folliculitis (inflammation of the hair follicle), which is also a precondition of saddle sores. The lesions are generally smaller (about one-fourth inch), and are first noticeable as small nodules. Individual lesions are quite painful, but may heal in about a week. As with other forms of *C. pseudotuberculosis* infection, contagious acne may spread and become generalized. Unlike the others, it spreads itself through the pus, which contaminates surrounding skin when the lesion ruptures. If the infection is allowed to spread, healing may take as long as four weeks.

How are *C. pseudotuberculosis* infections diagnosed?

Lesions of *C. pseudotuberculosis* may strongly resemble those which are symptoms of other disorders. Ulcerative lymphangitis, for instance, is manifested in nearly the same manner as the cutaneous form of glanders. A veterinarian should be consulted to isolate the organism from a pus sample.

How are C. _pseudotuberculosis_ infections treated and prevented?

The best treatment for all forms of the infection is thorough cleansing of the environment. Although proof has not been established, abscesses are apparently spread by flies, and contagious acne by infected grooming tools. Good sanitation measures and adequate fly control reduce the risk of infection greatly.

Immunizing has not proven effective, and antibiotics have been of only limited value. Given sanitary conditions, healing should take place after proper draining of the lesions is established.

PAPULAR DERMATITIS

What is papular dermatitis?

This is an inflammation of the skin (dermatitis) caused by a virus. It is referred to as a separate disease although it may be a variation of another viral disease known as horse pox (see page 345).

What are the signs of papular dermatitis?

Lesions appear as firm nodules of skin (papules) up to one-fourth inch in diameter, and do not contain any type of fluid or pus. Scabs form within a week and drop off, leaving hairless areas of skin. The papules may occur anywhere on the body, but usually localize around the girth region, preventing the use of a saddle. Papular dermatitis only affects the skin and has no effect on the rest of the body.

How is papular dermatitis treated?

There is no effective treatment for the dermatitis but it will usually heal spontaneously in about three weeks. Saddles, harnesses, and stalls may need to be disinfected to control the spread of the virus.

WARTS (PAPILLOMATOSIS)

Where on the horse's body do warts usually occur?

Warts appearing on the skin (cutaneous) are usually confined to the nose and lips. They are rarely more than 1 centimeter in diameter (less than ½ inch), and the number of warts can vary from two or three to a hundred or more, sometimes covering the entire muzzle. They develop as solid outgrowths of the skin's outermost layer, the epidermis, and have a rough, dry, hairless surface. Warts may also develop as outgrowths of mucous membrane and can form on the pharynx or esophagus, on the clitoris of the mare and on the penis of the stallion and gelding. The medical term for a wart is papilloma, a growth of epithelial tissue.

Are horses of all ages affected by warts?

Warts usually appear in young horses up to three years of age. Older horses are thought to have an immunity acquired by an apparent or inapparent infection with warts when they were young.

How are warts caused?

Warts are caused by a virus that is infectious only for horses; warts cannot be spread from horses to other species.

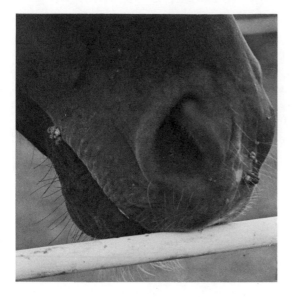

Fig. 17-31. Typical warts on the muzzle of a young horse.

Can warts be spread among horses?

Warts are common when young horses are kept together, and may be spread when colts nuzzle each other. The exact mechanism of transmission is unknown, but it seems that the virus usually enters the skin through small wounds or abrasions. Colts often nuzzle objects such as boards and fences that can cause skin breaks on the muzzle and allow entry of the virus. The virus may then be spread when the colts nuzzle one another. Halters and curry combs that become contaminated by infected animals can spread warts. Fences, feed troughs, and walls of stables may become contaminated, but it is not known how long the virus can live on those surfaces.

How are warts treated?

Warts on horses are often left untreated because they cause little inconvenience and usually disappear spontanteously about three months from the time they are first noted.

Various treatments, such as salves and ointments, are available but their efficiency is difficult to measure because of the tendency of warts to regress spontaneously. Tissue vaccines, prepared from the horse's own wart tissue and given in two injections one to two weeks apart, may be of some value. Occasionally, warts are surgically removed by a veterinarian but care should be taken to avoid causing scar tissue and depigmented areas on the muzzle. Warts should probably not be removed in the early stages of development since the growth of remaining warts may be stimulated and the warts may recur.

Can warts be prevented?

If warts are present in a group of horses, close contact between infected and uninfected animals should be avoided. Fences and stables should be cleaned and disinfected with a strong lye or formaldehyde solution to destroy the virus.

Vaccinations are sometimes used but they may not be worthwhile because their effectiveness is questionable. Horses become immune to the virus after an infection and are rarely re-infected.

SARCOID

What is a sarcoid?

A sarcoid is a tumor composed mainly of connective tissue which appears on the skin as the most common tumor of horses. The growth was first named sarcoid because of its resemblance to a sarcoma, a type of tumor often consisting mainly of connective tissue. The resemblance is in appearence only, since the manner of growth of a sarcoid is quite different and its effects on the horse less serious.

What does a sarcoid look like?

At first a sarcoid may resemble a papilloma (wart, see page 401), as a thickened and roughened bulging of the skin. There is growth of the epithelium and of connective tissue at this early stage, but soon the connective tissue develops more rapidly and the epithelium becomes thin and breaks. An ulcer, or erosion of the surface of the growth, may then form. As the tumor grows, it may become infected by bacteria and show signs of inflammation. Superficially, it often resembles inflammatory granulation tissue, which is composed mainly of capillaries and connective tissue and appearing as small, rounded red granules. The growths are very firm and fibrous and may reach the size of a man's fist.

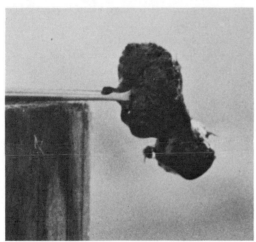

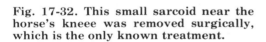

Fig. 17-32. This small sarcoid near the horse's kneee was removed surgically, which is the only known treatment.

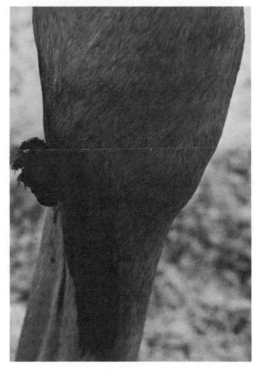

Where on the body do these growths occur?

Sarcoids are usuallly found on the head, especially at the base of the ears. They often occur on the shoulder, belly or sides of the body or in any skin lesion. Sarcoids on the lower legs usually appear at the site of wire cuts, bruises or breaks in the skin. The granulation tissue which then forms as the wound heals may include some sarcoids. The growths are often multiple, with several sarcoids growing together and adding to its resemblance to granulation tissue. The growths can be transferred from one part of the horse's body to another, possibly by rubbing an affected part of the body against unaffected skin. The lesions only affect the skin and do not spread to internal organs.

Can sarcoids be transferred from one horse to another?

Sarcoids have experimentally been transferred from one horse to another, suggesting that the tumors may be contagious to some degree. The growths have been spread throughout horses in a herd, not through direct contact with an affected horse, but probably through contact with an infectious agent such as a virus.

Does a virus cause the tumor?

The cause of sarcoids is still unknown, but the method of transmission suggests that a virus is responsible. Sarcoids are similar to papillomas (warts), which are known to be caused by a virus. Injection of bovine papilloma virus into the horse's skin will cause a sarcoid-like growth to develop, suggesting that the tumor may be caused by a virus.

How are sarcoids treated?

Sarcoids are difficult to treat and the results are often unsatisfactory. Surgical removal by a veterinarian may or may not be successful. Since the growths are often attached to the skin with branching strands of epidermis, complete removal of the entire mass is often difficult and the tumors may recur in the same site. It has been suggested that a sarcoid not be removed until it has reached its maximum size or is growing very slowly, since the tumor may actually be stimulated by surgical interference early in its development. Some sarcoids may be left untreated, unless they are in a position where they may interfere with the bridle or saddle or where they are susceptible to injury.

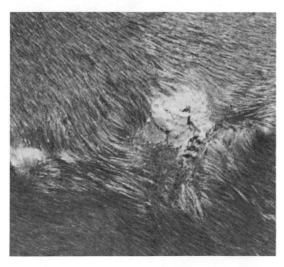

Fig. 17-33. Sarcoids may regrow once they are removed, as this one is doing.

NEOPLASMS OF THE SKIN

What is a neoplasm?

A neoplasm (tumor) is an independent, new growth of tissue, which acts as a parasite on the horse. Its difference from surrounding tissue is not that it uses different cell matter, but that it grows more rapidly than the surrounding tissue. The new tissue growth serves no function, and there are no natural limitations to its growth.

What causes a neoplasm?

As with tumors in humans, no cause has yet been established for most types. Sarcoids and warts are exceptions to this rule, and it is generally accepted that they are caused by viruses. It has also been observed that some tumors have their beginnings at the site of a wound, where the new cell growth begins as part of the otherwise normal healing process.

Are tumors harmful?

A benign tumor is one which grows slowly, looks much like the tissue in which it is growing, and has a definite "border." Unless this kind of tumor interferes with the functioning of an organ, it is not particularly dangerous.

Malignant tumors are called cancerous in human beings. They grow rapidly, infiltrating the body through a process called metastasis. If metastasis occurs through the lymph glands, malignant cells may break off and be carried by the lymph vessels to surrounding areas, where they again grow. This process is called embolism. If the cells simply grow along the vessel walls and pass through the walls to surrounding tissue, this is called permeation. The cells may also be metastasized though the bloodstream, which carries the malignancy to the lungs. The process of metastasis makes the tumors very difficult to isolate and potentially fatal.

What kinds of neoplasms occur often in a horse?

The sarcoid is encountered in the horse more frequently than any other neoplasm. It, like most other tumors, grows more often around the head than any other part of the body (see Sarcoids, page 403).

The melanoma is very prevalent among white or gray horses. It derives its name from the fact that it involves the melanoblasts, which are the cells that produce skin pigment. Melanomas are generally located on the bottom side of the tail, and on the areas just beneath the tail. They are usually black in color. If they are benign, they usually grow rather slowly and remain localized. A malignant melanoma spreads rapidly through the body and causes death more quickly than most other neoplasms.

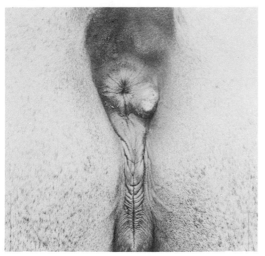 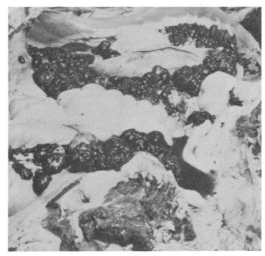

Courtesy of VETERINARY SURGERY, Edition VII, E. R. Frank,
Burgess Publishing Co., Minneapolis, Minn.

Fig. 17-34. The melanomas under the tail of this horse may or may not be malignant. If they are, they can metastasize quickly, as shown in these internal organs.

Squamous-cell carcinoma grows less swiftly, but it is malignant. In addition to the usual locations in and around the eyes, nose and mouth, this tumor may form on the head of the penis, on the penis sheath, or in the vulva of a mare. Its external growth may resemble a cauliflower, or it may affect inner tissue more strongly, appearing on the surface as an ulcer.

What other neoplasms are potentially harmful?

The limbs of the horse, particularly on the outside of the fetlock joint, may be subject to a condition called "bloody wart." This is usually a neoplasm of the connective tissue in the skin, properly called a fibrosarcoma. The popular name comes from the fact that the tumor is often covered with blood, since it is in a location where it is easily injured. Fibrosarcomas metastasize very quickly, and pose great danger to the horse.

Lymphosarcoma does not often affect the horse, but when it does it may easily be recognized. There are normally multiple nodules under the skin, where metastasis has taken the cells through the lymph system. The horse loses appetite, and becomes weak and listless.

How are neoplasms diagnosed?

If the skin shows the ulcers or external growths which characterize neoplasms, a veterinarian should be consulted immediately. A procedure called a biopsy, in which neoplastic cells are removed for microscopic examination, should reveal whether or not the tumor is malignant.

How are neoplasms treated?

The only known method of treatment is surgical removal of the neoplastic tissue. However, this procedure has several difficulties. Benign tumors of any sort are generally well separated from surrounding tissue, making removal generally simple. Problems arise in that a tumor which has remained benign may suddenly turn malignant when "stimulated" by surgery. If the tumor does not grow back after being removed, chances for recovery are good.

Of the malignant neoplasms, squamous-cell carcinoma offers the best hope of recovery. This is because it is generally localized, and does not metastasize quickly. The prognosis for this type of affliction is fair. Other malignant neoplasms are generally fatal, due to the speed with which they spread.

SUMMER SORES

What are summer sores?

They are wounds that do not heal in the summertime because of infestations of *Habronema* larvae. (See Stomach Worms, page 509.) The medical term for this is cutaneous habronemiasis.

How do summer sores begin?

Any wound that penetrates the skin can become a summer sore if stomach worm larvae get into it. House flies are normal carriers of these larvae. If the flies that land and feed on a wound happen to be harboring stomach worm larvae, they deposit them on the wound in the process. The larvae burrow into the wound in an attempt to complete their life cyle, causing itching and keeping the wound in a state of proliferative inflammation.

What do summer sores look like?

They are generally very round and tend to look like a ball of proud flesh. They can be as small as a pea to as large as a part of a softball.

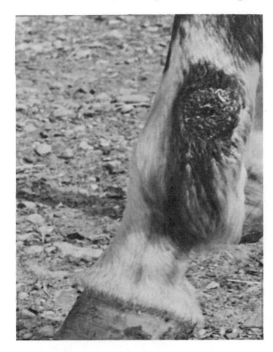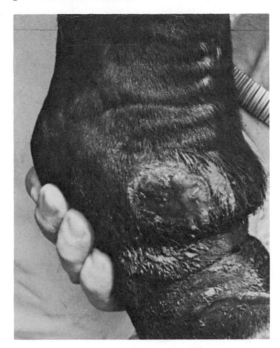

Fig. 17-35. Since the area around the fetlock joint is frequently subject to cuts and scrapes, it is also a common site for summer sores.

Do summer sores go away in the winter?

Usually they go into a resting state in the winter and may heal over if the lesion is not very large. Sometimes they stay healed, but usually the larvae become active again the next spring and the sore returns.

How are summer sores treated?

There are two basic methods of treatment, either of which must be administered by a veterinarian. Traditionally, the infested part of the summer sore has been surgically removed. Since it is extremely difficult to get out all of the fly larvae, and because reinfestation is likely, this method has not had great success. A newer method of treatment involves careful intravenous administration of a highly refined form of an anthelmintic (worm-killing) product called Neguvon.® The toxic effects of Neguvon® to the horse are countered by immediate prior injection of its antidote. This procedure entails some risk, but the use of precise, timed dosages has produced good results.

There have been many different summer sore remedies prepared and used for topical application over the years. Some seem to show a degree of effectiveness, but there is no real evidence that any of them are consistently effective in true *Habronema* cases.

Will effective fly control help prevent summer sores?

Yes. The fewer flies there are available to carry *Habronema* larvae the less chance there is for a summer sore to develop.

ONCHOCERCIASIS

What is onchocerciasis?

Onchocerciasis is a general term, applied to several disorders which involve the larvae of *Onchocerca cervicalis*. These are parasitic nematodes which live in the ligamentum nuchae (ligament at the back of the neck) in horses. The larvae themselves occur in the skin or in the lymph vessels.

What causes onchocerciasis?

Actually, it has never been clearly established that larvae of the *O. cervicalis* are directly responsible for the areas of inflammation in which they are generally found. It is possible that their presence only contributes to a condition which already existed. They are most commonly found in areas of the face, neck, shoulders and breast that show signs of dermatitis. Eye infections, fistulous withers, poll evil and nodules of the fetlock may also be associated with the larvae.

How is onchocerciasis diagnosed?

Since dermatitis is the most common companion of the larvae, signs of that disorder are most often present: that is, redness, swelling, the formation of lesions, and eventual drying of the skin. The actual presence of the larvae can only be diagnosed by biopsy or removal of a sample of infected skin, and should be done by a veterinarian.

How is onchocerciasis treated?

The larvae may be killed by a drug known as caricide, administered in the feed. This should be given only in dosages prescribed by a veterinarian. There may have to be simultaneous treatment with corticosteroids to avoid the skin irritation due to the massive presence of dead larvae. The treatment must be repeated periodically, since it has no effect against the adult nematode. Treatment which is appropriate for the accompanying disorder is usually helpful. Very few horses die due to the presence of *O. cervicalis,* and the prognosis is generally good.

RINGWORM (GIRTH ITCH)

What is ringworm?

Ringworm is the common term for infection by any of a group of fungi that affect keratin-bearing tissues such as skin and hair. Most of these dermatophytes (skin fungi) have a characteristic circular pattern of spread, giving rise to the name "ringworm." There are several types of ringworm which can only be distinguished by a veterinarian.

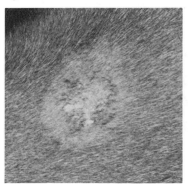 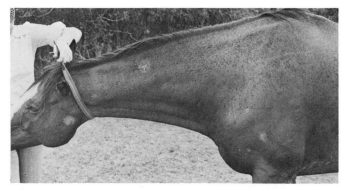

Fig. 17-36. This sort of round lesion is typical of a ringworm infection.

What are the signs of ringworm?

Round, scaly or crusty patches that are hairless or have short, broken-off hairs are characteristic ringworm lesions. There may or may not be itching and the rings sometimes run together to form irregular blotches of scales. Lesions may originate on the head, neck, base of the tail or forehead and spread to any part of the body. The central part of a lesion may be healing and growing new hair while the active, outer part of the lesion is still spreading.

What is the treatment for ringworm?

Ringworm often clears up if left alone, but the infection spreads very easily and is usually best treated topically on a daily basis for one to two weeks with iodine, glycerine, a captan wash, or Thiabendazole ointment. Oral administration of griseofulven may be prescribed by the veterinarian in cases that do not respond to topical medication.

Is ringworm contagious?

Yes. Ringworm is highly contagious and can be contracted by humans. Fence posts, grooming equipment, rats, blankets, almost anything can carry the fungus from one host to another. Anything coming in contact with a ringworm lesion should be disinfected or burned.

Can ringworm be prevented?

Good grooming, separation of affected animals, careful cleaning of grooming tools and equipment and overall good nutrition and condition are the best measures for preventing ringworm in a stable.

Are there any other skin conditions that might be mistaken for ringworm?

Yes. Some allergy rashes look very much like ringworm infection and could easily be mistaken for it. There also are cases of uneven shedding of hair, possibly from changes in hormone balance (usually in mares), that look much like ringworm. Uneven shedding is a peculiarity that is self-correcting and need not be treated. There are many skin cases that are just called "a fungus" without investigation. This can obviously be in error much of the time. For instance, girth itch may be due to a fungus, mechanical irritation or an allergic reaction.

MYCETOMAS

What are mycetomas?

Mycetomas are swellings caused by a fungus that appears in the skin or mucous membranes.

What do the swellings look like?

There may be one or more individual mycetomas varying in size from less than one-fourth inch up to ten inches. The swellings may be scattered over the surface of the body, but often occur in the skin above the coronary band, on the tail, in the mucous membranes of the nose and in a castration wound. The lesions usually abscess, forming pockets of pus containing the fungus. They may appear as reddish-gray nodules just under the outer layer of skin known as the epidermis, surrounded by white fibrous tissue. When a lesion is surgically excised, the fungus appears as small dark granules on the cut surface of the lesion.

How does the fungus enter the skin?

The fungus is usually introduced by sharp objects such as thorns and splinters which penetrate the skin. Infection by the fungus may also occur when a castration wound or other surgical incision is contaminated.

Are mycetomas harmful?

Mycetomas appear to cause no damage other than to the appearance of the skin, and will often heal without treatment if they are not irritated frequently by rubbing.

Do mycetomas need to be treated?

The lesions should be examined by a veterinarian for diagnosis as other fungal infections of similar appearance are more dangerous to the general health of the horse, but treatment of mycetomas may not be necessary. They will usually heal spontaneously within a few weeks, but may be surgically removed if desired.

PHYCOMYCOSIS

What is phycomycosis?

A phycomycosis is an infection caused by any of several fungi in the class of fungi known as *Phycomycetes,* and is the most common type of internal fungal disease affecting the horse. The infection may be localized in one area or organ of the body or it may involve the entire body.

How does a horse become infected with the fungus?

The various fungi of the class *Phycomycetes* may invade the body in different ways; some may be present in moldy feed and may be inhaled or be taken into the body when the horse is fed. Some fungi are present in soil and decaying vegetation and may enter the skin through minor injuries or insect bites. Fungal infection often occurs at the site of a break in the skin caused by a thorn or wire cut.

What are the signs of this disease?

The infection may first be noticed as swellings on the skin with discharges of clear fluid. These lesions occur most often on the legs somewhere between the hock or knee and the hoof, but they may be seen on the abdomen, neck, lips or skin surrounding the nostril. The lesions on the abdomen may be as large as 10 to 12 inches in diameter. The horse often shows signs of difficulty in breathing when lesions are present in the mucous membranes of the nostrils. The infection may spread to the upper lip and interfere with eating. Lesions may also occur in the mucous membranes of the trachea and stomach.

What do the lesions look like?

The swellings form ulcers, or abrasions on the skin, and granulation tissue develops. This tissue is composed of small granules of connective tissue and blood vessels, and usually forms at the site of a skin wound. As the lesions progress, pus drains from small channels in the granulation tissue. Dead (necrotic) tissue can be seen in the granulation tissue as gray to yellow masses of hard tissue as large as three inches long and one-fourth inch wide. When the lesions are examined fungi are found within the necrotic tissue.

Does the infection spread from the skin to other parts of the body?

Infection by some species of the fungi may spread through the body in the blood or lymph by a process known as metastasis. The horse may then show signs of damage to certain organs, indicating a generalized infection. Some of the fungal infections do not metastasize.

Can the fungal infection cause permanent damage?

Horses are often permanently disabled by phycomycoses. Lameness develops as lesions on the legs enlarge and spread to the tissue around the leg tendons. The infection seems to cause an intense itching, and as the horse bites or licks the lesions in attempts to relieve the itching, he may cause further damage to the tissue. The skin in the area of the lesions is destroyed, making healing difficult.

Can the infection be treated?

Early diagnosis and treatment by a veterinarian is necessary in a phycomycosis. The infection must be differentiated from a similar condition known as summer sores (cutaneous habronemiasis, see page 406) and treatment must be begun early to prevent the disease from progressing further. The only effective treatment is surgical removal of the entire mass of tissue around the lesion. If the lesion is very extensive or has been present for a long time, surgery may be impractical and the horse may have to be destroyed. Horses left untreated may die. Minor skin lesions may heal within two weeks after surgical removal, but the fungal infections often recur.

BESNOITIOSIS

What is besnoitiosis?

Besnoitiosis is an infectious disease involving the skin and subcutaneous tissue, blood vessels, mucous membrane of the nose, and some other tissues. The disease in horses occurs in cutaneous and intestinal forms, but the cutaneous form is more common and more severe. Besnoitiosis was first reported in Africa in horses and does occur in other animals, but no cases of the disease in horses have been reported in the United States.

What causes besnoitiosis?

The disease in horses is caused by a species of protozoa, which are one-celled organisms, known as *Besnoitia benneti*. A similar species of the protozoa *Besnoitia* infects cattle but the disease is not transferable to horses.

How do the protozoa infect the horse?

The parasites are transmitted by various bloodsucking insects and invade the linings of small blood vessels. There they multiply before entering the blood stream. The parasites then enter new cells and repeat the cycle of development. About ten days after the parasites enter the body, cysts begin to form, as sacs containing the protozoa continue to multiply. The cysts may be from 0.1 to 0.5 millimeters (less than 2/100 inch) in diameter and are present in the blood vessels and connective tissue beneath the outer layer of skin known as the epidermis. The skin of a heavily infected animal may contain over a million cysts.

What are the signs of the disease?

The disease begins with fever, and the horse becomes very weak and dejected. The skin becomes scaly, hard, thick and wrinkled and may cause movement to be painful. The thickened skin may develop cracks which could allow bacteria or fly maggots to enter and develop infections. The cysts formed by the parasites rupture and cause considerable damage to the skin. Cysts may be visible in the nostrils and in the membrane covering the eyeball. The eyelids are thickened and the legs swollen, and there is a loss of hair. The mucous membranes of the mouth are pale and dry. The horse's appetite may be affected, adding to the animal's generally poor condition. These symptoms occur in varying degrees of severity, and the horse may be sick for seven to eight months. The disease often results in death.

How is the disease diagnosed as besnoitiosis?

A microscopic examination of scrapings of skin are made by a veterinarian to check for the presence of the protozoa. In the intestinal form of the disease, the horse's feces are examined.

Can the disease be treated?

There is no specific therapy available for besnoitiosis but the horse should be isolated and treated by a veterinarian for the specific symptoms present. Treatment should include preventing secondary bacterial infections. A change of environment by moving the horse to a higher altitude and a more temperate climate is usually helpful. A vaccination to immunize the horse against infection by the protozoa may eventually be developed since there is now a vaccine available for cattle.

MASTOCYTOSIS

What is mastocytosis?

Mastocytosis is a skin disorder of horses in which nodules appear under the skin. The nodules are characterized by the excess presence of a specific sort of cell, called a mastocyte.

What causes mastocytosis?

The cause of this disorder is not yet known. It is thought that it may originate in the subcutaneous (below the skin) layers, and it may possibly be a sort of neoplasm (tumor).

What are the signs of mastocytosis?

The nodules of mastocytosis may vary in size anywhere from one-fourth inch to two inches. They are common on the head, but may appear anywhere on the body, sometimes affecting outer layers of muscle. The lump may be covered normally, it may be hairless, or it may be ulcerated. In fact, the most distinguishing characteristic of the nodule is that when a biopsy (surgical removal of sample tissue) is performed, the excess presence of the mastocytes may be seen under a microscope.

How is mastocytosis treated?

Mastocytosis cannot be confirmed with the naked eye, so a veterinarian should be called to examine any nodules where it may be present. Surgical removal is generally used, but there is little evidence to indicate the success or failure of the procedure.

SPOROTRICHOSIS

What is sporotrichosis?

Sporotrichosis is a disease which causes nodules in the subcutaneous (under the skin) lymph nodes. It is only mildly contagious.

What causes sporotrichosis?

The cause of the disease is a fungus called *Sporotrichium schenkii*. It lives on the surface of wood or plants, and a horse usually becomes infected through a puncture wound from a splinter, barb or thorn. An affected horse may spread the disease by direct contact with another horse.

What are the signs of sporotrichosis?

Usually infection begins at the lymph node nearest the entry point of the fungus. The infection spreads quickly to surrounding nodes, and a series of small, painless nodules develop. The nodules eventually rupture, give off a small amount of bloody pus, and heal within three to four weeks. Other nodules have generally formed during this time, though, and the untreated infection can continue for months. There is seldom a large increase in temperature, but weight loss may accompany drawn-out cases.

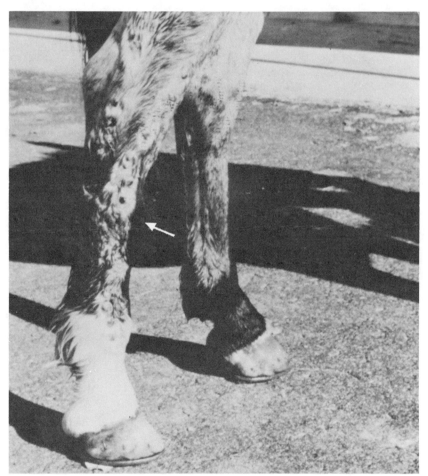

Courtesy of EQUINE MEDICINE AND SURGERY, Edition II, American Veterinary Publications, Inc., Wheaton, Ill.

Fig. 17-37. Sporotrichosis was the cause of these lesions, as established by laboratory analysis.

Another form of infection occurs rarely, in which nodules do not follow any system or pattern. Lymph nodes are not involved, no rupturing occurs, and the nodules are freely movable under the skin.

How is sporotrichosis diagnosed?

Glanders lesions are very similar to those caused by *S. schenkii*, but sporotrichosis spreads much more slowly. Only a biopsy (surgical removal and microscopic examination of sample tissue) will reveal the cause of any particular lesion, and this must be done by a veterinarian.

How is sporotrichosis treated and controlled?

A veterinarian should determine the extent of the infection, but mild cases have been successfully treated by daily application of tincture of iodine to the open lesions. More extensive cases call for the internal administration of iodides. Control consists of proper treatment of all cuts and abrasions, isolating and treating affected animals, and thorough sanitation. In general, the prognosis is good.

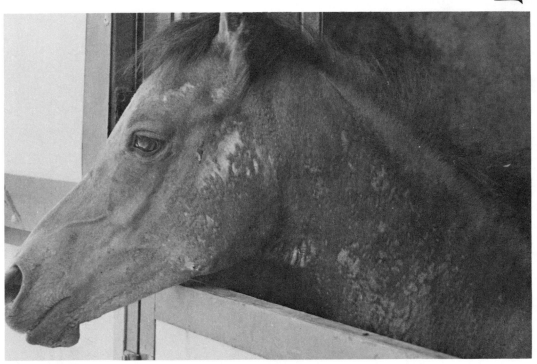

Fig. 17-38. This type of generalized skin problem shows the reason that skin scrapings and diagnosis by a veterinarian are so important. If the proper treatment is not used, these problems can take a great deal of time to clear up.

THE RESPIRATORY SYSTEM

ANATOMY

What is the purpose of the respiratory system?

Respiration is the process by which the horse takes on oxygen, and rids its body of carbon dioxide. In a final sense, this takes place in every part of the body. That is, the living cells take oxygen from the blood, and give back carbon dioxide. Of course, the initial step in the process involves the body making this exchange with the atmosphere.

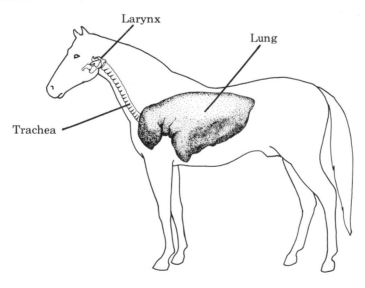

Fig. 18-1. Side view of the respiratory system.

How does the exchange of elements take place?

The actual exchange of elements takes place in the blood, as it flows through the lungs. In the horse, the right lung is responsible for more activity than the left, since the size of the left lung is limited by its closeness to the heart. To give some idea of the size of a horse's lungs, they are capable of holding an average of about 30 quarts of air. (An average man can hold about 5 quarts.) Seen from the side, they are shaped roughly like arrowheads, but their surfaces are molded around the internal structures that surround them.

Air enters each lung through a bronchus (tube) on the forward part of the lung. The main portion of the bronchus is an epithelial (covering tissue) structure, supported by rings of cartilage. Inside the lung, it divides into smaller branches called bronchioles, which are made only of the epithelium. The bronchioles end in tiny sacs, which look like bunches of grapes under a microscope, called alveoli. These sacs compose the body of the lung, and make it feel like a smooth sponge to the touch. Blood flows from small capillaries into the thin membranes of the alveoli, where a substance in the red blood cells called hemoglobin picks up oxygen from the surrounding air. Carbon dioxide is carried to the lungs as a separate element in the blood.

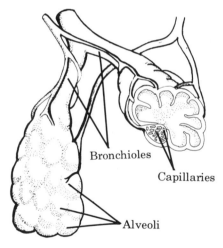

Bronchioles

Capillaries

Alveoli

Fig. 18-2. View of alveoli.

What draws the air into the lungs?

The lungs are filled primarily by the action of a dome-shaped muscle, located behind and beneath them, called the diaphragm. When air is exhaled, the internal organs behind the diaphragm push it into the lung cavity. For inhalation, the muscle contracts and draws the lungs into extension. The diaphragm is assisted in its action by the muscles of the thoracic cavity (chest area), and during hard breathing by the abdominal muscles.

What brings the air to the lungs?

The bronchi which provide each lung with air are divisions of one central "tube" called the trachea (windpipe). The bronchi and the trachea are lined inside with mucous membranes, and small cilia (hairs). These cilia protect the lungs from damage by "beating" constantly, which moves small particles back up the trachea. Rings of cartilage, open on one side, are contained in the epithelium of these tubes, and serve to keep them open. The upper end of the trachea is connected to the larynx, or "voice box."

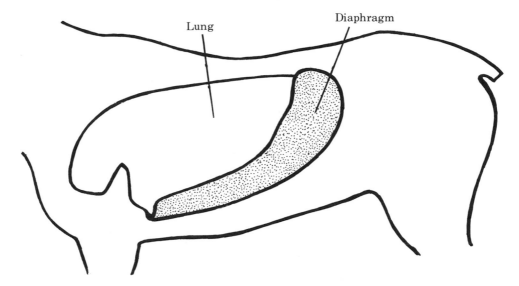

Fig. 18-3. Side view showing the location of the diaphragm.

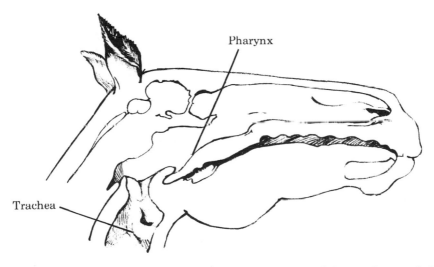

Fig. 18-4. Side view of head, showing the location of the trachea and pharynx.

How does the larynx work?

The larynx is essentially a hollow "shell" made of cartilage, which fits over the top end of the trachea. Most of it is covered with the same mucous membrane and cilia that are present in the trachea. This covering does not extend to the vocal cords, however, which are two strong ligaments stretched over the opening of the larynx. The horse's voice is heard when the cords are tightened, and air moves by rapidly enough to set up vibrations. In addition to this function, the vocal cords are strong enough to act as a valve to prevent air from leaving the lungs. This is normally done so that the thoracic cavity will be more solid when "pushing" with the abdominal muscles. Pushing of this sort is used in defecating, urinating, and giving birth.

The upper end of the larynx opens into the pharynx, which is a chamber that also contains the upper end of the esophagus (swallowing mechanism).

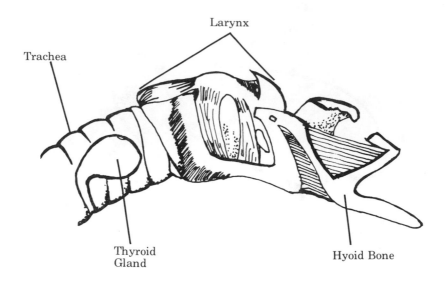

Fig. 18-5. Side view of the larynx, which fits over the top end of the trachea.

What purpose does the pharynx serve?

The pharynx, seen from the side, is shaped roughly like a funnel, with the small end toward the larynx and the epiglottis. It is built on a framework of cartilage held together by ligaments, and is moved by muscles. The bottom "slope" of the funnel is made of an epithelium-coated muscle called the soft palate. Its other side is at the back of the mouth. At the bottom of the soft palate, it is overlapped by a soft flap of cartilage, called the epiglottis, which is part of the larynx. Most of the time this overlapping effectively separates the mouth from the pharynx and allows the free flow of air into the larynx. When the horse swallows, however, the epiglottis flips over the opening of the larynx, the soft palate moves up, and food is admitted into the pharynx. It then passes into the epiglottis, which opens into the pharynx just above the larynx.

This entire mechanism separates the processes of breathing and eating very efficiently. It also makes breathing through the mouth very difficult and complicated.

The side walls of the larynx are furnished with small slits which are openings of the eustachian tubes. These tubes lead to the middle ear, and their presence assures that air pressure is equal on both sides of the eardrum. (See Head and Neck, page 332.)

The top end of the funnel leads to the entryway of the respiratory system, the nasal passages.

What purpose do the nasal passages serve?

The most obvious function of the nasal passages is to admit air to the system. Warming of cold air, though, is another vital function that they perform. Delicate, scroll-like bones take up much of the nasal passages, and their thick covering of mucous membrane not only warms the air, but provides more cilia to remove particles (see Head and Neck, page 327). The external nostrils (nares) are built around crescent-shaped cartilages, and may be expanded to take in more air.

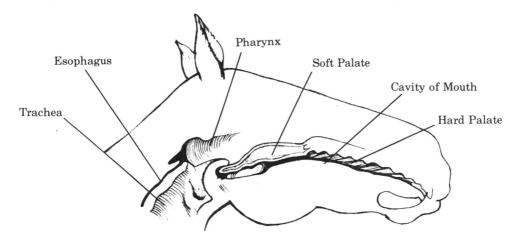

BREATHING

Fig. 18-6. Side view of the head, showing the position of the epiglottis during breathing. Notice that the larynx is open, and the mouth is separated from the pharynx.

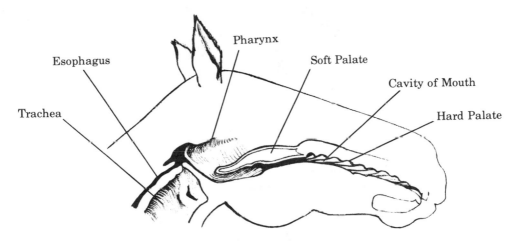

SWALLOWING

Fig. 18-7. Side view of the head, showing the position of the epiglottis during swallowing. Notice that the opening to the larynx is covered by the epiglottis and food passes from the mouth to the esophagus.

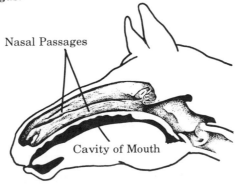

Fig. 18-8. Side view of the head, showing the location of the nasal passages.

HYDROTHORAX AND HEMOTHORAX

What are hydrothorax and hemothorax?

These conditions are the result of an accumulation of transudate (a body fluid which has passed through a membrane) or whole blood in the pleural cavity. Hydrothorax and hemothorax cause respiratory distress and collapse of the ventral portions of the lungs. They are similar to pneumothorax which is a disorder in which air gains entry into the pleural cavity.

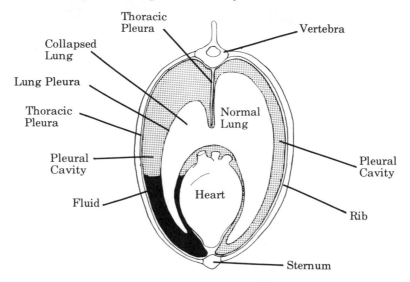

Fig. 18-9. Cross-section of the chest, showing a collapsed lung on the left, and normal lung on the right. Notice that fluid (as in hydrothorax) or blood (as in hemothorax) is present in the pleural cavity.

What causes hydrothorax and hemothorax?

Hydrothorax is most commonly caused by congestive heart failure resulting in a collection of fluids in the thoracic cavity. Hemothorax is the result of trauma to the thorax.

What are the signs of hydrothorax and hemothorax?

In both conditions there is labored breathing, but no fever. Percussion of the ventral thorax area gives a dull sound and, on auscultation (listening with a stethoscope), the heart sounds are faint. Acute hemorrhagic anemia may be present when extensive bleeding occurs in the pleural cavity. These conditions are always bilateral because the division between the left and right sides of the thoracic cavity is fenestrated (has holes in it) in the horse. If large amounts of fluid are present, there may be compression of the atria, enlargement of the jugular veins and an increased jugular pulse.

If signs of hydrothorax or hemothorax seem apparent, the veterinarian should be called to ascertain the primary cause and determine proper treatment.

Signs of the primary disease will be obscure, but quick recognition and correction is of utmost importance to the welfare of the horse.

How is diagnosis of hydrothorax or hemothorax made?

The veterinarian will diagnose either condition on the basis of the physical signs and, perhaps, clinical examination of thoracic fluid obtained by thoracentesis (putting a hypodermic needle through the body wall into the thorax and pulling some fluid out with a syringe). The two disorders can be differentiated from pleurisy by the absence of pain, toxemia, fever and sterility of an aspirated fluid sample.

What is the treatment of hydrothorax and hemothorax?

Thoracentesis with a trocar (a large, needle-like tube), performed cautiously to prevent circulatory collapse, can provide temporary relief. However, since the diseases are progressive, and since there is a great chance of damage to the lungs and heart by the trocar, the prognosis is poor.

The primary condition can and must be treated by the veterinarian. If breathing is extremely labored, fluid can be drawn from the pleural cavity. This relieves the problem for only a short time before the fluid reaccumulates. Parenteral coagulants and blood transfusions will probably be considered by the veterinarian in cases of severe hemothorax.

PNEUMOTHORAX

What is pneumothorax?

Pneumothorax is a disorder in which air gains entry into the pleural cavity. This is different from hemothorax or hydrothorax in which fluid accumulates in the pleural cavity, although the cause, effect and treatment for all three are similar.

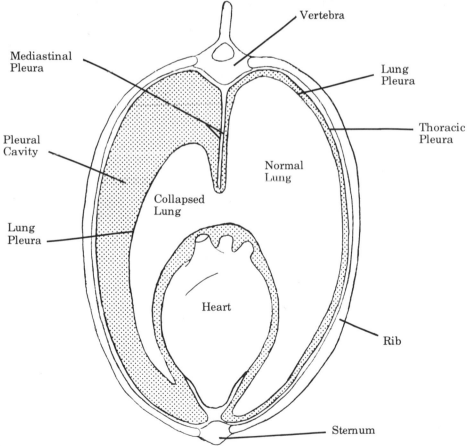

Fig. 18-10. Diagram of cross-section of the chest, showing the condition of pneumothorax. Notice that air has accumulated in the pleural cavity of the collapsed lung on the left.

How does air get inside the pleural cavity?

Pneumothorax is usually caused by either an injury or a lung disorder. A puncture wound of the thoracic wall, such as by a sharp foreign object, will provide a means for air to enter the pleural cavity.

A ruptured lung will also cause pneumothorax. (Air in the lungs escapes into the pleural cavity.) A lung can easily be ruptured, as in the case of a fractured rib where the broken end of the rib punctures the lung. Weakness in the lungs caused by a pulmonary disorder may lead to a spontaneous rupture, particulary if the horse exercises or coughs excessively.

What are the signs of pneumothorax?

The major sign is a sudden onset of inspiratory dyspnea (difficulty inhaling). This will be accompanied by pain and the horse may be in a state of shock. In addition, there will be a partial collapse of the lung and interference with the pulmonary circulation due to the pressure change within the pleural cavity.

The severity of the symptoms depends upon the amount of air in the cavity and the persistence of the opening that allows air to enter. A large amount of air usually causes both lungs to collapse because, in most horses, there is not a complete separation between the right and left pleural cavities. In most instances the disease progresses rapidly.

What is the treatment for pneumothorax?

A veterinarian should be called immediately because of the extreme seriousness and rapid course of the disease. The initial treatment is to surgically close the thoracic wound as quickly as possible and aspirate air remaining in the pleural cavity. If the disease is due to a ruptured lung or internal laceration (as in the case of a broken rib), very little can be done to prevent further entrance of air.

In either situation the attending veterinarian will probably require that the horse remain as quiet as possible, with *no* exercise. Also, it is a common practice to administer antibiotics in an effort to prevent complications such as pleuritis and pneumonia.

What is the prognosis for pneumothorax?

The prognosis is unfavorable unless the opening allowing the entry of air is promptly closed either surgically or spontaneously. Some small openings may close spontaneously, in which case the horse usually recovers within a month. If the puncture site has been surgically closed, the prognosis will depend upon the amount of air in the pleural cavity and whether or not complications develop. Small amounts of air can be absorbed quickly, but large amounts are likely to be fatal due to the tendency of both lungs in the horse to collapse.

In cases where an internal opening allows the continual entry of air, dyspnea usually increases in severity and death occurs within a few hours.

OBSTRUCTION OF THE NASAL PASSAGES AND UPPER RESPIRATORY TRACT

What areas of the respiratory tract are included here?

Obstructions of the nasal passages, the pharynx, larynx, or trachea are included in the upper respiratory tract.

Do obstructions cut off all breathing?

Obstructions may be complete or partial, depending on their location and cause. Partial obstructions make it difficult for a horse to breathe and more severe obstructions can make it impossible.

What causes obstruction of the respiratory tract?

There are many causes of obstructions in the upper respiratory system, but the most frequent ones are foreign growths or objects, abscesses, polyps, inflammations and strangles. Also, improperly administered intravenous injections may cause cellulitis (inflammation and swelling) that interferes with breathing.

What are the signs that a horse has an obstruction in the respiratory tract?

Depending on the type of obstruction, there may be a nasal discharge, reduced efficiency at work and difficult breathing. Large growths or foreign objects may cause difficulty in breathing even when the horse is at rest, but most breathing problems show up when the horse is exercised. Reduced endurance, loud respiratory sounds or labored, irregular breathing are signs of anoxia (lack of air) when the horse is exercised.

What type of treatment is available for this condition?

The veterinarian will have to determine the cause of the obstruction before treatment can be started. However, if there is a great deal of difficulty in breathing when the horse is at rest, the veterinarian may have to perform a tracheotomy (install a breathing tube) before other treatment can be administered. Corticosteroids and adrenalin may be used if the obstruction is due to swellings in the respiratory tract. Foreign objects may be removed with long forceps, but extensive nasal obstructions are not usually treatable, due to the construction of the nasal passages. (See Anatomy, Respiratory System, page 418.)

INJURIES TO THE TRACHEAL RINGS
COLLAPSED TRACHEAL RINGS

What injuries involve the tracheal rings?

The tracheal rings may be torn or fractured by wounds, or by dry, coarse feeds and little moisture, causing them to collapse and interfere with the passage of air.

What are the signs of injury to the tracheal rings?

This type of injury may cause the horse to show signs of difficulty in breathing. The breathing difficulty may be due to inflammation, swelling and pain associated with the neck injury. In some cases, the tracheal rings collapse and do not cause visible signs of breathing difficulty. Usually the collapsed rings can be palpated.

How are tracheal rings repaired?

The veterinarian will probably decide to surgically repair damage to the tracheal rings, especially if they are collapsed and interfering with air flow to the lungs. This repair procedure will usually be done under local anesthetic with the horse standing. Vinyl supports can be used to support damaged or collapsed tracheal rings, but surgical intervention is usually not helpful if a long section of the trachea is damaged.

ROARING

What is roaring?

Roaring (laryngeal hemiplegia) is commonly known for the whistling or roaring sound that can be heard. This sound is a sign of a paralysis of one or both intrinsic muscles of the larynx. It occurs on inspiration, and may be accompanied by dyspnea (difficulty in breathing) in severe cases.

The intrinsic laryngeal muscles normally draw the arytenoid cartilage and vocal fold outward during inspiration. If one or both recurrent nerves do not work properly, these structures are drawn aside insufficiently, leaving an obstruction to vibrate as air passes. This vibration makes the roaring noise. There is no resistance to the air flow on exhalation.

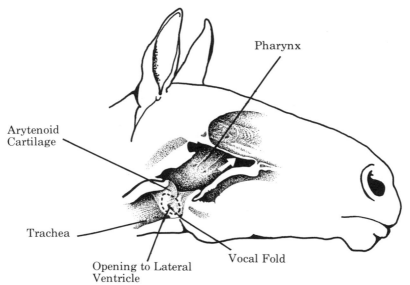

Fig. 18-11. Side view of the structures involved in roaring. (Arrow points into nasal cavity.) Dotted line indicates shape and size of lateral ventricle.

In most cases, only the left recurrent nerve is affected. All horses are subject to roaring, though it is more common in light breeds. Although no reason has been found for it, roaring is found more in geldings and horses than in mares. It occurs more at three to six years of age, probably because this age group is asked to do more strenuous work. Many cases are post-pneumonic.

What are the causes of roaring?

Degeneration of the recurrent laryngeal nerve is the immediate cause. Reasons for this degeneration are many. One theory is that because the left recurrent laryngeal nerve passes around the aorta and is subjected to the strong aortic pulsations, it is constantly irritated and possibly injured by this position. This accounts for over 90% of the cases being on the left side.

The majority of cases are related to a recent lengthy respiratory infection such as strangles, pneumonia, rhinitis, etc. Tests show that *Bacterium viscosum equi* may be a cause. Other possible causes include injuries to the nerve from an overextension of the head, an allergic reaction, any obstructive growth in the area, and lead poisoning or certain plant toxins. If toxins are the cause, roaring will cease when the poison is withdrawn.

What are the clinical signs of roaring?

Following a five-to ten-day incubation period, a harsh, dry cough appears spasmodically, accompanied by retching or gagging in an attempt to rid the throat of small amounts of mucus. Inspiratory dyspnea is sometimes present.

The condition is aggravated by activity or excitement. In mild cases, the signs will not be evident until the horse breathes deeply from strenuous exercise or is eating grain. The "roar" at this point will often be just a high-pitched whistling sound. Dyspnea is slight in early cases. The signs may show no change for a while, but usually become severe within a few weeks. Then the inspiratory noise will be easily heard after mild exercise and inspiratory dyspnea will be present. The signs will subside after a short rest period unless the case is severe or both nerves are affected. In these cases, inspiratory sounds can be heard even during quiet respiration. Affected animals tire quickly from severe dyspnea and are unfit for work.

How is roaring diagnosed?

The characteristic respiratory signs are generally sufficient for diagnosis in well developed cases. An endoscope, an instrument which allows the veterinarian to see the arytenoid cartilage and vocal cords, may be helpful in determining the problem.

With intermittent roaring, the veterinarian will have a harder time making a diagnosis since it is almost impossible to evoke signs during an examination. Some veterinarians feel that they are able to detect a depression between the arytenoid and thyroid cartilages on palpation of the larynx, an external sign that roaring is the problem. This depression is the result of atrophy of underlying muscles. Many affected horses will emit a characteristic grunt when frightened or when struck by a sudden blow over the ribs.

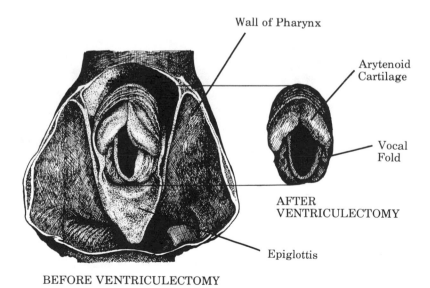

Wall of Pharynx

Arytenoid Cartilage

Vocal Fold

AFTER VENTRICULECTOMY

Epiglottis

BEFORE VENTRICULECTOMY

Fig. 18-12. Views of the opening of the pharynx before and after a laryngeal ventriculectomy, used in the treatment of roaring. After the surgical lesion has healed, the vocal fold and arytenoid cartilage are pulled outward.

Pharyngeal edema, tumors or cysts also cause odd respiratory noises similar to roaring, but these maladies produce sounds on both inhalation and exhalation. Endoscopic examination by the veterinarian can verify the diagnosis.

How is roaring treated?

Spontaneous healing of roaring rarely occurs. A laryngeal ventriculectomy to strip the affected ventricle is successful in restoring about 70% of roaring cases to usefulness. In this surgical procedure, the lateral ventricle is taken out. The desired result is healing of the lesion and contraction of the scar tissue, actually pulling the vocal chord and arytenoid cartilage outward. If the horse does not respond to this treatment, the veterinarian may decide to surgically retract the arytenoid cartilage.

HEAVES (CHRONIC ALVEOLAR EMPHYSEMA)

What are heaves?

Heaves (pulmonary emphysema, chronic alveolar emphysema or broken wind) is an abnormal distention and inability to empty the lungs of air caused by the rupture of some alveoli (tiny air sacks in the lung). Air which escapes from the alveoli can be trapped in "pockets" between them, which is the usual cause of inability to empty the lungs. Heaves are usually seen in horses five years of age or older, but it sometimes occurs in younger horses who have had respiratory infections. This respiratory disease is characterized by difficult breathing, a chronic cough, and generally poor condition. The symptoms are aggravated by exercise, dust and poor quality hay.

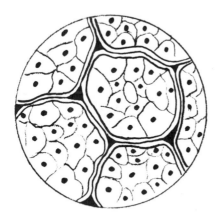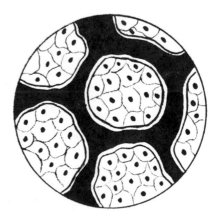

Fig. 18-13. Microscopic views of the alveoli. On the left, normal alveoli. On the right, air is trapped between the alveoli, so they cannot expand and fill with air.

What causes heaves?

The primary cause is, of course, the rupture of some alveoli in the lungs. The specific cause is unproven. The following are probable causes: (1) allergic reaction; (2) exposure to dust or molds; (3) the result of chronic bronchitis; (4) prolonged feeding on poor grade roughage; and (5) extreme exertion.

What are the signs of heaves?

At first the common signs of a cough and nasal discharge are the only evidence of a possible disorder. The first clue of emphysema is usually a shortness of breath and using the abdominal muscles to breathe after exercise. The horse may have been affected for a long time before the ailment is noticed. An increase of respiratory distress occurs often in dusty surroundings, and in hot weather or when feeding dusty hay. An attack may last a few days or several weeks.

As the disease progresses, not only do the labored breathing and coughing become more severe, but signs show up in the musculature of the respiratory areas. The nostrils dilate, the abdominal muscles become misshapen and, in advanced cases, the rectum may protrude during expiration. Dry or moist rales (rubbing sounds) may be present.

How does the veterinarian diagnose heaves?

The veterinarian will base his diagnosis on the clinical signs and the history of the case. The difficulty of diagnosis results from the similarity of heaves to other respiratory diseases such as bronchitis and pharyngitis. Diagnosis may be aided by the characteristic difficulty of expiration and the response to therapy.

What is the treatment for heaves?

There is no curative treatment for heaves. Palliative (to relieve the symptoms) treatments such as atropine, corticosteroids and antihistamines are sometimes used by the veterinarian to relieve distress. The affected horse should be stabled in a clean air environment away from high temperatures or otherwise foul air. No legume hay should be fed, and any hay offered should be clean and given in limited amounts.

INFLAMMATION OF THE AIR PASSAGES (LARYNGITIS, TRACHEITIS, BRONCHITIS, RHINITIS AND PHARYNGITIS)

How are inflammations of the air passages caused?

Inflammations of the upper respiratory tract are generally the result of infection. Laryngitis, tracheitis, bronchitis, rhinitis or pharyngitis occur as a secondary infection to another disease in most cases. Some horse diseases in which upper respiratory infection is characteristic are equine viral rhinopneumonitis, equine viral arteritis, equine influenza, infectious equine bronchitis and strangles. Other cases of upper respiratory inflammation are irritants such as the inhalation of dust, smoke, irritating gases, a lodged foreign body or the act of coughing.

What are the signs of upper respiratory tract inflammation?

Inflammation is rarely restricted to one area of the upper respiratory tract, although it may be more severe in one particular place. The signs are variable according to the site of location and according to the primary disease. Generally, however, a cough is the major sign. It begins as a harsh, dry cough, eventually becoming moist and painful as the condition becomes worse. Nasal discharge increases and becomes purulent, and the breath may have a fetid odor. Difficult breathing accompanied by rales, snoring, deepened respiratory movement and prolonged inspiration are common. The animal may stand with its head lowered and mouth open, and exhibit pain and difficulty in swallowing. In the acute stage, temperatures range from 103°-105° F. The animal has a loss of appetite, but a desire for water. Secondary bacterial infections or extensions of infection often lead to pneumonia.

How does the veterinarian make differential diagnoses in cases of upper respiratory inflammation?

Diagnosis is made on the basis of clinical signs, the history of the primary disease, and the response to therapy. Environmental factors must also be taken into consideration. Differentiation from pneumonia or various obstructions may be difficult and may require a complete examination of the respiratory system.

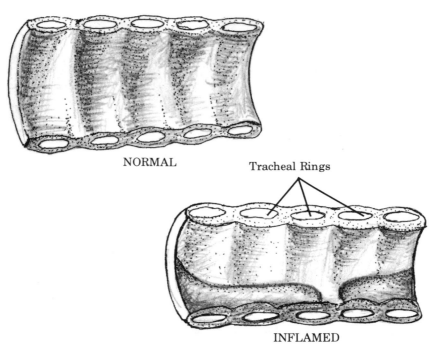

NORMAL

Tracheal Rings

INFLAMED

Fig. 18-14. Diagrams of the trachea showing normal and inflamed conditions. Notice the presence of pus, and the thickening of the epithelium in the inflamed state.

How are upper respiratory inflammations treated?

Identification and treatment of the primary disease is of first importance. Protection of the horse in a warm, dry, dust-free place is essential. The horse should be rested and fed soft foods. Antitussives for the cough, antibiotics or sulfonamides for infection, analgesics for the pain, or expectorants are all possible veterinary treatments. A tracheotomy, performed by the veterinarian, may be necessary if the obstruction is severe enough to hamper breathing drastically.

What is the prognosis in cases of upper respiratory inflammation?

In acute cases, the prognosis is good if treatment is administered quickly and consistently. Horses affected chronically tend to relapse and develop chronic bronchitis or bronchopneumonia. Chronic cases of pharyngitis and laryngitis can persist sometimes permanently unless properly treated.

PLEURITIS (PLEURISY)

What is pleuritis?

Pleuritis is an inflammation of the pleura, the membrane that encloses the lungs in the chest cavity. This inflammation frequently accompanies pneumonia and strangles if the infectious organisms spread from the lung tissue.

What causes pleuritis?

Most often, pleuritis is caused by the organisms that cause infectious pneumonia (see Pneumonia) or strangles. Less commonly, pleuritis may be caused by trauma or thoracic puncture.

What are the signs of pleuritis?

The first signs of pleuritis are a moderate fever, depression, lack of appetite, a reluctance to move and an anxious appearance. Anxiety is due to the pain of breathing, which causes the dry, inflamed membranes to rub and press against pain sensors in the pleura. Following this "dry" stage, a serous exudate appears which greatly reduces the pain. Since the membranes are moist and lubricated, less friction is caused. However, this fluid may be produced in excessively large amounts that can cause the lungs to collapse. The fluid may also cause compression of the heart, which can increase the collection of edema fluid. As the condition progresses, the fluid may be reabsorbed, but the fibrin deposits are left behind, forming adhesions between the pleura of the lungs and the wall of the thorax. These adhesions cause movement and breathing to be painful until continued movement breaks them down.

A shallow, painful cough is characteristic and breathing is painful, even after fluid makes movement of the membranes easier. Toxemia (presence of bacterial toxins) is often severe, especially if pneumonia develops. Death may be caused by a combination of toxemia and lack of oxygen due to the collapse of one or both lungs.

What is the treatment for pleuritis?

The primary aim in treatment of pleuritis is to control the infection of the pleura. Antibiotics and sulfonamides are used for this purpose, the specific drug being chosen after the exudate is examined. Aspiration (removal of fluid) may give relief from pressure, but should not be attempted routinely. Puncture of a lung is always possible and the fibrin frequently blocks the needle used to withdraw fluid. Mustard plasters or hot blankets placed on the chest may ease discomfort. The veterinarian will decide the extent of treatment which may include the placement of a temporary catheter to permit the escape of fluid.

PNEUMONIA

What is pneumonia?

Pneumonia is an inflammation of the lung with consolidation, i.e., the lungs become firm as alveoli are filled with exudate. It is usually accompanied by inflammation of the bronchioles and often by pleurisy.

In horses, pneumonia is often a complication of another weakening disease. In very young horses, pneumonia is generally acute, but in older horses it tends to be chronic and progressive.

Lung

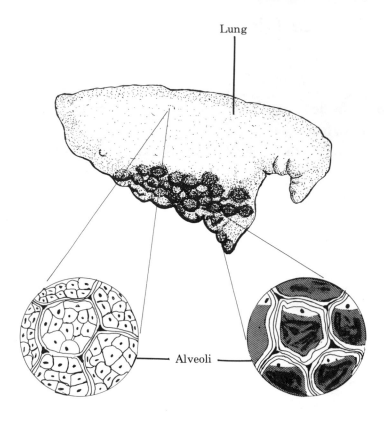

Alveoli

Fig. 18-15. Diagram of the lung and microscopic views of the alveoli. On the left, normal alveoli. On the right, the alveoli are filled with exudate, indicating pneumonia.

What are the causes of pneumonia?

Viruses pathogenic for lung tissue can enter the blood stream or the bronchi and cause primary pneumonia. Often the weakened condition of the lung tissue due to this "infectious equine pneumonia" allows a secondary invader to enter and begin growth, causing a secondary bacterial pneumonia. Other viruses and bacteria that cause upper respiratory diseases such as equine viral arteritis, equine rhinopneumonitis, equine influenza, and strangles can weaken the horse, especially in the bronchial and lung areas, making invasion by potential pathogens quite easy. These pathogens could not begin growth in healthy lung tissue. This type of pneumonia is a secondary bacterial pneumonia that enters through the bronchi (bronchial pneumonia, or bronchopneumonia).

Bacteria that cause a systemic disease in horses and a bacterium such as *E. coli, Salmonella spp.,* or *Actinobacillus equilis* (which localize in the joints) very frequently enter the lungs through the bloodstream. Since the animal is systemically weakened by the activity of the bacteria, these bacteria can then grow in lung tissue and cause pneumonia as a sequel to the primary septicemia. ("Foal pneumonia" caused by *Corynebacterium equi* is of this mechanism. A separate section on this disease is found on page 432.)

Gaseous, liquid or particulate matter can get into the lungs through the trachea and bronchi, causing inflammation of lung tissue which may allow present bacteria to grow on the inflammatory site, thereby starting pneumonia. A horse might breathe an irritant such as chlorine gas or accidentally "swallow some food or water down the wrong way" (as in Choke, page 493), or medicine could be put down the trachea via stomach tube or dose syringe. In some cases, a sizeable amount of medicine accidentally introduced into the lungs could lead to immediate severe shock and death. Any of these incidents will allow foreign material to get into the parenchyma of the lungs, causing irritation of the alveoli and leading quickly to a bacterial invasion and pneumonia of serious proportions. This mechanism leading to pneumonia is called aspiration or foreign body pneumonia.

Rarely, certain fungi such as *Cryptococcus neoformans* and *Histoplasma capsulatum* can cause lung abcesses, a form of pneumonia.

It is unusual, but sometimes there will be enough immature stages of "worm" parasites of the horse, such as *"Parascaris equorum,"* migrating through the lungs to cause sufficient lung damage to lead to secondary pneumonia.

What are the signs of pneumonia?

Affected horses will have rapid and shallow breathing and moist rales at the onset; labored breathing and dry rales in advanced cases. General signs include: 102°-105°F temperature, occasional nasal discharge, breath odor (odor of decay when pus collects in air passages, or putrid when pulmonary gangrene is present), loss of appetite, full and moderate accelerated pulse, depression and intermittent dry or moist cough. Cyanosis (a bluish discoloration of skin and mucous membranes) occurs only when large areas of the lung are affected.

In peracute (very rapid and severe) pneumonia there are often no clinical respiratory signs. Upon being exercised the horse may demonstrate rapid and shallow breathing. He will also be depressed and weak.

The clinical signs are fairly obvious with acute or subacute pneumonia. Sometimes navel infection or strangles may be apparent. Pleuritis rarely appears independent of pneumonia, but is described separately in this book.

How is pneumonia diagnosed?

It is hard to differentiate pneumonia from many upper respiratory diseases. The veterinarian will base his conclusion on a thorough physical examination and the history of the case. This will also enable him to distinguish various conditions which predispose toward pneumonia (such as congestive heart failure, anemia, and viral infections) from primary pneumonia. The presence of pneumothorax, hemothorax, hydrothorax or pleurisy makes diagnosis difficult because, like pneumonia, they blot out lung sounds.

In upper respiratory infections there are similar clinical signs of pneumonia, but the labored breathing is only inspiratory while pneumonia has sounds in both parts of the cycle. Depression, toxemia and coughing are generally more severe in upper respiratory diseases, also.

Pulmonary edema, embolism of the pulmonary artery, congestion and emphysema do not display the fever and toxemia that are characteristic of pneumonia. Otherwise, their signs are highly similar and often mistaken for those of pneumonia.

Auscultation (listening for sounds with a stethoscope) can be a valuable diagnostic aid since it can determine the stage of development and the nature of the lesion. Auscultation can also outline the area of lung tissue affected. Rales, heart sounds, chest movement and thoracic and tracheal percussion are all good indicators of the type of ailment present.

How is pneumonia treated?

After pneumonia has been diagnosed, affected animals should be separated from any others. The remaining horses should be examined for cases in early stages.

The veterinarian will treat the affected horses with anti-bacterial drugs for about a week. Enzymes alone or in combination with penicillin and streptomycin are of benefit in subacute and chronic cases because enzymes digest and liquefy the exudate. Corticosteroids may be administered in acute cases when shock is suspected or in more chronic cases when adrenal gland function has been exhausted. Supportive treatment includes expectorants and oxygen therapy.

The affected horse should be placed in warm, well-ventilated, but draft-free quarters. The animal should be encouraged to eat with plentiful fresh water and light nourishing food. Blankets during the fever period or intravenous electrolytes to prevent dehydration may be required. At least three weeks should be allowed for recovery with more rest time allowed after that before a return to training. Recovery is signaled by a normal body temperature and respiration rate, an improved appetite and increased alertness.

FOAL PNEUMONIA

What is foal pneumonia?

This is a disease caused by a *Corynebacterium equi* infection which results in a purulent pneumonia in foals. Foal pneumonia is relatively uncommon, but does occur more frequently in certain locations (or types of soil). In such areas, the disease may appear as an isolated case, or in small numbers. This specific bacterium was identified in the early 1900's and is thought to exist in soil, living on decayed matter. Exactly how the animal contracts the infection is not understood, but inhalation of the bacteria and entry by way of open wounds (including the umbilical stump) are possible modes of infection. It does not appear to spread directly from animal to animal. This particular infection usually occurs in foals under four months of age.

What are the signs of foal pneumonia?

In most cases this disease develops gradually, becoming well established before external signs are readily apparent. The signs are variable; affected foals may show very few signs of illness and maintain general physical condition until near death, or they may exhibit loss of appetite and condition for several weeks before respiratory symptoms are obvious.

Typically the disease is characterized by fever, rapid pulse and rapid respiration. Coughing usually accompanies the infection. Purulent nasal discharge, watery eyes and diarrhea are also frequently observed signs. With the commencement of evident respiratory signs, the disease generally follows a rapid course (one to two weeks) resulting in death.

How is foal pneumonia diagnosed?

The infection starts in the lungs and forms numerous suppurating abscesses. The lymph nodes, large intestine, liver, kidneys, brain and joints of the affected animal may also exhibit lesions characteristic of foal pneumonia. The preceding, however, are diagnostic aids at post mortem only.

For ante mortem diagnosis the veterinarian will obtain samples from the lungs of diseased foals. The samples are then cultured to establish whether or not *Corynebacterium equi* is present. Identifying the causative organism, *C. equi*, constitutes a positive diagnosis.

What is the treatment for foal pneumonia?

Successful treatment is heavily dependent upon early diagnosis and vigorous chemotherapy, both of which require veterinary attention. Conscientious nursing is also very important. Tetracycline and chloramphenicol are effective against *Corynebacterium equi* infections, but treatment can be frustrating because the bacteria tend to quickly become resistant to the antibiotics.

What is the prognosis for foal pneumonia?

The prognosis for this disease is poor, even when diagnosed in the relatively early stages. In fact, foal pneumonia has a high mortality rate and, unfortunately, there is no available immunization.

GLANDERS (FARCY)

What is glanders?

Glanders is a fatal, highly contagious, usually chronic disease of horses, although other species (including man) are also susceptible. Glanders is one of the world's oldest known diseases. The disease is characterized by nodules or ulcers in the respiratory tract and on the skin. At one time it was world-wide, but now it has been effectively controlled in many countries, including the U.S.A. Glanders is still of major concern, however, because it is commonly in the latent (non-active) form, making a blood test or the injection of a detecting agent necessary. Since horses are now transported quite easily, danger exists from infected horses brought into previously glanders-free areas, if the testing is not done on all horses coming from any area where the disease exists.

What causes glanders?

The organism which causes glanders is called *Actinobacillus (Malleomyces) mallei*. It is present in fluid from the ulcers it causes in nasal and skin tissue of infected animals. The nasal discharge gets into food and water which can then be ingested by other animals to spread the disease. *A. mallei* is not particularly strong, and is readily destroyed by heat, light and disinfectants. However, it can survive in water for about four weeks, and in other contaminated areas for as long as more than six weeks.

What are the signs of glanders?

The animal will begin to show signs about two weeks after exposure. Both the acute and chronic forms attack the respiratory tract.

The acute form is usually seen in asses and mules. There is high fever, cough and nasal discharge indicating bronchopneumonia. Ulcers appear rapidly on the nasal mucosa, and nodules develop quickly on the skin of the lower limbs or abdomen. Death due to septicemia (bacteria and toxins in the blood) occurs within a few days.

Chronic glanders occurs more frequently to horses, and lesions may be in the nasal passages, the pulmonary (respiratory) areas, or on the skin. The nasal and skin types commonly occur together. Nodules develop in the nasal septum in the mucosa and in the lower parts of the turbinates. The nodules eventually become deep, crater-like ulcers. Upon healing, these ulcers leave a characteristic star-shaped scar. Lymph nodes in the area are often swollen and filled with fluid in the early stages, and later adhere to the skin or deeper tissues. Nodules develop in the lungs in the pulmonary form, which may lead to pneumonia if they become extensive. If the nodules break down and discharge their contents into the small branches of the windpipe, the infection will spread to the respiratory tract above the lungs.

In the cutaneous or skin form the nodules appear along the course of the lymph vessels. These also form a crater-like ulcer which discharges a highly infectious pus. This form may occur from direct infection of the skin, or as a secondary infection to the pulmonary form.

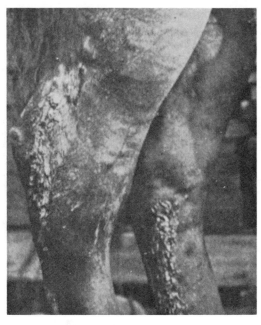

Fig. 18-16. Side view of the legs, showing pus discharging from lesions of cutaneous glanders.

Courtesy of EQUINE MEDICINE AND SURGERY, Edition II, American Veterinary Publications, Inc., Wheaton, Ill.

How is glanders diagnosed?

The most obvious signs of glanders are the nodules, scars and ulcers and the weakened condition of the animal. However, these signs do not develop until the later stages of the disease. Therefore, the specific diagnostic tests are needed for early detection.

What are the treatment and control procedures for glanders?

There is no method of immunization currently available. Even animals that have recovered from the disease do not have a solid immunity, and are carriers. Animals within an affected area should be completely quarantined. Those that demonstrate clinical signs should be destroyed, and all others should be tested at three-week intervals until tests show that all horses in the quarantined area are free of infection. Thorough disinfection of areas where infected horses have been will help to avoid spreading the disease.

Treatment generally consists of sulfadiazine given daily for 20 days. This has proven relatively effective.

MELIOIDOSIS

What is melioidosis?

Melioidosis is a bacterial infection similar to glanders. It occurs mainly in tropical countries in rodents and may, on rare occasions, affect man, horses, and other domestic animals.

How is the infection transmitted to horses?

The bacteria is primarily spread through food and water contaminated with feces of infected rodents. The bacteria lives in the soil and may enter the body through skin abrasions, insect bites, and inhalation. Infection probably occurs only when the horse's resistance has already been lowered by another illness or by being in poor condition.

How is the disease diagnosed?

The horse will have a high fever and show signs of a slight cough and nasal discharge. The bacteria invade the lungs, forming areas of dead (necrotic) tissue and causing a severe pneumonia. The infection may be confused with glanders, but melioidosis does not involve the skin or mucous membranes of the nose, and there is no enlargement of lymph nodes. Diagnosis by a veterinarian involves identifying the bacteria in a sample of nasal mucus.

How is the infection treated?

Treatment is usually ineffective. Some antibiotics may be helpful in controlling the infection, but there is a relapse when the medication is withdrawn. The disease is usually fatal and no useful method of prevention has yet been developed.

BORDETELLOSIS

What is bordetellosis?

Bordetellosis is an upper respiratory infection caused by the infectious organism *Bordatella bronchiseptica*. Very few cases have been reported in horses; the organism seems to prefer dogs, swine and laboratory rodents.

What causes bordetellosis?

Animals under stress (transport, bad weather) may develop bordetellosis. The presence of other organisms may weaken the horse sufficiently for exposure to *Bordatella* to cause infection. This bacteria is not normally present in the upper respiratory tract of horses.

What are the signs of bordetellosis?

The signs of bordetellosis develop gradually after a mildly elevated temperature (102°-103° F) is noticed. Within one or two weeks, animals usually develop a profuse nasal discharge followed by a persistent cough. Since there seems to be little systemic effect of *Bordatella,* the overall condition of the horse may remain good. This condition can easily become chronic if it is not treated, or if it is not treated properly.

How is bordetellosis treated?

Treatment of bordetellosis includes accurate diagnosis by the veterinarian. In order to determine the cause of the respiratory infection, a laboratory culture will be necessary. *Bordatella bronchiseptica* does not respond to penicillin or streptomycin. Tetracyclines and chloramphenicol are the only effective means of clearing up the infection. Affected horses should be separated from healthy ones because the disease is readily transmitted from contamination by nasal discharge.

PASTURELLOSIS

What is pasturellosis?

Pasturellosis is the term used to include the uncommon conditions caused by *Pasturella multocida* and *Pasturella hemolytica.* They are responsible for an acute septicemia that may be associated with pneumonia and other upper respiratory tract infections. Both organisms are usually found in the normal mucous membranes of horses and cause disease only when the horse is in a weakened or stressed condition.

What causes pasturellosis?

Since *P. hemolytica* and *P. multocida* are normally present in the horse, they do not have the ability to cause disease unless some other organism weakens the horse. Bacteria that cause pneumonia often weaken the horse enough to allow the pasturella to multiply and become strong enough to cause disease. The septicemia they cause is produced by the presence of pasturella in the blood and the toxic products that are released from large numbers of bacteria. Foals are especially susceptible to pasturellosis.

What are the signs of pasturellosis?

The signs of pasturellosis may include nervous signs such as tremors, incoordination, paralysis of the tongue and blindness. Most commonly, the signs are those of fever, weakness, hemorrhages in the mucous membranes and a lack of appetite. If the septicemia localizes in the lungs, the signs will be those of pneumonia (see page 429).

What is the treatment for pasturellosis?

The veterinarian may wish to do laboratory cultures to confirm the presence of pasturella, but they respond well to treatment with sulfonamides, streptomycin, tetracyclines and other broad-spectrum antibiotics, used in adequate amounts. Control of pasturellosis consists of preventing primary infections by good management and care.

TULAREMIA

What is tularemia?

Tularemia is a highly contagious disease of rodents (rabbits, mice) which may rarely be spread to horses. The organism, *Pasturella tularensis,* is transmitted by the bite of a tick and causes a highly fatal septicemia.

What causes tularemia?

P. tularensis does not require the presence of other organisms to be able to cause disease. It may be easily transmitted to adult horses, and young foals are very susceptible.

What are the signs of tularemia?

The signs of tularemia are fever (up to 107° F), stiffness and edema of the legs. In addition, foals may show signs of nervous affectation such as labored breathing and a lack of coordination. The septicemia may localize in the lungs, producing signs of pneumonia.

What is the treatment for tularemia?

Affected animals may be treated with oxytetracycline, streptomycin or chloramphenicol to reduce the septicemia. Control and prevention of tick infestations is the best means of preventing tularemia. Especially with young foals, stable hygiene should prevent tick problems.

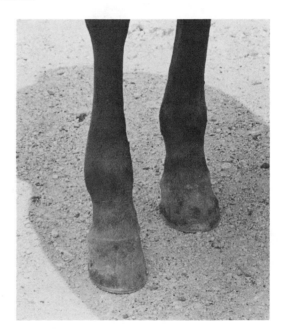

Fig. 18-17. Photograph showing edema of the legs.

CRYPTOCOCCOSIS

What is cryptococcosis?

Cryptococcosis is a fungal infection which in the horse causes lesions in the nasal cavity and lips, in the lungs, and in the meninges (membrane surrounding the brain and spinal cord). Cryptococcosis is not commonly diagnosed in the horse but is well known in man, and may also be referred to. as European blastomycosis.

What causes cryptococcosis?

The organism that causes cryptococcosis is a yeast-like fungus which is commonly present worldwide in dust, soil and manure. Both animals and man may be infected from these sources. Infection could possibly occur by inhalation of the virus or by direct transmission between animals or from animal to man, but the method of infection is not yet fully understood.

What are the signs of cryptococcosis?

There may be respiratory signs, such as a nasal discharge or difficulty in breathing, but for a diagnosis to be confirmed, a veterinarian must make a microscopic examination of gelatinous material taken from a lesion in the nasal cavity or lips. The lesions consist of a swelling and a replacement of tissue by the gelatinous capsules surrounding the fungus. Another noticeable symptom may be the enlargement of lymph nodes.

What is the treatment for cryptococcosis?

A medication used to treat cryptococcosis in man has not yet been proven to be of practical use in horses.

Surgical removal of the lesions in the lungs and meninges is virtually impossible, and there is no satisfactory medication for the infection. As a result, most cases are fatal.

COCCIDIOIDOMYCOSIS

What is coccidioidomycosis?

This is a fungal disease which occurs in many species of animals but rarely in a horse. Only a few cases in the horse have been reported, but there is a possibility that other cases of coccidioidomycosis have occurred without being recognized as such. The disease can produce signs similar to various types of respiratory diseases, and may be mistaken for mild respiratory infections that clear up spontaneously.

What are the signs of the disease?

The effects of the disease may be present for a few months before the infection is diagnosed. The affected horse is in poor condition and is weakened after a progressive weight loss during those few months. The horse may cough and show difficulty in breathing, indicating that the lungs are the organs primarily affected by the fungus. Lameness will be a sign of the disease if the infection involves an inflammation of the tendons and soft tissues of the leg. Lymph nodes in the area of the lungs may be swollen with pus and appear as swellings on the chest. Pus withdrawn from these swellings during diagnosis will aid in detecting the presence of the fungus, *Coccidioides immitis.*

How is this fungus transmitted to the horse?

Coccidioides immitis is present in the soil and has been found in arid sections of the southwestern United States, Mexico and several South American countries. The fungus can be inhaled with dust, or it may enter the body through skin abrasions or through the mouth into the digestive tract. The most common method of transmission appears to be inhalation into the lungs, where the infection causes inflammation of the lung tissues. The inflammation can progressively spread through the blood or lymph to other organs of the body, including the liver and spleen. One affected horse was reported to have died from a ruptured liver.

Is the disease fatal?

In the reported cases, the affected horses either died or were destroyed because the disease had progressed to an irreversible stage. Diagnosis of the condition is difficult and the condition is usually not detected until the later stages. If the lymph nodes of the chest are swollen, pus drawn from the swellings may be found to contain the fungus, confirming the diagnosis. If there are not such visible signs, diagnosis depends on the horse's reaction to an injection of coccidioidin, a solution containing by-products of the fungus. There is no effective treatment and no vaccine is available to prevent the infection.

EQUINE INFLUENZA

What is equine influenza?

This is an acute respiratory disease syndrome that spreads rapidly through groups of horses. Although many horses are infected, very few die from this disease. The incidence of equine influenza is world-wide.

What is the cause of equine influenza?

This disease is caused by any one of a group of related viruses. There are at least two different viruses within this group known to be responsible for equine influenza. In 1958, Czechoslovakian researchers identified one type of influenza and it is now termed A-equi-1. The other known type of equine influenza virus, A-equi-2, was identified in Miami in 1963.

How is equine influenza spread?

This disease is spread chiefly by inhalation of infective material. A cough accompanies influenza infections, aiding its spread in situations where horses are concentrated. Another factor in the rapid spread of equine influenza is the short incubation period (one to three days) of the disease.

What are the signs of the disease?

Equine influenza can vary from a mild, almost unnoticeable disease to a severe one. Factors influencing the severity of the infection include age of the horse, general physical condition of the horse and specific type of virus present. However, equine influenza is rarely fatal except in very young or very old horses.

After a short incubation period the onset of this disease is sudden. A fever, usually ranging from 101°-106° F, is the first sign. The fever commonly lasts for about three days. One of the major signs of influenza is the characteristic cough. It begins as a dry, hacking cough soon after the onset of fever. Within a few days the cough becomes moist and less frequent and, as a general rule, persists for several weeks. Depending upon the severity of the disease, other signs which may be present include a watery nasal discharge, weakness, stiffness, loss of appetite, depression and dyspnea. The actual illness normally lasts from two to seven days.

Influenza alone is a relatively mild disease. Most serious problems associated with equine influenza stem from secondary complications. Naturally, the viral respiratory infection leaves the horse in a weakened state. This is particularly true of very young horses in which bacterial pneumonia is sometimes a fatal complication. Other complications possible in horses of all ages include secondary bacterial infections, chronic bronchitis, pneumonia, emphysema and myocarditis.

Why does equine influenza have a "characteristic" cough?

The particular type of cough associated with this disease is due to the manner in which equine influenza viruses act. These viruses quickly attack ciliated epithelium (the lining of the upper respiratory tract) causing the dry, frequent cough. The epithelium soon sloughs, resulting in the moist and less frequent cough. At this stage there are many small wounds in the epithelium, providing numerous sites for secondary bacterial infections. Without complications, the cough persists for about three weeks because it normally requires about three weeks for regeneration of a functional, new respiratory epithelium.

Can equine influenza be easily diagnosed?

Because equine influenza closely resembles other respiratory diseases, such as viral rhinopneumonitis and viral arteritis, the veterinarian will use laboratory examination to conclusively diagnose equine influenza. Nasal discharges and blood samples are submitted to a laboratory for analysis.

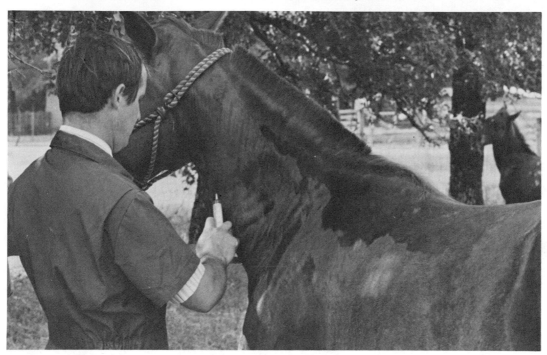

Fig. 18-18. The veterinarian may draw a blood sample to determine the presence of the virus in equine influenza.

What is the treatment for equine influenza?

Sensible nursing is extremely important because influenza responds poorly to most forms of treatment. The horse should be rested until the cough completely subsides to promote and aid healing of the respiratory epithelium. This may require from three weeks to several months, depending upon the severity of the infection and the healing ability of the individual horse.

Complications are best prevented by providing clean, well-ventilated quarters in addition to restricting exercise. It is advisable to consult a veterinarian, especially concerning protection of very young horses that may be highly susceptible to secondary bacterial infections. He may prescribe antibiotic therapy as a preventive measure.

There is an influenza vaccine which affords protection against both viral types. This should be used, upon veterinary recommendation, in situations where horses are kept in concentrated numbers and influenza is likely to be a problem.

EQUINE VIRAL RHINOPNEUMONITIS

What is viral rhinopneumonitis?

Rhinopneumonitis is an acute viral infection that usually affects young horses after weaning, and it generally occurs in the late fall or early winter. It is characterized by fever, a reduction in white blood cells, and inflammation of the mucous membranes of the respiratory tract. Secondary infections which affect the respiratory tract are predisposed by rhinopneumonitis. This disease gained notoriety as "viral abortion" because abortion often results when pregnant mares are affected. Some animals may be carriers.

What are the signs of rhinopneumonitis?

Signs include high temperature (102°-105° F) which lasts two to five days after the appearance of a nasal discharge, swelling of the eyelids, congestion, coughing and loss of appetite. The nasal discharge and coughing may last one to three weeks, and all signs increase with vigorous exercise.

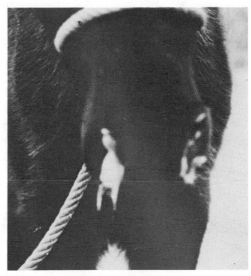

Fig. 18-19. A pony showing a nasal discharge, which may be a sign of viral rhinopneumonitis.

Courtesy of W. L. Anderson, D.V.M.

At four-or five-month intervals, reinfection may occur, but in such mild form that there are no visible signs, fever or complications.

Secondary streptococcal or staphylococcal infections may result in a pus-containing exudate coming from the nose and other signs of inflammation of the pharynx and larynx. These complications make the disease more serious, but most cases recover in 10-21 days. Young foals may develop a secondary pneumonia.

How is rhinopneumonitis transmitted?

Rhinopneumonitis is caused by a herpes virus (the herpes class of viruses characteristically affects cells of the skin and mucous membranes). During the febrile (fever) period, the virus is present in droplets of expectorate (mucus from the lungs or trachea), blood and possibly feces. The virus may be transmitted by contact exposure or inhalation or ingestion of infected material. Aborted fetal membranes, placental fluids and the fetus all contain the virus. Without this tissue the virus lives only two weeks, but it has been shown to live several weeks when dried on horse hair or oily burlap.

Infection has not been known to spread to the stallion through sexual intercourse. A mare may safely be bred at the second heat following an abortion caused by rhinopneumonitis, since the virus is shed with the fetus at the time of the abortion.

What is the relationship of rhinopneumonitis to abortion?

Pregnant mares who have not previously been exposed to the disease usually abort several weeks to several months after the virus has spread through the young horses. About 86% of the abortions occur in the last three months of gestation. The abortion usually proceeds without warning, complications or undue stress to the mare. Labor, delivery and expulsion of the afterbirth occur quickly.

How does the veterinarian diagnose rhinopneumonitis?

Rhinopneumonitis is hard to diagnose in the early stages because there are so many respiratory infections in horses with similar signs. A mild respiratory infection of young horses, abortions in convalescent mares and lesions in the aborted fetuses go together to form a group of signs characteristic of rhinopneumonitis. The viral phase, consisting of nasal discharge, fever and lowered white blood cell count, may go unnoticed. The disease would then not be apparent until after development of secondary bacterial infection, which is characteristic of the disease among broodmares.

What is the treatment for rhinopneumonitis?

There is no treatment which will alter the primary infection, but antibacterial therapy may prevent the onset of secondary infection. This antibiotic treatment should be continued for four to six days during and after the fever period. Any affected animal must be rested. Foals infected prenatally, but born alive, usually do not respond to treatment.

How is rhinopneumonitis prevented and controlled?

If the veterinarian advises that a particular area may be subject to rhinopneumonitis, vaccinations for the horses may be obtained and new horses should be quarantined for two weeks and vaccinated. In the case of an abortion that is suspected of being due to rhinopneumonitis, the veterinarian will probably send the fetus and its membranes to a laboratory for examination. He will also advise as to the proper methods for disinfection of the foaling area and isolation of the mare.

VIRAL ARTERITIS

What is equine viral arteritis?

Equine viral arteritis is an infectious disease of horses. It was recognized in 1957 as a specific disease rather than a "form of influenza" or "pinkeye," as previously believed. The general characteristics of viral arteritis are infection of the respiratory tract and frequently, abortion in pregnant mares. As the name implies, this disease is caused by a virus.

How is the disease spread?

The virus can be spread in a number of ways, including direct contact, ingestion of contaminated material, inhalation of droplets containing infective material (i.e., spread by coughing and sneezing), etc. Viral arteritis is easily transmitted among groups of horses because nasal secretions, saliva, blood and semen of infected horses contain the virus. In addition, the tissues of aborted fetuses harbor large amounts of the virus. There is an incubation period of two to ten days after exposure to the disease.

What are the signs of viral arteritis?

The early signs of this disease are fever (102°-106° F) and a watery nasal discharge. Other signs include excessive lacrimation ("watery eyes"), nasal congestion and conjunctivitis (inflamed eyelids). A laboratory examination will reveal that the infected horse has a lowered white blood cell count.

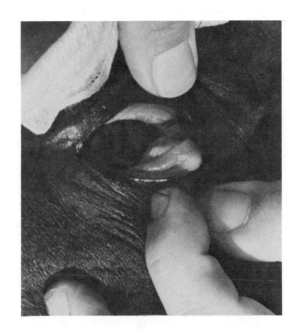

Fig. 18-20. View of a horse's eye showing conjunctivitis, typical in a case of viral arteritis.

Signs frequently include weakness, depression, loss of appetite, difficult breathing, coughing, colic and diarrhea, and edema of the eyelids and legs. Petechial hemorrhages may appear on the nasal mucosa and inner surface of the eyelids.

In most cases the signs persist for one to two weeks, although a longer period is usually required for edema, if present, to subside. Abortion generally occurs late in the course of the disease or in the early stages of recovery (12 to 30 days after exposure). Abortion due to viral arteritis is not characterized by either forewarning signs or retained placenta. Outbreaks of viral arteritis commonly result in an abortion rate of about 50%.

Complications due to secondary bacterial infections can be a sequel to viral arteritis. Pneumonia is a common example.

How does a veterinarian diagnose viral arteritis?

On the basis of external signs, viral arteritis is very similar to several other respiratory diseases. For this reason a laboratory examination is required to conclusively establish the presence of the specific virus. Recovery of the virus from aborted fetal tissues is one method to diagnose viral arteritis in the laboratory.

The name "arteritis" comes from the particular type of arterial damage that this disease causes. Although not visibly apparent, viral arteritis results in degeneration of the middle layer of arterial walls, especially in the small arteries. Hemorrhage and blood clots, depending upon the extent of arterial damage, may occur. An autopsy peformed by a veterinarian will reveal the type and extent of arterial damage in an individual horse.

How is viral arteritis treated?

As a general rule, veterinarians recommend absolute rest for several weeks after the signs of the disease have subsided. Comfortable, warm, draft-free quarters with a plentiful supply of fresh water and good feed are also important factors in aiding recovery. It is a common practice to maintain the horse on antibiotics for a prescribed period of time to either prevent or combat secondary bacterial infections. After the convalescent period, work must be resumed very gradually.

Do most horses make a sound recovery from viral arteritis?

Yes, if the disease was properly treated and complications were minimal. Although viral arteritis is an acute infection, few horses die as a result of the disease itself. In fact, the greatest loss is usually incurred by the high rate of abortion in broodmares. Severely affected animals, however, may continue to have impaired circulation and related problems after convalescence due to residual arterial damage.

An effective vaccine is available to prevent the disease in areas affected by viral arteritis.

ADENOVIRAL INFECTION

What is an adenoviral infection?

This is a respiratory disease caused by adenoviruses, a group of viruses affecting the upper respiratory tract and conjunctiva (membranes lining the eyelid). Certain types of bacteria may also be involved in the infection. Adenoviral infections in horses have been reported in the United States, England and Australia, and have all occurred in Arabian foals that were less than three months old.

What are the signs of this disease?

The first signs to be noticed are mucus discharges from the nose and eye. The disease is characterized by other signs of pneumonia, including coughing and a difficulty in breathing. Fever is present, with the body temperature varying from the normal 100.5° F to 106° F, and the pulse and respiratory rates are elevated. The eyes may have a glazed appearance, but vision is not affected. The foal is thin, has a rough haircoat, and tires easily.

How is the disease diagnosed?

Diagnosis by a veterinarian involves recognizing the signs of pneumonia present and identifying the virus responsible for the infection.

How is the infection treated?

Treatment so far has been ineffective since all reported cases of affected foals

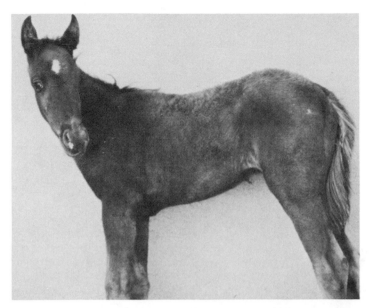

Courtesy of EQUINE MEDICINE AND SURGERY, Edition II, American Veterinary Publications, Inc., Wheaton, Ill.

Fig. 18-21. Foal with adenoviral infection. Notice the discharges from the nose and eye, and the generally poor condition.

have been fatal. Attempted treatment of the viral infection involves controlling secondary infections by bacteria and fungi. Blood transfusions from the dam may be helpful if the mare's blood contains high levels of antibodies against the virus. Affected foals should be stabled in a warm, dry, dust-free stall.

19

THE CIRCULATORY SYSTEM

ANATOMY AND FUNCTION

What is the circulatory system?

The heart, blood vessels, blood, lymph nodes, lymph vessels and lymph make up the circulatory system. This system is responsible for transporting nutrients and oxygen to every part of the body and collecting waste products that are formed in the body tissues. There are three specific divisions of circulation in the circulatory system—systemic circulation, pulmonary circulation and lymphatic circulation.

How is the heart structured?

The heart is a cone-shaped muscular organ that propels blood by alternate muscular contraction and relaxation. It lies in the center of the chest cavity of the horse between the left and right lungs opposite the third to the sixth ribs. This organ is divided into right and left sides and contains four cavities. The upper chambers of the heart are the right and left atria, which function as receiving chambers for blood coming from large veins. The right and left ventricles are the lower chambers of the heart and function as pumping chambers, propelling blood into the large arteries leaving the heart. Due to the pumping function, the ventricles are larger than the atria. Also, because the left ventricle serves to pump blood throughout the body, it is larger (more muscular) than the right ventricle. These four chambers are separated from one another and the rest of the circulatory system by muscular walls and valves.

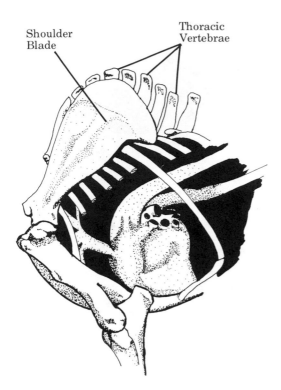

Shoulder
Blade

Thoracic
Vertebrae

Fig. 19-1. Diagram showing the location
of the heart within the chest cavity.

On each side of the heart, between the atrium and the ventricle, is a large valve called the atrioventricular valve (A-V valve). The A-V valve separating the left atrium and the left ventricle is also called the bicuspid valve because it is structured with two flaps (cusps). ("Mitral valve" is another term for this same valve.) The A-V valve separating the right atrium and right ventricle is made up of three flaps and, as a result, is commonly called the tricuspid valve. Both these major valves fall open, allowing blood to enter their respective ventricles as the ventricles relax. Then, as the ventricles contract, the blood within is forced against the A-V valves, closing them, which forces the compressed blood to find another route out of the ventricles.

There is another type of valve in the heart, called semilunar valves because their flaps are shaped like half-moons. On the left side of the heart is the aortic semilunar valve which separates the left ventricle and the aorta. The pulmonary semilunar valve is located on the right side of the heart, separating the right ventricle and the pulmonary artery. These valves are passive in action. The pressure of the blood opens or closes them, depending on what side the pressure comes from.

The walls of the heart are composed of three layers: pericardium, myocardium and endocardium. (The pericardium is further divided into two layers, the visceral pericardium and the parietal pericardium. The visceral pericardium (epicardium) is on the heart wall. The parietal pericardium surrounds the heart loosely, thus forming a sack or "bursa-like" arrangement which separates the heart from the other organs of the thorax.) The center layer of the heart wall is the myocardium (myo = muscle/cardium = heart). The endocardium (endo = inside/cardium = heart) is the inner layer of the heart wall. This is a very thin layer which lines the chambers of the heart, covers the heart valves and smoothly fuses with the linings of the blood vessels entering and leaving the heart.

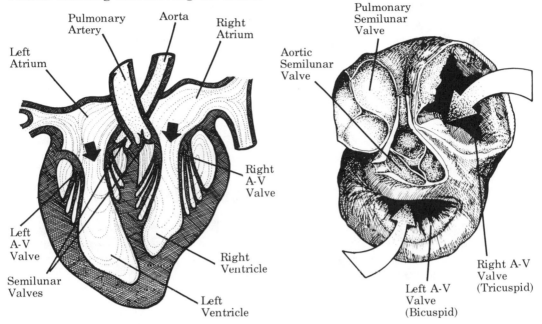

Fig. 19-2. Filling of the ventricles of the heart. Notice that the A-V valves are open and the semilunar valves are shut. Arrows indicate direction of blood flow.

Fig. 19-3. View of the bases of the ventricles. Notice that the A-V valves are open as the ventricles are filling.

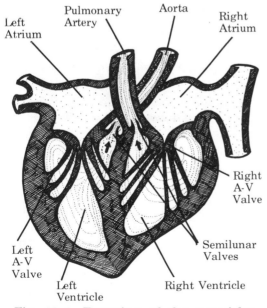

Fig. 19-4. Emptying of the ventricles through the semilunar valves leading to the pulmonary artery and aorta.

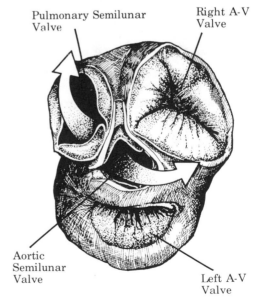

Fig. 19-5. View of the bases of the ventricles. Notice that the semilunar valves are open as the ventricles are emptying.

What are the different types of blood vessels?

The system of blood vessels carries blood to and from the tissues of the body in a continuous, circular path. One very large artery, the dorsal aorta, carries the blood away from the left ventricle of the heart, branching into smaller and smaller arteries as it progresses through the body. The blood goes through smaller arteries and arterioles, eventually going into networks of tiny vessels called capillaries. Continuing the journey, the blood flows through the capillary beds, where the tiny vessels merge, forming larger and larger veins. The merging veins carry blood into two extremely large veins, the cranial (head) vena cava and the caudal (tail) vena cava, entering the heart at the right atrium. From here, the blood falls into the right ventricle and is then forced by myocardial contraction into arteries branching and going to the capillaries in the lungs. From these capillaries, the blood (after oxygen and carbon dioxide exchange) is forced into venules and then into larger veins for transport into the left atrium and then again into the left ventricle where the circular path had begun.

How are the branches of the various vessels named and where are they located?

In general, there is one major artery, vein and lymph vessel going to each part of the body which usually takes the name of the part of the body it is going through. It serves little purpose to increase the reader's understanding of the inner workings of the horse to describe these vessels and their names in detail.

Are arteries just simple tubes?

No. Arteries (and arterioles) have a specialized structure for their function of carrying blood to the body tissues. They are constructed with thick walls of elastic connective tissue with some muscle fibers. These muscular walls help maintain the pumping force from the heart (control blood pressure) and also aid in controlling the amount of blood flowing at a given time. The continuous expansion and contraction of the arterial walls can be felt externally and is called the pulse. In the horse at rest, the pulse normally is between 32 and 44 beats per minute.

What is the structure and function of capillaries?

Capillaries are microscopic vessels with extremely thin walls. They form a network of connecting tubes between arteries and veins. The vital exchanges between food and oxygen carried by blood coming to the tissues, and waste products carried by blood leaving the tissues, take place in the networks of capillaries. The thin capillary walls are semipermeable (partially penetrable) membranes, which means that they allow only selected materials to pass through their walls.

In the pulmonary circulation, the capillaries allow waste products that are expelled through the lungs to pass out, and oxygen and micro-amounts of other gases to pass into the vessels.

How are veins structured and what is their function?

Veins and venules function to drain blood from the capillary beds, returning it from the various body tissues and transporting the blood back to the heart. Regardless of the specific division of circulation, veins always carry blood to the heart, just as arteries always carry blood away from the heart. Veins have thinner walls than arteries and are frequently larger and more numerous than their respective arteries. As a general rule, veins lie closer to the skin.

Very little arterial blood pressure is transmitted through the capillary beds to

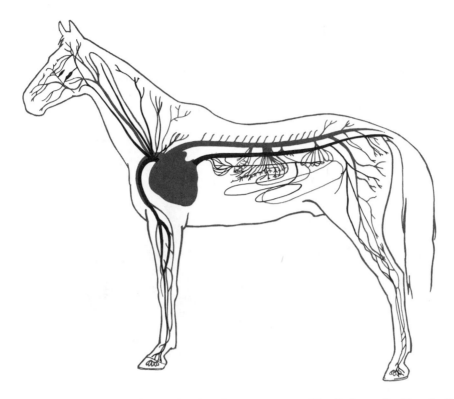

Fig. 19-6 Side view of the systemic circulatory system. The lighter shading indicates the arterial flow; the darker shading indicates the venous flow.

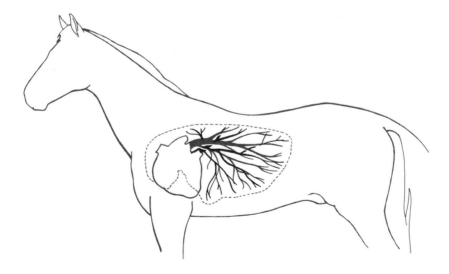

Fig. 19-7. Side view of the pulmonary circulatory system. (Dotted line represents the lung.) The lighter shading indicates the arterial flow; the darker shading indicates the venous flow.

help in the return of blood to the heart, so the veins are equipped with one-way valves, similar to the semilunar valves of the heart. The valves open to allow blood flow only toward the heart and are scattered at frequent intervals throughout the

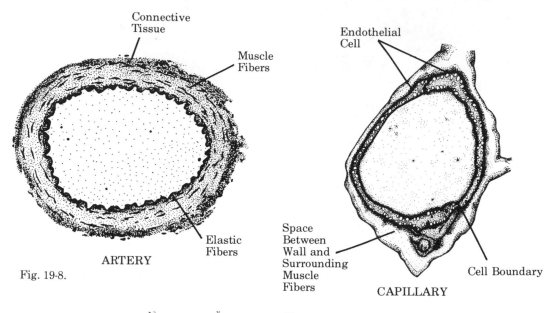

Fig. 19-8.

ARTERY

CAPILLARY

Fig. 19-9.

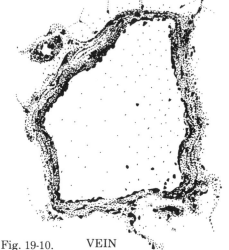

Fig. 19-10.   VEIN

Fig. 19-8. Microscopic view of a cross-section of a distributing artery, showing the three layers of the wall.

Fig. 19-9. Microscopic view of a cross-section of a capillary, at a much larger magnification than the artery (19-8) and vein (19-10). The wall of the capillary is extremely thin.

Fig. 19-10. Microscopic view of a cross-section of a companion vein to the artery in 19-8. The wall consists of three layers, like the artery, but the layers of the vein are less well-defined. Notice that the vein has a thinner wall and a larger interior than the artery.

venous system to prevent blood from flowing back toward the capillary beds. Most veins are situated between masses of muscles so that the muscular contractions of normal movement "squeezes" the veins and forces blood back to the heart. In fact, because of the one-way valves, anything that applies pressure to a segment of a vein aids in the return flow of blood. Some of the additional factors that aid in pumping blood toward the heart are the pulsation of arteries, contractions of the diaphragm during respiration, and peristalsis during digestion. (The stocking up (swelling) of the lower legs of horses when exercise is restricted, such as in a stall or trailer, is due to a lack of muscular activity which, in turn, greatly inhibits the return flow of blood and allows fluid accumulation in the extremities.)

Do arteries and veins actually supply blood to the heart, or do they just carry blood to and from the heart?

The heart is a muscle and, therefore, needs its own blood supply. A system of coronary arteries and coronary veins supplies the heart to provide all needed nourishment to cardiac muscle.

What happens during one heartbeat?

The actions of the heart during one complete heartbeat are called the cardiac cycle. Simultaneously, blood enters the right atrium from the body (through the caudal and cranial vena cavae) and the left atrium from the lungs (through the pulmonary veins). The atria contract when they are full, opening the A-V valves. As this happens, blood flows into the ventricles, which are relaxed. When nearly full, the ventricles begin to contract. At the same time, the atria relax and the A-V valves are closed by the pressure of the blood from the contracting ventricles. While the ventricles are contracting, the pressure also opens the pulmonary and aortic semilunar valves, forcing blood from the left ventricle into the aorta, and from the right ventricle into the pulmonary artery.

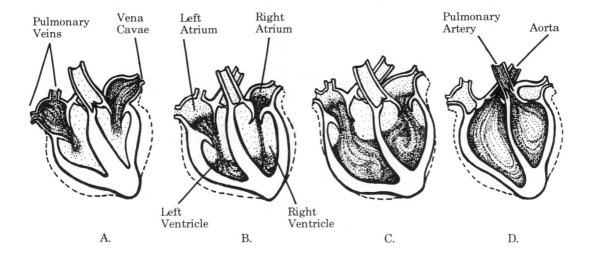

Fig. 19-11. Illustration of the steps involved in the cardiac cycle. A. Blood from pulmonary veins and vena cavae (caudal and cranial) has filled atria. B. Ventricles are being filled with blood from atria. C. Ventricles are nearly full as the atria contract. D. Ventricles are contracting, forcing blood into aorta and pulmonary artery. (Dotted lines indicate full capacity of heart.)

Diastole and systole are names for the actions of the heart's chambers. Diastole refers to the relaxation (dilation) of a chamber just before and during its filling. Systole refers to the contractions of a chamber in the process of emptying, which forces the blood onward.

A complex network of nerves supplies the heart to control its action. Once the nerve impulse triggers the heart, it goes through its orderly series of diastoles and systoles automatically. The process gives off micro-electric currents as the nerve network causes the total heart cycle. These currents can be measured and made to power a needle on paper causing a characteristic tracing. This procedure makes what is called an electrocardiogram (electric-heart-graph) or "EKG" for short.

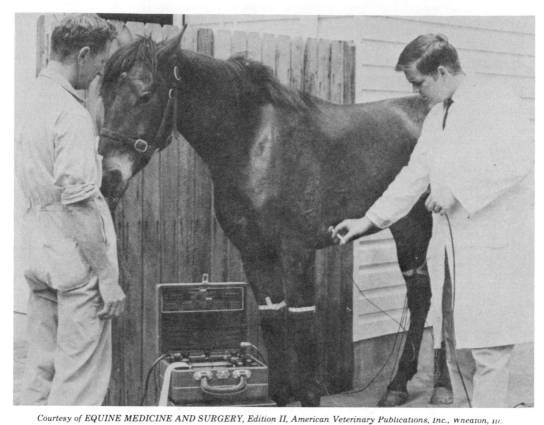

Courtesy of EQUINE MEDICINE AND SURGERY, Edition II, American Veterinary Publications, Inc., Wheaton, Ill.

Fig. 19-12. Recording an electrocardiogram. The horse usually is stood on a rubber mat.

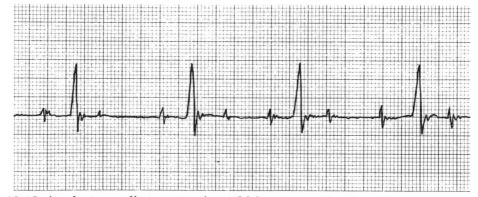

Fig. 19-13. An electrocardiagram tracing, which measures the electric currents of the heart.

THE BLOOD

What is blood?

This is a complex fluid with cellular components in suspension that circulates through the cardiovascular system. It is highly specialized to perform numerous functions.

What are the functions of blood?

Blood has the capacity for transporting a variety of materials. It carries nutrients absorbed from the digestive tract to all tissues of the body. Oxygen is transported from the lungs to the tissues, and carbon dioxide is carried back from the tissues to the lungs. The blood carries waste products from the cells to the kidneys for excretion. Hormones and factors by which the body fights disease are also carried by the blood. The clotting ability of blood helps insure that large quantities of blood will not be lost from injury to the vascular system. In addition, blood helps control the temperature of the body by transporting heat from deep structures to the surface of the body.

In summary, blood has many functions, including those that are respiratory, nutritive, excretory, regulatory (hormonal and thermal) and protective in nature.

What are the cellular components of blood?

Erythrocytes (red blood cells), leukocytes (white blood cells) and platelets (thrombocytes) are the cellular portion of the blood. These cells are formed in bone marrow—specifically, marrow in the ends of long bones and in flat bones, especially the ribs.

What is the function of erythrocytes?

Erythrocytes provide the blood with its ability to carry oxygen. A complex iron-containing compound called hemoglobin is responsible for this ability. Hemoglobin also gives erythrocytes their red color. Because of hemoglobin, the blood is able to carry about sixty times as much oxygen as the same amount of water can carry.

Erythrocytes are structured with thick edges and thin centers and, as a result, are provided with a greater surface area over which the oxygen exchange can take place. However, hemoglobin can combine with only a certain amount of oxygen.

Fig. 19-14. Views of a typical red blood cell.

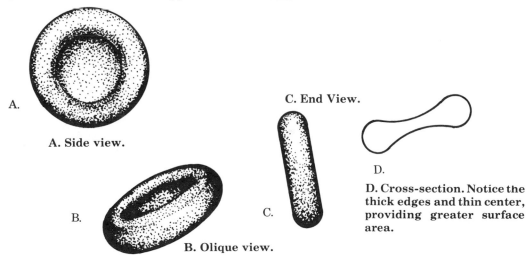

A.

A. Side view.

B.

B. Olique view.

C. End View.

C.

D.

D. Cross-section. Notice the thick edges and thin center, providing greater surface area.

One gram of hemoglobin can absorb only 1.34 c.c.'s (cubic centimeters) of oxygen. As blood goes through pulmonary circulation, oxygen is loosely attached by chemical bonding to hemoglobin in the red blood cells to be carried to the tissues. The chemical resulting from this bonding is called oxyhemoglobin. The fact that actual chemical bonding takes place here (in the lungs) has importance that will become apparent in some of the disorders described in this section. The oxyhemoglobin releases the oxygen in the capillary beds during systemic circulation.

In the blood, erythrocytes are continually wearing out and being replaced. The average erythrocyte in the horse has a life of four to five months, and then begins to disintegrate. Worn-out erythrocytes are removed from circulation by special cells in the liver, spleen, bone marrow and lymph nodes. Erythrocyte destruction takes place in the liver, and products which cannot be used again by the body (such as bile pigments) are excreted in the bile. A light horse normally has nine to twelve million erythrocytes per cubic millimeter of blood, while the number usually ranges from seven to ten million erythrocytes per cubic millimeter of blood in draft horses.

What is the function of leukocytes?

There are different types of leukocytes (white blood cells), including neutrophils, eosinophils, basophils, monocytes and lymphocytes. The main function of leukocytes is to combat infection in the body (see Process of Inflammation and Healing, page 8). Some, such as neutrophils, are most active in defense of acute infection, while others, such as monocytes, are most active in the face of less acute infections.

Fig. 19-15. An erythrocyte and various types of leukocytes:

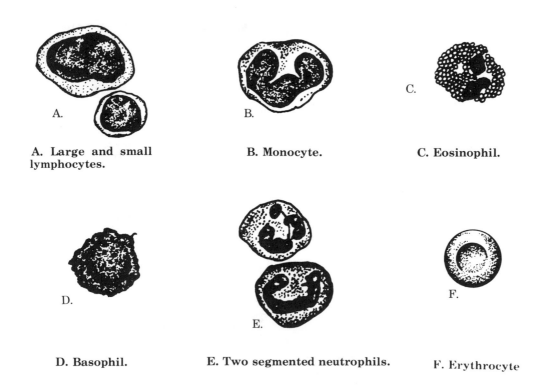

A. Large and small lymphocytes.

B. Monocyte.

C. Eosinophil.

D. Basophil.

E. Two segmented neutrophils.

F. Erythrocyte

Leukocytes, unlike erythrocytes, have independent movement. They are carried by the blood to general locations of infection and then can move to the actual site of the infection. Leukocytes fight infection by a process called phagocytosis—they literally engulf the invading bacteria and digest them. In the process, some of the leukocytes die. This material, in combination with dead tissues, is called pus.

The number of leukocytes circulating in the blood increases when infection is present in the body. Under normal conditions the horse has 8,000 to 11,000 leukocytes per cubic millimeter of blood.

What is the function of platelets?

Platelets, or thrombocytes, function to reduce blood loss when tissue is injured. Platelets are instrumental in forming the clot which "clogs" the damaged vessel to prevent further loss of blood.

What is the liquid portion of the blood in which the cellular components are suspended?

The fluid portion of the blood is called plasma and is about nine-tenths water. The kidneys are responsible for keeping this proportion of water in the blood at a constant level. Proteins and inorganic matter make up the other ten percent of plasma. Plasma proteins, including serum albumin, fibrinogen and globulin, aid in retaining fluid in the vessels. In addition, fibrinogen is a necessary component of the blood clotting mechanism, and globulin is instrumental in immunity and resistance to disease. Also, most of the carbon dioxide to be expelled by the lungs is carried from the tissues dissolved in the plasma.

How does blood clot?

Injured platelets release thromboplastin. Thromboplastin released in sufficient amounts causes prothrombin to change to its active form, thrombin. Thrombin then reacts with fibrinogen to form fibrin, which is the matrix for the clot. Erythrocytes, leukocytes and platelets become ensnared in the fibrin, forming a jelly-like clot which shrinks to form a true, firm clot and serum. (Serum is a term for the clear fluid that remains after blood has clotted. Basically it is blood with the cellular components and fibrin removed.)

THE LYMPHATIC SYSTEM

What is the lymphatic part of the circulatory system?

Lymphatic circulation is made up of the lymph, lymph vessels and lymph glands (nodes), including the spleen. The vessels and glands form a series of channels throughout the body to aid in filtering out and destroying substances that may be harmful to the body. Lymphatic circulation also collects nutrients from the area of the intestines and waste products throughout the body so that they may be properly directed.

What are lymph glands?

Lymph glands are masses of lymphocytes scattered throughout the body, along the paths of most blood vessels. These masses of lymphatic tissue are encapsulated, forming specific structures. The tonsils and the spleen are specialized lymph glands. Lymph glands serve as one of the first barriers against infection because they produce lymphocytes and antibodies, and by the action of the lymphocytes concentrated within them, act as filters of the lymph fraction of the blood that goes through them.

What is the spleen?

The spleen is a ductless gland located in the upper part of the abdominal cavity between the stomach and the diaphragm. The spleen is a sponge-like organ enclosed in a muscular capsule. It works like a sponge, serving as a storage area for blood, and constantly varies in size depending upon the amount of blood it contains. The spleen is also functional in the destruction of worn-out erythrocytes, releasing the iron from hemoglobin to be reused by the body.

Fig. 19-16. Illustration of the stages involved in the formation of a blood clot.

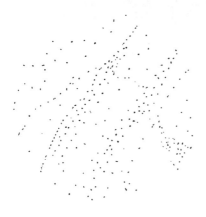

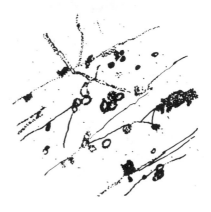

A. Area before clot has begun to form.

B. Threads of fibrin in first stages of clotting.

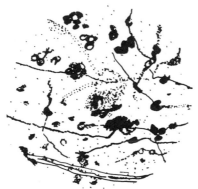

C. Cells entrapped in mesh of fibrin threads.

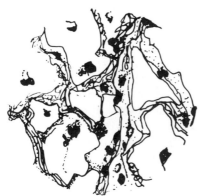

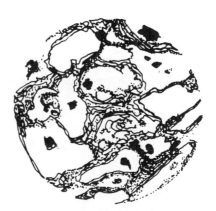

D. More cells, including erythrocytes, leukocytes, and platelets, entrapped in the fibrin.

E. A firm clot.

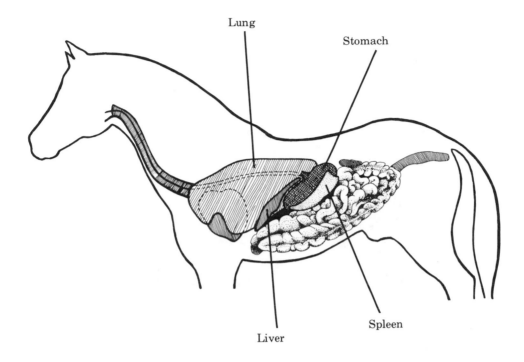

Fig. 19-17. View of the organs of the thoracic and abdominal cavities, showing the location of the spleen.

What is special about the tonsils?

They are unique in that they are the only lymph glands exposed to the outside environment. Inhaled air passes directly over the tonsils as it passes their location in the pharynx.

What are the lymph vessels?

The lymph vessels form a system of one-way channels and are structured with valves (like the veins), allowing the fluid to flow only toward the heart. Also, like arteries and veins, lymph vessels converge, becoming larger and larger until they finally empty into the cranial vena cava.

Where does lymph originate?

When nutrients and oxygen leave the bloodstream in the capillary beds, fluid also escapes. Most of this fluid is reabsorbed by the veins, but some remains out in the extracellular spaces. This excess fluid is collected by lymph vessels, and is called lymph as soon as it enters the vessels. Lymph is a clear liquid, very similar to blood plasma. After being filtered by lymph glands along the courses of the vessels, lymph is channeled into the return venous circulation at the cranial vena cava, and returned to the bloodstream. In summary, lymphatic circulation supplements the return functions of the veins.

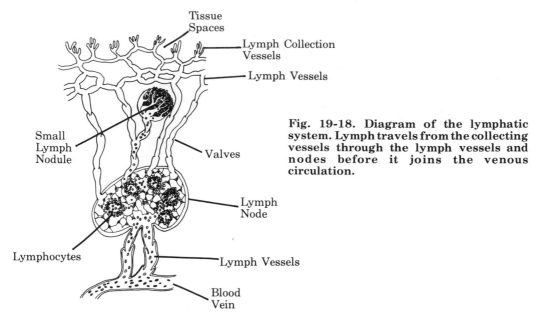

Fig. 19-18. Diagram of the lymphatic system. Lymph travels from the collecting vessels through the lymph vessels and nodes before it joins the venous circulation.

EPISTAXIS (NOSEBLEED)

What is epistaxis?

Epistaxis is simply nosebleed. It may appear from unexplained causes, but many times its appearance points to some other disorder.

What causes epistaxis?

Nosebleed is most often observed in race horses, just after a race. It does occur during a race at times, which may prove more hazardous to the rider than the horse, since horses have been known to react by making a very sudden stop. The bleeding comes from small fragile capillaries in the lining of the nasal cavity which expand and fill with blood as the horse becomes excited. As the race continues, blood pumps through the capillaries even faster, and heavy breathing rushes the air by the tissues at a rapid clip. The combination of these strains can occasionally put too much pressure on the capillaries, which then rupture. Epistaxis that is due to fragile capillaries may first be noticed when the horse is quite young. It sometimes ceases as the horse gets older, but can continue and become chronic.

Other cases of epistaxis may be caused by an external, forceful injury. For instance, it is not uncommon for the mucous membrane of the nasal passages, which is thickly lined with blood vessels, to be damaged by the passing of a stomach tube. Foreign bodies entering the passages or injuries to the facial bones can also be responsible.

Epistaxis that has no forceful cause often indicates an upper respiratory disorder. The mucous membranes of this area (including the guttural pouches) are subject to the lesions of viral infections, inflammation, weakening and rupture of the capillaries, tumors and parasites. Even a previous infection can weaken the tissue enough to cause bleeding.

A disorder that is not limited to the upper respiratory tract may also show up through a nosebleed. Equine infectious anemia and congestive heart failure are good examples of this.

How is epistaxis treated?

Since epistaxis may indicate that other problems are present, a veterinarian should be called. This may be an urgent requirement if the bleeding cannot be stopped quickly.

Epistaxis usually involves only one nostril, and the blood is dark red. If the horse does not recover spontaneously, the nostril may be packed with a tampon. Both nostrils may not be packed, as this would prohibit breathing. Cold packs may be applied if the site of the injury is not specific. Until the bleeding stops, the horse should be walked slowly rather than allowed to stand. When these measures are not effective, the veterinarian may choose to administer drugs which constrict the capillaries, or those that speed up blood clotting. Severe bleeding may call for a blood transfusion.

What are the long-range effects of epistaxis?

In most cases, epistaxis is a temporary disorder, and there is complete recovery. The outcome of epistaxis caused by another disorder depends, of course, on the successful treatment of the specific problem.

Bleeding from both nostrils that is bright red and frothy indicates hemorrhage in the lower respiratory tract, called hemoptysis. Bleeding in the lungs is difficult to stop, and the portions that have bled may become necrotic (die).

If the blood contains bits of ingested food, gastrorrhagia (hemorrhage of the stomach) is indicated.

PERICARDIAL DISEASE

What is pericardial disease?

Pericardial disease usually refers to an inflammation of the fibrous sac surrounding the heart (the pericardium) known as pericarditis. The inflammation also involves the epicardium, the outer surface of the heart.

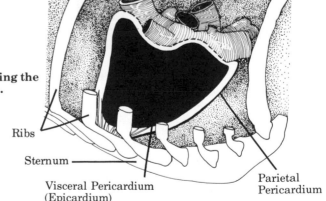

Fig. 19-19. View of the heart showing the structures involved in pericarditis.

Ribs

Sternum

Visceral Pericardium
(Epicardium)

Parietal
Pericardium

What causes pericarditis?

Pericarditis is usually secondary to various respiratory infections in the horse such as strangles and tuberculosis. Occasionally, the inflammation may be caused by violent activity, such as a hard collision with another horse, or by an injury from a nail or piece of wire that pierces the pericardium. In these cases, the pericardium may rupture and cause further damage to the heart, resulting in death within a short time.

How does pericarditis affect the function of the heart?

In pericarditis, fluid accumulates between the pericardium and the heart wall. This creates pressure on the heart and interferes with the return of venous blood to the heart by compressing the atria and right ventricle. These chambers, which receive the venous blood, are then prevented from expanding and completely filling with blood. This results in congestion, or engorgement, of the veins, which can lead to congestive heart failure.

What are the signs of pericarditis in the horse?

In the early stages, the horse feels pain, avoids movement and lies down carefully. The horse's back is arched, breathing is shallow and there may be signs of pneumonia. The pulse rate is increased and the body temperature is raised from a normal 100.5°F to 103°-106°F.

Pericarditis can often be diagnosed by detecting unusual heart sounds. There may be a scratching or grating sound caused by the surface of the heart rubbing against the inflamed pericardium. The heart sounds which are normally present may be muffled, due to the accumulation of fluid between the heart and pericardium.

How is pericarditis treated?

The condition must be diagnosed by a veterinarian so the underlying cause can be treated. Treatment involves the administration of antibiotics to control respiratory infection. Surgical treatment to drain the fluid from within the pericardial sac is rarely attempted and is usually not successful. If a foreign object has penetrated the pericardium, it must be removed.

MYOCARDIAL DISEASE

What is myocardial disease?

The myocardium is the muscular layer of the heart which is located between the smooth, inner lining known as the endocardium, and the outer surface, the epicardium. Myocarditis is an inflammation of the myocardium which sometimes occurs in horses. Other conditions which are less common include myocardial lesions involving the degeneration of tissue and necrotic (dead) areas of tissue known as infarcts.

What causes myocarditis?

Myocarditis occurs in various infectious diseases and may develop as an extension of inflammation of the endocardium or of the pericardium, the sac surrounding the heart. Myocarditis often occurs as a manifestation of tuberculosis and other bacterial respiratory infections, such as strangles.

What can cause other myocardial lesions?

Purpura hemorrhagica, a disease of the blood (see page 475), sometimes results in degeneration of fatty tissue and hemorrhage of the myocardium. Hemorrhages and necrotic areas of the myocardium also may occur in equine infectious anemia (see page 480). Myocardial infarcts may occasionally result from blood clots formed by migrating strongyle larvae, a type of parasitic worm larva.

Myocardial damage has recently been observed in some horses that were administered a drug for muscular relaxation during castration and other short surgical procedures. The affected horses showed either a decrease in their performance ability or sudden death. Examination of the heart after death revealed small hemorrhages in the myocardium.

What are the signs of myocardial disease?

The signs of myocarditis and other myocardial lesions vary, and inflammatory changes usually cannot be distinguished from other types of myocardial damage. Myocardial disease is often undetected until the horse's body is examined after death. Signs of myocarditis resulting from an infectious disease may not be observed until weeks after the infection is recognized.

Signs of myocardial disease include an increased heart rate and various irregularities in the rhythm of the heartbeat, such as missed beats. Abnormal heart sounds (murmurs) may be present, and an electrocardiogram may reveal certain abnormalities. There may also be signs of congestive heart failure, and sudden death sometimes occurs.

Can myocarditis be treated?

When the condition is secondary to another disease, treatment should involve controlling the underlying infection. In later stages of heart failure resulting from myocarditis, treatment is often ineffective or impractical. Since myocarditis sometimes goes undetected, treatment in these cases is impossible.

ENDOCARDIAL DISEASE

What is endocardial disease?

The endocardium is the membrane lining the inner surface of the heart, composed of endothelial cells and connective tissue. Inflammation of the endocardium can involve the surface wall or the heart valves, resulting in a condition known as endocarditis.

What causes endocarditis?

Endocarditis is usually caused by a bacterial infection, which may be an extension of respiratory bacterial diseases such as strangles. The inflammatory condition may also result from an allergic reaction, or from the presence of strongyle worm larvae in the bloodstream.

How does the disease interfere with the normal function of the heart?

Endocarditis usually causes malfunctioning of the heart valves controlling the openings of the heart. Lesions may develop on the valves and interfere with the normal passage of blood through the heart. Blood vessels connecting with the heart can then become engorged or congested, resulting in congestive heart failure.

How do these endocardial lesions develop?

In the process of inflammation, the endothelial cells of the endocardium are destroyed and sloughed off. A clot forms on the raw surface left by the damaged endothelium and continually grows in size. The clot contains fibrous tissue and may develop into large (over an inch) cauliflower-shaped growths, or small wart-like growths. These nodules of tissue are not serious if they develop on the wall of the endocardium, but lesions on the valves interfere with normal function. The growths can obstruct the passage of blood or prevent the valves from closing properly. In the later stages of endocarditis, further malformation of the valves may occur in which they become shrunken, distorted, and often thickened along the edges. This later distortion is caused by the contraction of the fibrous scar tissue that formed earlier.

Are there visible signs of endocarditis in the horse?

The horse usually suffers a loss of condition, involving a weight loss and weakness, and easily becomes exhausted during exercise. The heart rate is increased and there is a moderate fever. The mucous membranes of the mouth and nose often appear pale and there may be signs of pneumonia and arthritis. On examination, the veterinarian will hear a murmur (abnormal heart sound) caused by turbulence as the blood flows past the defective valves. Signs of endocarditis may be present for as long as several weeks or months, or the horse may die suddenly without previous signs.

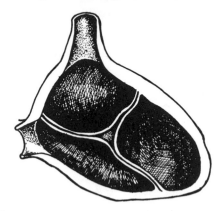

Fig. 19-20. Normal appearance of a valve of the heart.

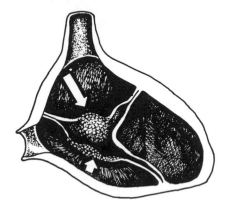

Fig. 19-21. Incomplete closure of a heart valve due to fibrous growths (arrows) as a result of endocarditis.

Can endocarditis be treated?

Treatment involves controlling the infection causing the condition. It is usually not very successful since the drugs may be unable to penetrate the thick endocardial lesions and get to the pathogenic bacteria. In addition, the pathogen may be resistant to many of the available antibiotics. The heart rarely fully recovers since the valves may be permanently distorted and similar types of clots and lesions may have formed in other organs of the body. Endocarditis is often recognized at too late a stage for treatment to be effective.

CARDIAC ABNORMALITIES

When should heart trouble be suspected?

Heart trouble may be suspected when a horse reacts to hard work or exercise by exhaustion or an unusual difficulty in breathing. The heartbeat may seem extremely rapid and irregular, or the horse may collapse or faint after exertion. Fainting often indicates a cardiac abnormality known as a heart block, which causes the heart to miss one or more beats. The horse may show incoordination and a trembling of the legs. Stumbling and lameness that have no obvious cause may be due to a circulatory disorder. Fading on the racetrack, which occurs when a horse slows down or pulls back after it has been running hard, can be due to an abnormal heart condition.

What kind of abnormalities affect the heart?

Cardiac abnormalities may be classified as either structural or functional. Structural abnormalities are relatively rare in the horse and involve defects which usually cannot be corrected. Congenital heart defects are usually structural. Functional cardiac abnormalities are more frequent and can often be treated. They are usually caused by a faulty nerve supply to the four chambers of the heart (right and left atria and ventricles). The two nerves controlling the action of the heart synchronize the muscular contraction of the right and left sides of the heart, causing the valves on one side to open and shut at the same time as the valves on the opposite side. When the two sides of the heart are not synchronized, due to an inefficient conduction of nerve impulses, the heartbeats become irregular.

What does the horse's normal heartbeat sound like?

In man, the normal heartbeat consists of two sounds, usually described as "lub-dup" (S1-S2). The horse's heartbeat is basically composed of the same two sounds but four heart sounds may often be heard in normal horses and described as ba, lub-dup, bup (S4,S1-S2,S3)

What causes these heart sounds?

The fourth heart sound is caused by atrial systole, the contraction of the right and left atria, forcing blood into the right and left ventricles. This sound occurs just before the first heart sound caused by ventricular systole (contraction of the ventricles). The third heart sound in the horse is caused by rapid filling of the ventricles with blood from the atria. It occurs just after the second sound, that of the closing of the semilunar valves of the ventricles. The semilunar valve of the right ventricle leads to the lungs through the pulmonary artery, while the semilunar valve of the left ventricle leads to the rest of the body through the aorta.

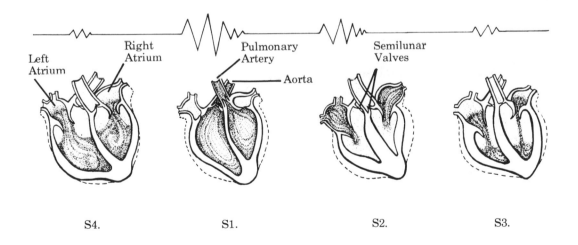

Fig. 19-22. Illustration of the actions causing the heart sounds. S4. Atrial systole. S1. Ventricular systole. S2. Closing of semilunar valves. S3. Filling of ventricles. (Dotted lines indicate full capacity of heart.)

Do variations of these heart sounds ever occur?

All four sounds may not be audible in normal horses; a lack of one or two heart sounds is not an abnormal condition if the rhythm of the beats is still regular.

Variations in a particular beat, such as a slight increase in the intensity of the first sound, may occur in normal horses. Abnormal sounds or sounds that are out of place are referred to as murmurs and usually indicate some type of cardiac abnormality.

What causes heart murmurs?

A heart murmur is the sound of an abnormal blood flow through the heart valves. Various kinds of murmurs may be caused by a backward flow or leaking of blood through the valves known as regurgitation, incompetence, or insufficiency. Murmurs may also be due to stenosis, which is a narrowing of a valve orifice or of a vessel leading to or from the heart. Murmurs in the horse are often difficult to evaluate since they may be present in the normal horse during systole (contraction of the heart) and diastole (dilatation or enlargement of the heart chambers as they fill with blood).

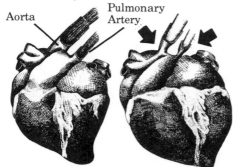

Fig. 19-23. Stenosis (arrows) of blood vessels carrying blood away from the heart, resulting in an abnormal blood flow. On the left, normal appearance of the heart.

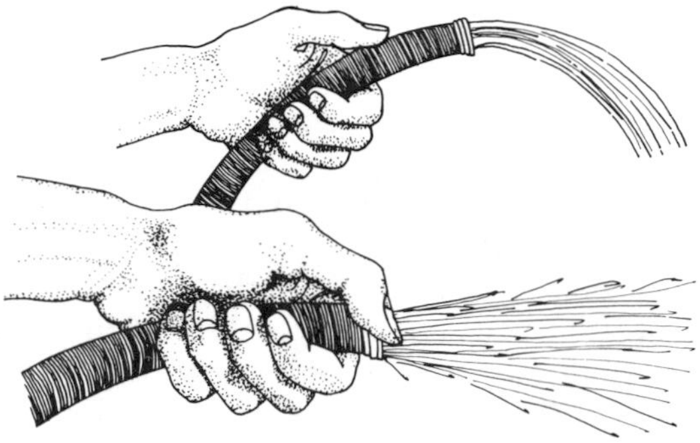

Fig. 19-24. Above, normal flow. Below, the flow is changed by narrowing the opening of the hose (or heart valve orifice).

What are some examples of heart murmurs?

One type of abnormal heart sound may be caused by atrioventricular insufficiency, in which the valve between the atrium and ventricle is deformed. The defective valve will fail to close completely at the proper time, allowing blood to flow back into the atrium as the ventricle contracts (systole). This regurgitation causes a murmur which can be heard during ventricular systole, beginning with the first heart sound and extending to the second. Other murmurs may be due to regurgitation at the semilunar valves of the ventricles.

Murmurs due to stenosis involve a narrowing of the valves or of the vessels connecting with the valves. There may be obstructions such as nodules of fibrous tissue on the valves or vessels, narrowing the passage for the blood. The murmurs usually occur between normal heart sounds.

When are the actual heart sounds abnormal?

The heart sounds themselves may sometimes be weak or very intense, and slight variations in intensity may sometimes occur in normal horses. An abnormally weak first sound may indicate tired or weak heart muscle resulting from a toxic disease, or it may be an early indication of heart failure. A weak second sound may indicate a fall in blood pressure which can occur when the horse has been weakened by illness. An increase in blood pressure, especially within the kidneys, may cause an accentuated second sound. An accentuated first sound may occur when an obstruction is present in the atrioventricular valves, and it may be associated with hypertrophy (enlargement) of the heart muscle.

Is an enlarged heart harmful?

Enlargement of the heart can involve two types of development known as dilatation and hypertrophy. Hypertrophy is an increase in the thickness of the heart wall, and may not be harmful to the horse's health. A normal horse's heart muscle will develop, becoming larger and stronger, in response to work and training. Horses that are continually overworked or kept in racing condition too

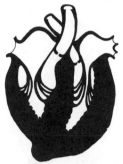 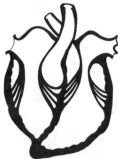

Fig. 19-25. Enlargement of the heart. In hypertrophy, the heart wall becomes thickened. In dilatation, the chambers of the heart enlarge, causing the wall to be thin and flabby.

HYPERTROPHY   DILATATION

long may develop abnormally large hearts. A hypertrophied heart then has no room for expansion within the pericardium, the fibrous sac enclosing the heart, and is subjected to abnormal pressure as it expands against the unyielding pericardium. The heart muscle will eventually tire and lose its efficiency when it works beyond its capacity in trying to overcome the increased pressure.

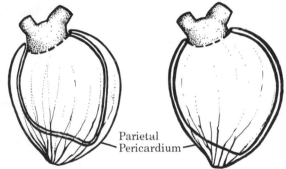

Fig. 19-26. The effect of hypertrophy. On the left, normal appearance of the heart within the pericardium. On the right, an abnormally large heart, which leaves little room for expansion within the pericardium.

Parietal Pericardium

How does dilatation affect the heart?

Dilatation is an abnormal enlargement of the chambers of the heart, causing the muscle wall to be thin and flabby. Both hypertrophy and dilatation may occur in response to excessive hard work, or to a stenosis (constriction) or insufficiency (leaking) of the heart valves. When blood leaks back through the valves, the ventricles may compensate by dilating in order to hold a larger volume of blood than usual. This would allow a certain amount of blood to leak backward, and still allow the normal amount of blood to be pumped out through the valves.

Do cardiac abnormalities ever affect the rate and rhythm of the heart?

These are usually functional abnormalities and include increased rates, decreased rates, arrhythmia (irregularity) and gallop rhythms. Increased and decreased rates may sometimes be normal responses to changes in the rates of nervous impulses in the heart. An increase in heart rate may be a normal response to excitement, pain, or increased body temperature. An abnormally rapid rate of contraction may be a severe defect and although it can be treated, is often fatal. A decreased heart rate may be associated with heart block, a type of arrhythmia.

What is heart block?

Heart block is an irregularity in the rhythm in which one or more beats may be missed. It is caused by a defect in the nerve supply, which interferes with transmission of impulses from the atrium to the ventricle. Some heart blocks may occur in normal horses and will disappear when the animal is exercised. Heart blocks which are highly irregular in the number of beats missed and the time sequence may be signs of heart disease.

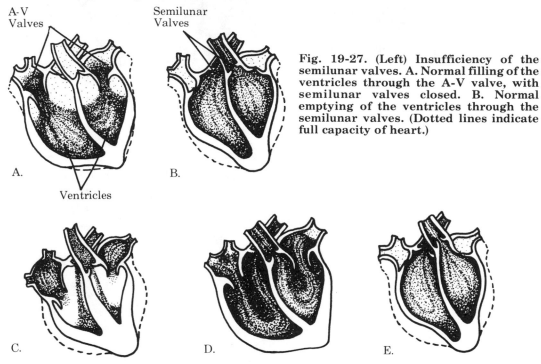

Fig. 19-27. (Left) Insufficiency of the semilunar valves. A. Normal filling of the ventricles through the A-V valve, with semilunar valves closed. B. Normal emptying of the ventricles through the semilunar valves. (Dotted lines indicate full capacity of heart.)

Fig. 19-27C. Insufficiency of the semilunar valves, causing blood to leak back into the ventricles. D. Ventricles filled with blood through the open A-V valves and the leaking semilunar valves. E. Contraction and emptying of the ventricles.

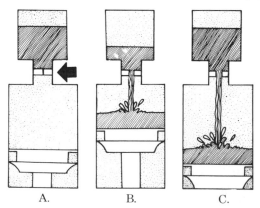

Fig. 19-28. A piston, used to demonstrate the principle of dilatation to compensate for insufficiency of the heart valves. A. The normal amount of fluid has been pumped upward through the valve (arrow). B. Fluid is leaking back through the valve into the bottom chamber. C. The piston is lowered, enlarging the bottom chamber (dilatation). More fluid can then be pumped through the valve, allowing some fluid to leak back while a normal amount of fluid is still present in the top chamber.

What are gallop rhythms?

This is a three-beat or triple rhythm that resembles the sound of a galloping horse. The third heart sound is more intense than usual, although it may be slightly accentuated in normal horses. It may be caused by an insufficiency of the valves or by some type of heart disease involving an inflammation of the walls of the heart.

Can cardiac abnormalities be treated?

Most structural defects, including congenital defects, cannot be corrected in the horse. Functional abnormalities may sometimes correct themselves spontaneously, and can often be controlled with various types of medication after proper diagnosis of the condition by a veterinarian. The horse should not be put completely at rest but should follow a schedule of light walking exercise for a long period of time until the heart has recovered its normal function.

CONGENITAL HEART DISEASE

What types of congenital heart disease affect the horse?

Congenital heart diseases usually involve structural defects at birth that cause illness or death in a few weeks. In other cases, the defect may not be observed until the horse is several years old. The heart may compensate for a structural defect by mechanisms such as dilatation or enlargement, when a defective valve is present. Congenital defects in the horse may involve various malformations of the heart valves, affecting the flow of blood in and out of the chambers of the heart and causing a murmur (abnormal heart sound). Other congenital defects include a patent ductus arteriosus and interventricular septal defects.

What is a patent ductus arteriosus?

In a normal heart, blood is pumped from the heart to the lungs through the pulmonary artery. In the fetus, blood is not required in the lungs since the lungs at this time are nonfunctional. Blood is diverted from the lung by means of the ductus arteriosus, a short blood vessel leading from the pulmonary artery to the aorta, which carries blood from the heart to the rest of the body. The opening of the ductus arteriosus will normally close a few days after birth. Occasionally, the opening does not seal shut and the defect is referred to as a patent (open) ductus arteriosus, resulting in the foal's lungs not receiving enough blood from the heart. A murmur can often be heard as blood passes through the opening.

What are interventricular septal defects?

These are structural defects in the muscular wall (septum) dividing the right and left ventricles of the heart. Interventricular septal defects and valvular deformities are the most frequent congenital abnormalities in the horse. In the developing heart of the fetus, the septum may fail to develop completely, leaving an opening between the ventricles at birth. Blood will then flow between the left and right ventricles, an abnormal condition which allows a mixture of the blood entering and leaving the heart. This results in a decreased amount of oxygen in the blood circulating throughout the body, a condition known as cyanosis. If the defect is not too severe, the foal may survive but fail to grow when young, or the foal may appear normal until maturity. Indications of heart failure may then be observed when the horse is older.

Can congenital defects be treated?

Most congenital defects require surgery, and for this reason, treatment is usually not attempted. The foal may survive only a few days, in the case of severe defects, or it may live for several years before the heart's efficiency is seriously affected.

VASCULAR LESIONS

What are vascular lesions?

The most common vascular lesions are aneurysms, thrombi and emboli. These are all conditions affecting the blood vessels which may occur separately, or in combination. Aneurysm is the term for a weakening and dilatation of a vessel wall. This weakening may be due to degeneration or inflammation of the vessel wall, or because of partial rupture. Development of an aneurysm usually is followed by formation of a thrombus, a blood clot made up of alternate layers of blood platelets and fibrous material attached to the vessel wall. Thrombosis may give rise to emboli (broken off parts of thrombi) which lodge in narrow branches of the vessels, downstream from the original mass. Emboli can cut off the supply to limbs or organs, resulting in tissue death, if there is no development of new blood supply to the affected part. The body usually attempts to develop "collateral" (alternate) routes of supply when one channel is blocked, but this may not form quickly enough to prevent necrosis (tissue death) and infection.

What is the significance of vascular lesions?

Vascular lesions are fairly common, though undiagnosed in most horses. They are due, in large part, to damage by *Strongylus vulgaris* (the principal large strongyle, see page 503) and are covered in detail in that section. When lesions interfere greatly with the blood flow, they may be the cause of lameness in the hindlegs, colic or death.

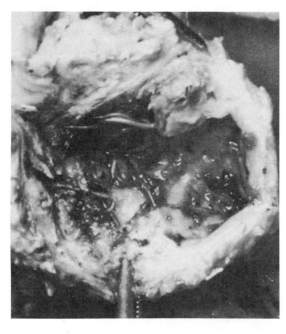

Fig. 19-29. Vascular lesions due to damage by *Strongylus vulgaris* larvae in an artery.

Courtesy of THE HORSE, by Peter D. Rossdale, M.A., F.R.C.V.S., published by The California Thoroughbred Breeders Association. Photo by Peter Rossdale.

Can vascular lesions be prevented?

Yes. Prevention of strongyle infestation greatly reduces the chances that aneurysm, embolism or thrombosis will occur.

POLYCYTHEMIA

What is polycythemia?

Polycythemia is a state in which there is an increase in the proportion of circulating red blood cells. It may be relative, due to a reduction in blood fluid, or absolute, due to an increase in the number of blood cells.

What causes polycythemia?

If polycythemia is due to a relative decrease in the amount of fluid circulating in the circulatory system, the condition may have several causes. Hemorrhage, excessive sweating, dehydration, diarrhea, restricted water intake, inflammation and shock, all allow the loss of fluids from the circulation. When fluids are not replaced, it makes the red blood cells appear more numerous and concentrated (called hemoconcentration). The condition of abnormally high red blood cell production, or true absolute polycythemia means that there has been an absolute increase in the number of red blood cells produced. Absolute polycythemia has not been reported in horses, but transient absolute polycythemia is frequent.

What is transient absolute polycythemia?

A transient absolute polycythemia means that there has been a temporary increase in the number of circulating blood cells. Race horses and other animals under stress have a temporary absolute polycythemia when they are excited. Excitement causes the spleen to release extra red blood cells to help carry oxygen to the tissue if "fight or flight" is necessary. Animals raised at high altitudes develop this condition to carry more of the thin oxygen found in high elevations.

What causes polycythemia?

Most frequently, polycythemia is caused by abnormal disorders that cause severe pain. The release of epinephrine is believed to be the reason for the increase in available red blood cells. Rare cases of chronic disorders of the heart and lungs may develop polycythemia to compensate for the decreased circulatory capabilities.

What are the signs of polycythemia?

If polycythemia is caused by another condition (dehydration, shock, etc.), the signs will be those of the principal condition. Temporary polycythemia may be distinguished by evaluation of blood samples by a veterinarian. In any case, polycythemia is important as a sign of other conditions.

What is the treatment for polycythemia?

Polycythemia is only treated if it is secondary to a treatable condition. If it is due to dehydration or shock, fluid therapy will probably be administered by the attending veterinarian.

HEMOPHILIA

What is hemophilia?

Hemophilia is a hereditary defect in the clotting mechanism of the blood. When a colt with hemophilia gets a cut or bruise, the bleeding is very difficult to control.

Fig. 19-30. Sex-linked Inheritance of Hemophilia.

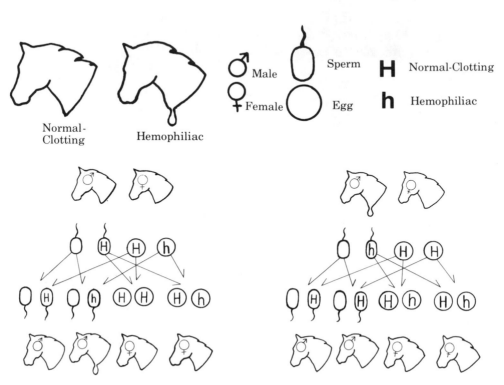

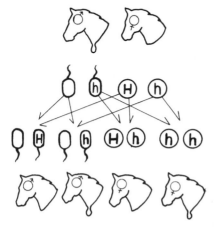

A. Normal-clotting carrier mare bred to normal-clotting stallion, producing a hemophiliac male foal and a female carrier (of the recessive hemophiliac gene, h).

B. Normal-clotting mare bred to hemophiliac stallion.

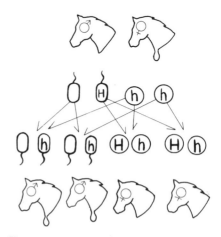

C. Normal-clotting carrier mare bred to hemophiliac stallion.

D. Hemophiliac mare bred to normal-clotting stallion

Fig. 19-30.   Matings B., C. and D. are highly unlikely situations, since hemophiliac male foals rarely survive to become stallions, thus preventing them from ever being bred and producing hemophiliac female foals.

What causes hemophilia?

The cause of hemophilia is a lack of one of the clotting factors (factor VIII). In horses, it appears to be caused by inheritance of a sex-linked recessive gene. This trait is relatively uncommon and is expressed (shows as a disease) only by males. Mares may carry the recessive gene, but it does not cause hemophilia in the mare. When she is bred and produces a male foal, the foal has a 50% chance of inheriting the disease.

What are the signs of hemophilia?

When a foal is affected with hemophilia, there may be difficulty with continued bleeding of the umbilical stump. Any tissue damage may cause large hemorrhages under the skin, into joints or internally. Weakness and swelling of hematomas are often the first visible signs. The internal and joint hemorrhages are crippling and eventually fatal.

What can be done to treat or control hemophilia?

Hemophilia can be treated with whole blood transfusions or plasma to replace the missing factor. This is only a temporary aid, however, because the colt will never be able to produce the clotting factor on his own. Since the condition can never be cured, euthanasia is usually recommended by the veterinarian if the laboratory tests show an absence of the necessary factor.

In order to prevent hemophilia, carrier mares should not be used as broodmares. If a mare has produced a foal with hemophilia, she is identified as a carrier and should not be bred again, unless the owners wish to take the chance of having to destroy an affected foal.

THROMBOCYTOPENIC PURPURA

What is thrombocytopenic purpura?

Thrombocytopenia is a reduction in the number of platelets circulating in the blood. Thrombocytopenic purpura is a rare disorder characterized by hemorrhages from the lack of platelets.

What causes thrombocytopenic purpura?

In horses, thrombocytopenic purpura is usually a secondary condition caused by bacteria or viral infections, especially equine infectious anemia. The lack of platelets may be due to reduced production of platelets in the bone marrow or to increased destruction of platelets by the spleen.

What are the signs of thrombocytopenic purpura?

The signs of thrombocytopenic purpura may be edema and hemorrhage of the mucous membranes and the tissues beneath the skin. These signs may occur in association with the signs of infection of the bone marrow, aplastic anemia or as a response to massive hemorrhage and the exhaustion of available platelets.

What is the treatment for this condition?

In humans, thrombocytopenic purpura is usually treated with corticosteroids, removal of the spleen, and the administration of whole blood. This treatment has been attempted with horses with some success. Since this condition is quite rare, it must be referred to a veterinarian for diagnosis and laboratory determination of platelet counts.

NEONATAL ISOERYTHROLYSIS (JAUNDICED FOALS)

What is neonatal isoerythrolysis?

Neonatal isoerythrolysis is a severe hemolytic anemia (red blood cell destroying) disease of newborn foals. Since jaundice is one of the signs, it is often called foal jaundice. This disease is similar to Rh sensitivity in human infants.

What causes the destruction of red blood cells?

During pregnancy, some of the foal's blood may pass into the mare's circulation. If the foal has inherited a blood type that is different from the mare, her blood will treat the foal's erythrocytes as foreign bodies. Antibodies (produced by the mare) to fight the antigen (the foal's blood cells) are stored and concentrated in the mare's first milk, the colostrum. When the foal receives colostrum, the antibodies absorbed through the intestine begin to attack and destroy his red blood cells. Antibodies may coat or clump red blood cells and cause them to be removed by the foal's spleen and liver. Rupture of the red blood cells is also caused by antibodies from the mare.

How does a mare become sensitized (produce antibodies)?

In isoimmunization, mares can be sensitized by their foals if some placental disease allows the passage of blood from the foal to the dam. Normally, this does not occur, which is why the foal is not affected when it is born. There is no transplacental (across the placenta) transfer of antibodies in horses. All of the antibodies are contained in the colostrum.

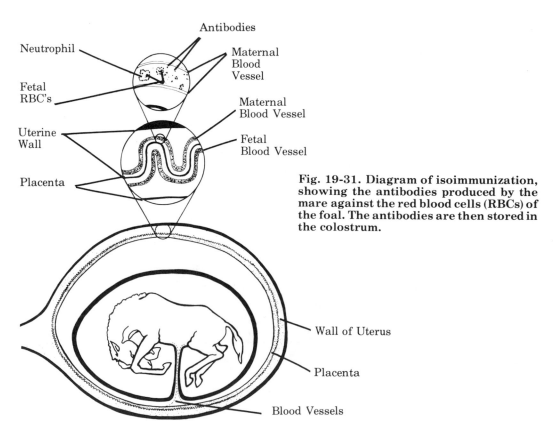

Fig. 19-31. Diagram of isoimmunization, showing the antibodies produced by the mare against the red blood cells (RBCs) of the foal. The antibodies are then stored in the colostrum.

Blood transfusions of incompatible blood or the use of vaccine that contains horse erythrocytes may cause the mare to produce antibodies.

What are the signs of this disorder?

Foals usually are quite healthy when they are born and nurse normally. Within 12 to 36 hours, however, they become dull, weak, do not nurse and they may collapse. Respiratory and heart rates are usually increased but the temperature may be normal or below normal. Mucous membranes may be pale for the first 24 hours, developing jaundice (yellowing) within 24 to 48 hours that gets progressively worse. The urine may vary from light yellow to deep red, depending on the severity and amount of red blood cell destruction. Death may occur from acute anemia within 12 to 36 hours. Frequently, foals survive only three to four days, but some may live for eight to ten days.

What can be done for foals with this disorder?

If possible, affected foals should be confined and given large volume transfusions of whole blood within 24 to 48 hours after birth. The veterinarian will want to perform blood tests on the mare and the foal, to determine the degree of damage to the foal's erythrocytes.

Where can blood donors be found?

The veterinarian can check available horses and find one whose erythrocytes are not affected by the mare's antibodies. Only one donor is usually necessary.

Can the foal ever nurse from his dam?

Most antibodies are removed from the mare's milk within 8 to 16 hours, if she is milked by hand every hour. After 48 to 72 hours, it is usually safe to return a foal to the mare's milk. A foster mare may be used, if one is available. Foals that are two or three weeks old may be safely transferred to the sensitized mare while her foal is suckled by the foster mare. If the foal is deprived of colostrum (none is stored or available), antibiotics will be necessary for four to six days as protection against infection.

How may neonatal isoerythrolysis be prevented?

If mares are known to be sensitized, they may be safely bred only to stallions whose blood is compatible with their own. Breeding of sensitized mares will always result in the production of antibodies. Foals from sensitized mares can be muzzled and given frozen colostrum, if the sire's blood type has not been matched with that of the mare. Blood tests of the foal's and mare's blood may reveal no clumping reaction, in which case the foal may be allowed to nurse. In any case, the foalings of known sensitized mares should always be attended, and the veterinarian alerted that a transfusion might become necessary, so he will have the necessary test equipment with him.

PURPURA HEMORRHAGICA

What is purpura hemorrhagica?

Purpura hemorrhagica is a disease of the horse characterized by extensive collections of fluid and blood in tissues beneath the skin (edema). These swellings occur primarily on the head and legs.

What causes purpura hemorrhagica?

Purpura hemorrhagica may be caused by an allergic reaction to the protein of streptococci, since it frequently occurs one to three weeks after a case of strangles, infectious arteritis or equine rhinopneumonitis. Damage to the capillary walls by toxins or an allergic reaction causes extravasation (escape) of blood and plasma into the tissues beneath the skin.

What are the signs of purpura hemorrhagica?

The signs of purpura hemorrhagica may develop slowly or rapidly, depending on the severity of the reaction. If the case is mild, edema may develop gradually over a period of several days. In more severe cases, swelling may be marked within two or three days. Appearing most frequently on the head and legs, swellings are often present on other parts of the body. These swellings vary in size, are cold, painless, "pit" on pressure and merge gradually with the normal surrounding tissue. Submucous hemorrhages are visible in the nose, mouth and often inside the eyelids.

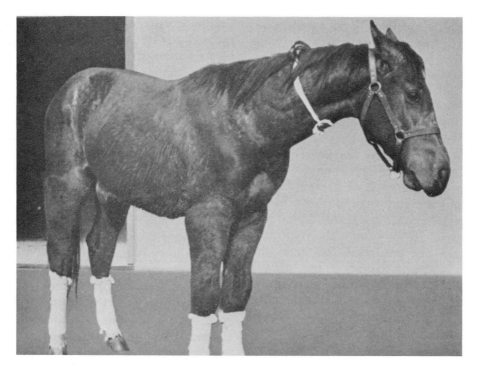

Courtesy of CLINICAL DIAGNOSIS OF DISEASES OF LARGE ANIMALS, Lea and Febiger Publishing Co., Philadelphia, Pa., W. J. Gibbons, D.V.M.

Fig. 19-32. A horse affected with purpura hemorrhagica. Notice the swellings of the face, lips, neck and legs. A tracheotomy has been done to facilitate breathing.

The skin may be tightly distended and ooze serum, especially over joints. Infection and sloughing of the affected skin and tissue are evidence of acute purpura. Severe forms of purpura hemorrhagica involve a progressive development of edema of the legs, eyes, upper respiratory passages and larynx leading to difficulty in breathing. Congestion of the mucous membranes may occur, and nasal discharges frequently contain serum and pus if tissue death has occurred in the upper respiratory passages. Affected horses have difficulty in moving, and they appear stiff and sore. As the disease progresses, urination may become difficult due to swelling of the prepuce. Appetite usually diminishes as the swellings spread and the animal becomes more reluctant to move its neck. Death is frequent (50% mortality) due to blood loss, asphyxiation or secondary bacterial infections.

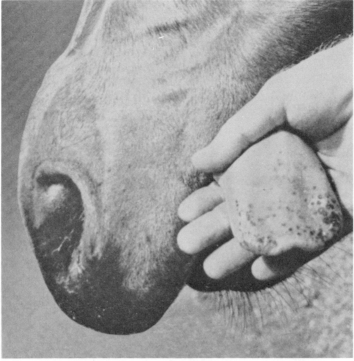

Courtesy of CLINICAL DIAGNOSIS OF DISEASES OF LARGE ANIMALS, Lea and Febiger Publishing Co., Philadelphia, Pa., W. J. Gibbons, D.V.M.

Fig. 19-33. Submucous hemorrhages in the tongue of a horse with purpura hemorrhagica. Notice the swollen nose and nasal discharge.

What is the treatment for purpura hemorrhagica?

There is no specific treatment for purpura hemorrhagica. Treatments have been aimed at reducing the allergic response (corticosteroids), combating the blood loss (transfusions), and fighting secondary infections (antibiotics). A tracheotomy may be necessary when breathing is obstructed by swelling of mucous membranes in the nose, pharynx and larynx. Bandaging and massage of the limbs is thought to be helpful, along with heavy bedding to avoid injury leading to further extravasation. Good nursing may reduce the mortality rate and facilitate recovery within two to four weeks. The recovery period may be longer if skin necrosis is extensive.

Can purpura hemorrhagica be prevented?

The only means of preventing purpura hemorrhagica is prevention of the diseases that lead to it. Also, continuing treatment with antibiotics for a week following infections of *S. equi* is recommended.

EHRLICHIOSIS

What is ehrlichiosis?

Ehrlichiosis is a non-contagious disease that is caused by a bacterium that invades the white blood cells. Most common in the foothill regions of Northern

California, it is important to distinguish ehrlichiosis from more serious disorders like infectious anemia, viral arteritis, leptospirosis and piroplasmosis.

What are the signs of ehrlichiosis?

This disorder is most acute in horses over two years old. In the acute form, signs of ehrlichiosis include fever (102°-107°F), depression, incoordination, lack of appetite, cool, painless edema of the legs and jaundice. Edema may include the belly and sheath. The testes of mature male horses may swell, then shrink. Fever and depression (and severe edema) can be present for up to two weeks. Younger horses usually develop only fever (less than one year old) or may show signs of fever and mild edema of the legs (one to two years old).

What is the importance of ehrlichiosis?

Since ehrlichiosis can only be positively identified by laboratory examination of a blood specimen collected during a period of fever, the disorder must be diagnosed by a veterinarian in order to treat it properly. If other, more serious disorders are assumed to be ehrlichiosis, the horse could possibly die without proper care. Also, ehrlichiosis could weaken the horse, allowing other infections to develop.

What is the treatment for ehrlichiosis?

In most cases, oxytetracycline has inhibited the multiplication of the bacterium *Ehrlichia*. The natural means of transmission is unknown, but horses are relatively immune to infection for about two years following recovery from ehrlichiosis.

PIROPLASMOSIS

What is piroplasmosis?

Piroplasmosis is one of the names along with Texas Fever, Redwater Fever, Biliary Fever, Horse Tick-Fever and Equine Malaria, that is used to describe Babesiasis. Babesiasis is a protozoal disease carried by blood-sucking ticks to infect the horse. Horses in most tropical and subtropical regions of the world are subject to the disease. Piroplasmosis first appeared in the United States in Florida in August of 1961. It is now considered as being established in southern Florida and has been observed in scattered cases in several other states.

Piroplasmosis may be peracute, acute, chronic or inapparent, depending on the number and virulence (disease causing potency) of the parasites originally introduced.

What causes piroplasmosis?

Babesia caballi and *B. equi* are the two babesial species which cause piroplasmosis in horses. They develop and grow as parasites within the red blood cells causing destruction of parasitized cells, resulting in a hemolytic anemia.

Various species of ticks may serve as vectors (carriers) for piroplasmosis. The only tick recognized as a vector in the United States so far has been *Dermacentor nitens*, the tropical horse tick. Only certain species of ticks can carry this disease because Babesia must be able to grow and develop in a tick to be successfully carried by it. *B. caballi* is able to persist through several generations of *D. nitens* by passage through the eggs.

In some parts of the world, the disease is enzootic: that is, it is constantly present at a level that allows animals to develop a fairly high level of immunity. Horses in these areas that have shown no signs of infection have been known to suddenly develop them, usually after some kind of stress. However, the United States is an epizootic area, which means that virtually all horses are susceptible to piroplasmosis because there is not a constant presence of the disease to stimulate natural immunity.

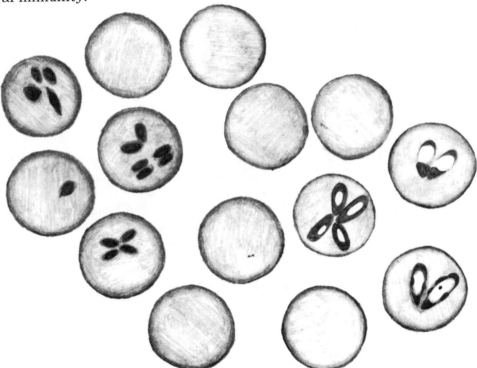

Fig. 19-34. Red blood cells, showing the babesial species which cause piroplasmosis. On the left, *Babesia equi*. On the right, *Babesia caballi*.

What are the signs of piroplasmosis?

Piroplasmosis may be obvious within 24 hours after the initial infection if a large number of parasites are introduced into a susceptible horse. However, the incubation period is usually 5 to 9 days after artificial infection, and 10 to 21 days after a tick bite.

Common developments concurrent in a case of babesiasis include pnemonia, digestive upset, kidney dysfunction and encephalitis. The characteristic signs of the disease include depression, appetite loss, swollen eyelids, a mucous nasal discharge, jaundice (yellowing of the mucous membranes) and sluggishness. The body temperature will usually rise to between 103° and 106°F., but fever may be absent. The horse may be thirsty, show colicky signs, and suffer from either diarrhea with bile-stained feces or constipation. The urine will usually be reddish-brown due to the destruction of many red blood cells, but true hemoglobinuria (presence of free hemoglobin in the urine) is infrequent. Sometimes the horse will secrete blood-stained tears or have edema of the head, limbs and lower parts of the thorax and abdomen. Weakness in the hindquarters often occurs, evidenced by a staggering gait. The pulse will become fast, weak and irregular.

How is piroplasmosis treated?

First, a diagnosis must be made on the basis of laboratory analysis. After piroplasmosis has been confirmed, a chemotherapeutic agent such as Euflauine, 5% solution, may be used by the veterinarian. The antibiotic oxytetracycline has also been found to be fairly effective against Babesia species. Many different drugs have been used with variable success, but therapy is most effective when begun in the early stages of the disease. However, it is not known whether any treatment will completely eliminate residual parasites, thus preventing the horse from being a carrier.

How can the spread of piroplasmosis be controlled?

There are three aspects to controlling equine piroplasmosis. One is, of course, aimed at controlling the vector, *D. nitens*. Another is finding out which horses are carriers through serologic tests. Thirdly, the carriers must be eliminated or treated with drugs to try to eradicate the residual parasites. Quarantine of horses in transport between countries is an important measure in piroplasmosis prevention.

What is the prognosis in cases of piroplasmosis?

In acute cases the horse may be dead within 24 to 48 hours. In areas where the horse population has no immunity by vaccine or previous infection, the mortality rate can be as high as 90%. Early, effective treatment can bring the mortality rate down to 5%. The 1961 Florida outbreak had a mortality rate of 15%. Most recovered horses will remain carriers for about 10 months, but possibly as long as four years.

EQUINE INFECTIOUS ANEMIA (SWAMP FEVER)

What is equine infectious anemia?

Equine infectious anemia (abbreviated E.I.A.) is an infectious disease of the blood that is caused by a virus. "Swamp fever" is characterized by a long, chronic illness which follows an acute attack. Horses which survive the initial attack of the disease become carriers of the virus, and can spread the disease to other horses.

What happens when a horse contracts E.I.A.?

It takes the virus between one and three weeks to cause any reaction in the horse. After this period, the virus is present in the blood in large enough numbers for the body to recognize its presence as a foreign substance (antigen). The body reacts by producing antibodies, which attempt to phagocytize (eat and digest) the virus. This reaction is responsible for the characteristic anemia in E.I.A. Complement, a system of enzymes, is produced in antigen-antibody reactions and is attached to or coats the living red blood cells, damaging them and causing them to break or rupture much earlier in their lifespan than is normal. After a short period, the virus is even found living in cells of the liver, spleen and lymph tissues. The most serious aspect of this disease is the fact that the antibodies are unable to eliminate the virus from the body of the horse. If it is unable to kill the horse, it persists in the blood as long as the horse lives.

What are the signs of E.I.A.?

Acute. The first sign of acute E.I.A. is a sudden fever, often reaching 105°F or higher. Rapid weight loss, anemia and hemorrhages of the mucous membranes usually accompany the fever (which may vary) for 10 to 30 days, when the horse usually dies.

Subacute. Horses with less acute virus infections may have several bouts of fever, each of which may last up to a week, with normal periods in between febrile (fever) periods. Weight loss is more obvious in longer infections, when the horse may become depressed and quit eating. Anemia and swelling of the legs and lower abdomen may be severe in these subacute cases. (Death usually occurs in these cases within two or three months.)

Chronic. If the horse develops chronic E.I.A., there will be similar periods of intermittent fever, mild anemia and weight loss. Lost weight may be regained during the periods when the horse appears to be normal. Death may occur at any time during a recurrent attack of fever. Any E.I.A. infection can become asymptomatic, that is, without outward signs of disease.

Can infected horses be recognized?

No. Infected horses that do not show signs of E.I.A. are often assumed to be healthy, normal horses.

Is there any way to determine the presence of E.I.A. virus in a horse?

Yes. A highly reliable test, the Coggins test, can determine the presence of E.I.A. antibodies in a blood sample.

How does the Coggins test detect E.I.A. virus?

The Coggins test is valid only if the blood sample is drawn and submitted by a veterinarian. Blood serum is removed from the sample, and placed on a dish of sterile gel, which contains a known positive sample of serum in three alternate positions around a center well of E.I.A. antigen. Two other horses can be tested on the single plate in the remaining wells. The reaction of an antigen with antibodies forms a line of clumps or precipitates where the two meet on the plate of gel. Three positive reactions are always present to compare the three test horses against. If a positive reaction occurs, the test is usually repeated to be sure of the results because horses are often destroyed on the basis of this test.

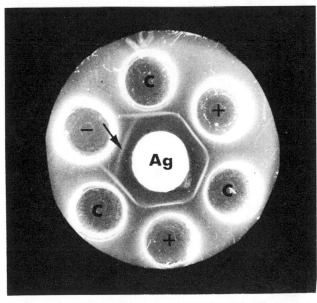

Fig. 19-35. The Coggins test for E.I.A. The center well (Ag) is filled with antigen, and the six outer wells are filled with serum. The wells marked (+) contain sera that react positively; this is reflected by the precipitin lines. The well marked (-) contains a negative serum, having a nonspecific precipitin line that is not continuous with the positive control lines.

Courtesy of EQUINE MEDICINE AND SURGERY, Edition II, American Veterinary Publications, Inc., Wheaton, Ill.

Can E.I.A. be controlled?

Yes. Since the disease is transmitted by any mechanism that transfers blood from one horse to another, there are means of controlling its spread. Control of biting flies and mosquitoes around stable areas, care in sterilization of surgical instruments, tattoo and hypodermic needles (or use of disposable needles) will help to prevent outbreaks of E.I.A. in areas where control is possible. Isolation of new animals until a negative Coggins can be obtained is also wise. Infected mares should not be used as broodmares, due to evidence that the virus may be transmitted to the foal through the placenta before birth, and through the milk after the foal is born.

PHENOTHIAZINE TOXICITY

What is phenothiazine toxicity?

Phenothiazine is a common element in horse wormers. Infrequently, some animals may react strongly to this drug, developing signs of anemia, abortion or photosensitization.

What causes phenothiazine toxicity?

The most important cause of toxic reactions is poor physical condition. Heavy parasite infestations or poor nutrition makes an animal more susceptible to a toxic reaction from phenothiazine. Refinement of phenothiazine also affects its toxicity, more refined forms being less likely to cause a reaction than the more crude forms of the drug. Very large doses of phenothiazine may cause this reaction in healthy horses.

What are the signs of phenothiazine toxicity?

Frequently, the signs of phenothiazine toxicity are those of anemia: depression, dullness, lack of appetite, paleness of mucous membranes, the presence of blood in the urine and (occasionally) abdominal pain. Some red discoloration of the urine is normal due to the conversion of phenothiazine into a dye. These signs usually begin one or two days after the phenothiazine is given. In some cases, the horse may become very weak and go into a coma. Prompt veterinary treatment is necessary to reverse severe anemia.

Other signs of a toxic reaction may include photosensitization (light sensitivity, page 386) or abortion.

What are the effects of phenothiazine?

Phenothiazine produces a poisoning effect on the red blood cells, causing them to break easily. In those cells which do not rupture, the phenothiazine causes the hemoglobin to condense and move to the edge of the red blood cell, forming a bulge (Heinz body). This abnormality of the red blood cells will help the veterinarian to determine the cause of the reaction if blood for a laboratory test is drawn from the affected horse.

How is phenothiazine toxicity treated?

If the toxic reaction is not severe, the veterinarian may decide not to treat the condition. In cases where treatment is necessary, blood transfusions and fluids are usually administered intravenously. Further exposure to the drug should be avoided once a sensitivity has been shown.

EPIZOOTIC LYMPHANGITIS (ULCERATIVE LYMPHANGITIS)

What is epizootic lymphangitis?

Epizootic lymphangitis is a rapid-spreading, usually fatal disease, which probably no longer occurs in the United States.

What causes epizootic lymphangitis?

Histoplasma farciminosum, which causes the disease, is a fungus that grows in the soil. It usually enters the body through abrasions on the skin, and may be picked up by contact with an infected animal or contaminated soil, fences, harness or grooming tools. When the site of infection is the eyes or nasal passages, flies are generally the carriers. The disease may also affect the lungs, which indicates that *H. farciminosum* may also be pathogenic (disease-causing) when inhaled.

What are the signs of epizootic lymphangitis?

The usual sign of epizootic lymphangitis is that the lymph vessels thicken and stand out from the skin, developing nodular lesions at varying intervals. The nodules develop into abscesses, which rupture, giving off a thick, yellow, oily pus, and become open wounds. These usually appear on the lower limbs, in areas where there have been saddle sores, or around the eyes.

Mucous membranes of the eye itself may be affected, as well as those of the mouth, nostrils and genitals. If the infection spreads to the lungs, the horse is unable to breathe properly, and a thick, yellow fluid comes from the nostrils.

Signs of infection do not show until about two months after exposure to the organism, and at that time the disease spreads rapidly to horses nearby. In the final stages, the horse loses appetite, temperature increases, and a general weakness may be noted.

How is epizootic lymphangitis diagnosed?

The external signs of epizootic lymphangitis are virtually identical to signs of several other disorders. The presence of *H. farciminosum* must be established before concluding the diagnosis, and this must be done under laboratory conditions.

How is epizootic lymphangitis treated and controlled?

There is no known treatment for epizootic lymphangitis, and it is usually fatal. The owner of an affected horse, after consulting a veterinarian, may wish to consider having the animal destroyed for the sake of controlling the spread of the disease. If at all possible, the body should be incinerated, flies should be controlled, all items in contact with affected horses should be disinfected, and stalls should be kept quarantined for six months.

THE DIGESTIVE SYSTEM

ANATOMY AND FUNCTION

What is the function of the digestive system?

The digestive system is responsible for the intake (ingestion and grinding) and subsequent breakdown (digestion and absorption) of foods. The nutrients contained in these foods are utilized for energy, growth, body repair and storage. Digestion takes place through muscular action, enzyme action, and bacterial fermentation. The digestive process is complete when usable nutrients are assimilated and undigested food residues and waste products are excreted.

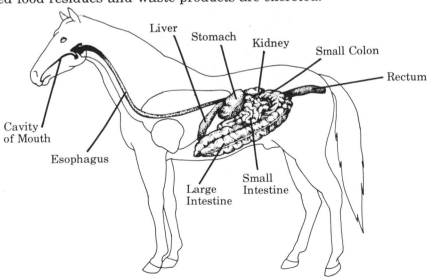

Fig. 20-1. This is a simple view of the horse's digestive tract, showing the various organs involved in digestion.

How is the digestive system organized?

The digestive tract of the horse consists of a muscular tube called the alimentary canal (digestive tract), which begins at the lips and terminates at the anus, and several associated organs. The alimentary canal consists of the mouth, pharynx, esophagus, stomach, small intestine, cecum, large colon, small colon and rectum. Associated organs which aid in the total digestive process are the teeth, tongue, salivary glands, liver and pancreas.

The alimentary canal is about 100 feet long in the mature horse. It changes diameter abruptly in several places, enlarging at the stomach, narrowing at the small intestine and enlarging again at the cecum. The tract is lined with mucous membranes, most of which contain glands to secrete digestive fluids.

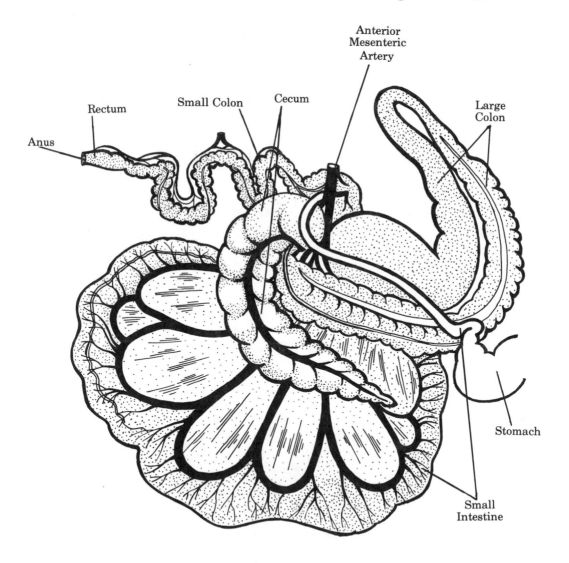

Fig. 20-2. A spread-out view of the gastro-intestinal tract. Notice the fan-shaped mesentery that supports the intestines.

What is the function of the mouth?

The digestive process in the horse begins at the mouth. The mouth is bounded in front by the lips, on the sides by the cheeks, above by the hard palate, and below by the tongue and the mucous membranes beneath it. The soft palate extends backward from the hard palate to act as a tube permitting the passage of food and water between the mouth and the pharynx but not from the pharynx into the mouth.

The lips pick up loose food and pass it back into the mouth with the help of the tongue. The incisor teeth are used to grasp and nip food when grazing. The mouth of the adult horse contains 12 incisor teeth, premolars and molars. The male will usually also have two canine teeth in each jaw while the mare may or may not. The molar or cheek teeth grind the food into small particles while it is mixed with alkaline saliva from the three pairs of salivary glands: the parotid, the submaxillary and the sublingual. The parotid glands are the largest and are located below the ear and behind the jaw. The submaxillary glands are located, one on each side, partly under the parotid gland and partly inside of the jaw bone. The sublingual gland is beneath the tongue and can be felt just beneath the skin between the bony ridges of the jaw. The mature horse secretes up to 10 gallons of saliva each day.

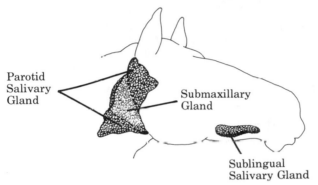

Fig. 20-3. Location of the salivary glands in the horse. The submaxillary salivary gland lies beneath the parotid salivary gland.

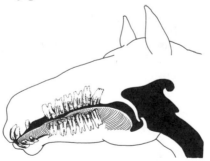

Fig. 20-4. This illustration shows the tongue and the teeth, the first structures of the digestive system

The horse is normally a slow eater and will take up to 15 or 20 minutes to eat a pound of hay or 5 to 10 minutes for a pound of grain. Hay absorbs four times its weight in saliva; oats absorb slightly more than its own weight. Saliva acts as a digestive juice on the sugars and starches in the food and lubricates the food for swallowing, which is initiated by the lever action of the tongue flipping a ball of food towards the pharynx.

In drinking, the horse uses his tongue like a piston on a suction pump to draw water back just as man does in drinking from a straw. Each swallow takes in about a half pint. The horse's ears will draw forward as a reflex action at each suction and fall back during the swallowing phase of each gulp.

What is the structure and function of the pharynx?

The pharynx is the muscular passage which separates the mouth from the esophagus. Food moves by muscular action through the pharynx to the esophagus. Being part of both the respiratory and digestive systems, the pharynx also provides an air passage between the nostrils and the larynx. The soft palate, at the back of the mouth, acts as a trap to prevent food, water and air from returning to the mouth from the pharynx. For this reason, the horse can neither breathe nor vomit through the mouth. Any food unable to pass down the esophagus due to obstruction or illness will return through the nostrils rather than through the mouth.

What is the function and structure of the esophagus?

The esophagus is a tube about five feet in length which connects the pharynx to the stomach by way of the neck through the thoracic (chest) cavity and diaphragm. The esophagus can be seen in the groove along the lower left side of the neck by watching as a horse swallows food or water. The circular muscles of the esophagus force food and water down by waves of constriction called peristalsis. This muscular action cannot work in reverse. Due to the acute angle at which the esophagus enters the stomach, excessive gastric pressure that would push food back up the esophagus in other species pushes the membrane flaps of the cardia (orifice where the esophagus enters the stomach) closed, thus preventing vomiting in the horse except on rare occasions involving certain severe forms of colic.

What is the function and structure of the stomach?

The stomach is a J-shaped muscular sac in the front part of the abdominal cavity close to the diaphragm. Openings from the esophagus and to the small intestine are rather close together so water tends to pass quickly out of the stomach, through the small intestine and into the cecum.

Considering the size of the horse, the stomach is relatively small. It can hold up to four gallons, but the first stage of digestion is more efficient when it is filled to about 2½ gallons rather than full capacity. Because of the small size of the stomach, it is best that food be given in small amounts at frequent intervals. (One should remember, when deciding how much to feed a horse at each meal, that the great amount of saliva mixed with the food increases its volume to nearly twice what has been measured out as the feed ration.) Solid food is acted on by digestive juices. In the stomach lining there are many cells that form and secrete primarily hydrochloric acid and the enzyme pepsinogen. Pepsinogen changes structure in the acid mediums within the lumen of the stomach to become pepsin, a protein-digesting enzyme. The hydrochloric acid changes the pepsinogen into pepsin and dissolves the mineral matter in the food. Food tends to enter the stomach in layers, with the end closest to the small intestine filling up first. Digestion begins as soon as food enters the stomach, but nothing starts to leave the stomach during feeding until it is two-thirds full because of a relaxation reflex that takes place during feeding. Then as more food comes in, a steady stream begins to pass out so that considerably more than the capacity of the stomach can be passed through at one bulky feeding. Total digestion and utilization of the feed is impaired in the case of a large feeding. Much of the food is deprived of the important early stage of digestion which changes feed from its natural state to a semidigested form called chyme in the stomach. When feeding is not excessive at one meal, the emptying process is slower, allowing more time for better mixture of the feed with gastric juices and more complete early digestion. The stomach is never completely emptied unless the horse goes without food for a couple of days. Drinking while digesting food can upset the layered food, resulting in a large amount of food being washed into the small intestine. Consequently, unless given free access to water at all times, a horse should be watered before being fed.

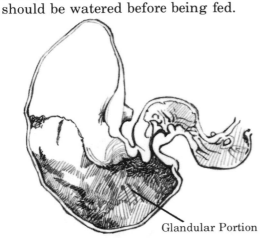

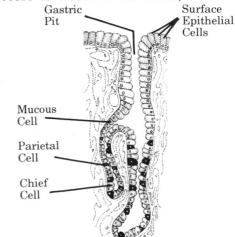

Fig. 20-5. Cut-away view of the stomach, showing the location of the glandular portion.

Fig. 20-6. Cross-section of the stomach lining, showing the structure of a typical gland.

What is the function and structure of the small intestine?

The small intestine is a muscular tube with an inner lining of specialized mucosal cells, which runs from the stomach to the cecum (first part of the large intestine). It is about 70 feet long, has a diameter of 2 to 3 inches, holds approximately 12 gallons, and is divided into three parts: the duodenum, jejunum and ileum. This division into parts is done for purposes of description in more detailed anatomy studies. The small intestine is located mainly in the dorsal (upper) part of the left abdomen. Most of it is suspended from the top of the abdominal cavity by a wide, fan-shaped fold of peritoneum called the great mesentery. The liver secretes bile, bile salts and other organic materials that have significance in the normal digestive process. The pancreas secretes juices which are carried into the small intestine through a duct that combines with the duct of the liver just before entry into the small intestine. It is in this part of the digestive tract that the major enzymatic breakdown of food occurs. This breakdown and absorption is accomplished mainly through the actions of the specialized secreting and absorptive cells of the mucosa that are arranged into villi (fingerlike projections) to increase the functional surface area. Proteins, sugars and fats then are absorbed and enter the blood stream through the walls of the small intestine. The remaining food matter, consisting mostly of fiber, moves on to the cecum and colon.

The enzymes that break down the partially digested food in the small intestine are of three types; protein-digesting, carbohydrate-digesting, and fat-digesting. The protein-digesting enzymes that first attack the chyme, trypsin and chymotrypsin, are formed in the pancreas in a non-active form and pass through the pancreatic duct and into the small intestine. Here they are activated by another enzyme into active protein digesters. Trypsin and chymotrypsin are not very effective in the breakdown of protein unless they are preceded by the action of pepsin on the protein in the stomach. This fact once again points to the validity of multiple small meals to enhance stomach digestion to increase total feed efficiency. The final breakdown of protein into amino acids is done by enzymes that are produced in the small intestine. Then the amino acids are transported through the absorptive cells of the intestinal villi and into the portal venous system, which carries them to the liver.

The carbohydrate-digesting enzyme amylase is formed in the pancreas and acts on starches, changing them to maltose, a sugar, in the small intestine. Maltose and other disaccarides (two-part sugars) that can be broken down by hydrolysis (the inserting of a water molecule) are hydrolyzed by absorptive cells in the small intestine into monosaccharides (one part sugars) and immediately absorbed by those cells and transferred into the portal venous system.

Fat-digesting enzymes are formed both in the pancreas and in the cells in the intestinal mucosa. They attack lipids (fats) and break them into smaller parts called fatty acids and monoglycerides by hydrolysis. These lipid parts are then absorbed by the absorptive cells and passed into the lymphatics for transport to the general blood circulation.

The mixing of chyme to achieve breakdown and absorption of nutrients is done by the muscular actions of the small intestine. There are several of these actions:

(1) segmenting contractions—intermittent contraction and relaxation of segments of the intestine. This has a kneading effect on the gut contents,

(2) pendular movements—this is the swaying to and fro of the suspended small intestine; another mixing movement,

(3) short propulsive movements—these are weak waves of contraction in the gut wall that go only one or two inches, then stop, then proceed again from where the first one ended. This has the effect of very slowly moving the chyme through the small intestine.

(4) peristalsis—waves of contraction all along the gut that propel the chyme rather rapidly through it. This is not a normal action of the healthy small intestine. It happens when the mucosa of the intestine is irritated, causing a diarrhea syndrome. This interferes with the normal digestive and absorptive process.

What is the function and structure of the large intestine?

The large intestine consists of four parts: the cecum, large colon, small colon, and rectum.

The cecum is about four feet long and holds about 7 to 10 gallons. It extends from the right flank forward and downward to near the diaphragm. It has a somewhat comma-like shape and the openings from the small intestine and the colon are close together. Since its contents are always predominantly liquid, this section of the large intestine is sometimes called the water gut. Chyme from the small intestine and much of the water drunk by the horse spend some time in the cecum, where they are mixed well together by contraction and relaxation of four longitudinal muscle bands called taeniae coli. This causes the cecum to form into saccules and then smooth out. During this process the bacterial population in the cecum further breaks down the chyme, resulting in the formation of fatty acids and some vitamins that are absorbed from the cecum and the large colon. The cecum and the colon have a mucosa that is very similar to the small intestine, but no villi are present, nor is there nearly as much secretion of specialized enzymes as in the small intestine.

The large colon, between the cecum and small colon, is about 10 to 12 feet long and about 8 to 18 inches in diameter. Some food digestion, mostly by bacterial fermentation and absorption, takes place here, as in the cecum. It can hold about 20 gallons of material and is usually distended with relatively fibrous contents that are liquified, but not as much as in the cecum. The large colon has only one taenia in some parts, while three and four are present in other parts. The small colon is approximately 10 to 12 feet in length and 3 to 4 inches in diameter. It extends from the large colon to the rectum. Since most of the moisture of the digested food is absorbed in the large and small colons, the remaining food residue is relatively soild and is formed into balls of dung by the small colon. The fecal balls are formed by the sacculating action of the small colon, which has two taeniae coli.

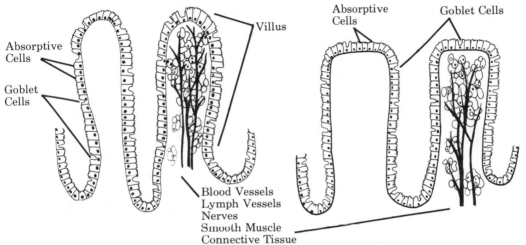

Fig. 20-7. Cross-section of the mucosa of the small intestine, showing the structures.

Fig. 20-8. A cross-section of the mucosa of the large intestine. Notice the similarity of structure in the glands of the small intestine.

The movements of the cecum and large colon for mixing and moving chyme are the same as in the small intestine, except that peristalsis is a normal action here and the sacculation action described above does not take place in the small intestine.

The rectum is a foot-long tract that reaches from the small colon through the pelvic cavity to the anus. It holds the waste material until it is passed out of the horse's body through the anal opening. This is the final part of the digestive tract.

The horse eats large amounts of cellulose which normal enzymes cannot digest but which bacterial action can break down into substances which can be absorbed. The cecum and the large colon are enlarged in order to hold more chyme to allow bacteria the greater amount of time it requires to act on the cellulose. Food moves very slowly in the large intestine.

Food-enriched blood is moved to the liver through a system of veins which join together to form the large portal vein. The liver, which is the largest gland of the body, weights from 10 to 20 pounds. The liver has three lobes and is a relatively flattened organ which is located at the front and top of the abdominal cavity. Part of it lies against the ribs and part against the diaphragm. The liver is the chemical processing plant for the body. It manufacturers bile and processes the digested proteins, sugars, minerals, and other food products. Its regulatory abilities allow the liver to either put these products to immediate use in general tissue metabolism, or to store them.

The pancreas is a relatively flattened organ that lies at the central top of the abdominal cavity just beneath and in front of the kidneys. It is formed of many lobules and ducts for the manufacture and secretion of the many enzymes described earlier in this chapter. Part of the pancreas called the Islet Cells of Langerhans manufacture a hormone, insulin, which is involved in the metabolism of sugar that has already been absorbed into the bloodstream.

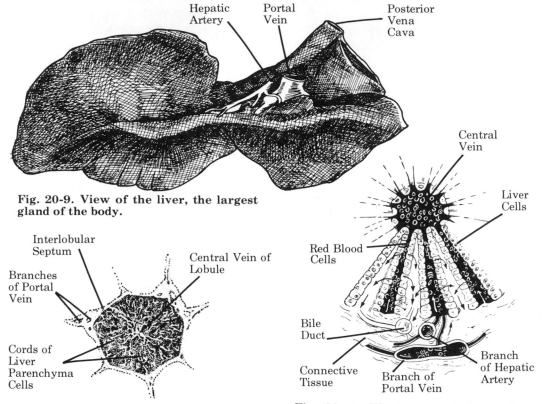

Fig. 20-9. View of the liver, the largest gland of the body.

Fig. 20-10. Illustration of a lobule of the liver.

Fig. 20-11. Illustration of the various structures of the liver lobule. Notice the direction of the flow for bile and blood.

DYSPHAGIA

What is dysphagia?

Dysphagia (difficulty in swallowing) is often a symptom of various disorders. This difficulty may be due to pain, mechanical obstructions, disturbed motor nerve function and brain damage.

What can cause dysphagia?

In some cases, the pharynx may be swollen and painful with inflammation caused by improper use of balling guns and dose syringes. Mechanical defects include cleft palate; a condition in which the nasal passages cannot be properly closed off when the horse swallows, allowing most of the milk (it is discovered soon after birth) to dribble out through the nostrils. In horses affected with strangles, the lymph nodes may be so swollen that they exert pressure on the esophagus, making swallowing very difficult and painful. Various poisons affect the nervous system (moldy corn poisoning, botulism, yellow star thistle poisoning) and cause difficulty in swallowing. Fractures of some bones (the hyoid, for example) can also cause dysphagia.

What are the signs of dysphagia?

If the inability to swallow is total or partial, there is usually a collection of food, saliva and exudate at the nostrils. Chronically affected horses lose weight and condition rapidly. In some cases, they may develop aspiration pneumonia from inhaling food and debris into the lungs. If horses are unable to swallow for more than a day, they usually spend more time around water, trying to drink.

Will these signs always be apparent?

Sometimes the signs of dysphagia are not easily recognized. In cases of brain or nerve damage, the horse may be so listless and disinterested in food that the inability to swallow is not noticed.

What is the treatment for dysphagia?

Treatment of nervous system disorders can only be supportive. The veterinarian will probably wish to administer fluids, electrolytes (salts and minerals) and easily digested food by a stomach tube. If abnormal growths are interfering with swallowing, the veterinarian may be able to remove them surgically. Often, a tracheotomy tube is used to make breathing easier for the horse if swollen lymph nodes make breathing and swallowing especially difficult.

CHOKE

What is choke?

Choke is a term that is used to describe an esophageal obstruction that may be partial or complete. The esophagus may be normal, of abnormal size, or have a constriction. At any rate, the horse is unable to get enough food or water to his digestive system. Death may be caused by perforation of the esophagus or degeneration and death of the tissues due to continued pressure.

What causes choke?

Many cases of choke are caused by medications that lodge in the esophagus. Bolets and tablets should be avoided, if possible, especially with Shetland ponies. These ponies have a very small, narrow esophagus that makes them prone to choke. Horses also choke on feed such as grain, dry hay and lush grass. Because of abnormal growths or structure of the esophagus, some horses are more prone to choke than others. Greedy eaters and horses with poor teeth who do not chew and moisten their food sufficiently may frequently develop choke. Spasms of the esophagus may account for some of the difficult to explain occurrences of choke.

What happens when something is lodged in the esophagus?

If the esophagus is blocked by feed or other material that is packed, inflammation does not usually occur for a day or two. However, irregularly-shaped foreign objects and some medications in bolus form (large pill) cause severe irritation, and inflammation rapidly contributes to the blockage. The swelling that accompanies inflammation and esophageal spasm wedges the irritating mass more securely, making it very difficult to remove or relieve the obstruction. Rupture of the esophagus may occur when inflammation weakens the tissues.

What are the signs of choke?

Horses with choke appear distressed and anxious. They may make repeated motions with the head and neck, arching the neck and then drawing the chin back to the chest or extending the head toward the ground. Shaking the head and pacing are anxious behavior that may be seen. Characteristically, the horse drools saliva and a mixture of food and saliva appears at the nostrils. This mixture coming from the nose may be mistaken for mucus or pus, much to the chagrin of the distressed horse. Owners have been known to make this mistake and treat the horse for strangles, causing it to die from a choke that otherwise could probably have been corrected by the veterinarian, had he been called promptly. If the choke does not spontaneously clear up after 18 to 36 hours, the horse usually becomes depressed and stops trying to swallow. He may stand quietly by the water source, sloshing or sipping water that returns through his nose. Since choke is sometimes caused by medicinal bolets or tablets, other signs of the original disorder may also be present. Colic, diarrhea, or respiratory infections are frequently associated with cases of choke. Pneumonia and dehydration may accompany chronic choke.

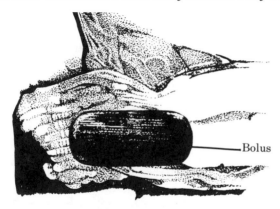

Fig. 20-12. This is an illustration of a bolus (large pill) that has become lodged in the esophagus. Notice the tissue swelling above and below the blockage.

Bolus

How is choke treated?

The veterinarian will determine the cause of the obstruction and decide on appropriate treatment. He may attempt to pass a stomach tube to push the obstruction down to the stomach. If the stomach tube passes through the area of the obstruction, it indicates that the choke is probably due to a foreign body, growth or spasm and will usually require surgery to remove. Food masses may be loosened by repeated attempts to pass a stomach tube, or water may be pumped in and withdrawn to help moisten and break up the mass. Spontaneous recovery from choke within two days is frequent, so it is difficult to evaluate the methods used to relieve obstructions of the esophagus. Chronic choke may require the administration of fluids intravenously, in addition to carbachol, pilocarpine or arecoline to increase salivation. Some veterinarians may suggest smooth muscle relaxants to help relieve spasms of the esophagus.

Can choke be prevented?

Horses that are prone to choke may be fed soaked feeds, which sometimes helps. Greedy feeders can be slowed down by placing smooth stones in the feedbox. If fresh water is available at all times, it may decrease the possibility of dry feed becoming lodged in the esophagus. Foals and Shetland ponies should not be given bolets or tablets, due to the small size of their esophagus. Dry, coarse hay should be avoided and the teeth should be properly maintained (see Dentistry, page 340).

CONSTIPATION

What is constipation?

Constipation is the inability to pass fecal material. In newborn foals, it is often caused by an inability to pass the meconium, hardened matter that has accumulated in the intestines before the foal was born. Frequently, adequate amounts of colostrum prevent constipation.

What are the signs of meconium retention?

Foals that are unable to pass the firm black, brown or green pellets of meconium within three hours or so after birth often show signs of colic. They may roll, strain and switch the tail and make frequent attempts to urinate. Many foals become depressed, cease to suck from the mare, and spend long periods lying down, showing signs of intermittent colic pain. The colic can become very violent, causing the foal to repeatedly stand and throw itself to the ground. Foals sometimes lie on their backs in odd positions and seem to obtain some relief from the pain in this way.

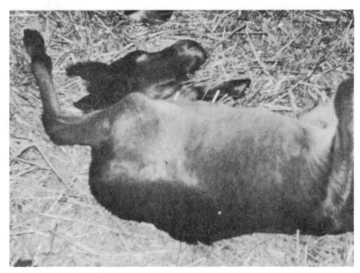

Photo courtesy of THE HORSE, by Peter Rossdale, M.A., F.R.C.V.S., pub. by The California Thoroughbred Breeder's Association. Photo by Peter Rossdale.

Fig. 20-13. Foals suffering from meconium retention show signs of colic and roll or lie in awkward positions.

What can be done to relieve constipation?

Many veterinarians advise repeated warm, soapy enemas to relieve constipation. A mixture of castor oil and mineral oil may be given by stomach tube to help lubricate the fecal matter.

If the constipation is due to a paralysis of the intestines, the veterinarian may treat the constipation as paralytic ileus (see Colic, page 513).

Constipation must be corrected quickly and surgical intervention is sometimes necessary. Surgical procedures should not be put off until the foal is critically ill, when it will have less chance of surviving the surgery.

ATRESIA COLI

What is atresia coli?

Atresia coli is a condition in which the small colon, or final section of the large intestine, is divided into two parts which do not join. One part begins at the rectum, and ends in a blind pouch one to three feet inside. The other section is from two to four feet long, begins at the large colon, and also ends in a blind pouch. This incomplete formation of the colon is a birth defect.

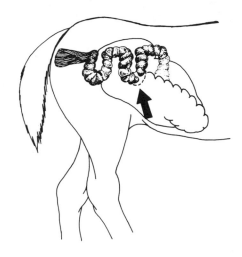

Fig. 20-14. Atresia coli is illustrated, showing the two segments of the large intestine which do not join.

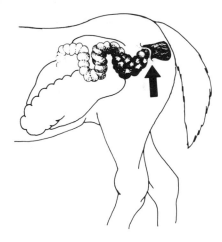

Fig. 20-15. Atresia ani, a less serious condition, involves the absence of an opening to the outside.

What are the signs of atresia coli?

An affected foal is in good health for up to 24 hours. It then develops what appears to be colic, which does not improve with treatment. A enema given to the foal does not result in defecation.

How is atresia coli treated?

Attempts have been made to anastomose (surgically join) the sections of small colon in affected foals. Usually too much of the intestinal tract is missing, and the foal cannot be saved.

In a related condition, atresia ani, the foal simply has no opening from the small colon to the rectum. No difficulty is usually experienced in correcting this problem surgically.

DISEASES OF THE LIVER

What are the major diseases of the liver?

Probably the most widely recognized sign of liver disorder is jaundice. Jaundice is not, strictly speaking, a disease, but an indication that something further is wrong. It discolors the mucous membranes and white parts of the skin to a yellowish tinge, and in advanced stages colors the urine either bright yellow, dark brown or black. This coloration is due to the excess presence of bilirubin (yellow bile pigment), and may be brought about by any of three different means. First of all, the bile duct, which carries bile from the liver to the intestines, may be blocked by a parasite (usually a bot or a roundworm). The bile then builds up in the liver, and is dumped into the blood. This may also be brought about by internal pressure, such as tumors, abscesses, etc. Secondly, the liver may destroy excessive numbers of red blood cells, such as in equine infectious anemia. One product of this breaking-down process is bile, which becomes excessive and is again dumped into the blood. Finally, jaundice can be brought about when some of the parenchymal (functioning) cells undergo necrosis (die), and bile cannot be eliminated from the system. This illness is known as hepatitis.

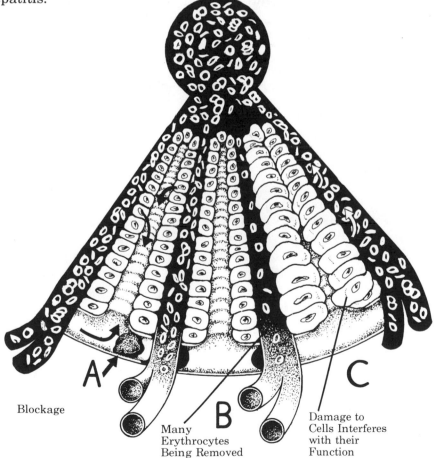

Blockage

Many
Erythrocytes
Being Removed

Damage to
Cells Interferes
with their
Function

Fig. 20-16. Causes of jaundice. A. Blockage of the bile duct. B. Destruction of excessive numbers of red blood cells. Fewer red blood cells are being returned to the circulation. C. Damage to the liver cell-hepatitis. Notice the swelling which interferes with the functions of the liver cells.

What causes hepatitis?

Hepatitis is a general term, used to describe the liver's reaction to an injurious agent. This process usually involves watery swelling of the tissue, change of the tissue into fat, necrosis, and, ultimately, regrowth of the tissue.

Hepatitis can begin in any part of the liver, and may progress through most of the organ. At any point in time, the degeneration may be in several different stages in different areas of the liver. The necrosis may be caused by infectious hepatitis, or by toxic hepatitis.

What is infectious hepatitis?

Infectious hepatitis occurs when an infective organism invades the liver, and is widely distributed through it. A horse's liver may be infected, for instance, by equine rhinopneumonitis. The organism may enter the liver through the bile duct system, from a nearby organ already infected, or through the blood. In foals, infection commonly enters through the umbilical vein when unsanitary conditions exist in the foaling stall.

What is toxic hepatitis?

Toxic hepatitis is brought on by the presence of poisons in the system. Although the microscopic appearance of the liver may be different from one affected by infectious hepatitis, the results are very much the same.

Substances poisonous to the liver have three known sources: chemical poisons, plant poisons and metabolic poisons. Chemical poisons include arsenic, copper, mercury and phosphorus, among others. It is of particular interest that tetrachlorethylene and carbon tetrachloride, both used as worming agents, are potential causes of hepatitis, when improperly used.

Plant poisons often involve plants from the genus Senecia, tar weed, or those of the genus Phyllanthus. Also suspect are lupines, vetches, velvet beans, other legumes, and the toxins produced by fungi or damaged feed.

Metabolic poisons are those produced by the body itself under given conditions. Gastroenteritis is believed responsible for these poisons, and they may accompany other serious infectious diseases. Certain vitamin deficiencies have been known to produce hepatitis, and it may be brought on by the toxemias of pregnancy.

If toxic substances that cause the hepatitis (particularly plant poisons) are not permanently removed, the condition may become chronic. When toxic hepatitis becomes chronic, it leads to cirrhosis.

What are the effects of cirrhosis?

A liver affected by cirrhosis produces large amounts of fibrous, connective tissue as a response to the ongoing hepatitis. Eventually, there is more connective tissue present than parenchymal tissue. Cirrhosis is usually brought on by repeated exposure to the same things that cause toxic hepatitis, but may result from chronic inflammation of the bile ducts, which produces a much more pronounced jaundice.

Due to the size of the liver, even the vast necrosis accompanying cirrhosis usually does not impair its ability to function. Instead, the excess connective tissue interferes with the flow of the blood through the liver, causing congestion in the digestive organs and spleen, and the buildup of yellow fluid in the sac surrounding the internal organs (peritoneum). Unfortunately, even the removal of the toxic substance is seldom helpful once cirrhosis has begun. The connective tissue seems to stimulate the growth of more connective tissue, and death ultimately results.

The possible existence of cirrhosis may first be suspected when the horse begins to demonstrate behavior characteristic of hepatitis and cirrhosis.

What behavior is characteristic of hepatitis and cirrhosis?

Hepatic disorders interfere with the normal functioning of the horse because of the liver's reduced ability to detoxify body poisons. As a result, nitrogenous substances, possibly ammonia, reach the brain and cause behavior which points clearly to liver problems. All behavioral signs are not necessarily present in mild cases; in acute cases they are usually quite pronounced.

Temperature is normal, but sweating persists. Urination and movement of the intestines for digestive purposes may stop altogether. Vision is usually impaired, and indigestion is common. If experience with hepatitis in humans holds true for horses, the animal is not in great pain, but is experiencing extreme mental depression. Typical reactions include restlessness, irritability, constantly walking in circles or straight lines, and pressing the head against solid objects or walking into them. Yawning, trouble breathing, lack of appetite and constipation may also be present.

Extreme reactions of this sort also accompany a disorder that is apparently related to toxic hepatitis, called serum hepatitis.

What is serum hepatitis?

Serum hepatitis is a necrosis of the liver with a high mortality rate, which appears to be linked to inoculations against certain illnesses. In reported cases, affected horses have been injected with encephalomyelitis serum, tetanus antitoxin, pregnant mare serum, African horsesickness antiserum or anthrax antiscrum, sometime within the six-month period before signs are noticed. Nearly 90% of the cases are fatal, bringing death in 12 to 48 hours. No theory concerning the exact cause of serum hepatitis has been proven.

Examination of the horse's liver after death reveals a typical "nutmeg" liver, indicating that all but a few of the liver cells have been replaced by blood cells. A liver with this appearance also accompanies congestion of the liver or congestive heart failure.

How are hepatitis-cirrhosis conditions treated?

If a form of hepatitis is suspected, a veterinarian should be called immediately. In the case of viral hepatitis, efforts are made to identify the infecting organism and to eliminate it from the system. If tests determine that the cause is a toxin, it should be eliminated from the area. Further treatment is aimed at reducing the blood ammonia level, and restoring the balance of blood glucose, electrolytes and water that are changed by the ineffective liver. Efforts should be made to guard against possible secondary infection.

Treatment of cirrhosis usually has no effect. The prognosis is fair to poor for cases of hepatitis.

INTERNAL PARASITES

What are the most common internal parasites of the horse?

The horse is host to a wide variety of internal parasites. Most common are the large strongyles *(Strongylus),* small strongyles, ascarids *(Parascaris equorum),* pinworms *(Oxyuris equi* and *Probstmayria vivipara),* intestinal threadworm

(Strongyloides westeri), stomach worms *(Habronema and Trichostrongylus axei),* tapeworms *(Anoplocephala),* and bots *(Gastrophilus).* Less common infestations (which will not be discussed here) occur with the lungworm *(Dictyocaulus arnfeldi),* eyeworm *(Thelazia spp.),* blood fluke *(Shistosoma),* liver fluke *(Fasciola hepatica)* and hyatid tapeworm *(Echinococcus)* found mostly outside the United States. Intestinal parasites are usually discovered in routine examinations of the feces, but they may produce visible signs in the infected animal.

What are the effects of internal parasites on the horse?

The effects vary widely with the species, but the most severe damage is caused by the large strongyles, especially *Strongylus vulgaris.* In addition to the number of infective parasites, the condition of the host determines how much damage will be caused. Very old or very young horses are the most severely affected by heavy parasite infestation, but poor condition in a mature horse contributes to parasite damage. Mature parasites may cause damage to the host by bloodsucking, tissue destruction, obstruction of passageways, production of toxins and by removing food from the digestive tract. Heaviest tissue damage in the horse is caused by migration of the immature larvae through the intestine, liver, spleen and arteries. The results of unchecked internal parasite infestations may be colic, enteritis, peritonitis or death. Visible signs may not be present until extensive, irreversible damage has been caused internally.

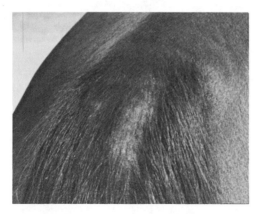

Fig. 20-17. Some horses may show no signs of parasite infection, but the rubbed-out tail on this horse is characteristic of parasite infection by pinworms.

How can internal parasites be controlled?

Specific treatments for parasite infections will not be given here because of the variability in effectiveness and resistance. Most commercial worming preparations are not effective either because their casual use by horse owners has permitted parasites to develop a resistance to them or because the preparation is not really effective in removing the type of parasite present. A veterinarian can mix highly efficient compounds and properly determine the effective dosages for the most efficient removal of internal parasites. A veterinarian can also recommend commercial preparations that are effective against the parasites in a particular horse.

What are the signs of strongyle infection?

The signs of infection include fever, lack of appetite, weight loss, depression, lethargy, colic, constipation and diarrhea. These can also indicate other disorders, so the veterinarian should be advised if the horse is not on a worming program that has been set up by a veterinarian.

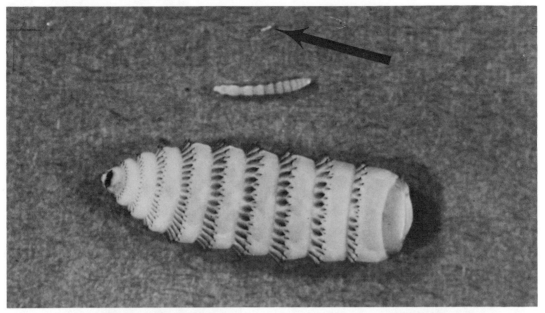

(Courtesy, Shell Chemical Company, Agricultural Division, San Ramon, California.)

Fig. 20-18. Shown are the three different stages of the bot larvae. First stage larvae, at the top of the picture, are the size that burrow through the horse's tongue.

Fig. 20-19. Pinworms cause irritation of the intestines and perineum in infected horses. Severe rubbing of the tail may cause breaks in the skin, which may result in secondary infections.

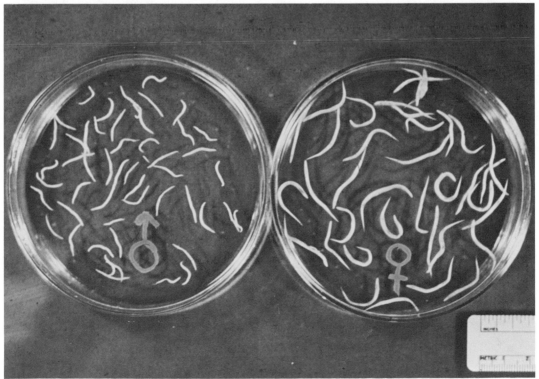

(Couresty, Shell Chemical Company, Agricultural Division, San Ramon, California.)

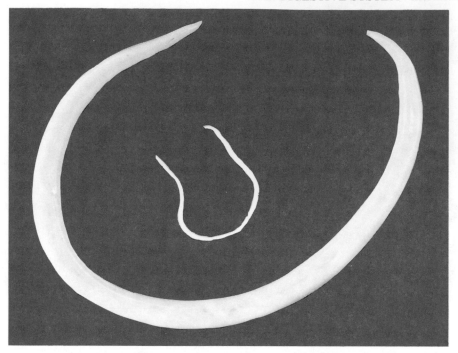

(Courtesy, Shell Chemical Company, Agricultural Division, San Ramon, California.)

Fig. 20-20. Development of ascarids is extremely rapid. The mature worm is actually 10 inches long.

Fig. 20-21. Large strongyles in the intestine. When these larvae are found in the anterior mesenteric artery, they can cause an aneurysm that may result in colic or death.

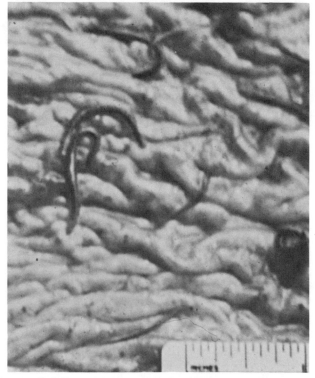

(Courtesy, Shell Chemical Company, Agricultural Division, San Ramon, California.)

What are the effects of strongyles?

There are two groups of strongyles, the large strongyles and the small strongyles. The red bloodworm, *Strongylus vulgaris,* is a member of the large strongyles, and causes the heaviest damage of all the internal parasites. Large strongyle larvae penetrate the intestinal mucosa in the posterior area of the small intestine, cecum and ventral colon, where they enter the small arterioles in the walls of these various organs. The larvae continue to migrate under the inner layer of the arteries (intima), traveling against the flow until they enter the larger arteries (ilial, cecal and ventral colic) and reach the base of the mesentery. Following this two-week journey, some larvae enter the aorta and travel to the heart or are carried to the renal and iliac arteries. In addition to the inflammation of the arterial walls caused by the larvae, thrombosis and embolism formation may occur. When the larvae remain in the anterior mesenteric artery and attach to the walls, inflammation causes a weakening and bulging of the arterial wall known as an aneurysm. If sufficient irritation is caused, there may be blockage due to the buildup of larvae, fibrin and cellular debris. Blockage of the iliac and mesenteric arteries may result in lameness and death of a portion of the intestine (infarction). It is not known whether the migrating larvae return to the intestinal mucosa, but that is where the mature worms are found. Large strongyles cause damage as adults in the mucosa of the cecum and ventral colon where they attach to the mucosa and suck blood.

Two other species of large strongyles, *S. edentatus* and *S. equinus,* cause less damage because their larval stages do not travel so extensively through the circulatory system. *S. edentatus* penetrate the intestinal mucosa and travel up the portal vein to the liver. The larvae damage the liver tissue with their enzymes in their passage to the hepatic ligaments, where they travel under the peritoneal lining of the abdominal cavity. Further migration brings them to the gut wall where they form edematous lesions on the mucous surface. They finally return to the mucosa of the ventral colon and cecum, where they become firmly attached. *S. equinus* migrate extensively in abdominal tissues and organs after they penetrate the cecal and colic mucosa. Following a period of encystation, the larvae migrate to the liver through the peritoneal cavity, then to the pancreas. Eventually, the larvae return to the intestine and attach to the cecum or ventral colon.

Small strongyles are not as destructive because their larvae do not migrate outside the walls of the intestine. Also, mature small strongyles of *Tredontophorus tenicucollis* and other species attach themselves loosely, if at all, to the intestinal mucosa and usually do not suck blood. Primarily, damage of small strongyles is limited to the craterlike openings and ulcerations left in the intestinal mucosa when the larval nodules rupture. This can cause severe diarrhea and constipation.

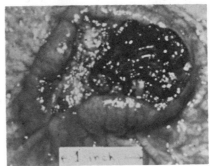

Fig. 20-22. Lesion of the intestinal mucosa caused by a small strongyle. These lesions cause irritation and inefficient digestion in the intestines.

(Courtesy, Shell Chemical Company, Agricultural Division, San Ramon, California.)

How do horses become infested with strongyles?

The sexually mature worms are attached to the large intestine where they lay eggs that pass out of the horse in the feces. These larvae can become infective in less than a week, or cooler weather may cause them to take several weeks to become infective. Infective larvae travel up stems and blades of grass where they are ingested by grazing horses. The ingested larvae then begin their various migrations through the host until they mature and repeat the cycle.

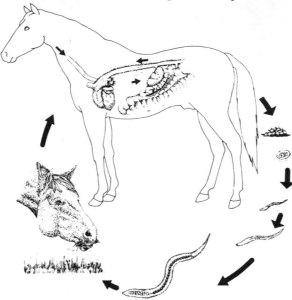

Fig. 20-23. Life cycle of large strongyles. 1. Mature worms are present in the large intestine of the horse. They lay eggs which pass out with the feces. 2. Larvae in the feces mature, become infective and crawl up stems of grass. 3. The horse ingests the larvae which travel from the digestive tract through the blood. Damage to the circulatory system is common. 4. The migrating larvae return to the intestines where they produce eggs and complete the cycle.

How long does it take for infective larvae to mature?

The larvae of *S. vulgaris* take approximately six months to migrate and mature, while the larvae of *S. edentatus* and *S. equinus* require eleven months and nine months, respectively. Small strongyles mature in six to twelve weeks, with some variance in species and conditions.

How can strongyles be controlled and prevented?

Depending on the area and conditions under which horses are kept, variable worming programs will be effective. The veterinarian can set up an efficient worming program, taking into account the frequency of reinfestation and general condition of the horses in question. Intervals between treatments must be carefully gauged because the larval forms are not harmed by anthelmintics (worm medicines).

What are the signs of ascarid infections?

The large roundworm *Parascaris equorum* (ascarid) is common in very young horses that have not acquired a resistance to them. Infected foals usually are rough-looking, have pot bellies, rough haircoats and slower growth than uninfected foals. Colic and diarrhea may also be signs of worm infections. Coughs in foals are commonly attributed to ascarid larvae in the lungs.

What are the effects of ascarids in foals?

Ascarid eggs are ingested in contaminated feed or water. These eggs pass to the intestine, where they hatch. From the intestine, larvae penetrate the intestinal wall and migrate through the portal veins to the liver and the lungs. After a period of growth and development causing destruction in these organs, larvae invade the respiratory passage and are coughed up and swallowed. When the larvae reach the intestines again, they mature and remain in the small intestine. Massing of worms is the primary danger of ascarid infection, sometimes causing rupture and peritonitis. Large numbers of worms are not required to cause intestinal rupture, but heavier infections increase the possibility considerably.

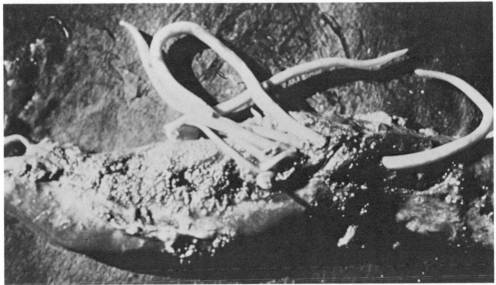

(Courtesy, Shell Chemical Company, Agricultural Division, San Ramon, California)

Fig. 20-24. Ascarids in the intestine. The presence of ascarids has caused a rupture of the intestine, a frequent occurrence in foals. Death is caused by the resulting peritonitis.

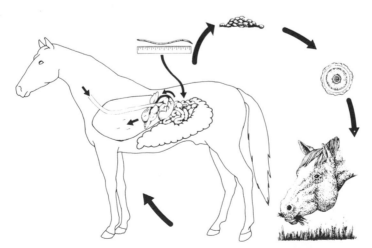

Fig. 20-25. Life cycle of ascarids. The larvae differ from those of the strongyles in that they do most of their damage in the liver and the lungs. From the lungs, ascarids are coughed up and swallowed, reaching the intestines to produce eggs which complete the cycle.

The largest parasite of the horse (mature worms are ten to twelve inches long), even small numbers of ascarids are dangerous, especially in very young foals.

How long does it take for ascarid infections to become mature?

Ascarids can complete a cycle of development in three months. Fatal ruptures of the intestine often occur in the fall in weanlings after being turned out in contaminated pastures.

Can ascarid infections be controlled?

Ascarid infections are fairly easy to control. Foals should be treated when they are eight to ten weeks old, and wormed at eight-week intervals until they are one year old. When they are yearlings, the emphasis should shift to strongyle control. Both infections are controlled by most strongyle compounds.

What are the signs of bots?

In spite of the absence of visible signs of infection, a horse is generally presumed to have bots if evidence of botfly eggs is found on the hairs of the throat, forelegs or on the lips. The various species of botflies *(Gastrophilus intestinalis, nasalis, inermis, pecorum* and *haemorrhoidalis)* lay their eggs in different areas of the horse, causing great agitation in many horses.

G. intestinalis is the most common botfly in the United States. This bee-like fly lays her eggs on the hair of the horse's fetlocks, forelegs, flanks and on the neck. The eggs must be stimulated by the warmth, moisture, and action of the horse's lips before they hatch and invade the mucosa of the mouth. They remain in the cheek or tongue for almost a month, then migrate to the stomach and attach to the mucosa. Visible signs of bot infection may be caused by the ulcers which form at the site of larval attachment. Many bot infections do not cause any visible signs and are tolerated quite well by the horse. The bots remain in the stomach, living on blood and tissue, for ten to twelve months. They then pass out with the feces, pupate in the soil for five to six weeks, and emerge as adult flies.

Other species found in the United States and Europe differ from *G. intestinalis* in the location they prefer for egg-laying and in egg-hatching requirements. Nose and throat bots lay eggs that do not require rubbing or licking in order to hatch. Other aspects of their life cycle are similar to those of *G. intestinalis.*

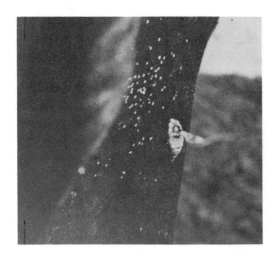

Fig. 20-26. Photograph of common botfly and eggs on the horse. These on the forelegs are deposited by the most common botfly, *G. intestinalis.*

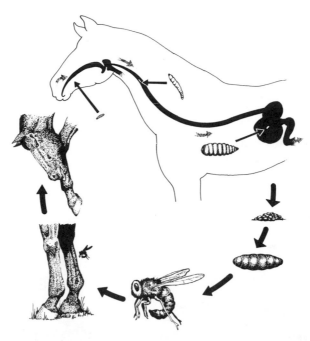

Fig. 20-27. Life cycle of the botfly. After the eggs are stimulated by the horse's mouth, the larvae hatch and invade the tongue and cheek mucosae. They emerge and travel to the stomach, where they attach and mature during the winter. Larvae pass out with the feces, pupate and hatch into mature bot flies in the spring and early summer.

RECOMMENDED WORMING PROGRAM

Age	Schedule of Administration	Parasites to Control
FOALS:		
60 days	60 days	Strongyles and Ascarids
120 days	60 days	Strongyles and Ascarids
180 days	60 days	Strongyles and Ascarids
220 days	40 days (Weaned)	Strongyles, Ascarids and Bots
December	Weanlings	Strongyles, Ascarids and Bots
February-March	Yearlings	Strongyles, Ascarids and Bots
November-December		Strongyles, Ascarids and Bots
MARES: (Brood and/or Barren)		
Pregnant	December, January or February February (one month before foaling)	Strongyles and Bots
Lactating	August 1	Strongyles and Bots
Post Weaning	October 15	Strongyles and Bots
STALLIONS:	On fecal examination every 60 days. A count of 50 eggs/gm. or more indicates need for reworming.	Strongyles and Bots

STRONGYLES: Relatively safe and effective Strongyle wormers: (1) Thiabendazole, (2) Mebendazole, (3) Cambendazole, (4)Pyrantel Tartrate, (5) Dichlorvos, (6) Phenothiazine*

ASCARIDS: Relatively safe and effective Ascarid wormers: (1) Piperazine, (2) Butonate, (3) Neguvon, (4) Butonate

BOTS: Relatively safe and effective Bot wormers: (1) Carbon Disulfide*, (2) Neguvon, (3) Dichlorvos, (4) Butonate

These compounds are found in many commercial (brand name) wormers. The horseman is urged to read all labels on commercial products, to determine if they are effective against the parasites present in his horse. Many of these compounds are available only to a veterinarian. However, they are reported to be the most effective means of controlling the various parasites.

---

*Not as safe and effective as other compounds, but are used.

How can bots be controlled?

Regular worming can remove larvae from the stomach, but it does not reach those that are still in the mucosa of the mouth. For this reason, worming programs that are administered only once in the late fall or early winter are inefficient. If the larvae are removed before they are mature, the cycle of production can be broken. Regularly removing the eggs by scraping or sponging them with warm water to hatch out the larvae helps keep the level of infection quite low. An effective worming program prevents bots "wintering" in the horse's stomach and drastically reduces the numbers of botflies produced in the spring. Proper disposal and spreading of manure also aids in controlling bots.

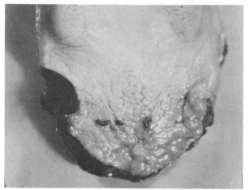

(Courtesy, Shell Chemical Company, Agricultural Division, San Ramon, California.)

Fig. 20-28. Bot larvae found in the base of the tongue.

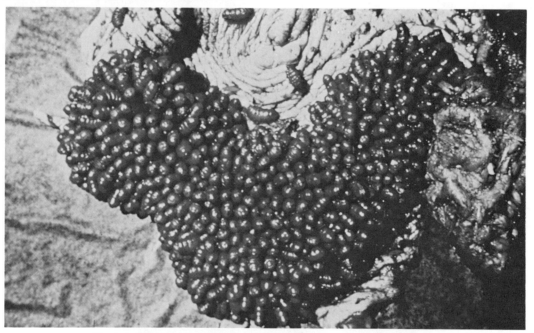

(Courtesy, Shell Chemical Company, Agricultural Division, San Ramon, California.)

Fig. 20-29. *G. Intestinalis* attached to the mucosa of the stomach.

What are the signs of pinworm infections?

Pinworms *(Oxyuris equi)* are most common in foals, but they may be found in mature horses. They cause anal irritation which results in the horse rubbing his tail. A "rattailed" appearance is characteristic of pinworm irritation. No other clinical signs are usually present.

What are the effects of pinworms?

Pinworms do not migrate or penetrate the intestinal mucosa. When the sticky eggs are ingested in feed or water, they mature in the intestines. Fragile, mature females migrate to the rectum and anus where they rupture and release their eggs. The eggs may pass out with the feces, or they may stick to and contaminate stable walls, fences and bedding. Pinworms are mature within five months after infection.

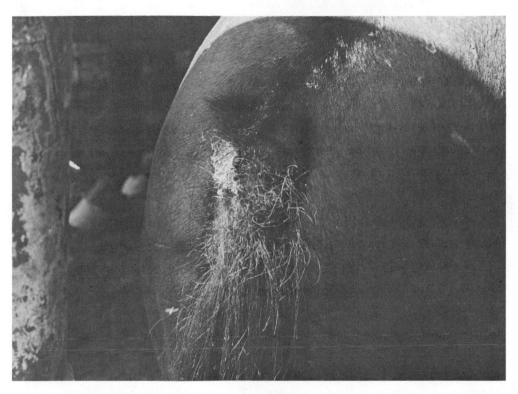

Fig. 20-30. The rattailed appearance characteristic of pinworm infections. This horse has caused a secondary infection by rubbing the skin open.

What treatment is necessary for pinworm infections?

Most pinworm infections are not treated specifically. They are effectively removed by most compounds used to treat other forms of parasite infections. If the regular worming program is effective, it will prevent pinworm infections.

What are the signs of threadworm infections?

Threadworms *(Strongyloides westeri)* are common in the small intestine of foals. They are primarily evident during the first six months of life and tend to disappear after the foal has reached this age. Some observers believe that *Strongyloides* infection causes diarrhea in foals, but there is little firm support for this theory. Infective larvae are transmitted to the foal in the mare's milk which is the only known means of transmission. Treatment of *Strongyloides* infections with Thiabendazole is required to remove the parasites completely.

What are the signs of stomach worms in horses?

The stomach worms *(Habronema muscae, Habronema majus* and *Draschia megastoma)* are found primarily in the stomach of the horse, rather than in the intestines. Infective larvae may also invade skin wounds and the eyes, causing "summer sores" and conjunctivitis (see Summer Sores, page 406). If the larvae invade the lungs, they result in pulmonary abscesses. When the larvae locate in the stomach, they produce abscesses that are very difficult to treat. Visible signs of stomach worm infections may be limited to gastritis or digestive upsets.

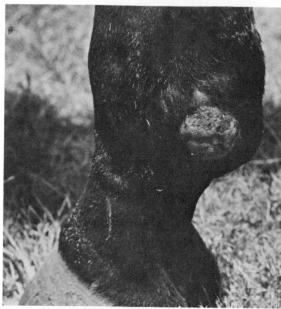

Fig. 20-31. A typical summer sore lesion. This sore has been recently cleaned, prior to removal of some tissue for laboratory analysis to determine the presence of *Habronema* larvae.

How can stomach worms be controlled?

Stomach worms are usually transmitted to horses by common houseflies or stable flies. These pests pick up the larvae from infected feces and deposit them in wounds and around the lips of horses. Stable hygiene and the control of flies is the best method of controlling stomach worms.

What are the signs of tapeworm infections?

Tapeworms *(Anoplocephala perfoliata, A. magna)* cause no visible effects if the infection is light. Heavy infections, which are quite rare, may result in digestive disturbances and poor condition. In a few cases, *A. perfoliata* have been responsible for perforation and severe ulcerations of the cecum.

Orbatid mites, present in pastures in some localities, are a necessary intermediate host of tapeworms. The tapeworms develop in the mites for two to four months and are then ingested by horses. Specific treatments for tapeworms have not been developed.

Other parasites are found in the horse, but they are relatively rare in domestic animals. Their diagnosis usually requires laboratory analysis which will be initiated by a veterinarian.

COLIC

What is colic?

Colic is a disease complex, not a specific disease. Specifically, it is abdominal pain which may be caused by a wide variety of disorders. They will be dealt with here as separate disorders which are recognized by the signs of abdominal pain (colic).

What causes colic?

The primary cause of abdominal pain in colic is distension of the stomach or the intestines. This distension may be caused by an accumulation of gas, fluid or feed due to an obstruction (blockage) of the digestive tract or to improper action of the peristaltic movements which force material through the tract. Pain is also produced when the peritoneum is stretched during attacks of "colic."

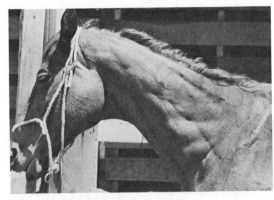

Fig. 20-32. Some colics may be caused by the chronic distension that results when a horse constantly swallows air. This "cribber" or "wind-sucker" shows the cording of the neck muscles that results when he forces air into his stomach.

What causes distension of the stomach and intestines?

When obstructions or lack of peristaltic movements prevent the passage of material through the digestive system, pressure results in a reflex reaction which causes adjoining areas to contract in spasm. The distension also causes further secretion of fluid into the intestines, increasing the pressure and distension. Past a certain point, reflex attempts to clear the obstruction cease, and the fatigued muscles quit contracting. This is called paralysis of the intestines (paralytic ileus) and is a period when the horse may appear almost free from pain. The level of sensation and pain is greatly reduced because of the muscular fatigue and slower responses of the pain sensors in the stretched tissue. When this type of paralysis occurs, the horse can be poisoned by his own intestinal contents. The lack of movement in the intestines allows toxic materials and fluids to escape through the stretched intestinal walls and enter the abdominal cavity.

What are the effects of distension?

The first response the body makes to distension is increased secretion of digestive juices, which increases the distension and results in continuous or intermittent pain. This cycle is automatic and continues throughout the period of distension. It is this constant secretion and loss of fluids (see above) that causes dehydration and an imbalance in the chemical systems of the body. This feedback reaction and fluid loss begins a systemic body reaction of collapse called shock (see page 1). Shock is present in most cases of abdominal pain, and is treated as a separate syndrome by the veterinarian, since it is frequently the cause of colic deaths.

What are the signs of abdominal pain?

In the horse, abdominal pain is usually sudden, expressed by sweating, rolling, kicking, or biting and looking around at the belly and violent pawing. Occasionally, a horse may sit on its haunches (like a dog) or appear drawn up or bloated in the belly. There may be muscle tremors and occasional straining; male horses may stretch out and relax the penis without urinating. When horses are down, they may thrash violently or assume unusual positions with all four legs up in the air.

Depending on the cause of distension, the pulse may be elevated (over 100 per minute) and breathing will be rapid and shallow. Temperature varies with the source of pain, but is usually below normal due to shock.

When the signs of pain are acute and the cause of distension is not removed, death often occurs within 12 to 48 hours. Rapid diagnosis and treatment are vital.

Fig. 20-33. Stretched-out position is one that colicky horses frequently assume. Notice the drawn-up appearance of the flank and abdomen.

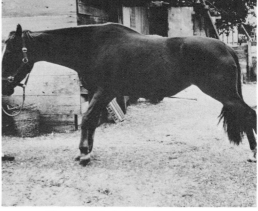

(Courtesy W. L. Anderson, D.V.M.)

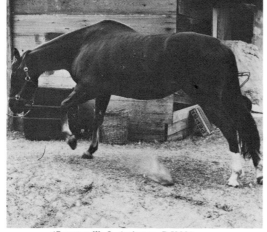

(Courtesy W. L. Anderson, D.V.M.)

Fig. 20-34. This horse is also pawing, another frequent manifestation of abdominal pain.

How is colic diagnosed?

The veterinarian must consider several disorders before making a diagnosis of colic. Since it is one of the most common disease complexes in the horse, early recognition and accurate differentiation are very important.

In order to differentiate between the causes of colic, the veterinarian may perform a rectal examination. This procedure should not be done by the horse owner due to the danger of damage to sensitive tissue structures. Intestinal contents and their positions will indicate to the veterinarian the presence or absence of intestinal motility and the location of the obstruction or impaction.

Another examination procedure that should only be performed by a veterinarian is the passage of a stomach tube. Stomach contents or gas can help the veterinarian decide the type of disorder and the severity of the condition.

Most veterinarians will note the pulse, respiration and temperature of an affected horse. The pulse rate should be less than 80 per minute for a favorable prognosis. A temperature that is below normal indicates the presence of shock which frequently accompanies colic. The presence or absence of intestinal sounds indicates excessive or absent intestinal movements.

Why is differentiation of causes important?

The veterinarian must differentiate between the specific lesions that can cause abdominal pain (colic), because the prognosis and treatment varies greatly with each. Generally, the prognosis is excellent when the pain is due to excessive activity of the intestines, good for pain due to impaction, and very poor for pain caused by twisting or intussusception of the intestines (unless surgery is immediate).

How is colic treated?

Pain must be relieved to prevent the horse from injuring himself, but the signs of the specific injury cannot be masked and interfere with correct diagnosis of the cause of pain. In order to achieve this, many veterinarians administer Meperidine, chloral hydrate or Pentazocine. Dipyrone has not been proved to be particularly effective in this respect. Mineral oil is the preferred lubricant because it does not cause excessive purgation. Drugs to stimulate peristaltic contractions are not normally used. If they are given, they are always preceded by administration of a lubricant to prevent unnecessary pain. Antispasmodics (atropine) are avoided unless there is definite evidence of peristalsis. These drugs may be overused by those who are not well acquainted with their actions. In most cases, intravenous saline solutions are required to maintain fluid levels in the affected horse. The dose rates may be very high and should be supervised by a veterinarian. Currently, very large doses of corticosteroids are being used to combat shock. Corticosteroids should not be used if surgery may be required to remove an obstruction or resection the intestine. Interference with the process of inflammation and healing with corticosteroids can cause the surgery to fail if infection cannot be controlled.

What is the most common cause of abdominal pain?

The most common (90%) colics in the horse are caused by parasitic obstruction and damage to the intestines. Strongyles cause severe damage to the intestinal arteries (see Strongyles, page 503), reducing (or blocking) the flow of blood to segments of the intestines. When the blood supply to a segment is reduced, the muscle tone (ability to contract) of the segment is seriously lowered. If the intestinal contents reach a weak segment of the bowel, they pass more slowly, causing distension of the bowel from the blocked portion back to the stomach. Distension and increased fluid secretion often are not sufficient to force the material through the weak area, resulting in a bout of colic from impaction.

Is this the only way parasites cause colic?

No. Parasites can also cause colic if they become large enough or numerous enough to block a segment of the intestine. The many twists and loops of the intestines provide areas where mature strongyles can lodge and cause fecal material to block the intestinal tract. This physical obstruction causes distention and the accompanying colic signs.

What is colic caused by impaction?

Impaction of the colon or caecum occurs when material passes through the stomach in an undigested form and collects in the caecum or large colon. This can form a complete obstruction in the caecum, the small colon, or the pelvic flexure of the large colon. Impaction of the caecum is more serious than impaction of the colon, but the two conditions often occur together. Retention of the meconium (material collected in the colon during fetal life) in newborn foals is a common example of impaction of the large colon.

What causes impaction?

Impaction may be due to poor overall condition (lack of muscle tone in the gut), poor quality roughage, defective teeth, and feeding at overly long intervals. Mild cases of parasite infestation can cause enough damage to partially or completely reduce the blood supply to sections of the intestine, causing an infarct (an area of tissue death due to the cut-off blood supply). These weakened sections cause a slowing down or stoppage of the intestinal contents and contribute to chronic constipation.

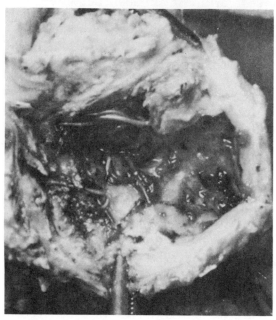

Fig. 20-35. The presence of strongyle larvae in the mesenteric artery leading to the intestines can result in embolisms which block off the blood supply to segments of the intestine.

Photo courtesy of THE HORSE, by Peter Rossdale, M.A., F.R.C.V.S., published by The California Thoroughbred Breeders Association. Photo by Peter Rossdale.

What are the signs of intestinal impaction?

Usually, the impaction builds up gradually, producing subacute abdominal pain for 8 to 12 hours. There will be mild signs of pain and only a slight increase in pulse and respiration. This is followed by an acute phase, if the impaction is in the ileocaecal area. The acute phase is characterized by an increase in the severity of the pain. Severe depression, patchy sweating, coldness of the extremities and violent rolling and struggling accompany the acute pain. At this point, the abdominal pain becomes severe and continuous, raising the pulse rate to between 80 and 120 per minute. There is also an increased respiratory rate of 30 to 40 per minute and a temperature of 103°F. Death usually occurs 36 to 48 hours after the onset of illness when the ileocaecal area (junction between ileum of small intestine and cecum) is impacted.

When only the colon is impacted, the disorder is more prolonged and less acute. Bouts of pain occur at intervals up to a half-hour and are of moderate severity. The horse does not eat, but he may lap or sip water almost constantly. Pulse rate does not usually rise past 50 per minute and the temperature and respiration may be unaffected. Feces are passed in small amounts which appear hard and covered with thick, sticky mucus.

How is impaction treated?

When impaction is diagnosed by the veterinarian, it must be carefully differentiated from gastric dilation, obstruction, spasmodic colic, enteritis and peritonitis. If the impaction is of the ileocaecal area, surgery is often required. Intravenous fluids are necessary to replace fluids lost in the distension. A large dose of mineral oil (with a wetting agent) is followed in two to three hours by a parasympathetic stimulant. This increases the intestinal contractions and causes severe pain. Rupture of the intestine may result from this treatment and is always carefully considered by the veterinarian. Death can also occur from exhaustion if the impaction is allowed to continue for several days.

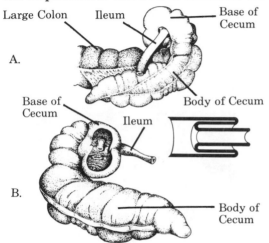

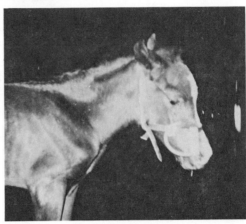

Photo courtesy of W. L. Anderson, D.V.M.

Fig. 20-36A. Diagram of the colon and cecum which may become impacted and cause colic.

Fig. 20-36B. Diagram of intussusception. The opened portion of the cecum reveals a section of the ileum which has telescoped into the base of the cecum.

Fig. 20-37. Foal with nasal tube taped in place. This facilitates treatment that must be repeated every 4 hours for meconium retention.

Retention of the meconium in foals may be treated with small doses of mineral oil and infusing mineral oil or glycerin into the rectum with a 12-inch rubber tube. Treatment should be repeated at 4-hour intervals until the foal recovers. Some cases may require removal of hard masses by traction with blunt forceps, or surgical removal.

How else can the intestines be obstructed?

Acute intestinal obstructions may be caused when the intestines are twisted and the passage of fecal material is physically cut off. This may occur when a loop of bowel slips through an opening in the mesenteric tissues and cannot slip back (like a hernia) or when a horse rolls violently and causes the intestines to tangle or twist. In young foals, a loop of intestine is very likely to slip inside an adjacent section, causing the intestines to fold up like a telescope. Telescoping of the intestines is called intussusception, which is the most frequent cause of colic in foals.

What are the causes of acute intestinal obstructions?

When obstructions occur in the intestines, the severity of the condition depends on the size of the obstruction and the amount of damage it immediately causes. If the twisting interferes severely with the blood supply to the affected area, or there are toxic substances in the isolated loop of intestine, the damage will be very serious. The mechanism of distension and circulatory collapse (shock) has already been discussed, but the toxic contamination of the abdominal cavity is equally important. Since veins are cut off more easily than arteries when the mesentery is twisted, the pressure from the arteries forces fluids to escape from the circulatory system. These fluids spread toxic materials from the intestinal contents throughout the abdominal cavity. Accumulated toxins from the strangulated tissue add to the tissue death and gangrene in the cut-off portion of intestine. Acute shock and septicemia occur in acute colics, but dehydration and chemical imbalances may be more important if the circulatory damage is less severe.

What are the signs of acute intestinal obstruction?

When the obstruction is acute, the signs of constant abdominal pain are pronounced. There is rolling, pawing, sweating, increased rate and depth of respiration, and the pulse rate is usually over 100 per minute and weak. Affected horses show no interest in food or water. An absence of feces indicates acute obstruction, with few or no sounds of movement from the intestines. The body temperature usually falls as the horse goes into shock and collapses. Death often follows within 12 hours, usually before 24 hours.

Fig. 20-38. Photograph of twisted intestines. Notice the knotting of the segment.

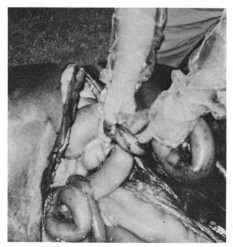

Photo courtesy of W. L. Anderson, D.V.M.

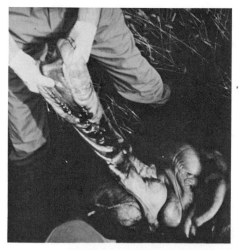

Photo courtesy of W. L. Anderson, D.V.M.

Fig. 20-39. After the twist is straightened out, the dark areas show the portions that have died from the pressure and lack of blood.

How can intestinal obstruction be treated?

Treatment of acute intestinal obstruction is completely beyond the horse owner. In addition to the difficulties of diagnosis (even a veterinarian can have trouble distinguishing between mesenteric thrombosis and intestinal tympany), intestinal obstructions can only be removed by surgery. Colic drenches and treatments are completely useless in these cases. Rapid diagnosis by a veterinarian is essential.

Can this type of colic be prevented?

In many cases, obstruction occurs when the horse is rolling because of abdominal pain caused by impaction or spasmodic colic. *Veterinarians caution against allowing a colicky animal to roll because the already-distended loops of intestine tangle more easily than the normally relaxed bowel.* Obstruction colic in foals (intussusception) can be prevented by making sure that they nurse or receive a meal within an hour or two after foaling. The presence of food in the intestine prevents telescoping of the intestinal segments.

What is gastric dilatation?

Gastric dilatation is dilatation (stretching) of the stomach. It is accompanied by acute abdominal pain and increased peristaltic efforts.

What causes gastric dilatation?

Acute gastric dilatation may be caused by a sudden, complete obstruction of the pylorus by a foreign body or by a spastic contraction, or by gross overeating and drinking. Since the cardia (entrance of esophagus into stomach) is easily occluded, the stomach is very susceptible to dilatation. The condition is most serious when the dilatation is caused by overeating grain, which results in putrefactive breakdown (fermentation) of the protein. Oats contain enzymes which start their own digestive process, so they do not have to reach the intestines to begin producing toxins. Chronic dilatation may be caused by cribbing or wind-sucking (distension with air) and stomach ulcers.

What is the effect of acute gastic dilatation?

In animals other than the horse, acute gastric dilatation causes vomiting. Due to the location of the cardia, vomiting is rare in horses. If vomiting occurs, it is projectile (takes very little effort), and most of the material passes through the nostrils. It often accompanies gastric rupture. Since horses cannot voluntarily relieve the pressure through the cardia by vomiting, gastric secretions accumulate and increase the stomach contractions. Stretching of the stomach walls and strong peristaltic waves cause severe abdominal pain. The stretched stomach walls allow some fluids to escape, usually causing shock and dehydration. Shock depresses respiratory, vasomotor and cardiovascular functions in addition to the toxic state that is caused by the release of protein waste products through the stomach walls. Rupture of the stomach may occur and cause peritonitis. When the dilatation is chronic, the digestive process is inefficient due to poor muscle tone and the appetite is usually poor because the stomach never has hunger contractions.

What are the signs of gastric dilatation?

Acute gastric dilatation may last for two to three days and is usually characterized by vomiting. If the horse does vomit, it is usually a terminal sign (followed shortly by death). The pain is usually severe and is accompanied by rolling, sweating, sitting on the haunches and kicking or biting at the belly. Severe dehydration may cause looseness of the skin and shrinking of the eyes. Laminitis (see page 59) often follows grain engorgement and complicates the treatment.

The signs of chronic dilatation are mild, recurrent pain, scanty feces, and a gradual loss of body weight. Feces are passed in small quantities and are usually soft and pasty.

How is gastric dilatation treated?

After the veterinarian has ruled out enteritis, gastritis and obstruction, there are two methods of treatment for gastric dilatation. He may attempt gastric lavage, passing a large tube down to the stomach in an attempt to siphon off the accumulated fluid and contents. This is often unsuccessful if the dilatation is due to grain engorgement because the mass is too pasty to pass through the tube.

Another method is administering mineral oil and a wetting agent, followed by a parasympathetic stimulant (intestinal activity stimulant). Parasympathetic stimulants should only be administered by a veterinarian because of the danger of causing the over-distended stomach to rupture.

Most cases require administration of intravenous fluids and drugs to relax the pylorus. Soft, palatable, concentrated foods may reduce the frequency and severity of attacks of abdominal pain in chronic cases.

What is gastritis?

Gastritis is an inflammation of the stomach that results in improper motility of the stomach and intestine, and vomiting in rare instances.

What causes gastritis?

Gastritis may be caused by frosted or frozen feed, coarse roughage, moldy hay, various poisons, salmonellosis, bot larvae and stomach worms. These agents cause inflammation and increased motility in the stomach.

What are the effects of gastritis?

Increased secretion of mucus protects the mucous lining but it also delays digestion and allows the stomach contents to ferment. Abnormal digestion causes further inflammation, which may spread to the intestines. Acute gastritis primarily involves an increased peristalsis which causes severe abdominal pain and rapid emptying of the stomach. Chronic gastritis slows down digestion and may result in chronic gastric dilatation.

What are the signs of gastritis?

Appetite is usually reduced but the horse may sip or lap water almost continuously. There is a rank smell to the breath and the feces are pasty and soft. Abdominal pain may be present, depending on the degree of inflammation and ulceration of the mucous membrane. Rarely, the horse may vomit forcefully if the gastritis is severe enough.

Chronic gastritis is characterized by an emaciated appearance caused by lack of appetite and poor digestion.

How may gastritis be treated?

The veterinarian must determine the cause of gastritis in order to treat the condition. In addition to treating or removing the cause of inflammation, the veterinarian will recommend withholding food. Fluids may need to be replaced, and a gastric sedative will probably be given to quiet the inflammation. When the horse is convalescent, medication can help stimulate normal stomach motility. Harsh purgatives should never be used because they would irritate the damaged mucosa. Bran mashes will help the horse regain appetite and normal stomach function.

What is spasmodic colic?

Spasmodic colic occurs more often in horses with excitable temperaments. More highly-strung horses are predisposed to this condition.

What causes spasmodic colic?

Spasmodic colic may be caused by anything which excites a horse. Lightning, thunderstorms, preparations for racing or a horse show, and drinks of cold water while the horse is hot after work may all cause colic in a susceptible horse.

What is the effect of spasmodic colic?

The heightened sensitivity of an excitable horse causes the parasympathetic tone of the intestines to increase, giving the horse a "nervous stomach" effect. This heightened muscle tone increases the strength of the contractions, causing distension and pain in alternate segments of the intestines. Increased gastric secretions also add to the discomfort.

What are the signs of spasmodic colic?

The signs of spasmodic colic begin abruptly and are characterized by short attacks of abdominal pain. Intestinal sounds are increased and may be heard some distance from the horse. During the intermittent attacks of pain, the horse may roll, paw and kick, then shake and stand relaxed until the next bout of pain. Patchy sweating and a slightly elevated pulse (60 per minute) are also characteristic of this disorder. If no treatment is given, the signs will usually disappear within several hours.

How is spasmodic colic treated?

Although spasmodic colic will usually disappear spontaneously, failure to call a veterinarian to treat it may result in serious injury to the horse. Enteritis is often confused with spasmodic colic, and intestinal obstruction may remain untreated if it is erroneously diagnosed as spasmodic colic. Treatment of the excessive contractions may involve the use of a spasmolytic (atropine) followed by mineral oil given by stomach tube. Promazine and mineral oil are frequently used in treatment of spasmodic colic.

What is colic enteritis?

Enteritis colic is an inflammation of the mucous membranes of the intestines which causes decreased absorption and increased secretion of fluids. It is often called "sand colic."

What causes enteritis colic?

Enteritis may be caused by any irritant; bacteria, chemical agents, internal parasites, and sand, all may cause inflammation. Specifically, *Escherichia coli* proliferate when the horse is in a weakened condition, particularly when the fluid content of the feces is increased. Race horses in training and other highly medicated horses may develop irritation because the normal balance of intestinal flora is upset by antibiotics and vitamins. Accidental poisoning or the excessive administration of harsh purgatives may also irritate the digestive system. Strongyles and ascarids are highly irritating to the intestines and frequently cause enteritis. Acute or chronic enteritis may occur when horses graze on poor, sandy pasture or are fed on the ground. Sand may be picked up with grass roots or in grain on sandy ground. The accumulation of sand in loops of intestine can cause severe irritation.

What is the effect of irritants in enteritis colic?

The effect on the mucous membranes varies with the irritant. Severe hemorrhages, a mild mucous inflammation, or extensive erosive or necrotic enteritis of the intestinal mucosa may follow irritation. Inflammation first causes the intestines to shed the outer layer of skin, which is peeled off by the increased activity and contraction of the intestinal segments. With this outer layer gone, the absorption of fluids and nourishment is impaired, while the speed of the contractions results in the evacuation of fluid contents (diarrhea). This failure to absorb fluid and protein in the intestines causes dehydration and shock. If enough of the epithelium is shed from the intestinal walls, toxic products and bacteria may enter the blood, causing severe shock and dysentery. When the enteritis is chronic, the intestinal wall thickens for protection and increases the production of mucus. Since the intestinal contents do not undergo complete digestion, there is a foul odor to the feces from the partial breakdown and fermentation of proteins and carbohydrates.

What are the signs of colic enteritis?

If the inflammation is acute, the increased contractions cause distension and pain, manifested by rolling and kicking at the belly. Pain is vague and intermittent (if it is present) in chronic enteritis.

Diarrhea is characteristic of acute enteritis. Depending on the degree of inflammation, blood, mucus and shreds of membrane from the intestines may appear in the fluid feces. The horse will be disinterested in food, but may drink large amounts of water. If shock is present, the heart rate may be increased. Acute cases may die within 24 hours, but chronic enteritis can persist for months.

How is abdominal pain caused by enteritis treated?

When the veterinarian decides that the cause of abdominal pain is inflammation of the intestines, he must also determine the cause. Treatment includes the removal of the causative agent from the intestine, usually by a bland purgative (mineral oil). Accumulations of sand are removed by treatments once a day with mineral oil for a week or more, or by treatments at half-hour intervals for eight hours.

Fluids must be replaced intravenously, and astringents and sedatives may help relieve pain. If possible, sedatives and spasmolytics are avoided, however, because they interfere with the ability of the intestines to remove the irritating substance. Especially in young animals, the replacement of fluids is the most critical factor in successful treatment of enteritis colic.

What is flatulent colic?

Flatulent colic is often called "gas colic" because it is often accompanied by the passage of much gas or flatus.

What causes flatulent colic?

The accumulation of gas in loops of intestine cause distension and acute abdominal pain. Highly fermentable green feed produces large quantities of gas, if it is eaten in large amounts. If the excessive gas in the intestines is primary (due to green feed), the distension builds up gradually because gas is periodically released. Most commonly, tympany (gas distension) is secondary to obstruction in the large or small intestine. Secondary tympany (due to obstruction) causes constant pressure and serves to depress the vital functions of the horse. Interference with respiration and circulation (shock) are common, and contribute to death in terminal cases.

What are the signs of flatulent colic?

Severe pain is associated with this type of colic because of the marked distension of the intestines. The abdomen is usually distended visibly and loops of intestine may be seen through the skin. Affected horses may paw and roll violently.

What is the treatment for flatulent colic?

In some cases, the veterinarian may have to insert a long needle (trochar) into the intestine to relieve the pressure. This procedure should be avoided if the case is not otherwise terminal because contamination of the peritoneum and accompanying peritonitis is likely to result from trocharization. Mineral oil with an antiferment (formalin, chloroform) and a sedative are administered to help relieve the obstruction and pain. Since most cases are secondary, the obstruction must be diagnosed and removed by the veterinarian if eventual recovery is to occur.

What is peritonitis colic?

Abdominal pain may be caused by inflammation of the peritoneum (the lining of the abdominal wall).

What causes this type of abdominal pain?

The most common cause of inflammation of the peritoneum is contamination from a perforating lesion of the stomach or abdomen, usually from bots or stomach worms. Passage of infection through the devitalized, weak intestinal walls in cases of intestinal obstruction and actual ruptures of the digestive tract are also sources of inflammation. The use of a trochar is likely to cause contamination.

What is the effect of peritonitis?

Inflammation is accompanied by the accumulation of a fluid exudate, the development of adhesions, toxemia or septicemia and paralytic ileus (see obstructive colic). In acute peritonitis, toxins produced by bacteria are readily absorbed through the peritoneum and spread through the circulatory system. Paralytic ileus is caused by a reflex inhibition of the digestive muscles when they are over-distended. This lack of movement in the intestines allows even more toxic substances to seep through the walls of the intestines with the escaping fluid, increasing the septicemia.

The formation of adhesions from the material in the fluid exudate is most important in terms of chronic repetition of the colic symptoms. If the horse is exercised and the local adhesions break down, the peritonitis can spread and increase in severity. These adhesions also interfere with movement of the intestines, preventing normal gut motility.

What are the signs of peritonitis?

The most constant sign of peritonitis is abdominal pain. This is shown by arching the back, standing motionless with a lack of desire to move, and breathing as shallowly as possible. If the horse goes down, he will be very reluctant to rise. The passage of urine or feces is painful and is avoided. Constipation makes the feces dark and mucus-covered. Appetite is completely lacking and the temperature varies between 103°-107°F. In cases where toxemia is present, death may occur within 24 to 48 hours. Less severe cases may be fatal in four to seven days, or they may recover during the same period of time.

What is the treatment for peritonitis?

Severe cases of peritonitis that are accompanied by toxemia involve administration of broad-spectrum antibiotics and sulfonamides to control infection and toxemia. If large quantities of exudate are present in the abdominal cavity, surgical drainage may be necessary.

ENTERITIS

What is enteritis?

Enteritis is an inflammation of the intestines marked by diarrhea, and is often secondary to an infectious disease.

What are the signs of enteritis?

The primary sign of enteritis is diarrhea. The feces will be loose, ranging from watery to a heavy "batter-like" consistency, and may contain mucus, dead parts of the intestinal lining, and blood. They will have a foul odor, and coloration will range from black to white.

The affected horse will generally show signs of abdominal pain, anxiety and depression. This may range from switching the tail and drawing up the rear limbs to rolling, kicking the belly and acting colicky. Appetite may be normal or poor, but there is nearly always increased thirst due to dehydration.

A mature animal may be only mildly affected, but continued diarrhea can lead to dehydration. As the disease progresses, the intestines lose their capacity to absorb nutrients from food, leading to constipation, depression, weakness and finally coma and death. In foals, the unprotected intestinal system becomes quickly infected, often resulting in septicemia and death in a few hours.

The duration of the illness may range from 24 hours, for acute enteritis, to several months for chronic enteritis.

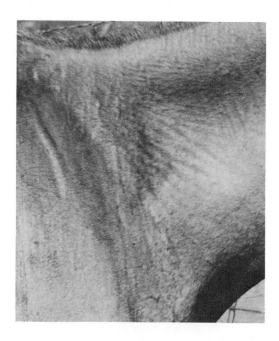

Fig. 20-40. Dehydration characteristic of enteritis. Notice the wrinkling and loss of elasticity of the skin.

What causes enteritis?

In newborn foals, enteritis is frequently caused by unsanitary conditions in the foaling stall. Infection may commonly result from bacteria (such as *Escherichia coli*), fungus, protozoa, and occasionally from viruses. The foal is especially vulnerable during the period immediately after birth, when the intestinal system is not yet protected by colostrum obtained by the foal from the first nursing. Such bacteria may enter the system through a navel which was not treated with iodine immediately after birth, or orally, if the foal is allowed to consume feces.

The danger to foals from enteritis continues after birth. Since the intestines are sensitive and not fully protected by antibodies and disease-resisting flora for some time, any sudden change in the system can lead to infection. Intestinal parasites, for instance, which mechanically damage the mucosa are a frequent source of trouble. Another cause is over-consumption of feed and fluid. This may be anticipated if the foal becomes overexcited when first separated from the mare, and overeats during the next feeding. Overexertion due to unrestricted exercise in exciting circumstances can likewise bring on this condition.

Generally, animals of any age can get enteritis from the following causes: (1) a sudden change in feed or ingestion of damaged feed, (2) an increase in fluid intake, (3) prolonged administration of antibiotics (particularly in foals), (4) eating toxic substances such as chemical fertilizers or toxic plants, and (5) large intake of sand, soil or feces.

How is enteritis diagnosed?

The presence of diarrhea is generally sufficient evidence of enteritis, but a veterinarian is needed for confirmation, and to find specific causes and institute appropriate treatment as quickly as possible.

How is enteritis treated?

First the premises must be examined to determine the specific cause of infection, followed by laboratory procedures. Unsanitary conditions are eliminated to prevent further infection, and damaged feed and foreign or toxic substances are removed.

Foals are commonly given antibiotics for treatment of bacterial infection and this may be indicated as well for mature animals. Replacement of lost fluids and electrolytes is necessary for horses of all ages, but is most critical with foals. When foreign substances must be removed from the intestines, a non-irritating purgative may be used, such as mineral oil given by stomach tube. Mature horses may require daily doses of one to two pints for a week or more to complete the process. If the intestinal irritation is due to incomplete chewing, the teeth should be checked and defects corrected.

How can enteritis be prevented?

It cannot be overstressed that foaling stalls must be sanitary. In fact, foaling outdoors in a clean, warm, dry, sunlit place can be an effective safeguard.

Prevention for mature animals consists of constant, good quality feed at regular intervals, avoidance of toxic substances, keeping teeth in good shape, controlling parasites and immunization against infection.

COLITIS X

What is Colitis X?

Colitis X is a highly fatal, noncontagious disease that occurs sporadically or in groups of horses. Knowledge concerning the disease is scant; it is of unknown cause and uncertain incidence. Death occurs three to forty-eight hours after the onset of signs. Horses from one to ten years of age may be affected, but adult horses are most often the victims. The disease is characterized by severe diarrhea and shock.

What causes Colitis X?

No viral, bacterial or other infection has been discovered as the definite cause of Colitis X. It has been related to spontaneous exhaustion shock, in that animals transported great distances have been known to demonstrate Colitis X, as have horses suffering from exhaustion due to excessive work. Other stresses that appear to predispose toward Colitis X include lack of food and water or a previous debilitating disease. It has been suggested that a bacterial toxin, *E. coli* endotoxin, is a cause since it produces similar signs and lesions.

What are the signs of Colitis X?

There is a sudden onset of severe diarrhea, depression, a rapid (100 per minute) pulse, abdominal pain and difficult breathing. There will be rapid dehydration, sweating, dilated pupils, and an initially high body temperature that gradually becomes subnormal. The horse will become very weak and will probably die within a few minutes after collapsing.

Sometimes death occurs so quickly that not all signs are evident. Necropsy shows that the cecum and colon are distended with a foul-smelling fluid and mucus. The submucosa may be greenish-black and blood stained or more completely blood-filled.

How is Colitis X diagnosed?

Colitis X can be diagnosed from its signs, although it may be difficult before death to distinguish it from an acute intestinal obstruction or acute arterial closure caused by *Strongylus vulgaris* larvae. Even with postmortem examination, Colitis X may still be confused with intestinal inflammation due to salmonella infection or arsenic poisoning. However, Colitis X is a more common disease than any of these others. Therefore, the veterinarian may prefer to offer it as a tentative diagnosis until laboratory examination can prove otherwise.

What is the treatment for Colitis X?

The disease is usually so peracute, and death follows so rapidly, that treatment is not possible. Treatment may be attempted by the veterinarian if a diagnosis is made quickly enough. In that case, he will administer therapy directed at relieving the shock and dehydration, with large intravenous inputs of various saline solutions, plasma extenders and corticosteroids.

PERITONITIS

What is peritonitis?

Peritonitis is an inflammation of the peritoneum that can be local or general, acute or chronic. It can be caused by microbial or chemical agents and it is accompanied by abdominal pain.

What causes peritonitis?

There are three major causes of peritonitis: (1) penetration of the abdominal wall; (2) escape of material through the gastrointestinal wall; and (3) systemic disease.

Penetration of the abdominal wall is the most frequent cause. It is the result of accidents such as landing on fences or from faulty surgical technique.

Escape of material through the gastrointestinal wall follows such things as ruptures, parasite damage, breeding accidents, inexpert palpation or rough use of an enema tube.

Peritonitis is secondary to a number of diseases such as strangles, influenza, viral arteritis and African horse disease. Primary peritonitis is the result of bacterial multiplication, toxin absorption, fluid and gas collection within the peritoneal sac, intestinal obstruction, or abdominal adhesions (the growing together by scar tissue formation of various structures within the abdominal cavity that should be free of one another).

What are the signs of peritonitis?

There are a number of signs of peritonitis. Obviously, the nature of the disease causes severe abdominal pain and contractions. The horse will show signs of shock such as depression, elevated temperature, high pulse rates, low blood pressure, congested mucous membranes and constipation followed by profuse diarrhea and dehydration despite the consumption of large amounts of water. The horse will assume a rigid stance and be reluctant to lie down. There will be a loss of appetite and a loss of condition and possible anemia. The horse will usually demonstrate restlessness and groaning. If it is a mild case of peritonitis, the signs will be less obvious. Recovery will come about uneventfully except for the development of adhesions. A severe case will result in death within a few hours to a few days.

How is peritonitis diagnosed?

Whenever a horse exhibits abdominal pain without obvious cause, peritonitis should be suspected, since it is often a secondary disease. Determining the cause by physical and laboratory exam and a complete history of the case will be helpful in making a diagnosis.

How is peritonitis treated?

A perforation of the abdomen (or of any internal organ) will require surgery. If there is an infection, it must be identified by the veterinarian and treated specifically. Generally, this treatment will include broad-spectrum antibiotics or a sulfonamide. The presence of fibrin and formation of extensive adhesions suggests the administration of digestive enzymes to try to break down the fibrin. If the peritoneal cavity collects large quantities of exudate, it may need to be drained. The development of severe anemia will require blood transfusions. The veterinarian will probably decide to alleviate pain with analgesics or tranquilizers for the comfort of the horse, and also to try to cut down on the tendency toward shock.

SALMONELLOSIS

What is salmonellosis?

Also called paratyphoid, salmonellosis is basically an enteritis (inflammation of the small intestine) caused by the bacterium *Salmonella typhimurium*. Various forms of salmonellae cause the disease in all animals, including man. The condition can be mild or severe, from the healthy carrier state to the peracute septicemia in which death is almost a certainty. A strain of salmonella, *Salmonella abortivoequina,* causes abortion in mares, testicular lesions in males and septicemia in newborn foals.

What are the signs of salmonellosis?

Infected horses show little or no interest in food but may drink water freely. Depending on the severity of the infection, fever can range from a mild 103°F to the acute 108°F in septicemic animals. In addition to fever, diarrhea is usually present, variable in its severity. The presence of mucus in the feces is common in salmonellosis, and in severe cases they may contain blood and sloughed mucous membranes. Most horses show signs of severe abdominal pain and there may be straining attempts to urinate or pass feces. If septicemia (penetration of the mucous membranes and entry into the blood by the salmonella bacteria) does not occur, the animal will appear dehydrated from the persistent diarrhea. In *S. abortivoequina,* abortion occurs between the 4th and 8th months. The foal is usually born dead or dies of septicemia shortly after birth. There may be no overt symptoms of illness, or the fever, diarrhea and colic pain of salmonellosis may be present.

What causes salmonellosis?

The disease is most frequent in animals under stress. Long hauls which exhaust horses, pregnancy, heavy parasitic infections, rigorous worming, and administration of gastro-intestinal irritants predispose a horse to development of salmonellosis, though the organism may have been present for some time in the animal.

Stress causes debilitation of the horse, allowing the salmonella to greatly multiply, resulting in abscesses and necrosis (tissue death) in the mucous membrane lining of the intestine. The presence of this massive infection in the horse's body is responsible for the congestion and thrombosis (blockage) of the blood system of the intestines, and spread of the infection to the liver, lungs, spleen, joints and the membranes of the brain.

How is salmonellosis diagnosed?

A veterinarian can diagnose salmonellosis from the animal's history, clinical signs and bacterial culture of several samples of feces, collected over a period of days. Carrier animals may discharge salmonella sporadically, so frequent sampling is necessary to establish the presence or absence of the infecting organisms. Blood tests may help confirm the veterinarian's diagnosis of salmonellosis, and sources of infection should also be tested.

How is salmonellosis spread?

The bacteria are present in the feces of infected and carrier horses, and contact with the feces is the usual means of transmission. When feces of rats or birds contaminate feed and water, infection may occur. Man can contract salmonellosis, and helpers in foaling barns have been instrumental in spreading the infection through improper sterilization of instruments and foaling areas.

What is the treatment for salmonellosis?

Treatment usually consists of parenteral (intravenous or intramuscular) administration of broad spectrum antibiotics and sulfonamides for the systemic infection, and nitrofurans and neomycin sulfate orally for the intestinal infection. Putting the oral medication in water is effective because the dehydration of diarrhea makes the animal very thirsty. The veterinarian may also give fluids intravenously to restore the acid-base imbalance and fluid level in dehydrated horses. Foals may require blood transfusions for the anemia caused by the massive infection. Surviving horses will be carriers of the disease, since attempts to remove the bacteria completely are fruitless.

Can salmonellosis be prevented?

Control of salmonella is difficult because of the nature of its spread. Proper manure disposal, fly control and feed storage are essential. Isolation of new horses, foals, carriers and infected animals is helpful in preventing total infection of a group of horses or foals. Healthy animals should be kept separately and pens and stalls disinfected to prevent re-infection with fresh bacterium. Major changes in feed which would disrupt the intestinal flora should be accomplished gradually. Resting animals frequently while traveling, and avoidance of possibly contaminated public drinking troughs can help protect traveling animals. Vaccination is available for *S. abortivoequina* and various other strains of salmonella. The veterinarian will determine by culture the vaccine that will be most effective. Breeding farms usually vaccinate if salmonellosis has been present in any foals or outside mares to prevent large outbreaks of infection.

TRICHOMONIASIS (PROTOZOAL DIARRHEA)

What is trichomoniasis?

Intestinal trichomoniasis in horses is an infectious disease characterized by a sudden severe diarrhea. It can occur in horses of all ages, but usually affects colts that are two to three years old.

What causes trichomoniasis?

The disease is thought to be caused by a species of the protozoa *Trichomonas;* trichomoniasis in horses is often referred to as protozoal diarrhea. A specific

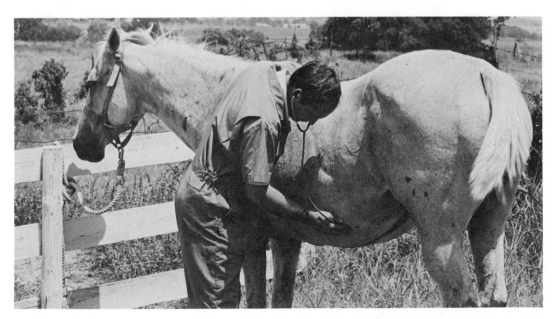

Fig. 20-41. Veterinarian listening for typical sounds in clinical examination of a possible case of trichomoniasis.

trichomonad known as *Trichomonas equi* has been isolated from the intestines of affected horses. *T. fecalis* has been found in human feces and possibly can infect the horse.

How does the horse become infected with the protozoa?

The method of transmission is unknown but experiments have eliminated rats, cockroaches, and flies as possible carriers of the protozoa. Contaminated feed and water troughs have also been eliminated as possible sources of infection. The disease is not spread among horses since only one horse in a group is usually affected.

Trichomoniasis is usually seen in horses that have been subjected to stress, such as injury, surgery, and illness, including strangles and other respiratory infections. These horses are treated with large doses of antibiotics, some of which could temporarily change the intestinal flora, the bacterial and protozoal population normally present in the intestine. Trichomonads may be normal inhabitants of the intestine, although they are usually not detected in the feces of normal horses. They generally do not cause disease, but when the intestinal flora is altered by large doses of antibiotics, it is possible that they multiply and cause signs of trichomonad diarrhea. The trichomonads can be found in large numbers in the feces of affected horses.

What are the signs of the disease?

Diarrhea is the first sign in all horses and begins as large amounts of greenish, watery feces, passed at frequent intervals. The content of the feces is normal, with no blood or mucus present. Abdominal sounds that resemble water splashing can often be heard.

Some horses may show no signs of illness other than the diarrhea. More severe cases may involve a fever as high as 104° to 108°F (from the normal 99.5° to 100.5°F), and a rapid pulse. The horse may show signs of abdominal pain, sweating and weakness. The appetite may remain near normal, but the horse still loses weight and is dehydrated.

How is protozoal diarrhea treated?

The horse should be examined by a veterinarian for the presence of trichomonads in the feces. If the condition is diagnosed and treatment is begun within eight hours after the diarrhea is first noticed, the horse's chances of recovery are good. Treatment involves medication to control the protozoal population, and fluids given intravenously to prevent further dehydration. A tranquilizer may be given if there is abdominal pain. A solution containing water mixed with feces from a healthy horse should be given through a stomach tube to restore the normal intestinal flora. When treatment is begun in time, the horse may recover within three to five days. Mild cases of protozoal diarrhea may recover spontaneously (without treatment) within three to four weeks.

Can the disease be fatal?

Trichomoniasis is sometimes fatal in severe cases within 24 hours. Other cases, if not treated soon enough, can result in a chronic condition, in which the horse does not completely recover from the disease. The horse has a continued mild diarrhea, with soft feces the consistency of cow manure. In these chronic cases, the appetite is often normal but the horse may still become very thin and weak.

HYPERPARATHYROIDISM (CALCIUM/PHOSPHORUS IMBALANCE)

What is hyperparathyroidism?

This is a condition of increased activity of the parathyroid glands, which are located in or near the thyroid glands. The parathyroids secrete a hormone known as parathormone, which acts in connection with a thyroid hormone and vitamin D to maintain proper calcium levels in the body fluids. The two hormones and vitamin D regulate the absorption and secretion of calcium in the intestines, kidneys, and in the mammary glands during lactation. They also regulate the rate of accumulation and release of calcium from bone. In hyperparathyroidism, the parathyroids increase the secretion of parathormone, which results in defective bone formation, a condition known as fibrous osteodystrophy.

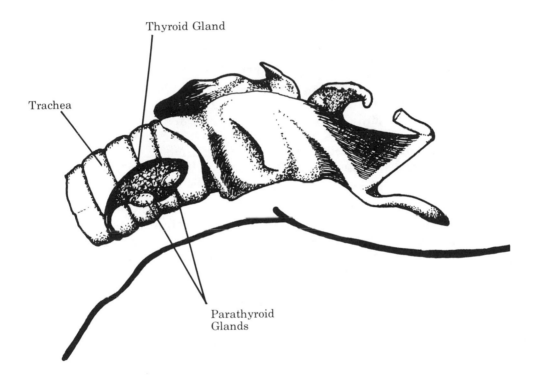

Thyroid Gland

Trachea

Parathyroid
Glands

Fig. 20-42. Fibrous osteodystrophy may be caused by a dysfunction of the parathyroid glands, located near the thyroid glands.

What causes an increased secretion of parathormone?

Primary hyperparathyroidism, in which the parathyroid gland is directly affected by disease such as tumors, rarely occurs in the horse. Hyperparathyroidism secondary to kidney disease is also rare in the horse. Secondary hyperparathyroidism due to a nutritional problem can occur in horses fed diets containing too much phosphorus relative to the amount of calcium. These unbalanced diets include cereal hays combined with excess grain or grain by-products such as bran. Fibrous osteodystrophy (a type of defective bone formation) is often seen in horses on these diets without enough calcium supplements.

How do these unbalanced diets cause defective bone formation?

The entire process is not yet completely understood, but it seems that increased amounts of phosphorus in the diet, resulting in increased phosphorus levels in the blood plasma, tend to reduce the blood plasma levels of calcium. A decreased level of calcium in the body will stimulate the parathyroid glands to secrete larger amounts of parathormone. This hormone will then restore the amount of calcium to its normal plasma level by causing more calcium to be released from bone. Since calcium is necessary for normal bone development, this loss of calcium from the bone (demineralization) contributes to defective bone formation. Hard bone and red bone marrow are replaced by soft fibrous connective tissue (fibrous osteodystrophy), causing bones to become soft and deformed.

Does this process occur only while the bones are still developing?

Fibrous osteodystrophy caused by nutritional hyperparathyroidism can occur in all horses, but usually affects young growing horses between two and five years of age. These young horses have high calcium requirements for bone development, so the effects of a calcium deficiency are more noticeable in these than in older horses.

What are the signs of fibrous osteodystrophy?

In the early stages, the horse shows signs of a mild lameness and sometimes an arching of the back. The horse's joints may creak badly as it walks, indicating a relaxation of tendons and ligaments. The lameness may occur in different legs at different times. Horses with fibrous osteodystrophy seem to be more susceptible to injuries such as fractures and sprained tendons because of the bone weakness. Fracture of the lumbar vertebrae has been known to occur in affected horses.

Are lameness and injury the only signs?

Other signs may be observed at later stages, but the condition is usually treated before it progresses to the advanced stage. The bones of the head seem to be the most affected, causing the disease to be referred to at times as "big-head." The jaw and other facial bones become swollen, and may become enlarged enough to interfere with breathing. The ribs may become flattened and the long bones of the legs curved, with swollen joints. The horse may become thin and anemic as the red bone marrow, which is the site of production of red blood cells, is replaced by fibrous connective tissue.

How is the condition differentiated from other types of lameness?

Diagnosis may be difficult at first since lameness and leg injuries due to various causes are relatively common in the horse. Nutritional hyperparathyroidism should be suspected if several horses in a group show the same symptoms of lameness. Their diet should be examined for high phosphorus or low calcium levels.

How is the condition treated?

Hyperparathyroidism and fibrous osteodystrophy are treated by correcting the nutritional deficiency. The levels of phosphorus and calcium should be balanced by feeding cereal hay supplemented with alfalfa or clover hay, both of which have a high ratio of calcium compared to phosphorus. Limestone may be added to the diet of affected horses as a good source of calcium, without increasing the phosphorus in the diet. Bone meal is not as effective in treating affected horses since it contains a high percentage of both calcium and phosphorus. A recurrence of the condition can be prevented by feeding a balanced diet containing about 1.2 parts of calcium to 1 part of phosphorus.

ORGANOPHOSPHATE POISONING

How does organophosphate poisoning occur?

This type of chemical poisoning can occur when a horse is exposed to insecticides containing organic phosphate compounds. Horses may be exposed to insecticides when they are allowed to graze in areas that have recently been sprayed with insecticide. Spray used on cereal crops and in orchards may be carried by the wind and contaminate pastures where horses are grazing. Many accidental poisonings occur as a result of improper use of sprays, such as using too high a concentration of insecticide.

Can organophosphate poisoning result from insecticides applied to the horse?

Some pesticides, such as compounds used to control mites, may be toxic when used in high concentrations. Worming medications that contain organic phosphates may not be toxic in themselves, but can have harmful side effects when a particular muscle relaxant (succinylcholine) is used within a month after the horse has been wormed. Organic phosphates in the body after worming, or accidental exposure to a field insecticide, lower the horse's tolerance of the muscle relaxant which may be used to cast a horse for a castration or other minor surgery. Its effects are then prolonged and may result in death.

Organophosphate poisoning may also occur in horses that have been safely wormed with organic phosphate compounds, but have then had topical applications of an insecticide such as malathion. The additive effect of the organophosphates in the wormer and the insecticide may be large enough to cause signs of toxicity in the horse.

Are all organophosphate insecticides toxic to the horse?

The horse may not be affected by some insecticides, depending on their degree of concentration. Organophosphate compounds vary in their toxic effects, and will not cause poisoning if properly used.

What are some of these organophosphate compounds?

Parathion is a well-known compound, used extensively in controlling mosquitoes and plant pests in orchards and on field crops. Malathion is one of the safest of the organophosphate compounds, but may be toxic at high levels. Tetraethyl pyrophosphate (TEPP) is one of the most toxic of all organophosphate insecticides. It is for use only on plants and an accidental spraying of a 0.33% solution of TEPP on a horse could cause death within 40 minutes.

Ruelene is commonly used both as a systemic and contact insecticide in livestock and may be fairly effective as a wormer. It is not highly toxic and most livestock can tolerate a spray with a concentration of 2%. Orally, a horse can be poisoned by Ruelene at 20 milligrams per pound. Dichlorvos is a compound used on both plants and animals which may be toxic to the horse at an oral dose of 10 milligrams per pound. At proper levels, dichlorvos is a safe and effective worming treatment.

What is the mechanism of organophosphate poisoning?

Organophosphates may be absorbed through the skin, by inhaling the spray, or by eating contaminated vegetation. The compounds then cause signs of poisoning by inactivating cholinesterase, an enzyme that breaks down acetylcholine, a chemical compound responsible for transmitting nerve impulses. The amount of acetylcholine present in the tissues is then allowed to build up, which abnormally increases the activity of portions of the autonomic nervous sytem. This part of the nervous sytem regulates involuntary actions of cardiac muscle, smooth muscle and glands.

What are the signs of organophosphate poisoning?

The severity of the horse's reaction to organophosphate compounds varies according to their degree of toxicity. Signs of mild poisoning may only involve a fluid diarrhea. Varying degrees of severe poisoning may include diarrhea, abdominal pain (colic) and difficulty in breathing, as the bronchioles of the lungs constrict in response to the increased amount of acetylcholine. The pupils of the eye may constrict to the size of pinpoints, and the horse may salivate and sweat profusely. There are often signs of incoordination, muscle twitches and tremors, weakness and paralysis. In the advanced stages there may be convulsions and coma, resulting in death if the horse is left untreated.

How soon after exposure will these signs appear?

In the case of more toxic compounds, signs of poisoning can occur within minutes of the exposure and the horse may die within two to five minutes. With less toxic compounds, signs may not appear for hours, but if left untreated, the horse may die within 12 to 24 hours.

How is organophosphate poisoning treated?

Prompt administration of large doses of atropine or protopam chloride by a veterinarian is usually effective in treating this type of chemical poisoning. The effect of atropine is similar to that of cholinesterase, which was inactivated by the organophosphates. The transmission of nerve impulses by acetylcholine is blocked in certain areas of the body, allowing the smooth muscle in various organs to relax and the affected parts of the autonomic nervous system to return to their normal level of activity. The administration of atropine or 2-PAM should be repeated every few hours for 24 to 48 hours, depending on the horse's response. Slower acting poisons may require treatment for up to ten days. Horses with mild cases of poisoning may recover spontaneously within one to two days.

Horses that have been sprayed with organophosphate compounds should be washed with water and soap, soda or detergent to remove any residues from the skin.

LUPINE POISONING

What is lupine poisoning?

Lupine poisoning may be caused by several species of lupines, a member of the pea family. Since it is very difficult to distinguish the toxic from the non-toxic species, the specific names will not be mentioned here. Lupine poisoning causes a gastrointestinal irritation and diarrhea when the seeds are eaten.

What are the signs of lupine poisoning?

In addition to diarrhea, affected horses may show signs of depression, weakness, prostration and coma. Liver damage may occur and a lack of appetite is apparent. Photosensitization (page 386) has been reported in some horses, and incoordination is usually noticed. The horse may stand or wander aimlessly and may lift the feet abnormally high when he is walking. Death may be preceded by convulsions or coma.

How is lupine poisoning treated?

Few worthwhile treatments are available to the veterinarian if the horse appears to be affected with lupine poisoning. Recovery sometimes occurs if the horse is taken off the dangerous pasture before the signs develop to a recognizable degree.

CASTOR BEAN POISONING

What is castor bean poisoning?

The castor bean *(Ricinus communis)* is the source of castor oil. Horses may be poisoned by eating a very small number of beans which contain a plant poison called ricin. Castor bean poisoning is characterized by a severe, acute irritation of the intestines.

What causes castor bean poisoning?

The plant itself is not poisonous. Only the seeds contain ricin, the poisonous substance. Because the plants are attractive, they are often grown around barns and corrals in the southwest as ornamental shrubs. New or young horses may be attracted to the plants and accidentally eat the seeds along with the leaves. It often takes about 150 beans to cause death in horses, but as few as 20 beans have been known to be fatal.

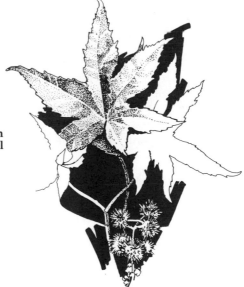

Fig. 20-43. Illustration of the castor bean plant frequently used as an ornamental shrub in the southwest.

How do castor beans affect the horse?

Unfortunately, the poison of the castor bean (ricin) is not affected by the digestive enzymes and acids in the horse's stomach and intestines. It acts upon the mucous membranes of the intestines, causing severe irritation and inflammation, and upon the nervous system. The nervous system degeneration is responsible for death, when it occurs.

What are the signs of castor bean poisoning?

Signs of severe enteritis are characteristic in castor bean poisoning. A period of time (a few hours to two or three days) passes before visible signs become apparent. When signs do appear, they are severe and rapidly become worse. The first indications of illness are usually dullness followed by incoordination. Sweating develops and becomes very heavy. Some horses may show signs of muscle spasms in the neck and shoulders, and the heartbeat is very strong. In fact, the whole body may shake with the force of the pounding pulse. Most horses develop a severe, colicky diarrhea unless the condition is fatal before enteritis is seen. Feces are thin and watery, without visible blood or clots. Signs of colic accompany the diarrhea (see Enteritis Colic, page 520). If the condition is not treated, the syndrome usually progresses to convulsions and death.

What is the treatment for this disorder?

Castor bean poisoning is more easily prevented than treated. Treatment relies upon the administration of body fluids and supportive therapy. The veterinarian may be able to obtain antiserum for castor bean poisoning, but it is very difficult to find.

SELENIUM POISONING (BLIND STAGGERS)

What is selenium poisoning?

Also known as "blind staggers," selenium poisoning causes nervous degeneration and gastrointestinal irritation.

What causes selenium poisoning?

In certain parts of the country, areas of soil contain more selenium than is normal. Also, some plants are more effective in pulling selenium out of the soil. If these plants (Astragalus, Stanleya or "prince's plume," Xylorrhiza or "woody aster" and oonopsis or "golden weeds") are found, it indicates that the soil has a high selenium content. Forage plants and common grains (oats, barley, wheat) may accumulate considerable amounts of selenium. Selenium is sometimes given as an antidote or preventative for enzootic muscular dystrophy.

What are the signs of selenium poisoning?

Poisoning may be acute or chronic, depending on the amount of selenium ingested and the period of access to selenium. Acute poisoning causes signs of blindness, head pressing, abdominal pain, fever, eventual paralysis, and death due to respiratory failure. Chronic selenium poisoning may be called alkali disease and causes signs of dullness, loss of condition, hair loss, stiffness and lameness. Hoof abnormalities are common and the hoofs may eventually be sloughed.

How is selenium poisoning treated?

Acute cases of selenium poisoning may be treated with potassium iodide, but most veterinarians find it ineffectual. A high protein diet provides some protection for horses in areas of selenium concentration, but removal from the area is the best treatment and preventative.

PHOSPHORUS AND ZINC PHOSPHIDE POISONING

What is poisoning caused by phosphorus and zinc phosphide?

This type of poisoning is rather uncommon in horses, but it is highly fatal.

What causes this type of poisoning?

Horses may be poisoned by phosphorus or zinc phosphide if they happen to ingest fireworks or rodent bait. Some cases have been reported when horses were allowed to graze on pastures that had been used as target ranges for artillery or other large munitions. (There are large amounts of phosphorus in gun powder.)

What are the signs of this disorder?

Acute signs of poisoning include violent colic, excessive salivation, intense thirst, convulsions and an odor of garlic on the breath. Shock is present. Chronic signs develop over a period of two to five days and include colic (abdominal pain), convulsions, coma and eventual death.

What treatment is effective for this type of poisoning?

Most treatments are not very effective, but the veterinarian may try administering copper sulphate, astringents, electrolytes and fluids. Mineral oil by stomach tube should not be used because phosphorus absorption from the intestines is aided by oily substances.

ARSENIC POISONING

What is arsenic poisoning?

Arsenic poisoning is one of the more common forms of poisoning in horses. Highly fatal, arsenic causes severe gastrointestinal irritation and mild central nervous system involvement.

What causes arsenic poisoning?

Arsenic is frequently used in dips or sprays for range horses, in weed killers and in rodent poisons. It is sometimes used in very small amounts as a feed additive in horses as a "tonic" to stimulate appetite and digestion. Affected horses may ingest the poison, or absorb it through their skin in cases where it is used as a dip or spray. When it is applied to the skin, it is much more toxic than when it is taken in through the digestive tract.

How does arsenic affect the horse?

The molecules of arsenic are capable of combining with certain elements in enzyme metabolism, interfering with the life-support system of cells in the intestines, liver, kidneys, spleen and lungs. This interference with metabolism causes the horse to lose large amounts of fluid through cell metabolism and the digestive tract.

What are the signs of arsenic poisoning?

Horses that have ingested or been in contact with toxic amounts of arsenic usually show no signs for several hours. One of the first signs of this disorder may be restlessness or acute colic. The signs of enteritis follow: diarrhea, rapid dehydration, a fast, shallow pulse (indicative of toxic shock), increased thirst and a total lack of appetite. In many cases, the mucous membranes will be red and congested. Severe diarrhea may be followed by a period of little or no activity of the gastrointestinal tract, then the diarrhea may resume. Convulsions and coma usually occur just before death.

What is the treatment for arsenic poisoning?

If the veterinarian is called at the first signs of discomfort, he may be able to help. In many cases, however, the veterinarian is not called in time to affect the fairly rapid course of this type of poisoning. Oily medications may be administered by stomach tube to try to prevent contact with the intestinal lining. Sodium trisulphate, astringents, BAL and fluids may also be used, if the veterinarian thinks they would be useful. The best form of treatment is prevention of arsenic poisoning. Dipping vats should be rigorously checked for the level of arsenic and horses should be well watered and cool before they are dipped.

21

THE URINARY SYSTEM

ANATOMY AND FUNCTION

What is the function of the urinary system?

The urinary system is responsible for collecting and removing the fluid waste materials in the body.

What is the general makeup of the urinary system?

The urinary system is composed of two kidneys, two ureters which lead to the urinary bladder, and a urethra which leads from the bladder to an external opening.

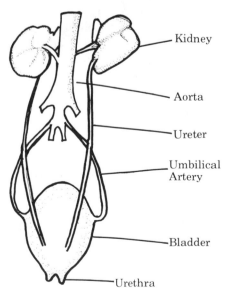

Fig. 21-1. This overall view shows the major parts of the urinary system.

Kidney

Aorta

Ureter

Umbilical Artery

Bladder

Urethra

What is the structure and location of the kidneys?

The kidneys are located one on each side of the vertebral column (spine). The heart-shaped right kidney lies near the seventeenth and eighteenth (last two) ribs and the bean-shaped left kidney lies further back. They are firmly attached to the dorsal (upper) abdominal wall by ligaments, connective tissue and the lining of the peritoneal (abdominal and pelvic) cavity. The kidneys of the horse weigh about one and one-fourth to one and one-half pounds each.

The kidneys, extensively supplied with blood and nerves, are structured in layers. The outermost layer is the capsule which encloses the entire kidney. Underneath this layer is the cortex which contains millions of small, round filters called glomeruli. Extending from the glomeruli is a complex system of tubules which make up the medulla (inner layer). These tubules are the structures for reabsorption of materials which can be recycled and used again by the body. The central portion of the kidney is a hollow cavity called the renal pelvis.

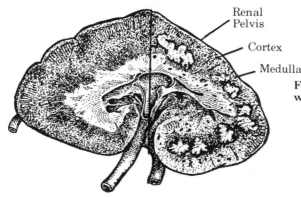

Renal
Pelvis

Cortex

Medulla

Fig. 21-2. A cross-section of a kidney, which shows its functional layers.

How does the kidney function?

The urinary system is important in eliminating fluid wastes (such as nitrogenous wastes, extra sugars and salts) from the body. As it purifies the blood, it also regulates the amount of a required substance in the blood. If an excess amount of a substance is present in the blood, it usually causes an increased release of that substance in the urine. Reabsorbing useful substances to the body such as salts, sugars, water and other nutrients is another key function. The kidneys are therefore an important regulator of homeostasis (a relatively regulated internal state).

The structure that regulates the volume and composition of fluids circulating in the body of the horse is the nephron. It is a system of capillaries and tubules which consists of: (1) a renal corpuscle (composed of a glomerulus and its surrounding double-layered tubule, Bowman's capsule), (2) a proximal convoluted tubule, (3) a loop of Henle, and (4) a distal convoluted tubule. Although it is not considered part of the nephron, the collecting tubules drain the distal convoluted tubule and eventually lead into the renal pelvis. The collected urine will then pass through the ureter (a tube that connects the pelvis of the kidney to the bladder) to the bladder.

The major site of fluid removal from the blood occurs in the network of capillaries found in the glomerulus. Blood pressure within the capillaries must be kept high to adequately filter out water and other small molecules. Large molecules such as fats, blood cells and protein usually are not extracted. Composing much of the renal cortex, the longest part of the nephron is the proximal convoluted tubule. The role of this segment is to reabsorb 85 percent of the water, sodium, chloride and bicarbonate needed to maintain homeostasis. In addition, the proximal convoluted tubule is believed to be the site that actively transports many of the sugars and protein components back into the blood. Henle's loop provides the connection between the proximal and distal tubules and aids in the concentration of acids that will compose urine. However, the final exchanges in the formation of urine occur in the distal convoluted tubule.

The final product that is drained by the collecting tubules is urine. It is composed of water, urea (the final waste product of protein foods), uric acid and various salts.

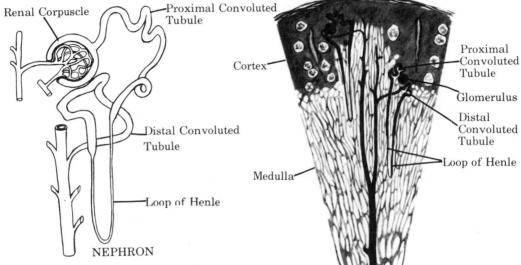

Fig. 21-3. There are thousands of these nephrons in each kidney. The structure inside the renal capsule is a glomerulus.

Fig. 21-4. A section of a kidney, showing two nephrons in black.

How does the bladder work?

Urine is drained in very small amounts through a muscular tube, the ureter, from the renal pelvis of the kidney to the urinary bladder. The bladder is a hollow, pear-shaped, muscular organ which serves as a storage chamber. The thick, muscular walls of the bladder become thinner as the organ expands. Depending upon the amount of urine it contains, the bladder varies both in size and position. The volume of the bladder varies with the individual horse, but normal capacity is three to four quarts of urine.

When the bladder is full, urine is discharged through the urethra. As the amount of urine in the bladder slowly increases, pressure increases on the pressure receptor nerve endings, causing a reflex contraction of the muscular wall of the bladder. However, the actual reflex action of releasing fluid is under voluntary nervous control. Infection or inflammation of the bladder, low temperatures or fright can falsely activate these nerve endings, creating the desire to urinate even though the bladder may contain only a small amount of urine.

SORE KIDNEYS

A horse is frequently thought to have sore kidneys when soreness is found over the loin region. According to all research, a "sore kidney," as such, is extremely rare. For the explanation of soreness and stiffness over the loins that is not due to bruising or muscle strains, refer to "Tying-up" Syndrome—Azoturia, page 626.

NEPHRITIS

What is nephritis?

Nephritis is an inflammation of the kidneys which is a rare disease of the horse. It almost always occurs secondary to another disease such as degeneration of the kidney known as nephrosis (see page 541). Prolonged nephrosis can sometimes result in glomerulonephritis, a type of nephritis primarily involving the glomeruli, which are coils of blood vessels of the kidneys. A more common nephritis of horses is purulent nephritis or renal abscess, which involves areas of pus formation within the kidney.

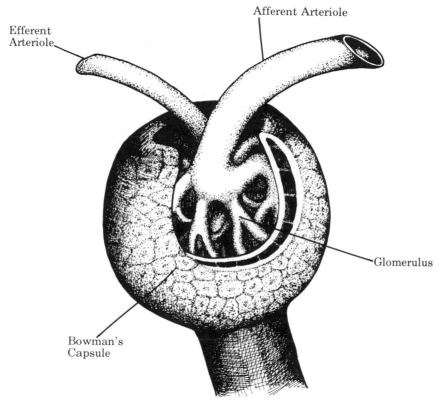

Fig. 21-5. A section of a nephron, showing a group of coiled blood vessels known as a glomerulus.

What are the signs of glomerulonephritis?

The first signs of this nephritis include swellings (edema) caused by an accumulation of fluids within the body tissues. The affected horse has an abnormally fast heart rate and difficulty in breathing after exercise. The tissue of the heart and lungs may occasionally be involved in the inflammatory process. The horse will pass little or no urine, indicating a retention of urine which has toxic effects on the body. In less severe cases, the horse may recover quickly and completely. In the chronic form, signs of glomerulonephritis may last for months. The horse then loses weight, becomes very weak and may suffer circulatory failure and die.

What causes purulent nephritis?

Purulent nephritis or renal abscess is caused by bacterial infections and may occur in foals with infection of the umbilical cord (see Navel Ill, page 569). Foal septicemia (blood poisoning) caused by infection with the bacteria, *Actinobacillus equuli,* mainly involves the formation of purulent lesions in the kidneys. Streptococcal infections, such as strangles (a respiratory disease), may spread to the kidneys and form renal abscesses.

How does purulent nephritis affect the function of the kidneys?

The bacteria responsible for the condition cause abscesses or purulent lesions to develop in the kidneys. These small masses of pus which obstruct blood vessels in the kidney are referred to as emboli. As a result, portions of the kidney may not be fully supplied with blood, and areas of necrotic (dead) tissue may develop. When the emboli are small, the unaffected areas of the kidney can usually compensate for the loss and allow the kidney to function normally, without showing signs of damage. If the emboli become large enough to block the blood supply to a large area of the kidneys, their function will gradually be lost.

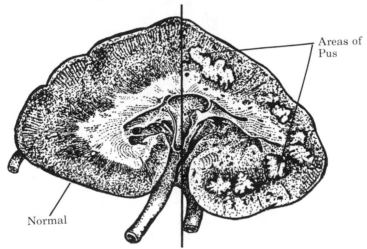

Areas of Pus

Normal

Fig. 21-6. Cross-section of a kidney, showing the pus formed in purulent nephritis.

How is nephritis treated?

Treatment is usually ineffective. In the case of purulent nephritis, the bacteria causing the infection should be identified by culture and sensitivity tests. Early treatment with the antibiotic shown to be effective in the sensitivity test will then aid in controlling the disease.

NEPHROSIS

What is nephrosis?

This is a condition involving inflammation and degeneration of the kidneys. The fatty tissue of the kidneys deteriorates and necrotic (dead) areas of tissue develop in the layer of epithelial cells lining the renal tubules. These tubules are minute canals throughout the kidney which reabsorb substances such as glucose and water from the blood that passes through the kidney. The tubules also secrete other compounds involved in the formation of urine by the kidney, and collect the urine where it can be further concentrated before being excreted.

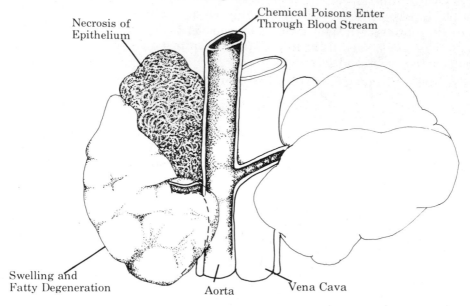

Necrosis of
Epithelium

Chemical Poisons Enter
Through Blood Stream

Swelling and
Fatty Degeneration

Aorta

Vena Cava

Fig. 21-7. Top view of the kidneys, showing the effects of nephrosis.

What causes nephrosis?

Nephrosis is caused by toxic substances brought to the kidney by the circulating blood and is usually associated with other types of kidney damage. The toxins may be produced by the body during some disease processes, or they may be chemical or plant poisons that enter the horse's bloodstream. Chemical toxins that can cause nephrosis by accidental exposure or by improper use in large amounts include mercury, arsenic, copper, carbon tetrachloride and tetrachloroethylene, the last two of which may be used as wormers. Various chlorinated-hydrocarbon insecticides such as toxaphene can cause kidney damage. Toxins produced by plants include poisons of young buds of certain species of oaks, certain mushrooms and moldy feeds. Bacterial toxins produced during some severe infectious diseases can cause major damage to the kidneys.

How is the function of the kidneys affected in nephrosis?

Portions of the epithelial layer of the tubules are destroyed and will be replaced by connective tissue. The affected tubules are then unable to function at a normal level, but the remaining unaffected tubules will tend to increase in size to compensate for the loss. If this occurs, the kidneys will then function well enough for the horse to live. When the amount of functional tissue destroyed is extensive, the horse will usually remain in poor condition and excrete large volumes of poorly concentrated urine. In less severe cases of degeneration, the kidney is sometimes able to regenerate some of the epithelial cells of the tubules.

How is the condition diagnosed?

A urinalysis can reveal abnormal contents in the urine, indicating nephrosis and malfunctioning of the renal tubules. Other signs may include a lack of appetite, a lower than normal body temperature, a slow heart rate and a small, weak pulse.

How is nephrosis treated?

Treatment by a veterinarian involves helping the kidneys maintain their normal function until the toxins have been removed from the bloodstream. Nephrosis will be fatal if large enough areas of the renal tubules are completely destroyed.

CYSTITIS

What is cystitis?

Cystitis is an inflammation of the bladder. The inflammation usually also involves the urethra, the canal carrying urine from the bladder to the outside of the body.

What causes cystitis?

The inflammation is usually caused by infection with bacteria such as streptococci, staphylococci, coliforms and corynebacteria. In the mare, cystitis can be an extension of infection in the uterus or vagina, which connects with the bladder through the urethra. Cystitis in the mare may also be caused by injury to the bladder during a difficult foaling. A common cause of cystitis in both sexes is the presence of a urinary calculus, or stone (see Urolithiasis, page 544) in the bladder, which irritates the mucous membrane lining the bladder. Infection of the bladder can occur when a contaminated catheter is used to empty the bladder or take a urine sample for urinalysis.

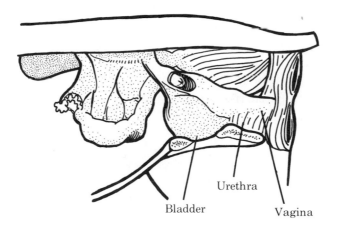

Urethra

Bladder   Vagina

Fig. 21-8. Side view of the mare's urogenital tract, showing the location of the bladder and urethra, which are involved in cystitis.

Cystitis has occurred in the southwestern United States in horses grazing on Sudan grass or Sudan hybrids during the growing stages from July to December. Sudan hay does not cause the condition.

What are the signs of cystitis?

The horse will urinate frequently, passing only small amounts of urine which contain blood and pus. After urination, which is painful due to the irritation of the urethra, the horse will remain standing in the same position and strain to pass more urine. In severe cases, there may be some abdominal pain which can be indicated by the horse treading with the hind feet, kicking or biting at the belly, and swishing the tail.

In cases of cystitis caused by Sudan grass, the mare may appear to be continually in estrus. The urethra and vagina are irritated by the infection, and there is a continuous dribbling of urine from the opening of the vagina. This leads to a loss of hair below the vagina and a discoloration of the hair inside the hocks. Affected geldings may lose hair on the abdomen as urine dribbles from the penis. As the disease progresses, there may be muscular incoordination of the hindlegs. The gait is weaving, and the hindlegs may buckle if the horse is moved backward, causing it to sit down or fall sideways.

How is cystitis treated?

In bacterial infections, the sensitivity of the bacteria to specific antibiotics must be determined. Administration of an effective antibiotic will then aid in controlling the infection. The treatment should be continued for 7 to 14 days to prevent a relapse. Full recovery is possible if the bacteria are completely destroyed, but small areas of infection may sometimes remain. In persistent cases of cystitis, the infection can spread to the kidneys, where it may cause enough damage to result in death. Horses with cystitis caused by Sudan grass rarely recover once the dribbling of urine appears, and may eventually die from severe kidney damage.

UROLITHIASIS (URINARY CALCULI)

What is urolithiasis?

Urolithiasis is a fairly rare condition in the horse involving the formation of solid masses of mineral substances somewhere in the urinary tract. These masses are known as uroliths or urinary calculi and are commonly referred to as stones. They may occasionally form in the kidney, but are more common in the bladder and urethra, the canal which carries urine from the bladder to the outside of the body.

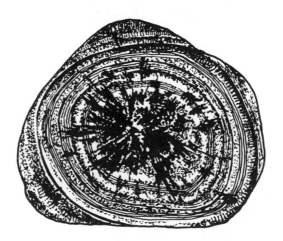

Fig. 21-9. This is a cross section of a calculus, showing the internal "rings" which are formed as the calculus grows.

Can all horses develop urinary calculi?

Calculi may form in all horses, but they usually do not create as much of a problem in mares. Small calculi which form in the bladder of the mare may be carried out with the urine through the wide, short urethra which empties into the large vagina. Calculi eliminated from the mare in this manner will then pose no problem, although large calculi, as wide as five inches, which cannot pass through the urethra may remain in the bladder. In the gelding and stallion, the urethra is long and narrow, and calculi may become lodged there after they leave the bladder in the urine. These urethral calculi can then obstruct the passage of urine out through the penis. Stones seem to occur most often in geldings, although the incidence of urolithiasis in horses as a species is low.

What causes urinary calculi?

Stones can occur in horses on diets consisting mainly of hay or pasture grasses which contain large amounts of salts of calcium, ammonium, and magnesium. The calculi formed will be composed mainly of calcium carbonate. Horses fed grain diets that are high in phosphorus may develop calculi composed of phosphates. Urinary calculi may occasionally develop as a result of a urinary infection and they may be associated with deficiency of vitamin A.

What are the signs of urinary calculi?

The horse may show signs of abdominal pain such as restlessness, kicking at the abdomen, and a swishing of the tail. The gait may be stilted and the horse may be reluctant to trot or gallop. The horse tries to urinate at frequent intervals, and may appear to be straining to do so. The amounts of urine passed are often small and they may contain blood or blood clots.

If a calculus obstructing the urethra is not removed, the urethra may be perforated or the bladder may rupture. The urine will then leak into the body tissues, causing a fluid swelling and a toxic condition which may result in death.

How is urolithiasis treated?

A veterinarian's diagnosis is necessary to differentiate the condition from various inflammations of the urinary tract. A catheter must be passed through the urethra to determine the location of the obstruction. The stone may sometimes be dislodged from the urethra by the catheter and be expelled from the body. Usually surgery is required to remove the calculus from the bladder or urethra, allowing complete recovery.

PERVIOUS URACHUS

What is pervious urachus?

Pervious urachus is a condition that develops when the urachus, a small ureter-like structure within the umbilical cord, fails to close up when the umbilical cord is severed. During the period before the foal is born, the urachus is the structure through which urine is excreted.

What are the signs of pervious urachus?

If the urachus does not close as the umbilical stump heals, the constant dripping of urine will keep the stump wet and unclean. The dripping of urine is most obvious when the foal is urinating. Infection can travel up the open urachus to the bladder, causing cystitis and other disorders.

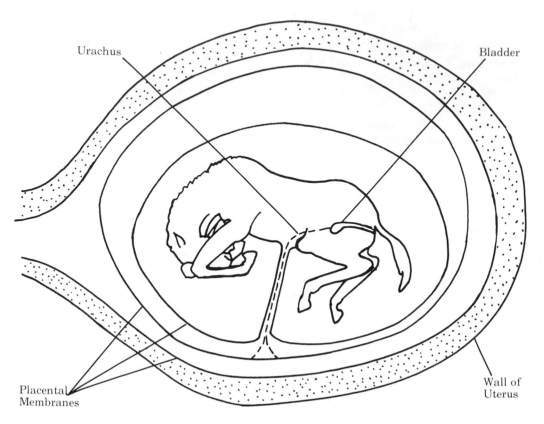

Fig. 21-10. The urachus, as shown in the diagram, extends from the bladder to the placenta through the umbilical cord. It is normally closed when the umbilical cord is severed after birth.

What is the treatment for this condition?

Most veterinarians believe that the umbilical stump should be cauterized every day with silver nitrate or strong tincture of iodine until the urachus closes. Tying the umbilical stump should not be attempted. Cleaning and cauterization should be done every day until the umbilical cord is completely dry.

22

THE NERVOUS SYSTEM

ANATOMY AND FUNCTION

What is the nervous sytem?

The nervous system is fundamentally a complex biological guidance system. It provides the horse with information about its external and internal environment, and it activates the body's response to the information.

Since the nervous system is so complex, the description of parts is very difficult. Anyone attempting to study the system should do so realizing that it operates as a complicated whole, so that rules about the system have frequent exceptions.

How is the nervous system controlled?

The nervous system is usually considered in two general categories: the central nervous system and the peripheral nervous system. The central nervous system consists of the brain and the spinal cord. Incoming data concerning the environment normally comes to one or both of these places, and the signal which activates the body's response originates here. Both the brain and the spinal column have the protection of bony enclosures. In the case of the brain, it is the skull. The spinal cord lies inside the spinal column. Both are further protected from damage by three tissue layers called the meninges. The outer layer is the dura mater which is tough and fibrous and contains capillaries. The middle layer is the Arachnoid mater, so called because it is like a spider's web. The spaces in the "web" are filled with cerebrospinal fluid to further protect the brain. Finally, the brain is closely surrounded by the pia mater, which is a thin, delicate membrane.

The cerebrum is the largest part of the brain, which has an outer layer of gray matter and an inner layer of white matter. The surface is covered with convolutions (folds). Intelligence, memory and emotion are directly controlled by the cerebrum, as well as the senses. It may also have secondary control over other parts of the central nervous system.

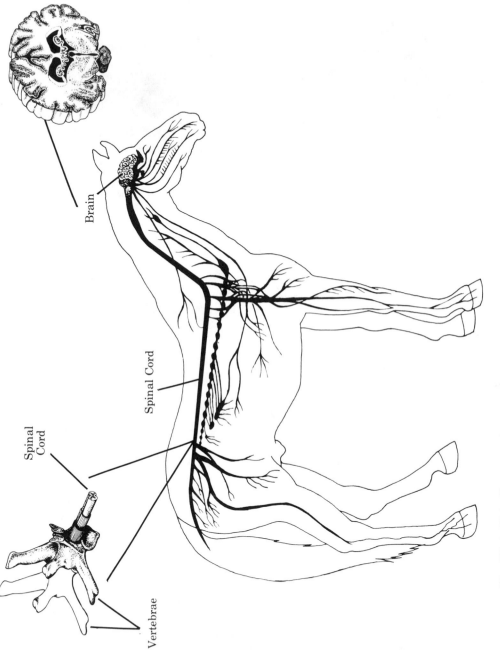

Brain

Spinal Cord

Spinal
Cord

Vertebrae

Fig. 22-1. This diagram of the central nervous system shows the brain in cross-section and the construction of the spinal cord.

The cerebellum is located slightly behind and beneath the cerebrum. It is responsible for muscular coordination and balance.

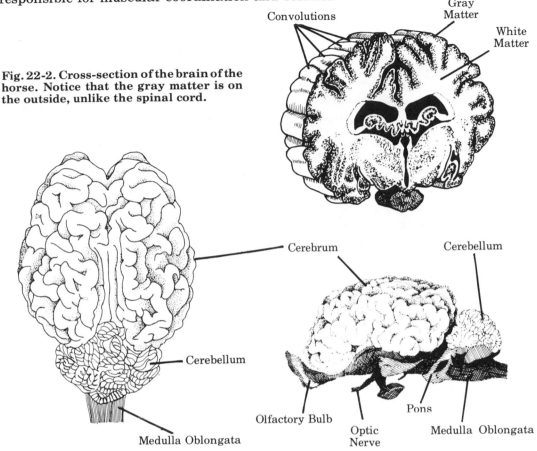

Fig. 22-2. Cross-section of the brain of the horse. Notice that the gray matter is on the outside, unlike the spinal cord.

Fig. 22-3. Dorsal view of the brain.   Fig. 22-4. Side or lateral view of the brain.

The brain stem, or medulla oblongata, is the slightly expanded upper end of the spinal cord. Its function is to control involuntary actions such as heart beat and circulation, respiration and body temperature.

The spinal cord of the horse is capable of many total responses to the environment in which the brain need not necessarily be involved. Its entire length is surrounded by the spinal column, and the same protective tissue and fluid that surrounds the brain. Unlike the brain, the gray matter of the spinal cord lies inside the white matter. The spinal cord is conveniently thought of as having five sections: the cervical, thoracic, lumbar, sacral and coccygeal. These section names correspond to the names of the spinal column sections in which they lie. One pair of nerves attaches to the spinal cord for each individual vertebra. The general function of the spinal cord is to make "unconscious" adjustments to changes in the environment. It also performs an intermediary function between the brain and other parts of the body.

The fundamental building block of both these organs is a highly specialized cell called the neuron. The neuron, like other cells, generally has one nucleus (center), but has two different types of fibers connected to the nucleus. The abundant presence of the cells in the brain and spinal column accounts for the grey color in certain areas. This denotes an area directly responsible for actions of the animal. The white areas of the brain and spinal column are composed fundamentally of nerve fibers that communicate the bioelectric impulses to the nerve cells.

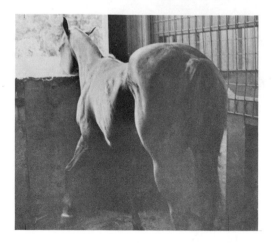 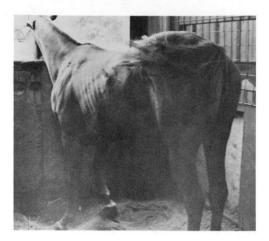

Fig. 22-5 and 22-6. This horse is weaving, a nervous activity that is thought to be caused by boredom. In humans, this type of repetition is frequently found in disturbed personalities.

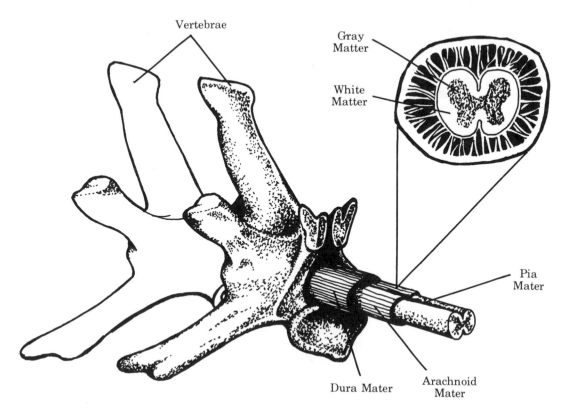

Fig. 22-7. Diagram of the three layers surrounding the spinal cord. The cross-section of the spinal cord shows the spider web appearance of the arachnoid mater.

The first type of nerve fiber is the axon. There is usually only one of these per cell, and it is comparatively thick, resembling a tree trunk. It is responsible for carrying impulses away from the cell. A cell may have several dendrites, which are smaller than axons and branch-like. They carry the impulse to the cell body. The axon of the cell may often be covered with a thin membrane called a neurilemma, or a lipoid (fatty) myelin sheath, or both. The myelin sheath is thought to serve not only as protection from physical damage, but as an insulator that preserves the chemical and electrical efficiency of the cell. Cells transmit signals to one another through a synapse, which is the junction of one cell's axon with another cell's dendrite. In many cases, these parts need not ever come in contact. The cells use a chemical combination of sodium, chloride, calcium and potassium to help "bridge the gap" between each other when sending or receiving an impulse. This same system is used in transmitting the bioelectrical impulse back to the affected part of the body from the cranial or vertebral centers. Nerves carrying impulses to these centers are called afferent nerves, those carrying impulses away are efferent nerves. The cells acting directly upon the activated portion of the body are called motor neurons.

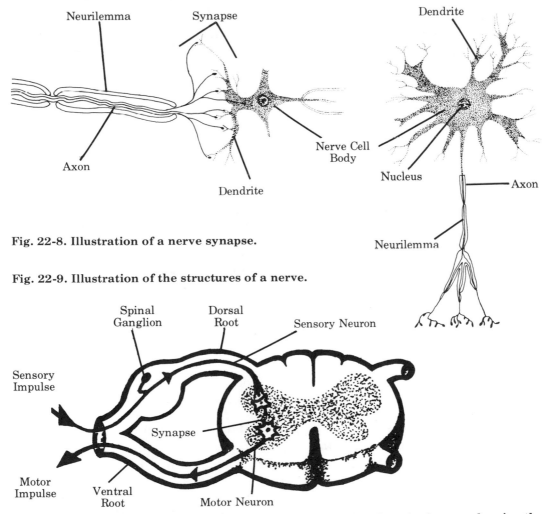

Fig. 22-8. Illustration of a nerve synapse.

Fig. 22-9. Illustration of the structures of a nerve.

Fig. 22-10. A diagrammatic cross-section of the spinal cord and a spinal nerve showing the elements of a reflex arc.

What are the nerves?

The nerves are often considered as a separate system, called the peripheral nervous system. In fact, the nerves are simply composed of bundles of axons and dendrites, and have the same color as the white matter of the brain and spinal column. Their function is to carry impulses to the neurons, most of which are located in the central nervous system.

The nerves are given general names according to locations, such as cranial nerves, cervical nerves, thoracic nerves, etc. Specific nerves have names that correspond roughly to their function, which may be sensory, motor, or both. For instance, there are twelve pairs of cranial nerves that emerge through foramina (openings) in the skull, one half of each pair serving one side of the body. The olfactory (smell), optic (sight) and acoustic (hearing) nerves are exclusively sensory. The oculomotor, abducent and trochlear (eye muscles), spinal accessory (shoulder and neck muscles) and hypoglossal nerves serve only motor functions. The facial nerves control portions of hearing, taste and facial expression. The pharynx muscle and another part of taste are activated by the glossopharyngeal nerves. The sensory and motor functions of the larynx are the responsibility of the vagus nerve.

There are forty-two pairs of nerves branching out of the spinal cord. They emanate from the spinal column in dorsal and ventral roots, which then come together to form a single nerve through the intervertebral foramina (openings between the vertebrae). One pair of nerves comes out between each two vertebrae. Each individual nerve has some roots in the dorsal (upper) section of the spinal cord, and some in the ventral (lower) side. The dorsal fibers function primarily as sensors, the ventral primarily as motor nerves.

This part of the system is characterized by the presence of plexuses, which are paired networks of nerves. Each half of the pair serves a member on its side of the body. The brachial plexus, for instance, serves the foreleg in the performance of motor functions. It is the combination of the last three cervical nerves and the first two thoracic nerves, and gives the appearance of a wide band. It then divides into twelve separate branches, some of which perform major functions. The radial nerve, for instance, innervates the extensor muscles of the elbow, knee and fetlock, pastern and coffin joints, and the lateral flexors of the knee. Damage to this single branch of the brachial plexus can result in a specific kind of lameness, known as radial paralysis or "dropped elbow."

The same basic function is performed for the hindlegs by the lumbo-sacral plexuses.

Does the nervous system affect internal organs?

The entire internal environment of the body is controlled by the autonomic nervous system, which is simply a specialized part of the nervous system already discussed. The nerves for this system originate in both the spinal and cranial areas. The autonomic nervous system is unique in that it has both a soothing and an activating function for each organ.

The parasympathetic nervous system is the subsystem that soothes, and it is constantly active in the resting animal. By lowering the blood pressure, constricting the bronchi (air passages of the lungs), and increasing digestive activity, it constantly makes minor changes to adapt to small internal and external stresses.

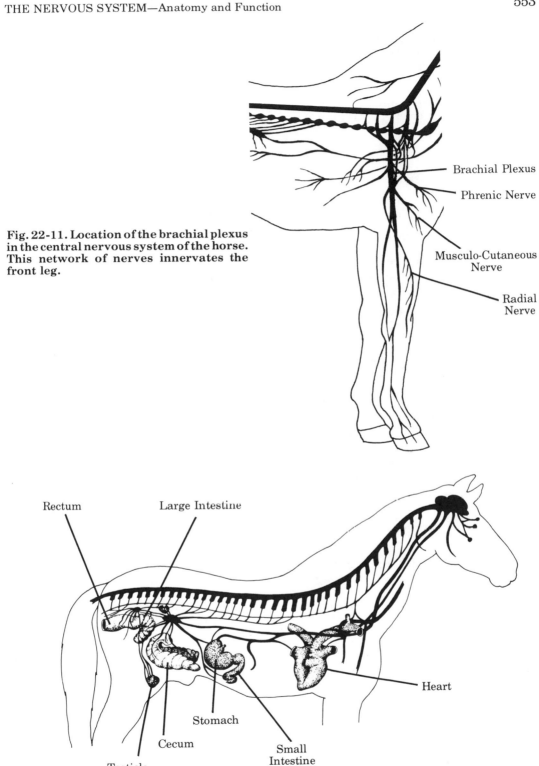

Fig. 22-11. Location of the brachial plexus in the central nervous system of the horse. This network of nerves innervates the front leg.

Brachial Plexus

Phrenic Nerve

Musculo-Cutaneous Nerve

Radial Nerve

Rectum

Large Intestine

Heart

Stomach

Cecum

Small Intestine

Testicle

Fig. 22-12. The autonomic nervous system, showing the way the various organs interconnect and react to stimuli.

The sympathetic nervous system also makes small adjustments, but is most active as the "fight or flight" mechanism. It reacts under severe stress to provide additional energy by increasing the heart rate, raising blood pressure, dilating the bronchi and diverting blood from digestive areas to the muscles.

Working in conjunction, these two parts of the autonomic nervous system maintain homeostasis (normal stability of the body's environment).

SHIVERING

What is shivering?

Shivering is a chronic neuromuscular disease of unknown cause. It usually affects heavy breeds that are regularly used for hard work, but has been seen in some light horses. Although the disease is still of concern in Europe where draft horses are used for work, it is a rare condition in the United States. Shivering generally attacks the hindlimbs. Hereditary influence has been suggested, but other theories place shivering as the result of neural lesions left from cases of influenza, strangles or other systemic infections. Trauma may also have some causative effect on the development of shivering.

What are the signs of shivering?

Not only does shivering make the muscles of the hindlimbs suddenly jerk, flex and pull in toward the abdomen during backing, but it also makes the tail rise in spasmodic jerks while the horse is moving backward. An advanced case of shivers may prevent the horse from moving back more than a few steps. The muscles of the hindlimbs and tail will shake and quiver. On occasion, an affected horse may raise one hindlimb and keep it elevated and shivering until the spasm passes.

In forward movement, the condition looks like stringhalt, except that the limb remains up and shivering until a gradual lowering begins rather than a series of fast jerking motions. Side moves are often awkward and spasmodic with the tail in a pumping motion.

Head, neck and forelimb muscle involvement occurs infrequently. Horses affected in such a manner will either thrust the forelimb to full extension and hold it just touching the ground, or flex up and in if the elbow extension muscles are shivering. Affected head and neck muscles will contract spasmodically.

How is shivering diagnosed?

Diagnosis of advanced cases is relatively simple since the signs are so uniquely characteristic. At this stage, an affected horse may be reluctant to lie down and have difficulty in rising again once down.

Since long periods can elapse between symptoms, routine examination may not reveal the disorder. However, careful observation and repeated performance tests will probably reveal the shivering. Since shivering is a nervous disease, excitement or irritation may bring on a demonstration of the signs.

Is there a treatment for shivering?

No treatment is known.

What is the prognosis for cases of shivering?

Although some working horses that are occasional shiverers may be able to perform for several seasons after being affected with shivering, the prognosis is generally poor. Shivering is a chronic and debilitating disease that increases in severity with regular work. Eventually the hindlimbs may become too stiff to use, although long rest periods will help the signs to subside.

EPILEPSY

What is epilepsy?

Epilepsy is a functional disorder of the brain, marked by convulsions which are of a short duration.

What causes epilepsy?

Some conditions of the brain such as inflammation, poisoning, or the presence of neoplasms can produce seizures resembling epilepsy. True epilepsy has no known cause, but may be a defect in the horse's developmental process. The role of heredity in the disease is uncertain.

What are the signs of epilepsy?

The only sure sign of epilepsy is the occurrence of repeated, sudden, characteristic seizures. Severe attacks are called grand mal seizures, which are evidenced by pronounced, unmistakable signs. The horse first becomes distressed, looks dazed, and begins to breathe deeply. Balance is then lost, the horse falls to the ground, and the muscles go rigid. The eyes remain open except for the third eyelid. Because the muscles that affect breathing go rigid, the horse is unable to breathe for some moments. When it appears that the horse is about to die from lack of air, there is a rapid jerking movement of the muscles, and hard breathing begins. The facial muscles may twitch, and grinding of the teeth and foaming at the mouth are common. The horse may pull its head to one side, and roll the eyeballs back in the sockets. Control of bowels and urinary function is lost. Finally, the jerking becomes harder but less frequent, and then stops altogether. This usually lasts from a minute to about thirty minutes, and may leave the horse too weak to stand for several hours. Some horses, though, are able to walk away immediately.

If the epilepsy is caused by organic brain disease, seizures may begin by affecting one side of the body at first, progressing to the other side. This is called Jacksonian epilepsy.

Petit mal (small) seizures are not normally violent, and may be mistaken for fainting. Sometimes the horse may be perfectly still, stare straight ahead and seem to notice nothing.

How is epilepsy treated?

If signs of epilepsy are evident, a veterinarian should be called immediately. Disorders which may lead to a "false" epilepsy should be identified and treated, and the horse's general health should be attended to in order to avoid further seizures. During an attack, efforts should be made to prevent the horse from injuring itself or others. Prolonged attacks may be shortened by the injection of sedatives, and bromides or barbituates may be used in true epilepsy to control future problems. While seizures of limited severity may be controlled, very severe seizures in young animals are considered hopeless since there is no known cure.

CONVULSIVE SYNDROME OF FOALS

What is the convulsive syndrome of foals?

The convulsive syndrome of foals has been reported in England and Ireland, where it is called "barker," "wanderer" or "dummy" foal syndrome. There are three stages of the disease, the "barker" syndrome being the most serious. Foals that survive the barker phase pass through the dummy and wanderer stages before they recover.

What causes the convulsive syndrome?

The cause of convulsive syndrome in foals is thought to be a lack of oxygen at the time of birth. This can be caused by human intervention (cutting the umbilical cord too early) or any trauma that causes an oxygen shortage to the brain such as broken ribs, crushing of the thorax (chest) and premature separation of the fetal membranes while the foal is in the birth canal.

What are the signs of the convulsive syndrome?

The signs of convulsive syndrome in foals usually are apparent within the first hour or so after birth. These signs include violent convulsions, a "barking" sound (like that of a small dog), blindness, and weakness. If the foal survives the convulsions, it will develop signs of a dummy or wanderer syndrome. These signs are aimless wandering, blindness, failure to respond to any stimuli and standing or lying quietly, as if the foal were completely alone. Affected foals do not suck in any stage of the syndrome.

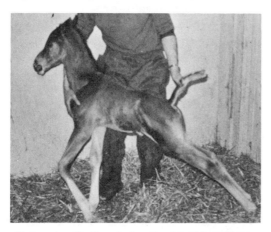

Fig. 22-13. Photograph of foal in convulsion. Notice that the head is held back and the hind legs are stiffly extended. Foals may convulse in standing or recumbent positions.

Photo courtesy The Horse, by Peter Rossdale, M.A., F.R.C.V.S., published by The California Thoroughbred Breeders Association. Photo by Peter Rossdale.

What treatment is available for affected foals?

If the foal is born with the acute form of the syndrome (barker), sedation may be necessary to prevent injury to the foal. Approximately 50% of the foals affected with the acute syndrome survive to pass through the dummy and wanderer stages. Foals that are affected with these forms of the syndrome at birth may need to be fed by stomach tube, as do barkers. Other than feeding the foal four or five times a day until it recovers (in three to ten days), treatment is unnecessary.

CONGENITAL HYDROCEPHALUS

What is congenital hydrocephalus?

Congenital hydrocephalus is the presence, at birth, of excessive amounts of cerebro-spinal fluid (CSF) in the cranial cavity. The pressure caused by this fluid usually results in compression of the brain, which may be accompanied by abnormal enlargement of the cranium.

What causes congenital hydrocephalus?

Internal hydrocephalus is the type that occurs most often. The choroid plexus manufactures CSF, and is located inside the brain. When the drainage system to the areas outside the brain is blocked, the fluid continues to accumulate, and compresses the cerebrum into a thin layer of tissue.

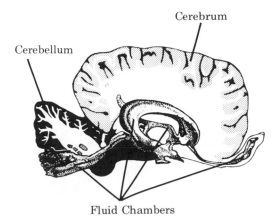

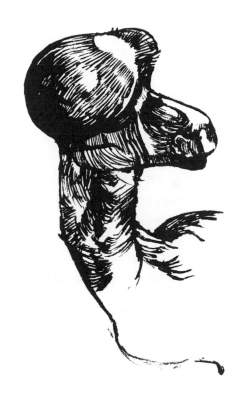

Fig. 22-14. This illustration of the fluid chambers of the brain shows how hydrocephaly is caused. A blockage in a fluid chamber will cause fluid to accumulate, creating pressure on the cerebrum.

Fig. 22-15. Illustration of a hydrocephalic foal. Notice the extreme enlargement of the brain area.

The other known form of hydrocephalus is external, meaning that the CSF is in the area around the brain, but cannot move to the spinal cord area or into the areas immediately next to the brain. In these instances, the brain is simply compressed by external pressure.

What are the signs of congenital hydrocephalus?

A sure sign of hydrocephalus at birth is the abnormal enlargement of the cranial cavity. Some cases are so severe that the skull of the foal must be crushed in order to make delivery, or it must be delivered by caesarean section (surgically). Foals that are seriously deformed in this way are usually either stillborn, or die shortly after birth. Less severe cases may live for a few days. Mildly hydrocephalic foals may appear lazy, drowsy, and unsteady on their feet. The head may be carried close to the ground. Most cases become steadily worse, although some have been known to remain stable and survive for some time.

How is congenital hydrocephalus treated?

At present, there is no known treatment for this condition.

INJURY OF THE CENTRAL NERVOUS SYSTEM

What causes injuries to the central nervous system?

The brain and spinal cord are subject to much the same injuries. Damage may be caused by a blow or fall which does not seem serious at the time of the accident. In some cases, little or no external damage is apparent.

What results from injuries to the central nervous system?

If a blow has caused a fracture which exposes the meninges (covering layers), a fatal, infectious inflammation may affect them and the underlying tissues. Even when the tissues are not exposed, they may be lacerated (cut), resulting in hemorrhage. Such internal bleeding often forms hematomas ("pockets" of blood) which can either put pressure on specific areas of the nervous tissue, or spread through the cerebro-spinal fluid. Local compression by a hematoma may impair some body functions, and bleeding into the cerebro-spinal fluid can cause non-infectious inflammation of the lining tissues (meningitis).

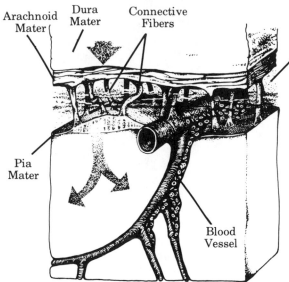

Arachnoid Mater Dura Mater Connective Fibers

Cerebrospinal Fluid

Pia Mater

Blood Vessel

Fig. 22-16. Hemorrhage anywhere in the central nervous system can affect the functions of various organs and muscles. Arrows indicate a blow which has stretched connective fibers and ruptured capillaries, releasing blood into the cerebrospinal fluid.

A blow without a fracture is often just as dangerous. It is true that nervous tissues are well protected by bone and the shock-absorbing system of tissue layers and fluid. However, when the shock-absorbing system reaches its limits, the protective bone acts as a hard boundary that the soft nervous tissue hits. This almost always causes unconsciousness and a shock of the tissues known as concussion. Unconsciousness may not result from a blow to the spine, but otherwise the results are much the same. When the nervous tissue makes its sudden stop against the protective bone which is opposite the site of the blow, hemorrhage may occur from the tearing of small blood vessels. The jar of the stop disrupts the flow of blood and lymph, and bruising (contusion) of the tissues is not infrequent.

Death from a blow to the head may be finally caused by extensive hemorrhages, but it is usually brought on by edema (swelling by fluid). This fluid usually comes to the injured area because the area has been deprived of oxygen or blood. As the pressure increases, the cerebrum may be forced into the space between it and the cerebellum, or the brain stem may be forced into the opening from the skull to the spinal cord. This process, called herniation, results in death.

Pressure on the spinal cord does not usually result in death, but causes paralysis of the areas innervated (activated) by the nerves posterior to (behind) the affected area. Since the pressure of edema does not cause death of the animal, local necrosis is more likely to be noted here than in the brain. The spinal cord liquefies when necrosis sets in, which results in irreversible paralysis.

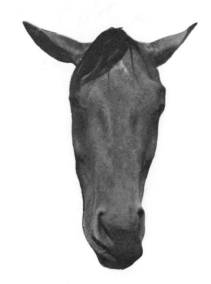

Fig. 22-17. Front view of facial paralysis. The lips are twisted to the left because the muscles on the right are controlled by a damaged nerve.

Can brain damage cause paralysis?

Brain injuries can also cause some kinds of paralysis, especially if the cranial nerves are damaged. There are twelve pairs of cranial nerves, responsible for sight, hearing, taste, and the activation of some muscles in the anterior (forward) portion of the body. Some of these nerves are easily injured, because they run close to the external surface. The facial nerve, for instance, runs around the posterior portion of the jawbone, where it may be easily crushed. This results in a characteristic drooping of the muscles on one side of the face. Little can be done to correct this situation, but good nursing has produced spontaneous recovery in cases where the nerve was not too severely damaged.

Another example of commonly observed cranial nerve damage is vagal paralysis. The vagus nerve, among other functions, activates the muscles that move the vocal cords aside during normal breathing. When the vocal cords do not move, a roaring or whistling sound is produced. This condition is popularly called "roaring" (see Roaring, page 424), and may be correctable by surgery.

What are the signs of central nervous system injury?

Brain injury may first be demonstrated by hyperirritability perhaps with convulsions. The horse may press its head against walls, and, as pressure increases, show signs of mental depression. Reflexes may be impaired, and the horse could settle into drowsiness and coma.

Injuries to the spinal cord may first be indicated by spastic movements of body parts acted upon by nerves posterior to the injury, and eventually these parts may have no sensation. Parts served by nerves in the immediate area of the injury may go limp, and this condition could become general as necrosis progresses.

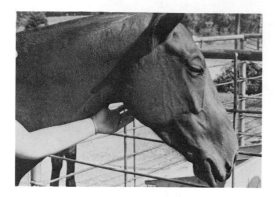

Fig. 22-18. Side view of facial paralysis showing the extreme looseness of the lips.

How are injuries to the central nervous system treated?

If damage to the central nervous system is suspected, a veterinarian should be consulted immediately. Most treatment is aimed at relieving pain and reducing swelling of the injured nervous tissues. Pain may be treated with narcotics, but great care must be taken to avoid further depression of vital functions. Edema may be relieved by the injection of certain drugs, but again, caution is advisable. Pressure may have to be released ultimately through surgery. In less severe cases, total rest may allow spontaneous recovery. The prognosis depends on the severity of the condition, but in general it is fair to poor.

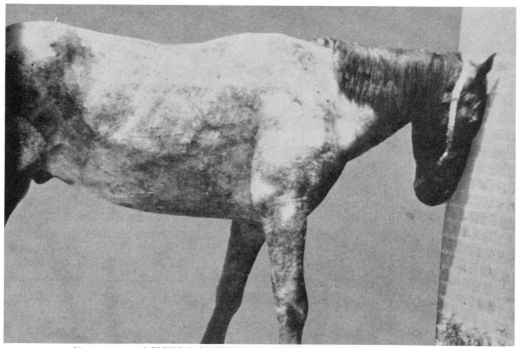

Photo courtesy of CLINICAL DIAGNOSIS OF LARGE ANIMALS, by W. J. Gibbons, D.V.M., Published by Lea and Febiger Publishing Co., Philadelphia, Pa.

Fig. 22-19. Head-pressing and bracing of the front legs are characteristic of a "dummy" attitude. This position is typical in many nervous disorders. This horse happens to have chronic hydrocephalus.

ELECTRIC SHOCK

What can cause electric shock in horses?

Electric shock can be caused by lightning during a thunderstorm when horses are in the pasture or in a stable unprotected by lightning rods. A horse may be accidentally electrocuted by coming into contact with an uninsulated wire that is conducting electricity. This may be due to faulty electrical wiring in the stable, or the horse may have chewed the insulation from the wire, exposing the bare metal conductor. Broken or low-hanging overhead high tension wires, which usually carry very high voltages, may cause electrocution. Improperly grounded electric hot walkers have also been a cause of electrocution in the horse.

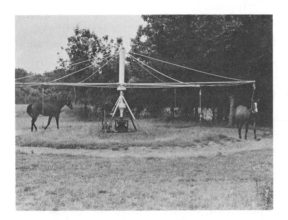

Fig. 22-20. Hot walkers must be properly grounded, with nylon or rope leads rather than chains to attach horses.

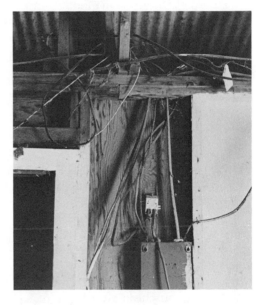

Fig. 22-21. Faulty stable wiring. If wiring can be reached by the horse or rodents, it should be in metal casing.

How much voltage is required to electrocute a horse?

Damage caused by an electric current passing through the body is usually due to high amperage (rate of flow) rather than high voltage (pressure). Animals can tolerate high voltage if the amperage is low. The electricity in most stables has an amperage of 15 to 30 amperes and a voltage of 110 volts, which can kill a horse that is well grounded. Lightning is electricity with high voltage, estimated at 1,000,000 volts.

Does a horse have to be struck directly by lightning or contact a wire to be electrocuted?

No. Electrocution can be caused by contact with trees, fences, barns, pools of water, or ground that has become electrified during a thunderstorm. Certain types of trees are likely to be struck by lightning, including oak trees and others that are tall, spreading, and have well-developed root systems just below the ground surface. Damp ground can act as a conductor for electricity passing along these roots, causing electric shock in horses standing near the trees. Different types of soil vary in their ability to conduct electricity. Loam is a good conductor, followed by sand, clay, marble and chalk. Shallow pools of water may become electrified when they are located above the roots of a tree that has been struck by lightning. Transmission wires falling into a pool of water will electrify the entire pool, and horses coming into contact with the water will be killed instantly.

Is electric shock usually fatal?

Most forms of electric shock are fatal. Since nervous tissue is a good conductor of electricity, an electric current causes a sudden shock to the central nervous system. Death results immediately from respiratory or cardiac arrest. The hair and skin of the dead horse may be singed or burned, indicating the severity of the shock. A mild electric shock causes a less severe nervous shock that can result in temporary unconsciousness.

What are the signs of electric shock in a horse that survives?

Horses that survive electric shock can make a complete recovery within several minutes or several months, depending on the degree of shock. Signs of nervous damage can vary from slight hyperexcitability to complete paralysis. Common signs include dizziness, affected vision, and a hypersensitivity of the skin.

How is electric shock treated?

Horses may recover from shock within a few minutes without treatment. In more severe cases, the horse should be provided with good nursing care but veterinary treatment may be required to help maintain the horse's normal body functions.

How can electric shock be prevented?

Lightning strokes cannot be avoided, but properly grounded lightning rods should be placed on all stables or barns where horses are kept. Electrical wires should be located out of reach of horses and fuse wires with an amperage higher than 30 amps. should be avoided. Any type of wire fence attached to trees, buildings and wood posts can conduct electricity during thunderstorms, and should be grounded. Metal fence posts in place of wooden posts at 150-foot intervals can be used to ground the fence, or metal rods may be driven into the ground beside the wooden posts at similar intervals. Electric hot walkers should be well grounded and the tie line on them should be of nylon rope rather than chain or steel cable.

WOBBLES (EQUINE INCOORDINATION)

What is wobbler disease?

Wobbler disease (equine incoordination, equine spinal ataxia, ataxia of foals, weak loin or jinxed back) affects the cervical spinal cord and vertebrae of young horses. It is a sporadic, nonparalytic disease marked by incoordination. Wobbles is not common, but affected horses usually cannot work. All breeds appear to be susceptible, but draft horses and mules are less often affected. Males contract the disease more often. The lack of coordination is generally developed by two years of age, although signs appear anywhere from three months to four years. Heavily muscled, well-nourished horses are stricken more often.

What causes wobbles?

Associated lesions (osteoarthritis of the vertebrae, narrowing of the spinal canal and degenerative lesions of the spinal cord) are well-documented, but the actual cause is unknown. Heredity has been suspected, but a definite genetic relationship has never been established.

Damage to the vertebrae, by disease or trauma, may result in subsequent dislocations and pressures on the spinal cord. This possibly accounts for the noted lesions of wobbles.

A relation has been drawn between the length of the horse's neck and the contraction of wobbles. A longer neck seems to have more chance of vertebral defect and resultant cord lesions. The large muscle development of male animals is also considered a contributing factor.

What are the signs of wobbles?

The characteristic sign is a lack of coordination marked by a wobbling gait. The onset of signs can be either gradual or sudden. If sudden, there was probably some previous incoordination compounded by trauma. Dragging of the toes, swaying or lurching of the hindquarters, and knuckling over in the fetlocks are all evidence of wobbles. Signs are usually exaggerated by backing, turning the horse from side to side, climbing and blindfolding. The horse's stance will be normal when at rest, except in the terminal stages of the disease and possibly during urination or defecation. The horse will move with forelimbs spread laterally to help maintain balance and hindlimbs over-extended.

The hindquarters of the affected horse will be weak. Although the wobbling will be most evident in the hindlimbs, it also affects the forelimbs and will eventually be noticeable there. Neck movements may be limited and painful. Occasionally the animal will go down and be unable to get back up again.

The disease is progressive and causes the horse to lose condition. There may be a period when the signs are arrested following the initial display of signs. However, very few cases have ever recovered.

How is diagnosis made in the case of wobbles?

The problem of diagnosis with wobbles is a matter of differentiating it from other diseases. Two diseases of note are Kumri and Brazilian Wobbles. Cerebrospinal nematodosis (Kumri) is a disease seen in the Far East with comparable signs. However, differences in the age incidence and the placement of lesions found at necropsy indicate a different cause. What is referred to as wobbles in Brazil differs in several respects and is thought to be the result of a nutritional deficiency. Overall, the distinctive characteristics of incidence and progression in wobbles set it apart from other maladies of incoordination.

What is the treatment for wobbles?

There is no effective practical treatment for wobbles at this time. Corticosteroids temporarily relieve the signs. However, correction of nutritional deficiencies, if any, may help to alleviate the disease. Yearlings with Brazilian wobbles may recover without treatment, gradually improving over a period of several months. They seem to respond better when kept in pastures 24 hours a day rather than being confined in stalls, and many recover fully enough to be successfully raced. In "true wobbles" there have been a few recoveries in response to surgical correction.

What is the prognosis for cases of wobbles?

Recovery is rare and the extent of debilitation is variable, but more than one "wobbler" has been known to recover and perform successfully. Any change for the better or worse will generally be determined in the first week after the onset of signs. While euthanasia is often recommended, some mares and stallions with only mild incoordination may continue breeding for years. Mares with Brazilian wobbles may show signs of incoordination only during the last quarter of pregnancy, and recover by the time the foal is weaned. The condition will reappear during following pregnancies, however, and gradually worsen until the mare either dies or is destroyed.

CEREBROSPINAL NEMATODOSIS (KUMRI)

What is cerebrospinal nematodosis?

Cerebrospinal nematodosis is a nervous disorder which is characterized by incoordination, imbalance, motor weakness and blindness. In the Far East, the disorder is called Kumri.

What causes nematodosis?

Cerebrospinal nematodosis is caused by the migration of the larvae of *Setaria digitala,* a long, thread-like worm that is normally a parasite of cattle. Horses are infected with the larvae by mosquitoes that have fed on affected cattle. Most common in late summer or fall, mosquitoes are the only means of infection for horses. The larvae burrow into the spinal cord and brain, causing signs after a latent period of 15 to 60 days that may be confused with those caused by "wobbles."

What are the signs of cerebrospinal nematodosis?

The signs of nematodosis may appear abruptly or gradually. There may be blindness, weakness (of the hindlegs, usually) or paralysis and incoordination. These signs may disappear gradually, or continue to degenerate. Most horses have some residual impairment of vision or nervous function.

What is the treatment of cerebrospinal nematodosis?

Diethylcarbamazine (caricide) has been very successful in preventing and systemically treating minor infections of *S. digitala.*

TETANUS

What is tetanus?

Tetanus is an infectious disease of the nervous system caused by the toxin of *Clostridium tetani.*

Soil is the natural habitat of the tetanus bacillus (rod-shaped bacterium) where most favorable conditions for growth occur in warm, heavily cultivated areas. With the exception of man, horses are the most susceptible of all animals to this disease. The incidence of mortality is 80 percent, yet of all bacterial diseases, tetanus can be most effectively dealt with by preventative measures.

How does *Cl. tetani* invade the horse?

The anaerobe, *Cl. tetani,* can be found in the feces of horses, in the intestinal tract, and the soil. It usually gains entry into tissues through a wound. The spore of *Cl. tetani* is nontoxic and requires favorable conditions for germination and eventual invasion into surrounding tissues. The absence of oxygen is the most important condition which is aided by a lowering of the blood supply to the area or the presence of foreign bodies in the wound.

Penetrating wounds of the foot are the most common sites of entry; however, any wound may be a site of infection. In newborn foals infection may result from contamination of the umbilical stump.

The route of spread of tetanus to the central nervous system is through peripheral nerve trunks or through lymph and blood. The toxin of *Cl. tetani* is quickly absorbed and bound to the nervous tissue. It destroys the orderly flow of nervous impulses from one nerve cell to another resulting in uncontrolled transmission of motor impulses. The effect of this destruction is general muscle spasticity and an exaggerated response to stimuli.

The veterinarian may encounter many cases of tetanus in which an obvious wound or site of inoculation cannot be found. This may be attributed to several points. For example, an insignificant wound that has healed over may still contain the spores necessary to generate tetanus. Also, the organism may have been carried by the blood into internal organs, or injury to intact mucous membranes, placenta, or fetal membranes may allow tetanus germ growth and production of toxin.

What are the effects of tetanus?

Tetanus may appear after an incubation period of anywhere from three days to a month or longer. The first signs will be those of stiffness around the head and neck region and a spastic closing of the third eyelid. Examination will reveal stiffness of the hind limb muscles and the muscles of the wound region. General stiffness is evident about 24 hours later with increased sensitivity of the skin and muscle spasms. The reflexes become exaggerated. Muscle spasms of the jaw make eating and drinking difficult; thus the term "lockjaw." The horse's ears become erect, the nostrils dilate and the tail becomes stiff and extended. The horse may be constipated and unable to urinate. Stiffness of the leg muscles causes the horse to assume a "sawhorse stance," making walking, turning and backing difficult. This stance may be confused with other diseases like strychnine poisoning and acute laminitis. Since all of these disorders are serious and progress toward serious

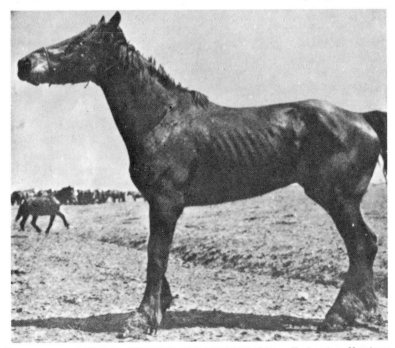

Photo courtesy of EQUINE MEDICINE AND SURGERY, Edition II, American Veterinary Publications, Inc., Wheaton, Ill.

Fig. 22-22. This photograph shows the characteristic position of a horse with tetanus.

damage to tissues or death, early examination and treatment by a veterinarian is important. Profuse sweating, rapid heart and respiration rates and congested mucous membranes are brought on by general spasms. The temperature will not rise much above normal except near the end of a fatal attack, when it may reach 110°F. Death usually occurs by asphyxiation due to spastic paralysis of respiratory muscles.

What is the treatment for tetanus?

The main considerations in the treatment of tetanus are the elimination of causative bacteria, the neutralizing and eventual elimination of the toxin and control of spasms.

Elimination of the bacteria may be attained through use of penicillin or tetracycline. This will make the environment less favorable for *Cl. tetani* growth and help control secondary infections. Tetanus antitoxin is routinely given but is essentially ineffective after the signs of tetanus appear.

Since there are no structural changes in the nervous system, supportive therapy can determine whether or not the disease will be fatal. This includes intravenous or stomach tube feeding when the horse cannot eat or drink; well-bedded, dark quarters big enough to protect against injury from convulsions; careful treatment of any skin lesions that are formed; and administration of enemas and catheterization in case of constipation and urine retention.

The control of spasms is of major importance. Mild cases may be treated by quiet handling and enclosure in a darkened stall, although sedation is almost always used. Further relief will involve treatment with tranquilizers and severe cases may require therapy with muscle relaxant drugs.

What are preventive measures for tetanus?

Immunity against tetanus can be provided through inoculation with toxoid or antitoxin. Toxoid is the injection of neutralized tetanus toxin to stimulate the horse to build its own antibodies. Antitoxin is the concentrated serum with tetanus toxin antibodies taken from another horse and administered as a preventive measure following wounds, surgery or foaling.

Active immunization is achieved through two injections of tetanus toxoid at four-to six-week intervals followed by annual booster injections. If a horse is immunized but wounded two or more months later, it might be wise for the veterinarian to administer another toxoid injection at that time. If not previously immunized, a wounded horse should receive the antitoxin which will give passive protection for up to two weeks.

Mares given toxoid in the last two months of pregnancy will pass on antibodies against tetanus to their foals through the colostrum. Active immunization may then begin for the foal at about six months of age. If the mare is not known to have received the toxoid during late pregnancy, the foal should be given antitoxin at birth.

BOTULISM

What is botulism?

Botulism is a form of food poisoning caused by the bacterium, *Clostridium botulinum,* commonly found in the soil and in the environment of decaying plant or animal matter. The toxins formed by these bacteria are the most potent poisons known.

What is the effect of *Cl. botulinum?*

Botulism toxins act on the peripheral nervous system by preventing transmission of nervous impulses, thus causing a flaccid (limp) paralysis. It is not certain if the toxins prevent the release of a transmission chemical at the nerve junctions or if they bind with it, preventing transmission of the nerve impulses.

What is the source of infection for *Cl. botulinum?*

On open range, animal carcasses may be chewed or eaten by animals with phosphorus or protein deficiencies. An animal carcass may have large numbers of *Cl. botulinum* in it. Horses may also be fed hay or grain contaminated by dead rats or other animals. Poorly maintained stock tanks are also a source of infection.

What are the signs of botulism?

Following access to the toxic material, the poisoned animal may develop signs within three to seven days. Signs include lack of fever and progressive difficulty in biting, chewing and swallowing food. The tongue and pharynx become completely paralyzed so that swallowing is impossible. Overall paralysis follows but death results from paralysis of the respiratory muscles. Some animals may die quickly without prior signs of illness; others may not eat or drink for a day or two. Botulism may be mistaken for equine encephalomyelitis or ragwort poisoning. In horses, botulism is rather rare, but it is usually fatal.

What is the treatment for horses with botulism?

General supportive treatment is indicated, but no antitoxin has been found that is economically practical. Purgatives to remove toxic material may be administered and animals may be fed by stomach tube. Treatment is usually attempted in cases where the signs develop slowly and some hope for recovery may be held.

Can botulism be prevented?

The best method of preventing botulism lies in careful inspection of hay and grain and proper storage conditions. Patrol of range areas to remove dead animals can prevent accidental poisoning of water sources. Vaccination is available from a veterinarian for the strain of *Cl. botulinum* found in the area's soil.

LISTERIOSIS

What is listeriosis?

Listeriosis is a rather recently discovered infectious disease caused by the bacterium *Listeria monocytogenes. L. monocytogenes* is highly infectious but it is not very pathogenic. That is, the bacterium has great power to set itself up in an animal, but does not have much power to initiate the disease it causes. Once predisposing factors such as poor nutrition reduce resistance within a host animal, *L. monocytogenes* becomes pathogenic. The disease takes the form of encephalitis, meningo-encephalitis, abortion or septicemia. Although it is not at all common in the horse, if the disease occurs, it is usually in the form of encephalitis (inflammation of the brain) in older animals, and abortion in the early months of pregnancy in mares. Foals contract listeriosis as septicemia, a widespread infection.

How is listeriosis spread?

There are thought to be several modes of transmission of *L. monocytogenes*. Oral transmission of bacteria is most likely, since the organisms are present in feces, urine, milk, aborted fetuses and uterine discharges. Anything contaminated by these materials can transmit infection.

What are the signs of listeriosis?

In the encephalitis form, loss of appetite, weakness and irritation when disturbed are early signs of listeriosis. The animal will gradually develop difficulties in feeding due to paralysis of the esophagus, and show other signs of neurological impairment. The severe cases press their heads against fixed objects, stand with heads held at awkward angles and circle in the direction of the deviation of the head one way only. Fever, an accelerated pulse and rate of breathing usually accompany the advancing infection. Facial paralysis on one side is the first visible sign of ongoing neurological destruction. Signs of septicemia are depression, weakness, fever, emaciation and diarrhea. Death will usually occur 3 to 10 days after appearance of the first signs of illness, and is due to respiratory failure.

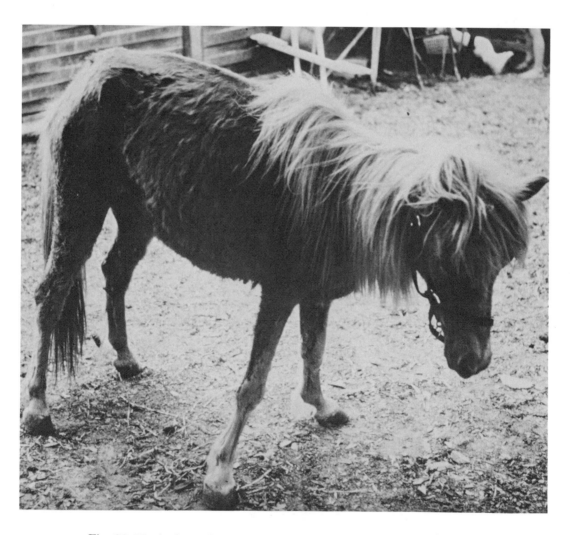

Fig. 22-23. Awkward stance common in encephalitis and listeriosis.

What is the treatment for listeriosis?

Penicillin, erythromycin, tetracyclines (chlortetracycline) and chloramphenicol have been proven effective in experimental infections, but are usually administered when the disease is too far advanced to be beneficial. Vaccines have not proven to be successful.

What are methods for controlling listeriosis?

Since it is rather uncommon and diagnosis can only be made by bacterial culture and identification, this will be the most difficult task. If a diseased animal is found and listeriosis is diagnosed, all possible methods of sterilization and sanitation should be observed. Special care should be taken by humans who handle infected fetuses or discharges, because the disease is almost always fatal in man.

SHIGELLOSIS

What is shigellosis?

An acute, highly fatal septicemia, shigellosis is also called navel ill, joint ill, polyarthritis and sleepy foal disease. These various names describe the manifestations of infection by the *Shigella equirulis (Actinobacillus equili)* organisms. It is estimated that shigella infections are the cause of about 25% of the foal deaths in this country.

What causes shigellosis?

The *Shigella equirulis* organism is found in the intestine and tissues of normal horses so deficiencies in colostrum, or failure to absorb immunoglobin through the intestinal wall during the first 24 hours after birth, are thought to be predisposing factors for the acute infection. The infection usually enters the body through the navel, although in utero infections are possible. Repeated infection of the foals from a single mare indicates the responsibility of the mother, in some cases.

What are the signs of shigellosis?

The signs of shigella are those of any acute infection: sudden fever, diarrhea, rapid respiration and lethargy are common. The "sleepy" appearance of a foal from birth and the loss of the suck reflex should be taken as a sign of grave illness. Walking in circles, bumping into walls, reversion to a comatose state after being aroused, and severe abdominal pain are all signs of a "sleepy foal." If signs are present at birth or soon after, death usually occurs within 24 hours. When signs begin several hours after birth and intermittent swelling begins in joints, foals usually die in two to seven days.

What treatment is recommended for shigellosis?

Following the veterinarian's diagnosis of the *S. equirulis* infection, streptomycin, chlortetracycline, chloramphenicol, and corticosteroids have all been proven useful against this type of infection. Penicillin is not effective against *S. equirulis*. Blood transfusions from the mare are helpful, and may provide antibodies that the foal lacks. Treatment, however, is usually not effective and the foal often dies.

What controls are available for shigellosis?

The best precautions are absolute cleanliness in the foaling stall and culling or treating mares who have delivered sleepy foals. Umbilical stumps dipped in iodine and dusted with appropriate fly powder are a good preventative of infection. Suspected mares should be watched carefully and their foals should be given the recommended antibiotics as soon as possible after foaling.

MENINGITIS

What is meningitis?

Meningitis is the term for an inflammation of the meninges (the three membranes that envelop the brain and spinal cord: the dura mater, the pia mater, and arachnoid). It is usually a complication of a pre-existing disease. This bacterial infection may affect the spinal cord (meningomyelitis) or spread to the brain (meningoencephalitis) or both.

What causes meningitis?

Streptococcus equi, the causative organism of strangles, is the bacteria which most often causes meningitis in horses. This bacteria travels through the bloodstream or within a continuous abscess. Horses have no primary meningitis like man. The infective organism is an extension of infection from elsewhere in the body.

Occasionally, meningitis is the result of penetrating wounds of the skull or an inflammation of the middle ear.

What are the effects of meningitis?

The part of the central nervous system that is affected and the severity of the inflammation determine the signs. These signs also change daily as the disease progresses. The spread of the inflammation in the nerve tissue initiates the signs of meningoencephalitis and meningomyelitis. The encephalitis type will show a consciousness level from hypersensitivity in the early stages, to dullness and eventual coma. The myelitis type will show a disturbance from incoordination to paralysis. Overall signs include incoordination, compulsive movements such as circling or pushing against objects, convulsions and generally high, but fluctuating, body temperature. The horse is in serious trouble if the pulse or respiration is varied from normal.

Streptococcus equi can cause brain abcesses of the cerebrum. This results in a drowsy horse who may demonstrate an unsteady gait, a tendency to fall, difficulty in rising, unnatural standing positions, and one or more joints collapsing repeatedly. Other possible signs are ear twitching, eye rolling, lockjaw, difficulty in swallowing, loss of appetite, urine retention and constipation.

Internally, meningitis causes local swelling and interference with blood supply to the brain and spinal cord. Defects of brain and spinal fluid drainage in acute and chronic meningitis result in increased intracranial pressure.

Is diagnosis difficult in cases of meningitis?

Parasites can cause lesions in the brain or spinal cord. The central nervous system can also be injured by fungal infections. These and any encephalitides will have signs similar to meningitis.

What is the treatment for meningitis?

Since the infection is bacterial, antibiotics or sulphonamides will be required by the veterinarian for treatment. Substantial doses will be given because of the incomplete passage of drugs into the cerebro-spinal fluid. Antibiotic treatment will continue for 7 to 10 days because of the frequency of relapses. If pain is severe, the veterinarian may administer analgesics (pain relievers). Intravenous electrolytes in large amounts may be helpful if the horse loses appetite. Sedation may be necessary in cases of convulsions, but the attendant must then tend the horse carefully to avoid pressure sores if it is down for any length of time.

In severe, acute cases the veterinarian may administer the antibiotics intrathecally (directly into the meningeal spaces). This is done on a last resort basis though, as inflammation of the arachnoid structures can result.

It is important to begin treatment early to save the horse from permanent nerve damage or death.

ENCEPHALOMYELITIS

What is equine encephalomyelitis?

Equine encephalomyelitis is a viral infectious disease which causes signs of deranged consciousness, motor irritation and paralysis due to degeneration of the central nervous system. There are several distinct viruses active in the United States; the primary ones are Eastern, Western and Venezuelan equine encephalomyelitis. These will be referred to as EEE, WEE and VEE respectively. A form of the disease, Japanese encephalitis, has a similar effect in the Far East, but is less virulent than WEE.

What causes equine encephalomyelitis?

All three viruses may be spread from animals to man, with mosquitoes as the primary means of transport. Wild birds, rodents and wild animals in all areas of the country are reservoirs of the disease, which enters the body of a mosquito when it feeds on infected creatures. While in the mosquito, the virus multiplies and becomes highly concentrated in the salivary glands. This infected mosquito then transmits the virus to a horse or a man, whichever is handy at its next feeding. In VEE, however, horses can spread the disease themselves since the virus is present in saliva and nasal discharges. The Eastern strain also produces a high level of infection in the blood which permits infection of non-carrier mosquitoes, increasing the epidemic aspect of the disease. Persons who handle animals with EEE should be aware that cuts or punctures of the skin readily admit equine encephalomyelitis virus. The various strains can only be diagnosed by laboratory examination of serum drawn by the veterinarian.

What are the signs of equine encephalomyelitis?

The signs of all three strains are highly similar. Following an incubation period of from one to three weeks, the first signs of infection are usually a marked depression and a high fever (104°-106°F) persisting for 24 to 48 hours. Nervous signs, hypersensitivity to sound and touch, periods of excitement, apparent blindness and wandering are followed by incoordination. Affected horses may show involuntary muscle movements such as yawning, tremor of the shoulder and facial muscles, erection of the penis and grinding of the teeth. Drowsiness and severe mental depression accompany the quiet period which follows nervous activity. The horse may eat and drink at this stage if food is placed in its mouth, or stand as if asleep with partially chewed food hanging from the mouth. This period is followed by a stage of paralysis in which the horse cannot hold its head up and rests it on some solid object. The lower lip will be pendulous with the tongue protruding. Weight may be balanced on the forelegs and the legs may be crossed. Some horses lean back on the halter when standing tied or press their head against a wall. Inability to swallow is usual, as is the suppression of urination and defecation. Complete paralysis marks the terminal stage, when the horse is down and unable to rise. Death usually occurs within two to four days from the first signs of infection. In VEE, however, horses may develop a severe, suddenly intense disease which affects the blood producing tissues and blood vessels. The same fever, depression and neurological signs follow, but there is a marked subnormal temperature just prior to death. Diarrhea also has been noted to occur in this form of the disease.

What is the treatment for equine encephalomyelitis?

Treatment is not usually effective because of the rapid course of the disease. In WEE, the disease progresses more slowly and there is a lower mortality rate (50%, as opposed to almost 90% in VEE and EEE) which permits more supportive treatment. Horses have been put in slings and blocks to keep them on their feet and fed by stomach tube in attempts to help them survive the virus attack. Protection from the flies and heat are recommended, as in maintenance of fluid and electrolyte balance. No specific therapeutic agent is known to influence the course of this disease.

How can equine encephalomyelitis be prevented?

Annual vaccination against the separate strains is required and can be provided by the veterinarian. Fly and mosquito control seems to be very effective, since most outbreaks do not extend to racetracks and stables where insect control is practiced.

BORNA DISEASE

What is Borna disease?

Borna disease is a meningoencephalitis (inflammation of the brain and the membranes that enclose it) caused by a virus similar to the one which causes Near Eastern Equine Encephalitis. It is rare in the United States, but it occurs frequently in Germany each spring.

What causes Borna disease?

The virus that causes Borna disease is found in food and water that has been in contact with soil that contains the Borna virus. Soil is contaminated by nasal discharges and urine from affected horses. Horses may be infected by ingesting the virus or by inhaling it. Some investigators feel that the virus is also spread by ticks, but not all veterinarians agree.

What are the signs of Borna disease?

The virus lives in the body for at least one month before visible signs are apparent. A moderate fever, paralysis of the pharynx, muscle tremors and a heightened sensitivity to noise or physical contact are all early signs of nervous system involvement. Most signs are hard to distinguish from those of WEE (see page 571).

What is the treatment for Borna disease?

Vaccinations are available and safe for prevention of Borna disease. In spite of treatment, 90% of horses affected with Borna disease die.

RABIES

What is rabies?

Rabies is a viral infection of the central nervous system that can affect any warm-blooded animal, although it is more common to certain animals. Its importance lies in the fact that it is highly fatal and transmissible to humans.

The rabies virus is carried in the salivary glands of the infected animal, then transmitted by a virus-contaminated bite wound. Farm animals are not widely affected by the disease. In the period 1960 thru 1970 there were 453 reported cases of rabies among horses in the U.S., or an average of 41 cases per year.

How is rabies transmitted?

The virus invades the central nervous system, the salivary glands, lacrimal glands, pancreas, kidney and adrenal tissues of the infected animal. Through the saliva the virus can be transmitted from animal to animal by means of a bite. Since the virus is carried via the nerve trunks to the spinal cord and eventually to the brain, the site of the bite determines the incubation period.

The rabies virus can be killed by most standard disinfectants. It will also die in dried saliva within a few hours. It is viable in the saliva of the animal for several days before the onset of clinical signs. The only known carriers that show no signs of infection are bats. Rarely is rabies transmitted other than by a bite.

Not all bites from rabid animals will result in an infection, because the virus is not always present in the saliva. Even if it is present, the virus may not invade the wound if the saliva is somehow wiped away. The spread of rabies also seems to be affected by seasonal movements of wild animals looking for food and mates. Seldom are domestic livestock the source of infection.

What are the signs of rabies?

In horses, the incubation period of rabies is from three weeks to three months. The earliest signs of the disease in horses are excitability and mania. The agitation is demonstrated by rolling. Their uncontrollable actions can become dangerous simply because of the horse's size and strength. These actions include biting, vicious striking, blind charges and sudden falling. The horse may bite and tear at any inflammation around the site of the original bite from the rabid animal.

Accompanying the violent and aggressive behavior are muscular spasms. In the final stages the horse will have difficulty in swallowing, paralysis of the hindlimbs and convulsions. Throughout the acute stage there is increased pulse and respiration rates. Postmortem lesions indicate encephalitis.

How is rabies diagnosed?

Since rabies occurs rarely in horses, the veterinarian must consider that the signs could be indicative of other encephalitides. A provisional diagnosis will be made on the basis of the incidence of rabies in that area and the history of any bites suffered by the horse. A horse suspected to have rabies should be isolated and kept alive as long as possible since the development of the disease is necessary for diagnosis. If the horse must be killed, the brain should be left intact for laboratory examination. The laboratory will be able to confirm a diagnosis of rabies.

Is there any treatment for rabies?

At present there is no antirabic serum. Immediate cleansing of the wound may prevent infection, but post-exposure vaccination is of little use since the animal generally dies before immunity has had time to develop. There is a series of rabies shots, especially known for their use in humans, which is effective after the bite but it must be implemented before the onset of signs. Usually, an animal is not known to have been infected early enough for this treatment.

Are there any preventative measures against rabies?

A number of commercially available vaccines can immunize horses against rabies. Again, these vaccines will not help an already infected horse. If rabies is known to have been diagnosed in a particular area, it is advisable that horses be vaccinated and that a program of observation and examination of the more common carrier animals such as dogs, cats, skunks, foxes and bats be initiated.

CHLORINATED HYDROCARBON POISONING

How does poisoning by chlorinated hydrocarbons occur?

Chlorinated hydrocarbons are commonly used in field or seed sprays and dusts against plant pests. This group of chemical compounds is also used in some insecticides applied as dusts, dips, and sprays to horses and other domestic animals. Poisoning can occur if horses are accidentally exposed to insecticides intended for plants. Toxic amounts of field spray may be inhaled or absorbed through the skin, or the horse may eat pasture plants or feed that have recently been treated with insecticides. Poisoning can result from improper mixing and high concentrations of insecticides intended for use on animals. Horses that are usually most susceptible to poisoning are those that are very young, very old, pregnant, weak or malnourished.

What are some of the chlorinated hydrocarbon compounds?

DDT is the most well known of the chlorinated hydrocarbons. It was used as an insecticide on animals and plants, but has been outlawed by the Federal Government in the United States because of environmental contamination. DDT poisoning in horses was rare if the chemical was properly used, and they were not harmed by sprays or dips containing 1.5% of DDT. DDT could be dangerous in very low concentrations if an aerial field spray of the compound contaminated feed or water. The toxicity level of chlordane for horses is similar to that of DDT. Chlordane is still legal for use around and under foundations, when used by licensed personnel for termite control.

BHC (Benzene hexachloride) and one of its products, lindane, were commonly used in dusts, dips and sprays for animals and some lindane products are still available. Sprays of 0.2 to 0.5% can safely be used on horses.

Methoxychlor is one of the safest and least toxic chlorinated hydrocarbon insecticides. It can be applied safely to horses and is practically nontoxic if used as recommended.

Aldrin, Dieldrin, Isodrin and Endrin were used as field or seed sprays and are too dangerous for use on animals. They are now legal for termite control by licensed personnel as in chlordane. Contamination of feed or water supplies can lead to accidental poisoning.

Toxaphene, which has a chemical structure similar to the chlorinated hydrocarbons, is an effective compound in dips or sprays against ticks and mites. It is actually classified as a chlorinated camphene. Like most insecticides used on horses, toxaphene is quite safe when properly used except for young foals, old or weakened horses.

What are the signs of chlorinated hydrocarbon poisoning?

The insecticides stimulate the central nervous system, affecting various nerves and associated muscles. Signs of poisoning appear within a few minutes to a few hours, and vary according to the type and amount of poison involved. In general, the affected horse first seems more alert. Then a twitching of the facial muscles, including those of the eyelids, begins, and this progresses until most of the muscles of the body are involved. Convulsions may then develop, lasting from a few seconds to several hours. Some horses may be seen standing in abnormal positions with their heads down between the forelegs or pressed against a wall or fence. Occasionally, an affected horse may become belligerent and go into a frenzy, attacking other animals or moving objects. Signs of poisoning often include a grinding of teeth and heavy salivation, and the horse does not eat. An affected horse may occasionally show no signs of excitability but instead be depressed and drowsy, eventually going into a coma.

Can this poisoning be treated?

Affected horses may die if the condition progresses, causing damage to the respiratory and circulatory systems. Some horses may recover suddenly and completely after nervous seizures lasting a few minutes or a few hours. When the poisoning is noticed in the early stages, veterinary treatment involves the use of sedatives if the horse shows signs of excitability or convulsions. If the horse is depressed and refuses to eat or drink, fluids should be given by injection or through a stomach tube. Calcium gluconate is an effective treatment for chlorinated hydrocarbon poisoning.

When poisoning has occurred by spraying, dipping or dusting, the horse should be washed with water and detergent to remove any residues of the compounds. If the horse has been poisoned by contaminated food or water, a non-oily purgative should be given to eliminate any chlorinated hydrocarbon compounds present in the stomach or feces.

STRYCHNINE POISONING

How does strychnine poisoning occur?

Accidental poisoning in the horse can occur from rodent and grasshopper poisons that contain strychnine. Strychnine is sometimes used in very small amounts in drenches as an appetite stimulant and in medications to improve nervous reflexes. Overdoses of these compounds occasionally result in signs of poisoning.

What are the signs of strychnine poisoning?

Signs of poisoning may appear within a few minutes but are usually delayed for at least an hour. At first there is a muscle stiffness and tremor, followed by convulsions which can be provoked by minor stimuli such as loud noises. During the convulsive seizures, which may last for three to four minutes, the legs are held rigidly and the eyeballs may protrude. The seizures progressively worsen, occurring after shorter intervals of relaxation, until death occurs from respiratory paralysis.

Can strychnine poisoning be treated?

A veterinarian should be called to control the horse's convulsions with sedatives. If the seizures can be controlled for a few hours, the strychnine will be excreted normally from the body within about ten hours after it has been absorbed, and the horse will soon recover.

ANTU POISONING

What is ANTU?

ANTU (alpha naphthyl thiourea) is a compound commonly used to kill rodents. Among horses that are accidentally poisoned by eating the rodent bait, older horses appear to be more susceptible than younger ones.

What are the signs of ANTU poisoning?

Weakness is the first sign of poisoning. The affected horse becomes progressively weaker, showing signs of incoordination and later being unable to rise after it has gone down. Fluid accumulates in the lungs, causing the horse to cough and have difficulty in breathing. The heart sounds are faint with a rapid, weak pulse rate. The body temperature drops below normal and there may be diarrhea in the late stages. The horse gradually goes into a coma and dies within a few hours after poisoning.

Can ANTU poisoning be treated?

There is no effective antidote for ANTU poisoning in a horse that has eaten a lethal dose (fourteen milligrams per pound). Half an ounce of ANTU can kill a 1,000 pound horse. Horses that accidentally eat smaller doses may recover, and after a few more mild poisonings of ANTU, they may develop a tolerance of over four times the original lethal dose.

FLUOROACETATE POISONING

What is fluoroacetate used for?

Sodium fluoroacetate is a chemical compound commonly used against rodent pests. It is highly toxic to all domestic animals and will cause signs of poisoning when the bait is accidentally eaten.

How does fluoroacetate affect the horse?

Fluoroacetate can affect the horse in two ways, involving an overstimulation of the central nervous system, which leads to convulsions, and a malfunction of the heart, which leads to heart failure. The cardiac effect is usually the major factor in deaths caused by the poison.

What are the signs of fluoroacetate poisoning?

Signs of poisoning appear within 15 minutes to several hours, depending on the dose. The first signs are nervousness and restlessness, with convulsions occasionally occurring. An affected horse is weak and cannot get up once it is down. The pulse becomes weak and rapid, often progressing to heart failure.

Is there any treatment for the poisoning?

There is no effective antidote for horses and a dose as small as one-fourth ounce can be fatal to a 1200 pound horse within a few hours. In mild cases of fluoroacetate poisoning, the veterinarian may attempt to empty the stomach by gastric lavage (washing out) to remove any remaining poison.

THALLIUM POISONING

How does thallium poisoning occur?

Thallium sulfate can be used against rodents, and poisoning can occur in horses that have eaten bait containing the compound. It has been shown to be toxic to most species of domestic animals, and appears to seriously affect mature animals more often than young ones.

What are the signs of thallium poisoning?

Thallium poisoning involves several body systems, causing various signs to be present. In affected horses, the major signs are nervous disorders, including tremors, depression, and paralysis. Usually there is difficulty in swallowing, leading to an apparent lack of appetite. The affected horse may salivate heavily and have severe diarrhea. Skin lesions may develop, causing a loss of hair from large areas of the body. Death can result from extensive damage to various internal organs, including the heart, lungs, liver and kidneys.

Can thallium poisoning be treated?

An antidote (dephenylthiocarbazone) that has been useful for other species of animals has not been very practical for horses. In cases of mild poisoning, symptomatic treatment of specific signs such as diarrhea and muscle tremors by a veterinarian can make it possible for a horse to recover.

PHENOL (CREOSOTE) POISONING

What is phenol poisoning?

Horses may chew wood that has been treated with creosote, causing burns in the mouth and digestive tract, or they may absorb phenol when they rub against creosote-treated wood. Small amounts of phenol exposure from chewing or rubbing against treated wood will not cause a problem.

What are the signs of phenol poisoning?

Acute phenol poisoning causes signs of nervous shock—depression, muscle tremors, coma, paralysis, convulsions and death. Chronic poisoning may cause paleness of the mucous membranes that have come in contact with the creosote, skin burns and progressive encephalitis (see page 571).

What is the treatment for phenol poisoning?

The veterinarian will probably suggest that the horse be removed from the creosote-treated area to prevent further exposure to phenol, and treat the horse for shock. Visible burns will be treated with a neutralizing solution, usually alcohol. After the burns are neutralized, they may be rinsed in saline solution and covered with wet packs moistened in the same saline solution. If the burns are extensive, antibiotics and fluids may be administered. Corticosteroids are also used to relieve stress in extensive or severe burns.

LEAD POISONING

What is lead poisoning?

Lead poisoning may be acute, caused by ingestion of a large quantity of lead at one time; or it may be chronic, caused by ingestion of small amounts over a long period of time. Stored in the tissues of the liver, cortex of the kidney and in the bones, lead may be gradually liberated from these tissues and excreted in the bile and urine if lead does not continue to be ingested.

What causes lead poisoning?

Lead poisoning has three main effects on the body: degenerative changes in nervous tissue, gastroenteritis, and peripheral nerve degeneration. Horses may ingest lead in flakes of paint, in plants that grow around old lead mines or processing plants and in plants that have been sprayed with lead compounds.

What are the signs of lead poisoning?

Although horses are not commonly affected by lead poisoning, they are very susceptible to lead when it is ingested. The most common sign is difficulty in breathing caused by paralysis of the laryngeal nerve. Paralysis of the pharynx may also occur, causing repeated cases of choke with regurgitation of fluid and feed through the nostrils. This frequently results in aspiration pneumonia, caused when the horse inhales food particles and fluid into his lungs. Some difficulty in moving may be noticed (stiffness), knuckling over at the fetlocks, and the hair coat may be harsh and dry. Occasionally, acute poisoning may cause signs of a lack of appetite, severe nervous depression, partial paralysis which increases to complete paralysis of the limbs, recumbency and abdominal pain. In some cases, convulsions may occur. Death may be due to pneumonia or due to paralysis of the muscles that control breathing.

What is the treatment for this type of poisoning?

Calcium versenate is sometimes given intravenously, but the veterinarian may administer magnesium sulfate in an attempt to remove the lead from the digestive tract. Although some horses may recover to a slight degree, severe lead poisoning does not usually respond to treatment.

Can lead poisoning be prevented?

Yes. Lead poisoning is fairly easy to prevent. Old barns and fences should be checked for the type of paint they carry. Old paints contained considerable amounts of lead and are the major source of lead poisoning in horses. Use of lead-free aluminum paints will prevent most cases of lead poisoning.

GRASS TETANY, LACTATION TETANY

What are grass tetany and lacation tetany?

Grass tetany and lactation tetany are closely related disorders of horses fed solely on rich pasture. Neither has been a serious problem since the days of the draft horse.

What causes grass tetany and lactation tetany?

Grass tetany occurs rarely in horses, and its cause is not well understood. It is known that after exclusively grazing on lush pasture, affected horses show hypomagnesemia (low magnesium in the blood) often accompanied by hypocalcemia (low calcium in the blood).

Lactation tetany is brought on by the same diet that causes grass tetany, but hypocalcemia is more often the cause. It is so named because it occurs most often to mares that are nursing, or that have recently weaned a foal. This is probably because the vital calcium is taken up in the production of milk.

Both disorders are probably related to the high crude protein content of the pasture. Calcium and magnesium are used in the digestive process to properly digest the protein, and as a result, only small amounts of them are available for maintaining other bodily functions.

What are the signs of grass tetany and lactation tetany?

Both afflictions bring on lack of coordination, muscle spasms and tremors, sweating, hard breathing and a thumping sound inside the chest. This thumping may be a violent contraction of the diaphragm.

Body temperature and appetite are not usually affected, but the horse cannot eat, drink, defecate or urinate during an attack. As the illness progresses, these symptoms become more intense. Within 24 hours the animal usually goes down, and death comes in about 48 hours.

Handling the horse, particularly when it is to be transported, increases the sickness by causing excitement. For this reason both conditions are sometimes called transit tetany, railroad disease or railroad sickness. Other names include staggers, grass staggers, wheat poisoning and eclampsia.

How are grass tetany and lactation tetany treated?

If the signs of these disorders are present, a veterinarian should be consulted immediately. Both are treated by the intravenous injection of calcium solution, which produces spontaneous recovery. Magnesium may also be injected, but is not used as often. If the case is diagnosed and treated properly, the prognosis is good.

ENCEPHALOMALACIA
(MOLDY CORN POISONING)

What is encephalomalacia?

Encephalomalacia is commonly called moldy corn poisoning. It results in liquefaction and extensive bilateral softening of the white portion of the brain.

What causes encephalomalacia?

The organism has not yet been isolated, but it is thought to be due to a toxin from the mold found on ear or loose corn. How the toxin travels to the brain is not sufficiently understood.

What are the signs of encephalomalacia?

Signs of toxicosis include muscle tremors and weakness, followed by loss of the ability to swallow and staggering. Affected horses may press their head against a wall or fence or walk in circles. Eventually, the animal becomes extremely depressed and dies. Death will usually occur within 48 to 72 hours after the appearance of signs, and may be preceded by jaundice (yellowing of the mucous membranes).

What is the treatment for encephalomalacia?

There is no effective treatment. Antibiotics seem to be of no use, and the causative toxin cannot be isolated to develop an antitoxin.

How can encephalomalacia be prevented?

Prevention is rather simple. Careful inspection of ear and loose corn when it is purchased and proper dry storage will prevent development of the contaminating mold. Moldy corn should never be fed, even in small amounts.

OLEANDER POISONING

What is oleander poisoning?

Oleander poisoning is rare in horses because they will not normally eat *Nerium oleander,* which is frequently grown as an ornamental shrub in California and the Southwest. Poisoning usually occurs when clippings are fed to horses where they are used to eating hay. The poison of oleander is similar to digitalis and its effects upon the horse are characteristically those of an abnormal or irregular heartbeat.

What are the signs of oleander poisoning?

As few as 30 leaves have been known to produce signs of poisoning and death in horses. The signs include profuse diarrhea and abnormal heartbeat. The mucous membranes turn slightly blue and the extremities are cold. Horses usually go down and struggle, but they may be able to rise again. Death usually occurs within 12 hours of ingestion of oleander, but the poison may take up to 24 hours to cause death.

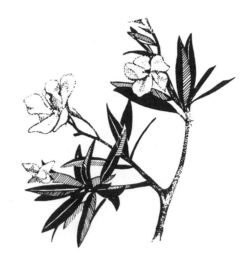

Fig. 22-24. Drawing of oleander. All varieties are poisonous.

What treatment is used for oleander poisoning?

The veterinarian may try atropine to treat affected horses, but no particular treatment has proved effective in oleander poisoning.

NICOTINE POISONING

How does nicotine poisoning in horses occur?

Nicotine poisoning in horses usually occurs when wild tobacco plants are eaten. Nicotine sulfate, derived from plants containing nicotine, has been used as an insecticide spray or dip and a wormer in other species of farm animals. Overdosing or improper use on horses could produce signs of nicotine poisoning.

What are the signs of nicotine poisoning?

Nicotine poisoning causes signs of a disorder of the nervous sytem including tremors, incoordination and then paralysis. The pulse and respiration become weaker and slower and death usually results from respiratory failure.

Can nicotine poisoning be treated?

There is no effective treatment for horses poisoned by the wild tobacco plant, and death may occur within a few hours after the plant is eaten. Horses affected with mild cases of poisoning caused by tobacco plants or improper use of copper sulfate may recover spontaneously. Treatment of copper sulfate poisoning may involve removal of the compound from the skin or stomach, artificial respiration and veterinary treatment for cardiac arrest and shock.

LOCOWEED POISONING

What is locoweed poisoning?

Locoweed poison acts upon the nervous system of the horse, causing signs that suggest that the horse is "loco" (Spanish for crazy). Some of the species of the leguminous plant *Astragalus,* which are common in the west, are believed to be the cause of this disorder. Although some *Astragalus* are also causes of selenium poisoning (see Selenium Poisoning, page 534), the substance that causes locoweed poisoning is thought to be an alkaloid.

What are the signs of locoweed poisoning?

Horses are very susceptible to this type of poisoning, and only need to eat about 30% of their body weight in *Astragalus* over a period of about a month in order to develop signs of poisoning. Horses that are affected stagger, wander aimlessly, act depressed and can become convulsive and fall to the ground. Other nervous signs include head pressing and running into objects. It is thought that some of the signs are due to affected vision, but that has not really been proven.

Can locoweed poisoning be treated?

No treatment is known for this type of poisoning.

BRACKEN POISONING

When is bracken poisoning most likely to occur?

Poisoning by bracken fern, or brake fern, usually occurs in the fall, when bracken is one of the few pasture plants that is still green. Horses will normally avoid the plant if other forage is available since it is fairly unpalatable. Poisoning can occur in horses fed meadow hay that contains bracken plants. The plant poison has a cumulative effect, and the fern must be eaten for at least 30 to 60 days before the horse shows signs of poisoning. Signs can appear two to six weeks after the horse has been moved from a pasture containing the fern.

What are the signs of bracken poisoning?

An affected horse first shows signs of weight loss and unsteadiness when walking. The horse sways from side to side, and becomes progressively more uncoordinated. It often stands with legs placed wide apart and its back arched. Muscle tremors develop and the horse may fall and be unable to get up. When the condition is allowed to progress to the final stages, the heart rate is usually rapid and there are severe muscle spasms.

How does the poison cause these signs?

Bracken poisoning has been found to cause a deficiency of thiamine (vitamin B1) in the horse. For this reason, the toxic substance in the plant is thought to be a thiaminase, an enzyme which inactivates thiamine. Bracken poisoning and other types of thiamine deficiency cause disturbances of the central nervous system, but the relationship between a lack of the vitamin and the nervous signs which develop is still unclear. Similar signs of poisoning, apparently caused by a thiaminase, can be seen in horses fed meadow hay that contains large amounts of another plant, Equisetum, commonly called horsetail or scouring rush.

How is bracken poisoning treated?

Affected horses respond to injections of solution of thiamine. Treatment is continued for 7 to 14 days until the horse has completely recovered. If the condition is left untreated, it can eventually end in death of the horse.

Can bracken poisoning be prevented?

Poisoning can be prevented by an alternative grazing plan, in which horses are allowed on a pasture containing bracken fern for three weeks and then are removed for three weeks. The plant poison cannot accumulate in the body in this short period of time and will cause no damage even if the fern is eaten in large amounts. This alternative grazing system also allows the fern growth to be controlled by close grazing or trampling, and the amount of bracken in the pasture can gradually be brought below dangerous levels. Burning pastures does not control bracken fern and there are no effective weed killers against the plant.

NIGROPALLIDAL ENCEPHALOMALACIA (CHEWING DISEASE)

What is chewing disease?

Chewing disease is a specific nervous disease of horses characterized by involuntary chewing movements and is known as nigropallidal encephalomalacia. Encephalomalacia is a softening of the brain, which in this particular disease is due to necrotic (dead) tissue in certain areas of the brain, the substantia nigra and the globus pallidus.

What causes the disease?

The disease, also called yellow star thistle poisoning, occurs when a horse eats large amounts of yellow star thistle in the late summer or fall when pastures are dry. The plant is fairly unpalatable, but the horse may eat it when there is no other

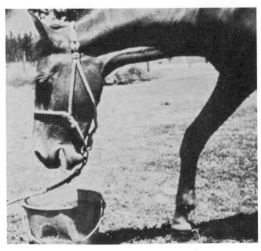

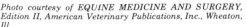
Photo courtesy of EQUINE MEDICINE AND SURGERY, Edition II, American Veterinary Publications, Inc., Wheaton, Ill.

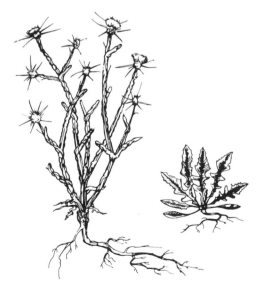

Fig. 22-25. Photograph of horse with yellow star thistle poisoning. Notice the hypertonicity of the facial muscles.

Fig. 22-26. Drawing of yellow star thistle, showing the plant in its stages of development.

forage available, and might eventually even acquire a taste for it. Signs of poisoning will appear after the horse has been eating the plant for one to three months and has consumed several hundred pounds of it.

Yellow star thistle is an annual plant, considered a noxious weed, found over much of the United States. It is most prolific in areas of California and other western states. The toxic substance of the plant has not yet been isolated, but feeding yellow star thistle to horses has been found to cause damage to the specific tissues of the brain already mentioned.

What are the signs of chewing disease?

The muscles of the face and lips are taut and rigid, giving the affected horse a "wooden" expression. The horse has difficulty in picking up food and in swallowing, due to paralysis of the muscles involved. The horse may push its head into water but be unable to drink. The mouth is held half open and the tongue is flicked in and out. The horse often appears to be chewing when there is no feed in the mouth. When feed is present in the mouth, the horse is unable to push the food back into the area of the molar teeth. Some affected horses show other signs of nervous disorders such as incoordination and slight convulsions. Horses with yellow star thistle poisoning lose weight and condition, since they are unable to eat or drink, and will die of starvation or thirst if not helped.

Is there a treatment for this poisoning?

The horse can be temporarily assisted in eating and drinking but there is no effective treatment. Recovery of the horse's normal functions is impossible because the damage to vital areas of the brain is irreversible.

Can yellow star thistle poisoning be prevented?

Horses should either be removed from dry pastures containing yellow star thistle or they should be provided with extra hay or supplemental forage to prevent them from having to eat the poisonous plant.

THE REPRODUCTIVE SYSTEM

FEMALE REPRODUCTIVE SYSTEM

ANATOMY

Which organs make up the reproductive system of the mare?

The mare's reproductive system is comprised of two ovaries, two oviducts (also called Fallopian tubes), a uterus, a vagina and a vulva. The ovaries are called primary sex organs, while the oviducts, uterus, vagina and vulva are termed secondary sex organs.

What are the ovaries?

The ovaries are essential organs of reproduction in the female and have two main functions. The ovary produces an ovum (the "egg") and also produces hormones necessary for normal reproductive functioning. Estrogen and progesterone are two hormones secreted by the ovary and absorbed directly into the bloodstream.

The ovaries are paired glands located one below and behind each kidney. They are suspended from the "roof" of the abdominal cavity in a fold of peritoneum along with the oviducts, uterus and vagina. This fold of peritoneum is called the broad ligament. The ovaries are structured in two layers, or made of two different types of tissue, the cortex (cortical tissue) and the medulla (medullary tissue).

What is the structure of the ovaries?

The medulla consists of loose connective tissue containing the blood vessels and nerves which supply the cortex. The cortex is made up of dense connective tissue and contains oocytes (immature egg cells) which have migrated from the surface of the ovary. A capsule called the tunica albuginea encloses the cortex and medulla of the ovary. The outer surface of the tunica albuginea is covered with a very thin layer of cells called the germinal epithelium.

What is the size and shape of the ovaries?

Normally, the ovaries of the mare are variable in size from about one and a half by three inches in a young mare to about one by one and a half inches in an old mare.

Most domestic animals have ovaries which are oval-shaped, but the ovaries of the mare are bean-shaped. This bean-shape is due to a depressed area called the ovulation fossa on the border of each ovary. In ovulation, the ovum almost always

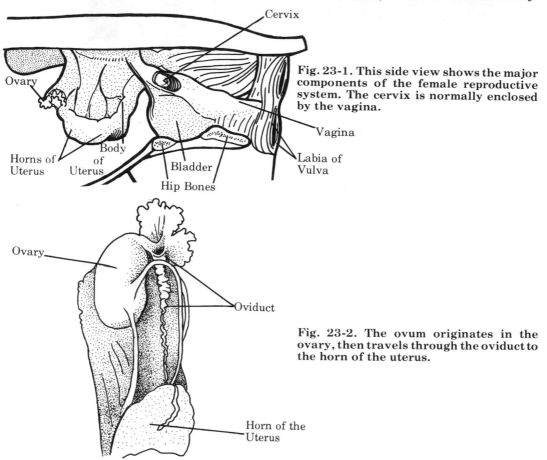

Fig. 23-1. This side view shows the major components of the female reproductive system. The cervix is normally enclosed by the vagina.

Fig. 23-2. The ovum originates in the ovary, then travels through the oviduct to the horn of the uterus.

passes from the ovary at the ovulation fossa. Medullary tissue is the inner layer of the ovary in other species but in the mare it extends to the surface over nearly the entire ovary. Cortical tissue is found only in the region of the ovulation fossa of the ovary of the mare.

How does the ovary produce ova?

Germinal cells migrate down from the germinal epithelium into the cortex of the ovary. Here the germinal cells clump together, forming primary follicles. In each primary follicle there is one large cell called an oocyte which will develop into an ovum. The ovum and other cells of a follicle increase in size, forming a fluid-filled sac within the follicular cells. At this stage the maturing follicle is referred to as a Graafian follicle. As the Graafian follicle grows in size, it pushes toward the surface of the ovary, eventually appearing like a blister on the surface of the ovary.

The follicle softens and then ruptures when it is mature, expelling the ovum. This process is called ovulation. In the mare, during each heat period, one follicle usually develops sooner than the others. Because of this, when the follicle ruptures only one ovum will be released, hence the mare normally gives birth to a single offspring.

The cells lining the cavity left on the ovary by the rupture of the ovum proliferate, enlarge and undergo fatty changes to become lutein cells forming a corpus luteum. The chief function of the corpus luteum is to secrete a hormone causing the cells lining the uterus to prepare for implantation and later, maintain pregnancy. If the ovum is not fertilized, the corpus luteum decreases in size until it leaves a small scar (corpus albicans) on the surface of the ovary. Then the entire cycle of follicle development and rupture begins again.

What are the oviducts?

These are small, paired tubes extending from each ovary to the uterus. The function of an oviduct (or Fallopian tube) is to carry ova from the ovaries to the uterus.

There are three parts of an oviduct. The infundibulum is the funnel-shaped end of the oviduct near the ovary which aids in guiding ova into the opening of the oviduct. This end of the oviduct is not completely attached to the ovary but is arranged like a tube and funnel, hooked on only one side and hung beneath the ovulation fossa. The ampulla is the tube-shaped portion of the oviduct, while the isthmus is the junction between the oviduct and the uterus.

The lining of an oviduct is highly folded and ciliated (covered with tiny, hair-like projections) for almost its entire length. The portion of lining that is not ciliated is made up of secretory cells. These secretory cells produce a large amount of fluid during heat. The fluid aids movement of the ovum and provides a suitable medium in which the ovum can exist and be fertilized by a sperm cell.

Both circular and longitudinal layers of muscles make up the wall of the oviduct. These muscular layers, action of the cilia and secretions of the lining combine to transport ova through the length of the oviduct. It usually takes about eight days for an ovum to travel through the oviduct.

How soon must an ovum be fertilized after ovulation?

An ovum is viable and fertilizable for only a matter of several hours after ovulation, so fertilization must take place in the oviduct.

What is the uterus?

The uterus is the organ of the female reproductive system responsible for accommodating the developing fetus.

The body, horns (cornua) and cervix (neck) are the three parts of the uterus. In the mare, the body of the uterus is well developed and the horns are relatively small, compared to other domestic animals. In a nonpregnant mare, the body of the uterus is usually about ten inches long and the horns are generally seven to eight inches long, relatively straight and blunted on the ends. The cervix is two to three inches thick and projects into the vagina one to two inches.

Three layers make up the wall of the uterus. An inner mucous membrane lining (endometrium), an intermediate layer of smooth muscle (myometrium) and an outer serous layer (peritoneum) form the uterine wall.

What is the structure and function of these three layers of the uterus?

The endometrium, or mucous membrane layer, has glands scattered throughout the folded lining. The thickness of this layer varies depending upon hormonal changes in the body. The endometrium thickens prior to estrus as a part of the "building up" process preparing for pregnancy.

The two muscular layers making up the myometrium are separated from each other by blood vessels and connective tissue. The inner layer of smooth muscle is circular and the outer smooth muscle layer is longitudinal, as in the oviduct.

The outermost layer of the uterus, the peritoneum, is a part of the membrane which lines the abdominal and pelvic cavities and encloses all of the organs in the region.

What is the function of the cervix or "neck" of the uterus?

The cervix is a strong, smooth sphincter (ring-like) muscle. The cervix functions like a valve in the reproductive tract. Most of the time it remains tightly closed, but it relaxes during heat and birth. During pregnancy the cervix secretes mucus, which forms a plug to seal off the uterus from the vaginal canal. This mucous plug helps guard against infection.

What are the vagina and vulva?

The vagina is the part of the birth canal between the uterus and the vulva. It is lined with mucous membrane and the walls are constructed of an inner, circular layer of smooth muscle and an outer, longitudinal layer of smooth muscle. The vagina forms a sheath for acceptance of the penis during copulation.

The vulva extends from the vagina to the exterior, forming the external opening of the reproductive system. Labia is the term for the external lips of the vulva.

Together the vagina and the vulva form a passageway for sperm at the time of breeding and for the new foal at the time of birth.

What is the reproductive cycle of the mare?

The estrous cycle is the interval between the beginning of one estrus (heat period) and the beginning of the next estrus. Mares are seasonally polyestrous; they cycle regularly during the breeding season of the year. This is controlled by hormones secreted by the ovary and anterior pituitary gland. Through the year most mares seem to go through three phases: a dormant stage, an adjustment stage, and a true breeding stage. These phases are related to the seasons of the year. Ambient temperature, length of daylight, and the type of feed or pasture are environmental factors that apparently control this "annual cycle."

The dormant phase is generally 2 to 3 months long and encompasses anywhere from late summer to early winter. The adjustment phase may last anywhere from 2 weeks to 3 months and occurs during late winter and early spring. This is followed by the "true breeding season" that runs from midspring through midsummer.

The estrous cycle can be divided into different phases. Proestrus, estrus and metestrus are three of these phases. Metestrus is followed by diestrus, anestrus or pregnancy. Proestrus is also called the building up phase. During this period a follicle is maturing on the ovary, under the influence of FSH (Follicle Stimulating Hormone), and increased growth is taking place in the rest of the reproductive system, under the influence of estrogen, preparing for estrus and pregnancy.

Estrus follows proestrus and usually lasts about five days. During this phase a mare will accept the stallion. Frequent urination and vaginal secretions are external signs of estrus. The cervix and the external genitalia (vulva) are relaxed in anticipation of ovulation. Ovulation occurs near the end of estrus and is followed by metestrus. During estrus the level of FSH decreases while the level of LH (Luteinizing Hormone) increases. LH stimulates corpus luteum formation.

Metestrus is also called the post-ovulatory phase. During this phase the corpus luteum functions, increasing the level of progesterone. Progesterone prevents further development of follicles on the ovary and subsequent estrous cycles.

Diestrus, anestrus or pregnancy may follow metestrus. If the ovum released at ovulation is fertilized, pregnancy follows; if it is not fertilized, diestrus follows. This is a short period between estrous cycles, during which the corpus luteum regresses in preparation for another cycle. Anestrus is the long period between breeding seasons when the ovaries are inactive.

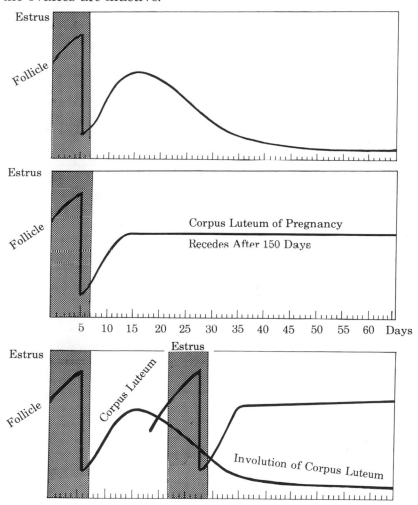

Fig. 23-3. The top graph in this chart shows the normal estrus cycle of a mare when no conception takes place. The second graph shows estrus with conception, and the third shows conception taking place during the normal cycle of estrus.

When does a mare begin to have estrous cycles?

Puberty refers to the time a mare becomes sexually mature, or begins producing ova. This usually occurs between ten and twenty-four months of age, with eighteen months being average.

HEAT DETECTION

Can mares be bred throughout the year?

A few mares will come in heat (estrus) at regular intervals throughout the year and may be bred successfully during any heat period. Most mares, however, can only be bred during a specific breeding season, and will often fail to conceive if breeding is attempted at other times of the year.

When is the breeding season?

The breeding season is generally considered to extend from midspring through midsummer. During this time, the mare usually has heat periods at relatively regular intervals, and ovulates (releases an egg from the ovary) every three to four weeks. Ovulation usually occurs toward the end of each heat period.

How long is each heat period?

The average length of each heat period is about five days, during which time the mare is receptive to a stallion. At the beginning of the breeding season, the heat periods normally last from seven days to two weeks. In the middle of the season, estrus may last five to seven days, decreasing to one to three days toward the end of the season in July and August.

Why do most mares come in heat only during the spring and summer of breeding season?

The estrous cycle of the mare is greatly influenced by seasonal changes, including the environmental temperature, the number of hours of daylight, and the type of feed or pasture present during the year. From the late summer through early winter, the mare is usually in a dormant phase of the estrous cycle. The ovaries are not producing ova (eggs) and there are no signs of estrus. In the late winter and early spring, the mare goes through a period of adjustment which may last from a couple of weeks to three months. At this time, the estrous cycle is irregular and there may be unusually long heat periods, but true, complete estrus with ovulation usually does not begin until later in the spring. The mare will then show regular signs of estrus and will be ready for breeding.

What are the signs that a mare is in estrus and is ready to be bred?

A mare in estrus will often show a change in behavior, become more docile and more responsive to handling. There may be signs of frequent urination, a raised tail, and a "winking" of the vulva as the lips of the vulva contract and relax. The most efficient way of detecting estrus in a mare is to bring her together with a stallion or a teaser to act as a stallion. Her reaction will determine whether or not she is in estrus and receptive to the stallion.

How does a mare in estrus react to teasing?

When a mare in estrus is teased, she will usually lean towards the teaser and stand in a breeding position, with hindlegs spread apart and tail raised. The lips of the vulva contract and relax, and the clitoris is exposed. The mare usually urinates at the sight or sound of the stallion or teaser. When the mare shows these signs, she will normally allow herself to be mounted and bred by the stallion.

How does a mare react to teasing if she is not in estrus?

A mare that is not in estrus will resist the male by kicking or biting. The male can be injured by the mare unless there is a teasing board or other obstacle separating them. The mare will usually whip her tail back and forth and resent being handled when the teaser is present.

Can the mare be examined for signs of estrus?

During the breeding season a mare can be examined by a veterinarian by rectal palpation or visual examination of the cervix. In rectal palpation, the ovaries are felt through the rectal wall. If the mare is in heat, a follicle containing the egg can usually be felt as a small blister on the surface of an ovary. Toward the end of estrus, the follicle ruptures, releasing the egg into the oviduct which connects the ovary to the horn of the uterus. Changes in the vagina and cervix may be evident when a speculum is inserted into the vagina to expose the cervix. When the mare is in estrus, the cervix is red and swollen and secretes large amounts of clear, thin fluid. The cervix of a mare that is not in estrus is pale and tight, with thicker secretions. The vagina and vulva of a mare in estrus will also become red, soft and moist. Because these changes may not be observed in all mares in estrus, teasing normally is the method of choice for detecting heat. In mares who show no visible signs of heat, teasing is especially useful.

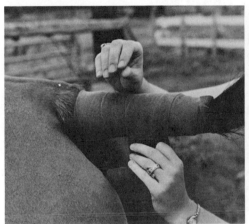 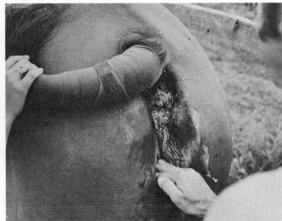

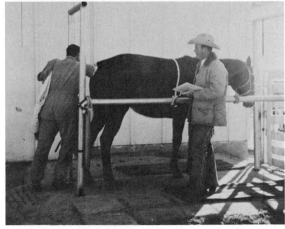

Fig. 23-4. To avoid the dangers of infection and internal damage, rectal palpation must be done properly. The tail should be wrapped, the external genitalia cleaned and lubricated, and the actual palpation performed by an experienced person.

Photo of palpation, courtesy of W. L. Anderson, D.V.M.

What is "foal heat"?

Almost all mares will show signs of heat between 2 and 18 days after foaling. This period of heat is referred to as "foal heat," and usually occurs 9 to 11 days after foaling. "Foal heat" is also commonly referred to as "nine-day heat."

Can mares be bred during "foal heat"?

In instances where foaling early in the year is desirable, mares are often bred during the foal heat to try to accomplish this. The mare should be bred only if she is in good condition after foaling, and even then the breeding may not be successful, though conception rates are fairly good at foal heat if everything is in order. A mare usually needs a longer time than the nine days before the foal heat for her reproductive tract to fully recover for another breeding. The foal heat appears to be a natural method of cleansing the uterus and vagina. It aids in the removal of possible sources of infection such as straw, and of blood and remnants of fetal membranes that may not have been expelled by the contractions of the uterus during foaling. If there weren't so much pressure for "early" foals, it would probably be well to allow mares to recover during the foal heat and be bred during the following heat period.

PREGNANCY TESTING

How is pregnancy in the mare determined?

Pregnancy in the mare can be diagnosed in several ways, but no one method is completely reliable. An accurate method is manual examination, accomplished by inserting the arm into the mare's rectum and palpating the reproductive tract through the rectal wall. Laboratory tests involving blood or urine samples of the mare are commonly used in later stages of pregnancy. Visual examination of the vagina and cervix is sometimes helpful in determining whether or not a mare is pregnant. A mare's change of disposition and reaction to teasing, to observe whether or not she has returned to heat, are sometimes included in a pregnancy diagnosis.

Is an absence of heat a method of determining pregnancy?

The absence of estrus in a mare is a poor indication of pregnancy because it is only 50-70% accurate. Most mares will not return to heat if they are pregnant, but occasionally a pregnant mare will show signs of heat and may even accept service from a stallion after she has conceived. Other mares may not conceive after breeding but still fail to return to estrus, in which case a lack of estrus would not be a sign of pregnancy. Estrous cycles in mares are often irregular and are not reliable guidelines for determining pregnancy.

How soon after breeding can pregnancy be determined?

A veterinarian who regularly uses rectal palpation can diagnose pregnancy as early as 19 days after the last service. The results may not be accurate at this early stage, partially because there can be a delay of up to five days from mating to ovulation and fertilization. Most mares are therefore checked between 25 to 42 days, and the exact stage of pregnancy can usually best be determined most easily between 25 and 30 days. Mares checked and found pregnant at 40 days should be palpated again at 60 days. This is usually recommended since in about ten percent of pregnant mares, the fetus dies between 40 and 60 days. Rectal palpation can be fairly accurate up to about 65 days, but between 70 days and 5 months the precise stage of pregnancy usually cannot be determined.

When is an examination of the cervix and vagina useful?

When rectal palpation is inconclusive, the veterinarian may find that visual examination of the cervix and vagina is helpful in diagnosing pregnancy between

18 and 30 days. A sterilized speculum is used to spread the vagina and provide a clear view of the cervix. The cervix in the pregnant mare is tight, causing the cervical opening to become smaller. The opening is filled with a mucus plug, which effectively seals off the uterus and protects it from infection through the vagina. About 20 days after breeding, the cervical mucus secretions are thick and waxy, forming a protective coating over the cervix. The cervix and the surrounding area of the vagina are pale, and the mucus secretions of the vagina are thicker. If further evidence is necessary, a microscopic examination of a vaginal smear can be useful in confirming a pregnancy.

When are laboratory tests used for pregnancy diagnosis?

Laboratory tests involving samples of blood and urine are not very popular because they cannot be used in early stages of pregnancy; rectal palpation can be used at least 20 days earlier than biological laboratory tests. Blood samples are not accurate diagnostic tests until the 40th day of pregnancy, since the gonadotropic hormones, which stimulate the ovaries, do not appear in the blood until this time. They are present in the blood serum from the 40th to the 120th day of pregnancy. The Friedman test with pregnant mare serum between the 45th and 100th day of pregnancy is 99% accurate. A urine test to detect the presence of estrone (an estrogen) is about 90% accurate any time after the 120th day of pregnancy.

How are these laboratory tests performed?

Several laboratory tests for determining pregnancy are available. The Friedman test is a common test which involves an injection of the mare's blood serum into a mature female rabbit. If the mare is pregnant, gonadotropic hormones will be present in the serum and cause one of the rabbit's ovaries to develop a follicle (the egg and its surrounding cells). This structure can be seen when the ovaries are examined after the rabbit has been destroyed.

Another blood test for determining pregnancy involves mixing the blood serum of the mare with rabbit serum containing anti-gonadotropin antibodies. If the mare is pregnant, the gonadotropin in the serum will neutralize the rabbit's antibodies and there will be no reaction when sheep blood sensitized to the hormone is added to the mixture. If the mare is open, the rabbit serum is not affected by the mare's serum and will cause the sheep blood to coagulate.

Estrone is present in the pregnant mare's urine after the 120th day of pregnancy. A chemical method to detect the presence of this hormone involves mixing urine with hydrochloric acid, benzene and sulfuric acid. A specific color change will be observed if estrone is present in the urine. Urine or blood tests are useful in confirming a diagnosis of pregnancy if rectal and clinical examination is inconclusive.

Can a rectal examination be performed only by a veterinarian?

A rectal examination should be carried out only by a veterinarian who is experienced in palpating mares. Careless palpation can cause the rectal wall to be punctured, resulting in peritonitis which can easily lead to death of the mare. There is also a good possibility of damage to the fetus which could lead to abortion. The fetus does not become firmly attached to the wall of the body of the uterus (implantation) until 49 to 70 days after conception. Rough handling of the reproductive tract before this time, especially before 35 days, could cause the embryo to be dislodged and reabsorbed or aborted.

Can pregnancies be misdiagnosed by rectal palpation?

Rectal palpation by an inexperienced examiner will probably result in misdiagnosis. A filled urinary bladder or a portion of the large intestine, felt through the rectal wall, may occasionally be mistaken for the uterus, or a fecal ball in a piece of intestine can accidentally be interpreted as an ovary. Pyometra, a condition of pus in the uterus resulting from an infection, may resemble a pregnant uterus and occasionally be misdiagnosed as a pregnancy. Palpation can be difficult in an older mare who has had several foals, since the uterus may contain much scar tissue and have developed thick walls. An enlargement of the uterine horn, indicating a developing embryo, may be difficult to detect and the fetus may not be felt until the 45th or 50th day. Pregnancy in a maiden mare is usually easier to diagnose, since the uterus is small, has good tone, and changes in the body and horns of the uterus can more easily be felt by the experienced equine practitioner.

What changes can be felt in the uterus during pregnancy?

The equine practitioner can detect changes in size, tone, contractility to stimulation by palpation, and texture. He has trained himself to be able to interpret these signs as to what they mean in terms of diagnosis of pregnancy and disease in the uterus of the mare.

How rapidly does the fetus grow?

The developing embryo at 18 to 25 days can be felt in a uterine horn as a swelling about the size of a pigeon's egg. At 25 to 35 days, it is approximately the size of a golf ball, increasing to the size of a hen's egg between 35 and 42 days. The embryo usually starts to enter the body of the uterus at about 50 days, and is about the size of a grapefruit. At 60 days, the embryo is the size and shape of a football, and is about halfway into the uterus. At 90 days, the entire uterus is enlarged and has begun to drop into the abdominal cavity, where it cannot be reached. At five months the uterus is out of reach, down in the abdominal cavity. After seven months, the uterus has enlarged enough to be reached and definite structures of the fetus can be felt as it continues to grow in size.

Can rectal palpation have an effect on the estrous cycle of an open mare?

Yes. It has been shown to cause irregular cycling and lower conception rates in mares that are promiscuously palpated.

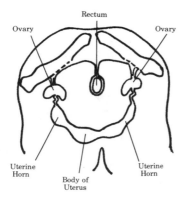
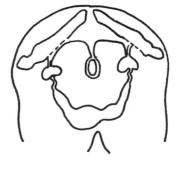

Fig. 23-5. These cross-section diagrams show the uterus of a non-pregnant mare, and the uterus of a mare about 60 days pregnant.

INFERTILITY AND ABORTION

What are infertility and abortion?

Infertility is simply the inability of a mare to conceive, or of a stallion to cause conception. Abortion is the birth of a foal before it is able to survive. (A horse is unable to survive outside the uterus before its 300th day.) The causes for both these problems are closely related and, in some cases, identical. The general causes are psychological problems, infections, hormonal disturbances, nutritional factors and mechanical anatomical problems. Of course, any particular case of infertility or abortion could be contributed to by factors from several of these groups.

What psychological problems can cause infertility and abortion?

While a mare may be uncooperative as far as breeding is concerned, actual infertility due to psychological problems is rare. If a mare is in good health and physically able to conceive but fails to do so, it may very well be that her estrus (heat) simply does not coincide with the breeder's wishes. Since the mare ovulates (has an egg ready to be fertilized) most often and for longer periods at about mid-summer, it is somewhat harder for her to conceive in mid-winter.

Another problem that may be partly psychological lies in the method of verifying estrus. It is common practice among breeders to palpate the ovaries by rectal palpation in order to determine whether or not a follicle (egg structure) is ready to be fertilized. Studies have shown that frequent, irregular palpation, especially when done by a non-professional, can prevent a mare from settling into a predictable estrous cycle, which can considerably impair conception.

The mechanism that regulates the frequency and duration of estrus is centered in the pituitary gland. It accomplishes this through the release of two hormones: luteinizing hormone (LH) and follicle-stimulating hormone (FSH). Some breeders have been successful in "prodding" the pituitary gland into action through the use of artificial lights. In theory, the day is "lengthened" for the mare by the use of these lights, and her system begins to react as if it were summer. There is considerable evidence that this method is effective, but it is certainly not a "cure-all" for barren mares with other problems.

Stallions are known for developing quirks in their breeding habits. They may bite the mare, refuse to mount, or ejaculate only after several covers, to name a few. Stallions may be completely uncontrollable, but this may be improved by professional handling and proper exercise. If a stallion is introduced to breeding by an experienced handler who uses a gentle, experienced mare for the occasion, problems are far less likely to occur. It should be kept in mind that current "hand" breeding practices are somewhat artificial, and cut the natural period of "courtship" short, which undoubtedly puts some initial stress on both horses. Any unnecessary, additional tension should be avoided. Pasture breeding eliminates most of these problems, but then man's control over cleanliness and infection is also eliminated.

Another problem with stallions involves sexual urge or "libido." Although there can be other causes for lack of libido, psychological reasons figure strongly. A young stallion in his first service may show no interest, and may have to be coaxed and guided repeatedly before understanding what is required of him. In some cases, this can take as long as a week of daily exposure. Stallions already in service may lose interest when used too often. This situation usually corrects itself if the horse is given sexual rest. If the horse is sound and normal but still shows no libido, he may be masturbating. There are several devices that may be put on the horse to prevent this habit, and their use generally solves the problem.

The role of psychological problems in abortion is uncertain, but it is not unusual to find abortions where there has been abnormal excitement. The presence of low-flying planes, the constant annoyance of dogs, rough handling and travel are examples of things to be avoided.

What kinds of infections affect fertility and abortion?

Probably the single most common cause of female infertility is infection as the result of pneumovagina (air in the vagina). Air tends to pass in and out of the vagina during estrus, but may do so at all times if there is a conformation problem. The problem may be brought about by stretching or tearing of the genital area during foaling, but some mares simply have a combination of a flat croup, high tail head, sunken anus and small, nearly horizontal vulvar lips, increasing the chances of infection. This conformation allows fecal matter to come in direct contact with the genital area, exposing it to bacteria. Cervicitis (inflammation of the cervix) and endometritis (inflammation of the mucous membranes of the uterus) are the common results. A variety of bacteria may be responsible, including *Streptococcus genitalium, Encapsulatus genitalium* (which causes the venereal disease Klebsiella), *Streptococci* and *Staphylococci*. Among the worst of these infections is pyometra, in which two or three gallons of an exudate containing pus may fill the uterus. The uterine wall becomes thin and weak, the mucous membrane thick and tough, and the mare usually does not recover breeding soundness.

Poor breeding practices may result in the passing along of these infections to the stallion. While it is common practice to wash the mare's vulva and buttocks before breeding, failure to wash the stallion's genitals both before and after may cause infection of every mare he services afterwards.

Bacterial infections usually lodge in the stallion's testicles and seminal vesicles. Orchitis (inflammation of the testes) is usually brought on by a streptococcus infection. Infection often occurs as the result of a wound, and the painful, sensitive swelling may involve other structures such as the vas deferens. The pain does not usually prevent the stallion from breeding, but the presence of pus in the semen makes the semen almost useless.

Inflammation of the seminal vesicles does not reduce fertility as greatly, nor does it seem to be transmitted to the mare. The foals conceived by affected stallions, though, may be weak and sickly, or may abort. The condition is temporary, and only symptomatic treatment is necessary, but affected animals should be given sexual rest for two months to avoid spreading the disease. Males and females are affected by the virus of coital exanthema. Lesions of the genital area characterize this disorder, which may form pustules and ulcers.

Stallions and mares may also experience general watery swelling of the genital area through a protozoal venereal disease called dourine. This infection does not occur with any frequency in the United States, but it is reported in much of the rest of the world. Discharge from the vagina and uterus is common in the female, while the fever, gradual paralysis and death may affect both sexes if left untreated.

In the mare, bacterial infections due to conformation problems can be avoided by a procedure called Caslick's operation. This involves suturing the upper vulvar lips together so that infectious fecal matter does not come in contact with the mucous

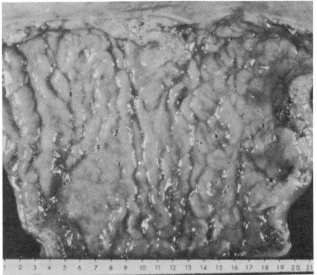

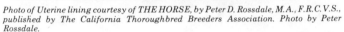

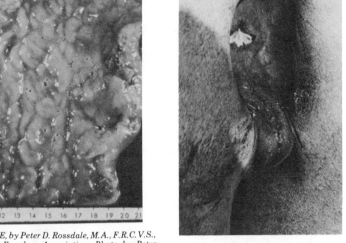

Photo of Uterine lining courtesy of THE HORSE, by Peter D. Rossdale, M.A., F.R.C.V.S., published by The California Thoroughbred Breeders Association. Photo by Peter Rossdale.

Fig. 23-6. A mare with wind-sucking conformation, as shown, is not uncommon. In such a mare, intercourse can introduce air (along with infection) into the uterus, as shown by these bubbles in the uterus lining.

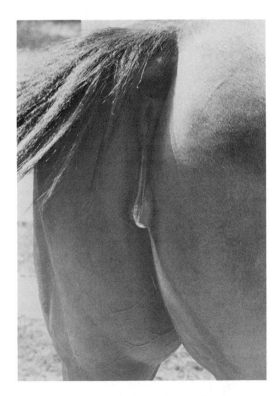

Fig. 23-7. This mare has an infection that results in external swelling of the genital area, and excess discharge. These signs indicate that the mare is unlikely to be able to conceive.

membranes. The infections themselves are sometimes combatted with a surgical procedure known as curettage, which involves a gentle scraping of the uterine lining. There is usually an antibiotic that can be used for each specific kind of

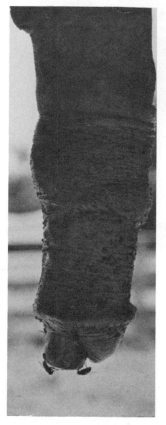
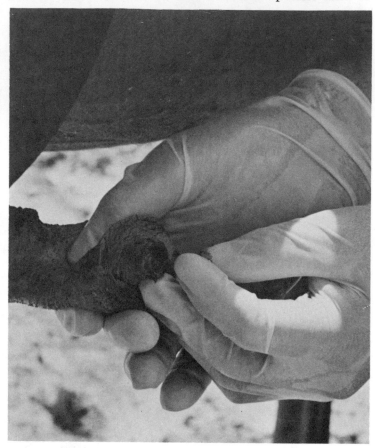

Fig. 23-8. Flies have caused serious infection at this horse's penis, which appears to also be affected by paraphimosis (inability to retract the penis).

infection, but unless the animal is allowed sexual rest and proper sanitary procedures are followed, reinfection invariably follows.

If by some chance an infected mare is impregnated, or if she becomes infected at breeding, the usual result is abortion. Bacteria which figure strongly are *Streptococci, Escherichia coli, Klebsiella* and *Staphylococci,* and they may cause abortion at any stage of pregnancy.

Equine Herpes virus (rhinopneumonitis) and arteritis virus may attack the fetus, and they are probably the most common cause of abortion. Arteritis causes an obvious illness in the mare prior to abortion, in which the eyes and nose discharge, and the limbs swell. Herpes virus infection of the fetus shows no external signs.

A fungus does not attack the fetus directly, but rather diminishes the placenta so that the fetus has no nourishment. Abortion usually occurs in the last half of pregnancy.

In general, the infections that cause infertility have a great deal to do with abortion as well. In fact, quite often the abortion may be directly traced to the fact that the mare suffered from pneumovagina.

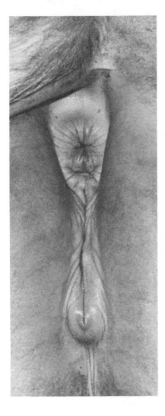

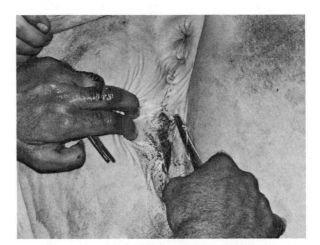

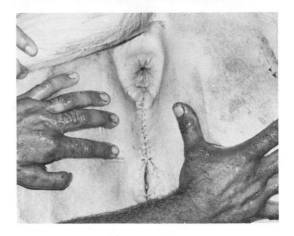

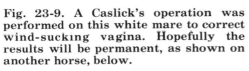

Fig. 23-9. A Caslick's operation was performed on this white mare to correct wind-sucking vagina. Hopefully the results will be permanent, as shown on another horse, below.

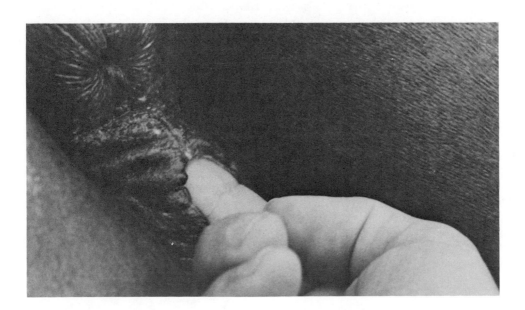

What hormonal problems contribute to infertility and abortion?

The mare's sexual growth and estrous cycle are controlled by the pituitary gland, through hormones known as follicle-stimulating hormone (FSH) and luteinizing hormone (LH). FSH stimulates the ovary to secrete the hormone estrogen, which produces the external signs of estrus and is needed to produce a follicle in the ovary. LH causes ovulation and the formation of a yellow body in the ovary. The yellow body produces progesterone, which is necessary for a normal pregnancy.

Many mares with normal hormone balance have been mistakenly injected with FSH when the real block to conception was infection. An experienced veterinarian should determine whether or not a mare has such an infection, in order to avoid such useless action. Much of the time, hormonal infertility in a mare can be detected by rectal palpation. Immature ovaries (which cause anestrus), absent or small follicles (which cause failure to conceive) and enlarged follicles (which accompany abnormal estrus) can all be detected in this manner. Much of the time, injection of the regulating hormones will restore the natural balance of the system in such cases.

In the stallion, FSH is thought to be responsible for the production of sperm, and LH for stimulation of the growth of certain cells in the testicles which produce testosterone. Growth of the penis and accessory glands, and the development of secondary sex characteristics are regulated by testosterone. Imbalance of these

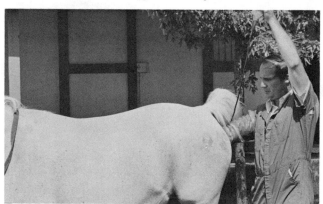

Fig. 23-10. One method of treating uterine infection is by irrigation of the vagina.

hormones can result in lack of sexual drive or low sperm count. LH injected into the system can often improve libido, and doses of FSH have significantly helped sperm counts.

Hormones are also critical in maintaining a normal pregnancy. The importance of progesterone has already been mentioned, but an imbalance of estrogen or cortisone can contribute to an abortion as well. Evidence from other species suggests that the secretion of the hormones corticotropin and cortisone by the fetus help to determine the time of birth. It is entirely possible that an imbalance in this mechanism could cause abortion as well. Recent research in England indicates that once a mare does abort, the presence of a certain hormone can inhibit her ability to conceive again for up to two months. Ulcer-like structures, called endometrial cups, form in the uterus and begin manufacturing a hormone (known as PMSG) on about the 35th day of pregnancy, and continue to do so until about day 100. If the mare aborts any time after the 40th day, the cups continue to manufacture the hormone, which seems to make conception impossible until after the 100th day.

What nutritional factors influence infertility and abortion?

Any animal that is markedly undernourished often cannot conceive or cause conception. In fact, the reproductive system will atrophy (wither) when an animal's intake drops below the survival level. Beyond the fact that an unhealthy mare usually cannot conceive, the effect of missing, vital elements on her fertility is not known. It is known that once conception takes place, the dietary deficiency is passed on to the foal. Foals born of a mare with dietary deficiencies are weaker, have lower resistance to infection and often have defects of conformation.

A stallion's fertility is very definitely affected by his diet. On a substandard diet, libido diminishes and sperm are produced in smaller quantities which are of increasingly abnormal form. Vitamin E has been reported to increase libido and sperm quality, and it has been shown that vitamin A is essential to sperm production.

One of the mechanisms of nature that protects the mare (and females of other species) is that if she becomes extremely undernourished while pregnant, she will nearly always abort the fetus.

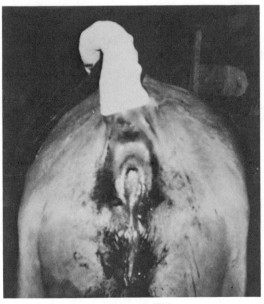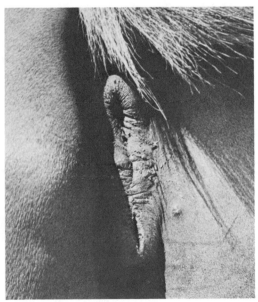

Photo courtesy of W. L. Anderson, D.V.M.

Fig. 23-11. The area between the rectum and vagina may be torn by the foal's sharp hooves when the mare is giving birth. The result is a recto-vaginal fistula. Even after healing, its appearance is distinctive.

What mechanical-anatomical factors influence fertility and abortion?

The importance of pneumovagina as a factor leading to infection has already been stressed. Other mechanical problems, though, can lead to the same kind of infection. Unattended foaling, for instance, can result in a recto-vaginal fistula, which simply means that the foal's hooves have torn the vagina so that it shares its opening with the rectum. This leaves the vagina in a constant state of infection, and unless the tear is repaired surgically, no conception can occur. Foaling is also known to produce cervical atresia (closure) when the cervix is injured in delivery and heals in a closed or partially closed position. This is rather difficult to correct, but there has been some success in opening the uterus with a device called a pessary.

Even if the uterus must remain partially closed, a mare with this condition can sometimes conceive by artificial inseminiation. Injuries that occur to the vagina during intercourse do not usually require suturing, but sexual rest should be allowed, and a "breeding roll" put between the mare and stallion during future services.

Particularly in old mares, sinking vagina can be a problem. This is a condition in which the cervix end of the vagina has dropped down and become filled with urine. This obviously also prevents conception, and must be allowed to heal by sexual rest or be repaired surgically.

Other inhibiting influences are those of age. The persistent hymen of the maiden mare, which is too thick to be broken in coitus, can prevent intercourse until relieved surgically. In old age, the lining of the uterus is no longer richly supplied with blood, and cannot sustain life as easily. So far, there is no known treatment for this.

Stallions may experience difficulty when one or both testicles fail to descend into the scrotum. Cryptorchidism, or failure of both testicles to descend, may cause increased libido, but the stallion is nearly always sterile. Monorchidism, or failure of one testicle to descend, may allow the horse to produce sperm. The failure of "retained" testicles to produce sperm is undoubtedly due to the fact that testicles must be below body temperature for sperm growth. This also accounts for reduced fertility when an inguinal hernia brings a section of intestine into or near the scrotum. Of course, such a hernia may discourage the stallion from mounting, due simply to the pain that it would bring.

The few abortions caused anatomically are usually related to a genetic or hormonal problem. If a mare conceives twins, a possibility which is genetically determined, she will probably abort. Although there are some rare exceptions, horses are thought to be generally incapable of carrying twins to full term. The failure of a placenta to attach to the uterine wall is thought to be determined by genetics or hormones. It has been speculated that this kind of natural abortion is a built-in mechanism for eliminating birth defects, but the fact that some horses are born with defects calls this theory into question.

Of course, there are plain and simple physical reasons such as a severe direct kick to the mare that disturbs the uterus, that account for some abortions. These, however, are not the norm. By far the greatest number of abortions that have their root cause in anatomy are brought about indirectly; that is, through improper conformation of the vagina, causing infection.

PREMATURE FOALS

What are premature foals?

The average gestation period for mares is 340 days. Foals born before they are 320 days old are usually considered to be "premature."

Are premature foals physically normal?

Foals born before they are 320 days old have a great chance of being born when they are not fully developed. The lungs are especially likely to be underdeveloped in premature foals. If the foal is born before 300 days' gestation, there is so little chance of survival that the birth is called an abortion.

What problems do premature foals face?

In many cases, premature foals are not breathing when they are born. They usually require oxygen and human assistance to maintain their body temperature. The body temperature of premature foals is usually two or three degrees below normal, which makes them very susceptible to drafts, infections and colds. Normal foals are fairly hardy, but a premature foal has to have some luck and assistance in order to survive.

What can be done to help premature foals?

If a mare shows signs of premature foaling, she should be brought inside to a *draft-free, absolutely clean* stall, although some authorities believe that a *very good* grass pasture is the best place for a mare to foal, if the weather is quite warm. With premature foals and the usual breeding practices, however, a premature foaling does not usually occur in pleasant weather.

The mare should be carefully watched and a veterinarian should be available to help if the foal is not breathing when it is born. No unusual complications occur in the birth process just because it is premature.

Oxygen should be given to the foal from a nasal tube. The veterinarian may want to leave a stomach tube in place if the suck reflex is not present in the foal. Antibiotics, vitamin supplements and blood transfusions are usually a good idea, even if the foal is given colostrum (the mare's first milk).

Do premature foals usually survive?

If the foal is born alive and lives for a day or two, it has almost the same chances for survival that a full term (340 day) foal has. Both premature and normal foals are susceptible to infections, lack of oxygen (the signs of which are seen several hours after birth), and many other disorders. Proper care and feeding of the mare, from the time before she is bred to the time of foaling, can often minimize the chances of a sick or disabled foal.

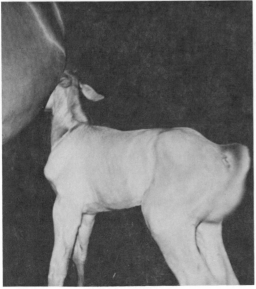

Courtesy of W. L. Anderson. D.V.M.

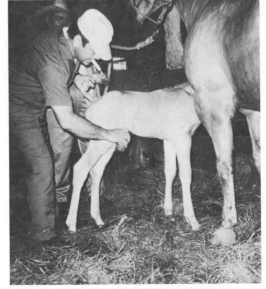

Courtesy of W. L. Anderson, D.V.M.

Fig. 23-12. Newborn foals are particularly susceptible to infection. They especially need the protection of colostrum in the mare's milk, and it is important that the stump of their umbilical cords be treated.

MASTITIS

What is mastitis?

Mastitis is an inflammation of the mammary gland or udder. This condition is very unusual in mares, but can be very inconvenient if a nurse mare is not available.

What causes mastitis?

Mastitis is most frequently caused by avocado poisoning. This occurs when horses are allowed to eat the leaves, bark or fruit of the avocado tree. In rare cases, infections of the udder can be caused by scratches or by infections carried by the foal to the mare.

What are the signs of mastitis?

Inflammation causes swelling, heat and a great deal of soreness in the udder of an affected mare. Non-infectious mastitis (caused by avocado poisoning) is characterized by a short (one week) period of inflammation. Milk production ceases and does not resume for the entire lactation period in cases of avocado poisoning.

What is the treatment for mastitis?

The veterinarian will probably use antibiotics or corticosteroids to control infection or inflammation. Nothing can be done to re-stimulate lactation if it stops, however.

MALE REPRODUCTIVE SYSTEM

ANATOMY

Which organs are involved in the male reproductive system?

The genital organs of the male horse include two paired testicles (testes), each with an epididymis, a vas deferens, and a spermatic cord. There are also various unpaired accessory sex glands and the penis.

What is the structure and function of the testes?

The testicles are specialized glands which produce spermatozoa (sperm) and testosterone (male sex hormone). A normal testicle is egg shaped, three to five inches long, and weighs about ten ounces in the adult stallion. The relative size of each testicle varies from stallion to stallion, but usually the left is larger than the right.

Each testicle is suspended within the scrotum by its spermatic cord which consists of the internal spermatic artery and veins, the cremaster muscle, an autonomic nerve supply, the vas deferens, and the tunica vaginalis propria which surrounds the other structures of the spermatic cord and the testicle itself. The tunica vaginalis propria is a thin layer of serous membrane (a thin, clear, flexible tissue) that is an extension of the abdominal peritoneum.

Each testicle has its own strong fibrous sac, the tunica albuginea. Inside it there is a soft, reddish-grey gland substance that is tightly packed which gives the normal testicle its turgid (firm) feel. This glandular tissue is composed of many minute winding tubes called seminiferous tubules that become larger and straighter as they unite with similar tubes. These tubules eventually join together to form the epididymis.

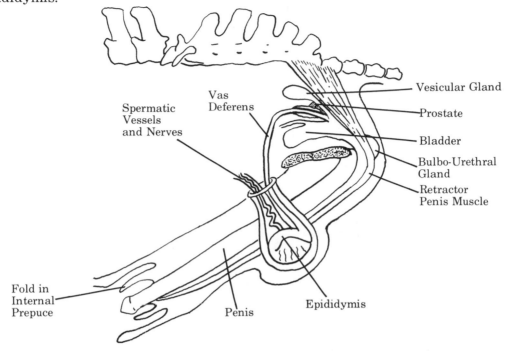

Fig. 23-13. This diagram illustrates the major portions of the male reproductive system.

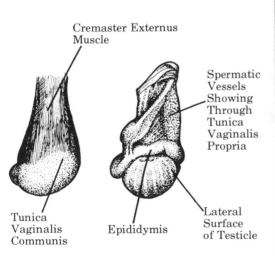

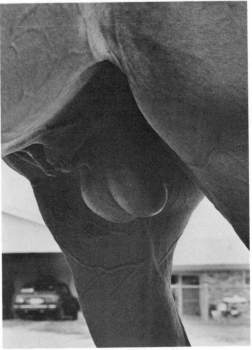

Fig. 23-14. The testicles are responsible for the production of sperm. They can be moved by the cremaster muscle, and the sperm leaves them through the spermatic cord. The photograph illustrates the typical egg shape of the testicles.

How is sperm manufactured?

The male hormone, testosterone, is secreted by the cells of Leydig located in the connective tissue between the seminiferous tubules.

The outside of these tubules is constructed of germinal epithelium containing constantly dividing male sex cells. As they mature, the older cells migrate toward the lumen (interior) of the tubules where they develop tails to become free-swimming mature spermatozoa. It takes approximately 21 days for spermatozoa to form and mature. If they are not ejaculated, the spermatozoa die and are absorbed. The production of viable sperm is only possible when the temperature of the testes is below that of body temperature.

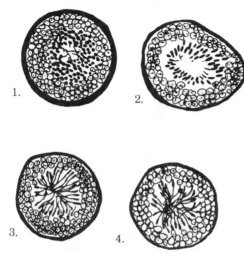

Fig. 23-15. A cross-section diagram of four stages of spermatogenesis, as it takes place in the seminiferous tubules.

What is the structure and function of the scrotum?

The scrotum is composed of thin, relatively hairless skin that is pliable so as to conform in size, shape, and location to the testes within. Since temperature control is so important to the maintenance of sperm life, fibro-elastic tissue and smooth muscle fibers called the tunica dartos run immediately inside the scrotum and help raise the testes close to the abdominal wall during cold weather and lower them during warm weather. This tunica dartos also passes between the two testicles to form the scrotal septum that divides the scrotum into two compartments, one for each testicle.

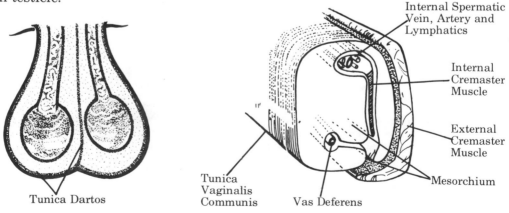

Fig. 23-16. These diagrams of the testicles show the tunica dartos, and give a closer view of the spermatic cord.

What is the structure and function of the epididymis?

The epididymis is a transport tube for sperm. It is a long, winding tube which connects the testicles with the vas deferens, and is divided into head, body and tail sections. The head attaches to the same end of the testicle as do the nerve and blood vessels. The body of the epididymis runs the length of the testicle while the tail continues as the vas deferens, which doubles back along the body of the epididymis and its head where it joins the spermatic cord. In addition to its transport function, the epididymis provides a nourishing fluid and acts as a reservoir for the sperm for 5-10 days during the 21-day maturation period.

What is the vas deferens?

This tube extends from the tail of the epididymis to the urethra, passing through the inguinal canal (passage from the abdominal cavity to the exterior) as part of the spermatic cord and continuing towards the bladder enclosed in the genital fold.

A muscular tube, the function of the vas deferens is to propel the spermatozoa from the epididymis to the ejaculatory duct in the prostatic urethra (the portion of the urethra surrounded by the prostrate gland) during ejaculation.

What is the cremaster muscle?

The cremaster muscle holds the other structures of the spermatic cord together and is capable of lifting the testes from the scrotum into the lower part of the inguinal canal.

What is the role of the urethra in the male reproductive system?

The urethra is a long tube extending from the bladder to the glans penis (end of the penis). It receives openings from the accessory sex glands and is enclosed in a layer of muscle which aids in the ejaculation of semen as well as in the expulsion of urine.

Which are the accessory sex glands?

The male accessory sex glands include the ampullae of the vas deferens, the seminal vesicles, the prostate gland and the bulbo-urethral (Cowper's) glands. Their function is to produce the majority of the components of the semen. While each gland apparently has a specific function of its own, little is known about their roles.

The ampullae of the vas deferens are well developed in the stallion. These glandular enlargements of the ends of the vas deferens contribute fluid to the semen.

In the stallion the seminal vesicles are hollow, pear-shaped paired glands which empty by way of the various ejaculatory ducts into the pelvic urethra just below the neck of the bladder. These elongated sacs are about six inches long and one to two inches wide. They are possibly the site of origin for the albuminous (similar to raw egg white) part of the ejaculate.

The prostate gland is an unpaired structure shaped like a walnut, that almost completely surrounds a portion of the urethra within the pelvic cavity. On each side of the urethra, multiple ducts open in two parallel rows to secrete a milky alkaline fluid which gives semen its characteristic odor. Possibly it is responsible for buffering the ejaculate, thus lengthening the life span of the sperm that has been deposited within the female reproductive tract. Advancing age may bring on an enlargement of the prostate, which impinges upon the urethra and interferes with urination.

Below the other sex glands are small paired glands called the bulbo-urethral (Cowper's) glands, located on either side of the pelvic urethra. Each gland is about two inches long and has six to eight ducts which open into the urethra. Its secretion probably is the first part of the ejaculate which cleans and neutralizes the lumen (inner tube canal) of the urethra.

What is the function of semen?

Semen provides nutrition to the spermatozoa, acts as a buffer against excess acidity of the female genital tract, and serves as a transport medium for the spermatozoa. There are an average of 120 million spermatozoa per milliliter (very nearly the same volume as a c.c. or cubic centimeter) of ejaculate in a range of 30 to 800 million per milliliter. The amount of ejaculate can range from 30-300 milliliters with 70 milliliters being the average.

What is the structure and function of the penis?

The penis, the male organ of copulation, is structured in three parts: the glans, the body, and the two crura, or roots, which attach to the ischial arch of the pelvis.

The glans penis is the enlarged free end of the organ. The horse has a free portion of the urethra, called the urethral process, projecting beyond the glans. Just above the urethral process is a small, inward sack-shaped cavity called the "diverticulum of the fossa glandis." This diverticulum is where smegma (secreted by the sebacious glands of the prepuce) collects, forming a putty-like mass that takes on the shape of the diverticulum it has filled. This mass, what horsemen refer to as a "bean," should occasionally be removed as part of the hygenic maintenance of the penis of the stallion or gelding.

Originating at the midline of the ischium of the pelvis, the two roots of the penis converge to form the bottom part of the penis. The upper part of the body of the penis is formed by the urethra, surrounded by the corpus cavernosum urethrae (a continuation of the erectile tissue of the urethral bulb between the roots of the penis).

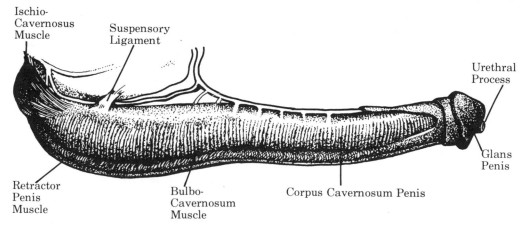

Fig. 23-17. Side view diagram of the penis. The projection on the glans penis is the urethral process.

Erectile (cavernous) tissue composes the internal structure of the penis. It consists of blood sinusoids (channels) separated by septa (connective tissue) which originate from the tunica albuginea, a heavy fibrous capsule surrounding the penis. In the stallion, there is a small amount of connective tissue in relation to the amount of cavernous (erectile) tissue, so the penis becomes enlarged all over.

Erection is achieved by the input of more blood into the penis than is allowed out through the veins. Contraction of the muscles of the penis constrict the veins to slow the outflow of blood. The increased blood volume swells the cavernous tissue, resulting in enlargement and hardening of the penis. After ejaculation, the muscles relax and the blood flow through the veins of the penis back into general circulation is allowed, causing the penis to relax and shrink back to its resting size. Both the brain and the spinal cord are involved in a complicated system of nerve control from the initial stimulus, through the muscular reaction, to the final relaxation. In the horse, erection is rather slow, but ejaculation takes only 10-15 seconds.

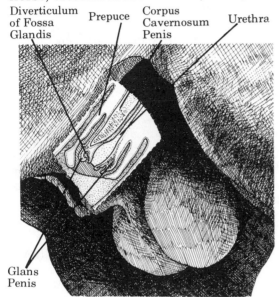
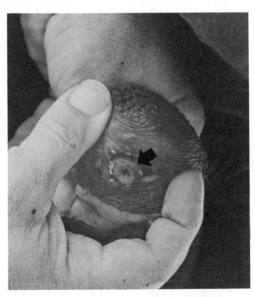

Diverticulum of Fossa Glandis   Prepuce   Corpus Cavernosum Penis   Urethra

Glans Penis

Fig. 23-18. This median section of the penis (and surrounding structures) shows the position of the prepuce when the penis is retracted. The photograph shows the urethral process and diverticulum of the fossa glandis, as labeled in the diagram.

What is the prepuce?

Surrounding the penis of the horse is a double fold of skin called the prepuce or the sheath. Its outer surface looks like skin, but the interior has a preputial and a penile layer. These layers are hairless and are supplied with large amounts of sebaceous glands which continually secrete a fatty, foul-smelling material called smegma. This material should be regularly removed with a mild soap and water every few weeks.

What is the function of testosterone?

The hormone testosterone is responsible for secondary sex characteristics of the stallion. These characteristics are demonstrated by the development of a crest (varied in size according to breed), less laying down of fat (both surface fat and marbling), and suppressed mammary development. Testosterone promotes sex drive and the development and functioning of the accessory sex glands.

SEMEN EVALUATION

When should a stallion be evaluated for breeding?

Before a stallion is bought, he should undergo a thorough examination for breeding soundness, including an evaluation of his semen. The quality of his semen should also be checked before each breeding season, far enough in advance to allow the stallion to be replaced, or to be treated and recover, if his semen is of poor quality. Semen evaluation can be especially useful in the case of young stallions who have not yet proved themselves in enough test breedings. Poor semen quality may be responsible for cases of infertility, even though the stallion displays enough libido and performs well.

Why should semen be checked before the breeding season instead of at any time of the year?

Evaluating semen close to the breeding season allows a more accurate estimate of the stallion's potential. Semen quality should be at its highest during breeding season. The volume and total number of sperm in each ejaculate is about half as large in the late fall and early winter as during the spring and summer. If a stallion's semen is evaluated at a time other than close to the breeding season, the variation in semen quality due to season must be taken into account.

What else besides season can affect semen quality?

Overuse of a stallion is a common cause of lowered semen quality. Some stallions can be used once or occasionally twice a day for at least a month, without reducing the sperm count. Other stallions may show signs of infertility if used as often as once a day.

Poor nutrition can be a cause of poor semen quality. There has been no evidence of a specific element of the diet required for a high semen quality, but a well balanced ration will help maintain normal semen quality.

Illnesses and infections, especially those that cause fever, affect the stallion's condition in general, resulting in a decrease in semen quality. Stallions should be allowed time to recover from the effects of an illness before being used for breeding.

The size of the testes has been shown to be directly related to sperm production in bulls and boars. This relationship possibly applies to stallions also, and should be considered in connection with semen evaluation.

A large amount of exercise is considered necessary by some people for stallions used only as studs. Although adequate exercise is essential to overall health, a lack of exercise has not been scientifically shown to be responsible for poor semen quality.

What measurements are used in evaluating semen quality?

There is some disagreement over which factors of semen quality are the most reliable determinants of fertility or reproductive efficiency. Predicting fertility on the basis of semen quality is not absolutely accurate, since other factors involving the sexual behavior of individual stallions must be considered in evaluating breeding potential. In an evaluation of a semen sample (sperm plus the accessory fluids), the concentration of sperm in the ejaculate is considered by some authorities to be the single most important factor in predicting fertility. Many factors may be involved, but a semen evaluation commonly includes four factors: concentration, volume, sperm morphology (examination of the sperm to detect abnormally shaped sperm) and sperm motility (activity).

How is a semen sample collected for an evaluation?

Samples should be collected when the stallion is in normal condition and has had at least one week of rest from sexual activity. A mare in heat is used as a teaser until the stallion has an erection. He is then allowed to mount the mare, and the ejaculate is collected into a condom or artificial vagina. The artificial vagina is a rubber tube encased in a warm water jacket to simulate the temperature and pressure of the mare's vagina.

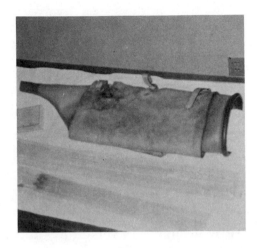

Fig. 23-19. An artificial vagina, used for semen collection.

Courtesy of W. L. Anderson, D.V.M.

Is the entire ejaculate used in a semen evaluation?

The ejaculate usually consists of three fractions, and an evaluation may include the entire ejaculate or it may exclude the last portion. Evaluations are sometimes made only from the dismount sample, which is collected from the penis as the stallion dismounts from the mare. A dismount sample can provide an estimate of semen quality, but it is not completely accurate since without the other portions of the ejaculate there is no measurement of the total volume or total number of sperm.

What are the portions of the ejaculate?

The first portion is a thin, grayish fluid which is secreted by the accessory sex glands. This fluid contains few or no sperm but adds volume to the ejaculate and cleanses the urethra before the rest of the semen is passed through it. The second fraction is the largest portion of the semen and contains most of the sperm. The last portion of the ejaculate is white and gelatinous, and may be absent or present in very small amounts in lighter breeds of horses and in stallions that are overused. This last portion is sometimes removed by filtration before the sample is evaluated for volume and other measurements. When this gel is present in small amounts, the total volume of an ejaculate will not differ greatly from the volume of the gel-free portion.

What is the normal volume of an ejaculate?

The volume of the complete ejaculate may vary from 60 to 300 milliliters. The normal ejaculate of lighter breeds is between 50 and 150 milliliters, although some horses that are breeding every day for a month or more may have a total ejaculate of as little as 30 milliliters. Stallions that are producing a low volume of semen may be rested for a few days to allow time for the volume to return to normal.

What is normal concentration of sperm?

The number of sperm per millileter can vary greatly, from about 50,000 per milliliter to 500,000,000 per milliliter. The concentration of sperm, combined with the volume of semen, will indicate the total number of sperm in the ejaculate. The total number of sperm and the motility are considered by some veterinarians and technicians to be the two most important measurements.

How is motility measured?

Motility of the sperm involves an estimate of the number of motile sperm and their type of movement. Some sperm move slowly in circles and some exhibit a rapid forward movement which is more desirable for traveling through the mare's reproductive tract to fertilize the egg. In a good sample, 90 to 95% of the sperm will be alive, with rapid, strong movement. A semen sample with a motility of about 70% is considered normal.

How is the fourth major measurement determined?

The sperm are microscopically examined for their shape and structure (morphology) to determine the percentage of normal sperm. A normal sperm is composed of an oval-shaped head and a long straight tail. Abnormal sperm are usually less efficient in fertilizing an egg. Sperm that are headless or tailless, with coiled, bent or small tails and several other variations are considered abnormal. An average semen sample should have between 70 and 80% normal sperm.

How accurate is semen evaluation as a prediction of a stallion's fertility?

There is still little information and some disagreement on the accuracy of semen evaluation. Estimates of volume, concentration, motility and morphology (as the percent of normal sperm) which are considered normal often vary greatly. Some stallions may have normal sperm counts and yet have little success as breeders while others may appear to have low quality semen and still be efficient. A stallion that is sterile due to a near complete lack of sperm in the ejaculate can easily be identified by a semen evaluation. Breeding stallions with poor quality semen should not be replaced merely on the basis of a semen evaluation. Individual stallions may still be efficient breeders, and superior sires may still be used in artificial insemination programs where breed regulations allow it. One can be confident that a stallion with sufficient libido and a good semen sample will be a good, fertile breeder.

ORCHITIS AND VESICULITIS

What are orchitis and vesiculitis?

Orchitis is an inflammation of the testes which may be accompanied by vesiculitis, an inflammation of the seminal vesicles.

What causes these inflammations?

Inflammation of the testes and seminal vesicles is usually secondary to a systemic infection, such as strangles. The infective agent is often streptococcus, but staphylococcus, pseudomonas or a coli bacteria can cause the same type of condition. Sometimes the testicles are inflamed due to trauma, which is not the case with the seminal vesicles, due to their location.

What are the signs of orchitis and vesiculitis?

Since the testes are easily available for inspection, the swelling and heat that accompany inflammation are readily apparent. The seminal vesicles, when the veterinarian palpates them, will be swollen and they may be very sensitive. In both cases, the semen will contain pus, abnormal sperm and the infective bacteria. The fertility of the stallion can be greatly decreased by orchitis or vesiculitis, but he will still be fertile enough to settle a mare.

Do these conditions inferfere with libido or breeding capability?

Yes. In some cases orchitis is painful enough that the stallion will refuse to breed. Vesiculitis can impair the stallion's ability to ejaculate, making him impotent, but these cases are uncommon.

Can a mare be infected by an infected stallion?

Very few mares develop vaginitis, cervicitis or endometritis from an infected stallion. They apparently harbor the infectious agent but do not succumb to it. If these mares are settled, they often have sickly, weak foals or abort.

How are these conditions treated?

Treatment by the veterinarian involves culturing the semen to determine the bacteria that is responsible for the inflammation. Systemic antibiotics and enzymes can then be chosen to clear up the infection. Sexual rest and application of cold water (for orchitis) are generally advisable. Some testicular degeneration always occurs with orchitis, but prompt treatment can minimize the residual impairments of fertility. Most important is the early recognition and treatment of these conditions to prevent chronic infections.

SCROTAL HERNIA

What is a scrotal hernia?

A scrotal hernia is a protrusion of a piece of the intestine into the scrotum.

What causes a scrotal hernia?

A scrotal hernia in its initial stage is called an inguinal hernia. This is because the piece of intestine forming the hernia comes down the inguinal canal, which is the passageway for the testicles to descend from the abdomen to the scrotum. A scrotal hernia occurs when the intestine descends the length of the inguinal canal and comes into the scrotum on one side. These hernias are most frequent in foals, because the inguinal ring, which restricts the size of the canal, is not yet fully developed.

What are the signs of scrotal hernia?

The most obvious sign of scrotal hernia is enlargement of one side of the scrotum. They may also be palpated through the rectum, which reveals them to be either reducible or irreducible. A reducible hernia is one in which the intestine can be moved back into its place in the abdomen; an irreducible hernia cannot be so moved.

An irreducible hernia can become strangulated or "pinched off." This commonly occurs when the inguinal ring tightens and traps the piece of intestine. Inflammation, infection and necrosis (tissue death) commonly follows. If not relieved, the condition leads to death. Strangulation is normally accompanied by obvious pain, great distress, and an altered gait.

How are scrotal hernias treated?

For the most part, scrotal hernias in foals are not treated unless they become strangulated. This is seldom the case, though, since they usually heal by themselves.

Scrotal hernias in stallions may cause infertility because the heat of the intestine raises the temperature of the testicle too high for sperm production.

If a scrotal hernia is diagnosed early, it may be possible to move the intestine back through the canal, manipulating through the rectum. If it is necessary to reduce the hernia surgically, the affected testicle is nearly always removed.

COITAL EXANTHEMA

What is coital exanthema?

Coital exanthema is a contagious disease which causes temporary sterility in the mare and can be spread from mare to mare by the stallion.

What causes this disease?

It is caused by a herpes virus. Herpes is a class of viruses that cause lesions on the skin and mucous membranes.

How is it transmitted?

Coital exanthema is easily spread by contact, either directly through sexual contact or indirectly from infected secretions on contaminated brushes, currycombs and sponges.

What are the signs?

In the mare many small blisters, one to three millimeters (about one-sixteenth inch) in diameter, develop on the mucous membranes of the vulva and vagina. These blisters become pustules and then small ulcers. Because of the lesions, the vulva is congested, swollen and very sensitive. There is a whitish discharge on the buttocks and tail, and the swollen vulva itches, causing the mare to stand with her back arched, to urinate frequently and to switch her tail. After a few days, the clinical signs decrease and the lesions disappear, leaving nonpigmented spots that may last several weeks.

In the stallion, small blisters will form on the glans, or tip of the penis, and then on the body of the penis. These will develop into pustules and ulcers in a few days.

How will this affect fertility?

Coital exanthema has only a temporary effect on fertility, with no permanent aftereffect. The disease is self-limiting in that the inflammation caused by the virus kills it off as the lesions progress through the various stages.

Does this mean that the disease does not need to be treated?

The infection could clear up after a time without treatment, but a veterinarian should be consulted at the first sign of lesions since they could be indications of some other more serious disease that requires treatment. In the mare, treatment should be symptomatic (just for relief of the signs), and the animal should be quarantined for two months. In the stallion, the affected areas of the penis should be treated by washing with a mild antiseptic solution and cauterizing with silver nitrate. The infected stallion should not be used for breeding until the lesions have completely healed since the disease is highly contagious. Infection does not result in permanent immunity to the disease.

How can coital exanthema be prevented?

The stallion should be checked before breeding for cleanliness and signs of lesions on the penis to prevent spread of the disease to the mare. Brushes and other equipment used on infected animals should not be used on other animals.

DOURINE

What is dourine?

Dourine is a venereal disease of horses. Although it has not been reported in the United States for a number of years, dourine still is found in Mexico and other regions of the world.

What causes dourine?

The trypanosome *T. equiperdum* causes dourine after an incubation period of 2 to 12 weeks. Transmitted by horses through coitus, dourine is a venereal disease that may be fatal.

What are the signs of dourine?

The first signs of dourine are fever, a lack of appetite, edema of the genitalia and a discharge from the vagina or urethra. If the disease is allowed to progress, urticarial (itchy) raised areas (placques) may appear on the side of the body. A progressive muscle paralysis may start at the front of the body and continue to develop until it reaches the hind legs. If the horse does not receive treatment, dourine is often fatal, or the horse may become a carrier without symptoms.

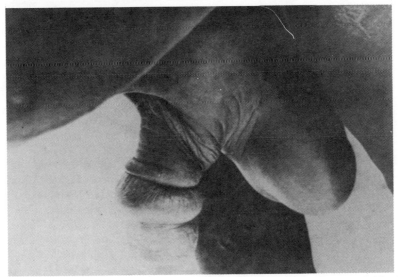

Courtesy of EQUINE MEDICINE AND SURGERY, Edition II, American Veterinary Publications, Inc., Wheaton, Ill.

Fig. 23-20. Dourine can cause edema on the female genitals as well as male. Even when the disease is not fatal, an infected horse is usually infertile.

What is the treatment for dourine?

Affected horses must be diagnosed by a veterinarian who will confirm the diagnosis with laboratory examination of spinal fluid or fluid from the area of edema. If dourine *(T. equiperdum)* is present, the veterinarian will probably treat the horse with a drug called antrycide. A single treatment is usually effective.

24

SYSTEMIC DISORDERS

NEONATAL BACTERIAL INFECTIONS

Foals are susceptible to many infections before and after birth. Many immunizing factors cannot pass through the placental membrane so the foal is born with insignificant levels of defense against infections. Two to four hours may pass before a normal-appearing foal makes its first efforts to nurse, and receives the protective antibodies in the colostrum. This is ample time for the development of infections from *Escherichia coli, Actinobacillus equuli, Salmonella abortus-equi, Streptococcus pyogenes, Salmonella typhimurium, Listeria monocytogenes, Pseudomonas aeruginosa, Clostridium perfringens* and *Corynebacterium equi,* all of which are frequently involved in neonatal infections.

What disorders are caused by these disease organisms?

The infecting organisms cause similar disorders in newborn foals. Most common are the septicemias caused by *Streptococcus pyogenes* (polyarthritis), *Salmonella typhimurium* (colitis), *Salmonella abortus-equi* (Salmonellosis), *Actinobacillus equuli* (Shigellosis), *Listeria monocytogenes* (Listeriosis) and the encephalitis and enteritis syndromes caused by *Escherichia coli* (sleepy foals) and *Clostridium botulinum* (shaker foals). Foal pneumonia, caused by *Corynebacterium equi,* is a characteristic respiratory disorder. Specific signs and effects are discussed under each disorder and will not be covered here. Needless to say, any suspected abnormality in a newborn foal should receive the attention of a veterinarian as soon as possible. Cultures and laboratory tests are often required before diagnosis of the causative agent can be made and the appropriate antibiotic treatment determined. Many of these organisms do not respond to penicillin, the common "home" remedy. This unsupervised treatment can result in unnecessary foal deaths which can be prevented by prompt professional diagnosis.

BRUCELLOSIS

What is brucellosis?

The disease is most common in cattle, where it causes abortions and sterility and is called "Bang's disease." A variety of strains affect different species of animals and humans, but the *Brucella abortus,* found in diseased cattle, occurs in horses and is found in the lesions of poll evil and fistulous withers. (See Fistulous Withers-Poll Evil, page 265.)

What are the signs of Brucella infection in horses?

Indications of infection by the Brucella organisms are those of general infection: variable temperature, dullness, stiffness and difficulty in moving around, and enlargements of the bursae (lubrication sacs) at the poll or withers may be present. If bursal enlargements are present, they may or may not be draining fluid.

What is the source of infection?

Brucella infections may be suspected among horses that run with cattle infected with Bang's disease. The infection may be spread by contact with contaminated placentas or recently aborted fetuses. Combinations of *Brucella abortus* and *Actinomyces bovis* (also found in cattle) have caused fistulous withers and poll evil in experiments with horses. It also seems to be a sequel to blows on the poll and withers which result in bone chips and tissue death.

How is brucellosis treated?

Vaccination with strain 19 has had some favorable effect, and antibiotics are widely used. For severe development of fistulas, surgical removal and drainage are considered the best method of treatment, combined with drug therapy.

Can brucellosis be prevented?

Separation of horses and cattle greatly lowers incidence of infections in horses. Vaccination with strain 19 has also been effective, as has treatment with antibiotics and anti-inflammatory drugs following blows to the head and withers.

LEPTOSPIROSIS

What is leptospirosis?

Leptospirosis is thought to be a contagious disease due to infection by one or several of the bacteria Leptospira. It is present in the blood of horses affected with periodic ophthalmia, which is the only visible aftereffect of a leptospiral infection. The infection eventually burns itself out and leaves a higher than normal serum agglutination titer (blood serum clumping level) in a test for leptospirosis. These organisms come to rest in the kidneys, where they live and are excreted for years, serving as a source of infection for other animals.

What are the signs of leptospirosis in horses?

If the animal is examined at the time of infection, the temperature will be elevated (103°-105° F) for two or three days, in addition to signs of depression, dullness, lack of appetite, jaundice, and an increase in neutrophils in the blood. These signs end on the seventh or eighth day following the onset of the infection, when serum agglutinens appear in the blood.

How is leptospirosis diagnosed?

Leptospirosis can only be positively diagnosed by a veterinarian, on the basis of two blood samples spaced seven to ten days apart, or the appearance of the organism in freshly collected urine.

What is the treatment for leptospirosis?

There is no specific treatment, but the use of antibiotics is generally considered prudent. Research has provided no evidence that they are effective in removing the bacteria from the kidneys or inhibiting development of periodic ophthalmia.

Are there any lasting effects of leptospirosis?

Other than a remote relationship with periodic ophthalmia (scarring of the iris of the eye) which may follow an infection with Leptospira, abortions in the middle or final third of pregnancy have been noted during the infection.

Can leptospirosis be prevented?

The only means of preventing infection by Leptospira is to maintain adequate hygiene around stable areas and to prevent contamination of outside water sources with infected urine.

ANTHRAX

What is anthrax?

Anthrax is one of the oldest diseases known to affect man and animals. In the horse, it is a suddenly-occurring, rapidly fatal septicemia. Man, who is affected by the bacteria less frequently than the horse, develops the disease as a localized, persistent cutaneous pustule (malignant carbuncle), although the disease is systemic if the bacteria spores are inhaled (Woolsorter's disease).

What causes anthrax?

The anthrax bacteria form a protective case (spores) when they are exposed to air. These spores spread in the air, in blood or fecal discharges, and in the hide and tissues of an infected animal. The anthrax spores can remain in the soil, unharmed, for years. Favorable conditions (over 60°F and humid) stimulate the spores to reproduce, contaminating soil and grass in infected areas. Horses ingest the spores from the ground and infected water or from feed grown on infected soil. Most frequently, sparse pasture conditions favor development of anthrax infections because there may be slight damage to the lips and mucous membranes of the mouth from dry, scratchy feed. These slight scratches and abrasions make it easier for anthrax bacteria to enter the blood stream. Infection also occurs by insect transmission of the spores from infected animals or carcasses.

What are the signs of anthrax?

The first case of anthrax in a herd is usually discovered after the animal is dead. Since the bacteria multiply and destroy tissue very rapidly, the active phase of the disease may only last 48 to 96 hours after an incubation period of one to two weeks. Horses commonly develop the acute form of anthrax which is characterized by septicemia with enteritis and colic, if the infection is ingested. Transmission by insect bites causes hot, painful swellings that appear on the throat, lower neck, the base of the chest and abdomen and on the prepuce. These swellings are accompanied by very high fever (up to 107°F), severe depression, stupor, staggering, lack of appetite and colic. Convulsions, the discharge of blood from the body openings and death follow within 48 to 96 hours.

620   SYSTEMIC DISORDERS—Malignant Edema

Is anthrax always fatal?

The acute form of anthrax is almost always fatal, but rare cases may develop a chronic form of the disease which involves local lesions of the tongue and throat. However, some animals may suffocate or choke to death from these. Horses may also develop localized lesions in wounds or abrasions, like the malignant carbuncles in human cases of anthrax.

What is the effect of the anthrax bacteria on the body?

Anthrax causes a severe septicemia which includes hemorrhages and damage to the spleen, liver and kidneys. Severe shock and massive edema from the origin of infection (the intestines or pharynx) may be the cause of death before septicemia develops.

How is anthrax treated?

Massive doses of antibiotics are currently used in the treatment of anthrax. Penicillin or streptomycin appear to be effective in the early stages of the disease. Treatment should continue for at least five days to avoid reappearance of the disease. Anti-anthrax serum is available but expensive. The best treatment for anthrax, however, is prevention.

How may anthrax be controlled and prevented?

The anthrax vaccines currently available are very effective in preventing anthrax. When these vaccines are administered to horses, large swellings often occur at the site of injection. It is best to allow horses to rest after vaccination, which should not be done in hot weather.

Outbreaks of anthrax require vaccination of all unaffected animals in the area and disinfection of contaminated stable areas. Persons who come in contact with infected animals must be particularly careful to avoid direct skin contact with the animals or their discharges. Infected carcasses should not be opened or autopsied. Tissue putrefaction and decay in the carcass will destroy the bacteria if fresh air does not reach the spores. Intact carcasses and contaminated soil and bedding material should be burned or buried at least six feet deep with quicklime added to aid decomposition. Careful quarantine of suspected animals and annual vaccination can greatly reduce the incidence of anthrax in a specific location.

MALIGNANT EDEMA

What is malignant edema?

Malignant edema (fluid infiltration and inflammation of tissues) is an acute wound infection caused by *Clostridium septicum* bacteria. These bacteria are frequently found in the soil and in the intestinal contents of man and animals.

What are the signs of a malignant edema infection?

Cl. septicum prefer deep puncture wounds that are surrounded by traumatized dying tissue. Surgical wounds (castration, firing, venepuncture) and accidental wounds are equally attractive to the bacterium, as are umbilical cords of newborn foals and the vaginal mucosa and vulva of mares who have recently foaled. Signs of the violent infection appearing 12 to 48 hours after injury are heat, the presence of swelling which pits under pressure and fever ranging from 106°-107°F. The swelling gradually becomes firmer and the skin appears tight and dark. If the wound is severely infected, froth may ooze from the opening or a blood tinged fluid may escape. These signs are followed by depression, weakness, muscle tremors, increased pulse rate and stiffness or lameness in the affected quarter. Mares who have infected foaling tears or who have been infected by stallion service may have a reddish brown fluid discharge or swelling extending down the perineal area. Reddening of the conjunctiva (mucous membranes) is a characteristic sign of severe toxemia (bacterial toxins in the blood). Death usually occurs within 24 to 48 hours following the appearance of signs of infection.

What is the treatment for malignant edema?

Malignant edema should be given emergency treatment due to the extreme toxicity of the *Cl. septicum* infection. Surgical drainage of swellings and large amounts of penicillin or broad-spectrum antibiotics given systemically are of prime importance. Treatment of the wound with hydrogen peroxide has been found to be useful and cold packs are used to limit the spread and absorption of toxins from the infected area. Fluids and whole blood may be administered by the veterinarian if the animal's condition requires them.

How can malignant edema be prevented?

Prevention consists of maintaining proper antiseptic wound treatment and hygiene in castration, foaling and surgical procedures. Penicillin should be routinely administered for deep, contaminated puncture wounds, and penicillin ointment applied directly into the puncture.

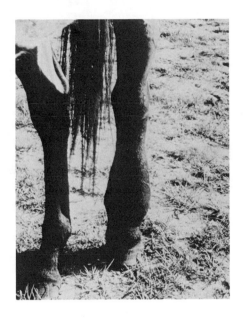

Fig. 24-1. Malignant edema of the hindleg. Notice the extreme enlargement of the whole leg.

TUBERCULOSIS

What is tuberculosis?

Tuberculosis is a contagious disease that is characterized by the progressive development of tubercules in various organs. Tubercules (firm, grayish-white tumor-like growths with a central core of pus) are most frequently found in the mesenteric lymph nodes, the spleen and the intestinal mucosa of horses. This disease is rare in horses because they are usually infected by the cattle bacterium *(Mycobacterium bovis)*, which has been almost eliminated in the United States.

What are the signs of tuberculosis?

The first sign of tuberculosis is usually loss of condition in spite of normal appetite and the availability of food. Many horses show a stiffness of the neck which may be severe. Additional signs may include a dry, shaggy haircoat, an upper respiratory tract infection, nasal discharge or a moist, short cough.

How is tuberculosis spread?

The bacteria that cause tuberculosis are present in the feces, urine, vaginal discharges, milk, saliva and exhaled air of affected horses. Other horses may be infected by contact with these discharges, although horses are slightly resistant to tuberculosis infection.

Is tuberculosis treatable?

Tuberculosis can be treated, but the disease is almost always chronic. The tubercules generally spread throughout the body, causing tissue damage and loss of function in various important organs (lungs, liver, intestines). Affected horses are sources of contamination for other horses, and are usually euthanized. Suspected cases should be reported to a veterinarian, who will be able to perform tests to determine whether or not the horse has tuberculosis.

TRYPANOSOMIASIS

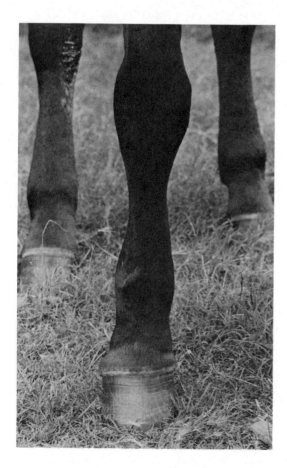

Fig. 24-2. This edema of the lower legs is typical of trypanosomiasis. Notice the involvement of the front and hind legs.

What is trypanosomiasis?

The term trypanosomiasis includes the diseases Nagana, Surra, Mal de Caderas and Murrina that are caused by the trypanosomes *T. brucei, T. evansi, T. equinum* and *T. Hippicum*. These diseases occur primarily in Africa, the Middle East, South America and Central America.

What are trypanosomes?

They are protozoa (one-celled animals) that are transmitted by tsetse flies and vampire bats. Some species do not spend a period of development in the fly or the bat, but *T. equinum* and *T. hippicum* infect, develop in, and may kill vampire bats.

What are the signs of trypanosomiasis?

The signs of these diseases include anemia, intermittent (irregular) fever and edema of the lower legs and abdomen. Affected horses may become weak, emaciated and they may avoid light. Death can occur after an acute illness or after a prolonged, wasting disease.

What is the treatment for trypanosomiasis?

Effective treatment includes fly control and the use of drugs that have a specific action against the trypanosomes, such as antrycide.

AFRICAN HORSESICKNESS

What is African horsesickness?

This is a highly fatal viral infection transmitted by biting insects to horses, mules and donkeys. It occurs in acute, subacute and mild forms. The horse is more frequently and more seriously affected.

The disease is most prevalent in low-lying swampy areas especially in late summer. The rate of incidence increases greatly following rains, particularly when hot and rainy weather alternate. The first frost usually stops the spread. Recovered animals are not carriers. Because of its high mortality rate and its ability to spread quickly, African horse disease is of concern to the western world.

What causes African horsesickness?

African horsesickness is caused by a virus that is present in all body fluids and tissues of affected animals throughout the duration of the disease. There are nine known immunological types and more than 42 distinct strains of the virus at present. They are only moderately resistant to drying and heating but can live in putrified blood for up to two years. Most manufactured vaccines include several strains of the virus.

Foals can gain immunity that will last about six months through the colostrum (first milk) from an immune dam.

What are the signs of African horsesickness?

There are four main types of African horsesickness. They are called (1) horsesickness fever or mild; (2) pulmonary or acute; (3) cardiac or subacute; and (4) mixed form.

(1) The incubation period for horsesickness fever can vary from two to four weeks. Characteristic developments include a slight loss of appetite, a redness of the membranes which line the eyelids, labored breathing and an increase in pulse rate. There will be a high temperature within one to three days following the onset of signs. This fever will drop back to a normal temperature as the horse begins to recover. This form of African horsesickness is most commonly the result of vaccination reaction or of an existing immunity that is partially overcome.

(2) Victims of the pulmonary variety of African horsesickness rarely recover. The course of the disease lasts four to five days. During this time the appetite stays good and the horse will appear normal until the last 24 to 36 hours. However, in the terminal stage the body temperature will rise to about 105°F with sweating, weakness, staggering and eventual collapse. The bronchi and upper respiratory tract fill with a fluid that looks frothy and comes out of the nostrils. This congestion causes severely labored breathing with coughing. The horse could be said to drown in its own fluids. Death is the result of a lack of oxygen.

(3) In the cardiac form, the areas of edema (fluid swelling) are in the head and neck. The incubation period is dependent on the virulence of the strain. The course of the disease lasts about two weeks. It is the most common type of African horsesickness found in areas prone to the disease. It is also the type in which recovery occurs most commonly, although the convalescent period is longer than convalescence of pulmonary form survivors. The cardiac form is manifested by fever, labored breathing, redness of the eyelid lining, restlessness, some abdominal pain, and a bluish discoloration of the mucous membranes of the mouth and tongue. The cardiac form of African horsesickness also damages heart function.

(4) The mixed form of African horsesickness has both pulmonary and cardiac signs. Rarely is this form diagnosed in life, but rather, it is discovered during necropsy.

How is African horsesickness diagnosed?

The clinical signs can give ample evidence of the disease to one who is highly familiar with African horsesickness and, consequently, capable of recognizing the disease readily. However, because of the recent spread of the disease into areas where it is not well known and because of the multiplicity of strains, laboratory analysis is the only sure way to confirm diagnosis.

African horsesickness may be confused with such infections as EIA and equine viral arteritis, but tests and specific examination of lesions make differentiation possible.

How is African horsesickness treated?

As of this date, no effective treatment has been developed. Careful nursing and symptomatic treatment may be of some help. Generally, the mortality rate is 90-95% in horses.

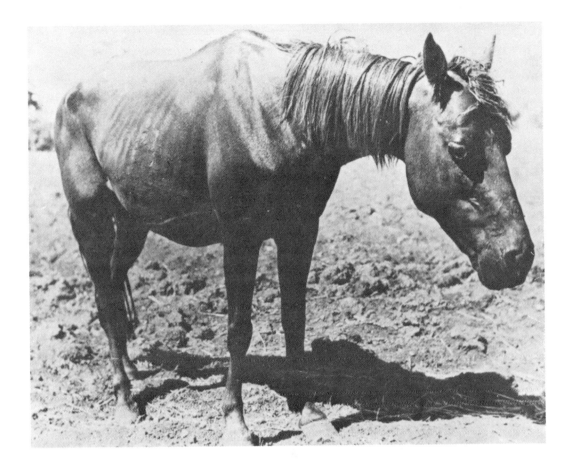

Photo courtesy of EQUINE MEDICINE AND SURGERY, Edition II, American Veterinary Publications, Inc., Wheaton, Ill.

Fig. 24-3. Typical attitude of horse with African horsesickness. Also notice the edema over the face, supraorbital fossae, and abdomen. Although this disease has not been reported in the United States, the rapid transportation of horses makes the spread to North America entirely possible.

What are the control procedures involved with African horsesickness?

Control is a most difficult and almost overwhelming problem. Widespread vaccination is the best solution so far, but the continuous natural development of new strains of African horsesickness makes absolute protection impossible.

Of course, guarding against insects is important, although only somewhat effective. Insect-proof stables, outdoor activities only in broad daylight, repellents, etc., are the control methods involved. Quarantines and strict transportation laws will help protect countries presently free of African horsesickness, but there is no guarantee that this will prevent the spread of the disease.

ASPERGILLOSIS

What is aspergillosis?

This is a fungal infection caused by any of various species of fungi of the genus *Aspergillus*. The fungi are common in nature, and may appear on feed and plants as white, fluffy mold.

How is the fungus transmitted to the horse?

Aspergillus fungi are usually inhaled from moldy hay or straw and may be taken into the body when moldy hay and other improperly cured feeds are eaten. The infection is most common in stabled horses, and may affect horses of any age. Horses that are in a weakened condition from a previous illness or that have been treated extensively with antibiotics seem to be most susceptible to infection. Antibiotics tend to alter the normal bacterial population of the intestine, allowing fungi from moldy feed to become established in the digestive tract.

What are the signs of aspergillosis?

Signs of the infection vary according to which organs of the body are involved. When the fungi are present in the digestive tract, diarrhea may be a sign of infection. Foal diarrhea due to heavy worm infestations can become persistent as a result of Aspergillus fungi multiplying and causing disease in the abnormal gut environment. In these cases, treating the diarrhea with antibiotics will probably only aggravate the condition. The fungi can infect the horse's guttural pouches (see Guttural Pouch Infection, page 337), causing a nasal discharge, nosebleed, difficulty in swallowing and various other signs. The lungs may develop abscesses and areas of dead tissue caused by the infection, leading to signs of respiratory disease. Abortion in mares can occur if the fungus invades the uterus either before or during pregnancy. The nervous system may be involved in the infection, causing such obvious signs as incoordination and a wobbly gait. Various other organs, including the liver and kidneys, are occasionally damaged by the fungi.

How is the disease diagnosed?

Since various nonspecific signs may be present, depending on the organs involved, diagnosis by a veterinarian is necessary to differentiate the condition from similar infections. Diagnosis may involve identifying the fungus in a sample of tissue, nasal or vaginal discharge, or feces.

Can the infection be treated?

No effective treatment is yet available. The disease can be fatal when vital organs are severely damaged, but horses with minor infections may recover spontaneously. Foals with persistent diarrhea may respond to treatment with an antifungal medication.

AZOTURIA OR "TYING-UP" SYNDROME

What is azoturia?

Azoturia is a condition associated with forced exercise after a period of rest ("Monday morning disease") during which feed has not been reduced. Upon resumption of exercise, the animal "ties up" or finds it painful to move.

What are the signs of azoturia?

The problem is characterized by profuse sweating, a rapid pulse, nervousness, a stiffness of gait and particular difficulty controlling the hindquarters, where the muscles are tense and painful. These signs begin 15 minutes to one hour after the beginning of exercise which is not necessarily vigorous. Myoglobin (muscle serum) may be found in the reddish-brown or black urine.

What is the difference between azoturia and the tying-up syndrome?

The causes are thought to be the same, but the syndromes differ in the degree of severity. A tied-up horse will show signs of stiffness and unwillingness to

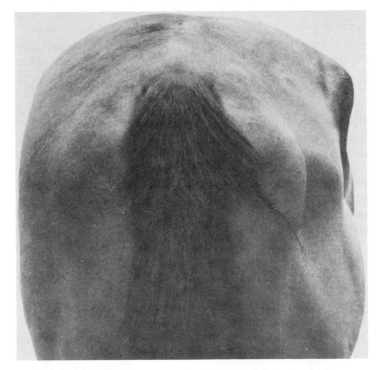

Photo courtesy of EQUINE MEDICINE AND SURGERY, Edition II, American Veterinary Publications, Inc., Wheaton, Ill.

Fig. 24-4. Atrophy of musculature over the right hip following a severe attack of exertional myopathy with myoglobinuria.

move, frequently some time after he has worked. This happens often with racehorses; during or after work, the stride may become shortened and appear stilted. The horse may or may not sweat excessively and the affected muscles of the loin and hindquarters feel tense and swollen when palpated. No treatment may be necessary, or the veterinarian may treat it with the same drugs as in azoturia. Kidney damage and muscle atrophy are not common in tying-up syndrome.

What causes tying-up or azoturia?

These conditions are said to be caused by an accumulation of glycogen, a carbohydrate storage compound, in the musculature. When the animal is exercised, the glycogen is broken down for energy and large amounts of lactic acid are formed and accumulated in the muscles. This lactic acid destroys the muscle cells, releasing myoglobin from the cells into the system. Usually, the acid is carried off by the vascular system and does no damage. It is the unusually large storage of available carbohydrates, and the inability of the blood to "wash" away the wastes formed (quickly enough) when they are produced in the muscles, that results in muscle fiber damage. The kidneys are not built to cleanse the blood of myoglobin, and kidney damage can result from these by-products of muscle damage.

What should be done with a severely or moderately tied-up horse?

If at all possible, the animal should not be moved, even to return to the stall. The veterinarian should be called while the horse is dried off and covered where he stands. Temporary shelter should be provided, if necessary, because serious damage is done if the horse is forced to move after the signs become apparent.

What is the treatment for azoturia?

The veterinarian will determine the severity of the case and treat the animal accordingly. Mild cases may require only a tranquilizer or sedative to relieve discomfort. Severe cases may be treated with muscle relaxers and sodium bicarbonate in solution to readjust the acid balance in the muscles. Keeping the horse standing is desirable, even if slings are required. Selenium and alpha-tocopherol are considered effective in treating and preventing recurrence of the disability. Also used are corticosteroids, thiamine, calcium borogluconate, physostigmine, insulin and various other drugs.

What is the prognosis for eventual recovery?

The prognosis is good for horses that remain standing, are not forced to move after the signs are noticed, and whose pulse returns to normal within 24 hours. If the horse does go down and remains quiet, the prognosis is still good if he can roll onto his sternum and prop himself up, and regains his feet after 24 hours or less. The prognosis is not good for a horse that remains restless while he is down, cannot roll upright on his sternum, or whose pulse does not return to normal after 24 hours.

What causes death in azoturia?

In severe cases, the renal (kidney) damage combines with the physical damage that happens when a horse lies down constantly and results in death. An autopsy will show muscles that are pale and bleached, their blood supply choked off by coagulation (clotting) in the small arteries.

Can horses have azoturia more than once?

One attack seems to predispose the horse to other attacks. Further attacks are not likely to be as severe, however, because owners are familiar with the apparent causes and recognize the signs more quickly than on the first occurrence.

Can attacks be prevented?

To a degree, yes, attacks can be prevented by careful regulation of diet. Reduction of a horse's feed during any periods of inactivity, gradual warm up before exercise, and careful cooling out procedures should decrease the incidence and severity of attacks.

When can the horse resume work?

After the pulse is normal, the horse should be rested 48 hours, on reduced feed, before light exercise is begun. Severely affected horses may be lame and show difficulty in moving, so the veterinarian will set a program for bringing the horse back to condition.

HYPERTHERMIA

What is hyperthermia?

Hyperthermia is heat exhaustion and heat stroke, both malfunctions of the body's heat-regulating mechanism.

What causes heat exhaustion?

Heat exhaustion is due to exposure to high environmental temperature, high humidity, and poor ventilation for prolonged periods. This causes the peripheral blood vessels to dilate, bringing about circulatory collapse and shock. The horse may be at light or heavy work, or may be stabled when this syndrome occurs. Horses may collapse hours after work, or after no work at all.

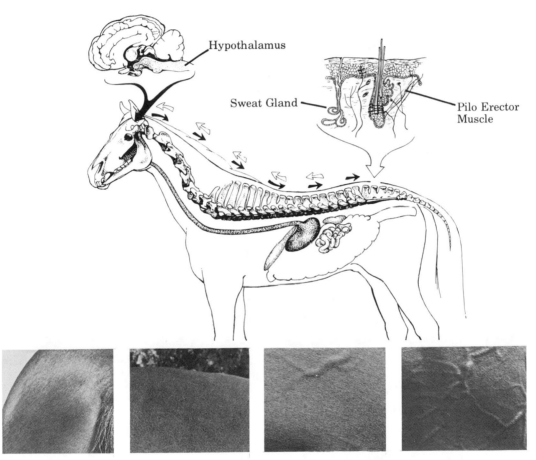

Fig. 24-5. Illustration shows the heat-regulating mechanism of the horse. Blood flow from the internal organs is controlled by the hypothalamus, as is the reaction of the vaso-dilator and pilo erector muscles of the blood vessels and skin. Heat is dispersed when the internal heat is brought to the surface of the skin.

1. Smooth hair. 2. Hair raised by pilo-erector muscles. 3. Normal appearance of blood vessels. 4. Distended blood vessles

What are the signs of heat exhaustion?

Most animals show signs of weakness, rapid breathing, muscular tremors and collapse. The pulse and body temperature may be moderately increased (105°-108° F) and the onset may be rather gradual. The animal sweats heavily.

What are the signs of heat stroke?

The principal signs are rapid, deep breathing and collapse. There may be a staring expression of the eyes. The body temperature rises considerably higher than in heat exhaustion (possibly up to 115°F), and the onset of collapse is more rapid. Sweating usually stops and heat stroke often results in death before treatment can be effective.

What are the differences between heat stroke and heat exhaustion?

Since most horses will sweat when subjected to conditions that cause heat stroke and heat exhaustion, one of the differences in heat stroke is the absence of sweating as the syndrome progresses. This is indicative of the advanced breakdown of the heat regulating mechanism of the body. Heat stroke is the more serious of the two conditions.

What is the treatment for heat exhaustion and heat stroke?

The most important factor is to reduce the body temperature by spraying with cold water, if possible. Standing the horse in ice water to constrict the vessels of the feet will help the circulatory system maintain adequate pressure for major body functions and will help prevent collapse. If the veterinarian can be called, he may administer fluids to replace those lost in sweating and in the failure of the peripheral circulatory system. Salicylates may also be given to draw fluids from the tissues into the blood stream and increase the volume of blood which carries heat from the skin. Fresh water should be made available and the horse should be placed where there is adequate ventilation, using fans, if necessary.

Can hyperthermia be prevented?

Yes. Care can be taken in conditioning animals, especially before performing work in the summer months. High humidity and temperature with the possibility of air stagnation should temper work periods, with frequent rest periods and water breaks. Salt must also be available at all times.

NUTRITIONAL MYOPATHY— WHITE MUSCLE DISEASE

What is nutritional myopathy?

Nutritional myopathy is a non-inflammatory degeneration of skeletal and heart muscle in foals. Although the disease is much more common in lambs, calves and pigs, it does occur in foals.

What causes nutritional myopathy?

The exact mechanism is not understood, but a deficiency of vitamin E and selenium appears to be the cause of this myopathy. It is thought that vitamin E prevents breakdown of the cells and their membranes, and selenium helps the body absorb vitamin E through the intestines and tissues. Absence of these two substances may allow the muscle tissues to degenerate.

What are the signs of nutritional myopathy?

Foals are usually affected between birth and seven months of age. If the deficiency is severe, myopathy may be acute, causing signs of difficulty in moving. Affected foals may quickly go down and be unable to rise. Death may follow within five hours in severe cases, resulting from pulmonary congestion, heart failure and edema. Less severe cases may show signs of gradually increasing stiffness of gait and stiff carriage of the head and neck. Some foals lose the ability to suck. If the deficiency is not corrected and the disease progresses, the foal will eventually go down and be unable to rise. Painful swellings beneath the skin may appear, due to accumulations of fluid and blood from the degenerating tissues. Difficulty in swallowing and sucking occur when the lingual and pharyngeal muscles deteriorate. This can result in inhalation pneumonia and starvation.

What is the treatment for nutritional myopathy?

Two injections of selenium, given a week apart, will most probably be recommended by the veterinarian. Vitamin E will also be given orally for three to five days. If this treatment is begun soon enough after the appearance of signs, recovery can occur. Some areas of the country are more prone to this disorder, due to a lack of selenium in the soil. In these areas, the veterinarian may wish to inject pregnant mares with selenium a month before they are due to foal, or he may give the foal selenium at birth. Selenium may be given to foals at monthly intervals if nutritional myopathy is anticipated because of area deficiencies.

HEREDITARY MULTIPLE EXOSTOSIS

What is hereditary multiple exostosis?

Hereditary multiple exostosis is a rare abnormality of the skeletal development. It is quite rare in horses, but has been reported in Quarter Horses and Thoroughbreds. Specifically, the disorder has been seen in a stallion and followed through numerous of his offspring. Research is currently being conducted to further determine the cause of the exostoses and the possibility of malignancy developing in the horse.

What are the signs of multiple exostosis?

The signs are usually present at birth or by the age of six months. Bony enlargements on both sides of the shoulders, ribs, hips and legs are characteristic of multiple exostosis. These lesions continue to grow and develop until the animal reaches maturity. No lameness or soreness seems to accompany the bony enlargements, which occur in various sizes and shapes.

What causes multiple exostosis?

From the pattern of appearance in a stallion's line, the condition appears to be hereditary, the result of a single dominant gene. Exostoses do not always develop near growth plates or areas of stress, but develop from small, gray-blue foci found on the surface of most bones of the body. These focal areas seem to be sites of early maturation of the bone cartilage which build up abnormal mounds of bone that are covered by the periosteum (bone membrane). In some human cases, the exostoses have been known to become malignant.

What is the treatment for this condition?

There has been no treatment reported, since malignancy has not been noted in the horse. Breeding to affected stallions might be discouraged if show animals are desired. The lesions can occur in areas that would also prevent the affected animal's use as a pleasure or working horse.

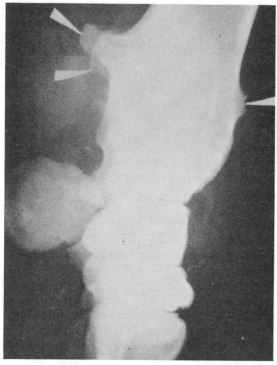

Fig. 24-6. Hereditary Multiple Exostosis. Pointers indicate the areas of exostosis on the distal end of the radius. Similar growths may occur at the distal end of the tibia; exostosis over the ribs also occurs.

Photo courtesy of LAMENESS IN HORSES, Edition III, O. R. Adams, Lea and Febiger Publishing Co., Philadelphia, Pa.

INSECT VENOMS

What are the effects of insect venoms on the horse?

The most toxic insect venom comes from bees and wasps. Some bee venom contains complex toxins that act upon the nervous system of the horse. Single stings may be fatal if the horse has been sensitized to the venom by stings in the past. Stings are most serious when they occur on the head, since the swelling may interfere with breathing. Serious swelling may also occur from numerous ant bites if the horse pushes his nose into an ant hill while grazing.

What are the signs of insect stings and bites?

The most obvious signs of insect stings or bites are the swellings that they cause. Usually, the reaction is just local swelling and discomfort. If large numbers of insects attack a horse, however, a generalized systemic reaction may occur. In rare cases, the horse may rapidly collapse and die. Swelling of the nose and lips may cause difficulty in breathing or eating and the pain of numerous bites may cause the horse to appear excited and restless. Severe reactions to insect venom include diarrhea, jaundice of mucous membranes, the presence of blood in the urine and a very rapid heartbeat.

What is the treatment for insect bites and stings?

Local treatment with weak ammonia or sodium bicarbonate may bring some relief. The veterinarian may use adrenalin or epinephrine to stimulate the nervous system if a general reaction occurs to the venoms. Antihistamines are often used. Surgery may be necessary to provide an airway for free breathing if swelling threatens to close the air passages.

SNAKEBITE

Do snakes frequently bite horses?

In certain areas of the country, snakebite is fairly common. The most aggressive snake in the United States is the rattlesnake. Snakebites from copperheads and moccasins are also common in the horse, and their venoms are very similar to that of the rattlesnake. The only other poisonous snake found in the United States is the coral snake whose venom is neurotoxic. Coral snakes are not widely distributed in the United States (Florida and the deep south only) and are not very aggressive, so their bites are rare in horses.

How serious is a bite from the rattlesnake?

Due to the curious nature of the horse that is bitten, most snakebites occur somewhere on the head, the most serious area in which a horse may be bitten. Bites also may occur on the legs or chest, but they are less serious there. The danger also depends on whether the horse was exercising just before the snakebite (exercise spreads the venom faster) and upon the size of the snake. Large snakes are capable of injecting more snake venom per bite. Rattlesnake venom, which causes the breakdown of blood and protein, gives rise to tremendous swelling in the region of the bite, often causing the nasal passages to be swollen shut. If veterinary help is not available immediately, this may be the most serious aspect of the snakebite.

What are the signs of a snakebite?

Snakebite is most frequent during the first warm days of spring and throughout the summer. The first sign of snakebite is usually extreme swelling around the bite. If the horse is bitten on the head, the whole nose may become edematous and the nasal mucosa may swell greatly. A bloodstained, frothy exudate may be seen at the nostrils, due to the passage of the exudate through the skin tissues. Swelling usually extends to the eyes, which may be swollen shut. The ears may be swollen and allowed to droop straight out to the sides. Involvement of the nasal passages causes loud, labored breathing. Most horses become extremely depressed and weak; Thoroughbreds and other well-bred horses are extremely susceptible to the effects of snake venom, which causes a rapid, weak heartbeat.

What treatment should be given to a bitten horse?

The best treatment is antivenin, which is expensive, but is developed to treat bites from snakes in each area of the country. Horses should not be ridden or trailered to the veterinarian, if possible, because exercise will help spread the venom through the horse's system. First aid includes making shallow incisions in the bite and using a suction cup to remove the venom (if the bite is discovered very soon after it happened). Tourniquets may be placed two inches above the bite (if on a limb) and loosened for two or three minutes every twenty minutes. Recovery often depends on obtaining rapid help from the veterinarian. The veterinarian will probably wish to give the horse a tetanus booster, wide spectrum antibiotics (to combat infection carried by snakes), corticosteroids to limit the inflammatory response, and fluids to support the horse and combat the shock that accompanies snakebite. Due to local infection and tissue damage from the venom and swelling, the area around the snakebite frequently sloughs, so aftercare by the veterinarian will usually be necessary. If treated quickly and properly, snakebite is rarely fatal.

CANTHARIDIN POISONING
(BLISTER BEETLES)

What is cantharidin poisoning?

Cantharidin is a poisonous substance that is found in the tissues of the blister beetle *(Epicauta vitatta)*. This poison is very irritating to the digestive tract and causes severe kidney damage.

How do horses come in contact with blister beetles?

Horses are poisoned with cantharidin when blister beetles are accidentally included in alfalfa hay. Some harvesting machines that cut and crimp the hay in one operation crush the beetles in the hay. They are then dried and baled with the alfalfa. Due to their feeding habits, hundreds of beetles may be trapped in a single "flake" or "block" of hay.

What are the signs of cantharidin poisoning?

If the horse eats more than a few beetles, the signs may be acute, including profound shock and death within a few hours. Lesser amounts of cantharidin causes signs of severe irritation to the mucous membranes of the mouth and intestinal tract. Affected horses may keep their noses in the water trough, playing with their tongues in the water to try and wash away the burning chemical. Colicky behaviour is common, and diarrhea may be present. Most horses that live longer than six to eight hours pass small amounts of blood-tinged urine frequently. There may also be clots of blood in the urine and feces due to the damaging effects of cantharidin on the intestines and kidneys. Sweating usually occurs and may accompany a fever of up to 106°F, with a rapid, thready pulse. Incoordination and

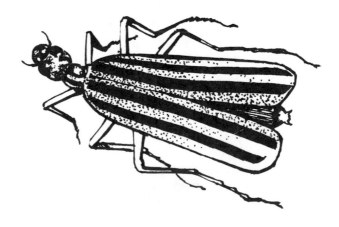

Fig. 24-7. Drawing of a blister beetle.

convulsions sometimes occur. Frequently, pulmonary edema develops, and froth appears at the nose and mouth just before death.

What is the treatment for cantharidin poisoning?

If the veterinarian is called in time, there are several things that can be done. Corticosteroids may be used to minimize shock and a protective coating may be administered by stomach tube, to prevent further absorption of the toxin. Oily substances should not be used, however, because cantharidin is soluble (mixes easily) in oil. Fluid therapy may be used to help maintain the chemical balance in the horse's body. Alfalfa hay should be regularly checked, particularly in the southwest, to prevent feeding blister beetles to horses.

FLUOROSIS

What is fluorosis?

Fluorosis is a chronic disorder caused by continuous consumption of toxic amounts of fluoride. Fluoride is normally found in small amounts in soils, water, vegetation and the air. Fluoride poisoning may be acute if excessively large amounts are ingested over a short period of time.

What causes fluorosis?

Fluorosis is usually caused by the ingestion of unnecessary amounts of fluoride over a long period of time. Since fluoride is stored by the teeth and bones, signs of fluorosis are first seen in the mouth. In order to store fluoride, the body allows this element to replace part of the calcium structure in teeth and bones. This takes place only in actively growing teeth—mature, already-formed teeth are not affected. If the fluoride is ingested in very large amounts, the fluoride acts directly on the tissues of the digestive system, causing severe gastroenteritis.

What are the sources of excessive fluoride?

In the United States, fluorosis is usually caused by the contamination of drinking water and pasture with excessive fluoride. Feed supplements may also cause fluorosis if the phosphates in them contain fluoride. In other countries, volcanic ash, industrial contamination and the feeding of phosphate rock supplements are causes of fluorosis.

Drinking water contamination comes from ground surface levels of fluoride or from fluoride-bearing rock beneath the surface. Phosphatic limestone is frequently the cause of surface and pasture contamination.

What are the signs of chronic fluorosis?

Since most horse's teeth are not frequently examined, fluorosis may first be discovered by the intermittent lameness it usually causes. The fluoride is most commonly deposited on the periosteal (outer covering) surface of the long bones of the legs and the jaw. This results in a disturbance of this layer and the production of painful, bony enlargements, characterized by abnormal bone tissue and lameness. Exercise or work causes this lameness to become more severe. Pain is evident, even if the horse is not worked, by shifting positions frequently and assuming unnatural or awkward leg positions. In many cases, the hair coat is poor (and sheds slowly), the skin is less pliable than normal, and tooth defects may be visible. Bony deposits on the nose result in a characteristic "Roman nose."

If the teeth were forming during excessive fluoride ingestion, there will be mottling, staining, incomplete development and excessive wearing-away (abrasion). The presence of excessive fluoride allows unusual brown or black discoloration. The mottled areas become pits, the teeth are brittle and appear dull and opaque (not translucent and shiny like normal enamel).

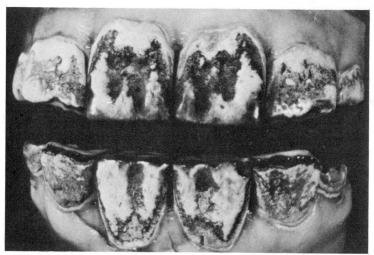

Courtesy of LAMENESS IN HORSES, Edition III, O. R. Adams, Lea and Febiger Publishing Co., Philadelphia, Pa.

Fig. 24-8. Permanent incisor teeth in a 5-year-old Thoroughbred mare with fluorosis. Notice the discoloration and abnormal abrasion and pitting of the enamel.

What are the effects of these signs?

The tooth discolorations are visible indicators of the abnormal bone and calcium structure in affected horses. Discolored teeth wear badly and tend to decay. Gum abscesses and abscesses of the jaw may be due to the poor teeth. In some cases, the teeth may wear so excessively that the horse is unable to chew food at all. Bony enlargements of the legs from fluoride deposits result in osteomalacia, osteoporosis and exostoses due to mobilization of calcium and phosphorus that are joined to the fluoride. Affected bones fracture easily, with little cause. Severe anemia may occur if bone marrow activity is affected. The coffin bone is often enlarged and roughened, increasing pressure within the foot and contributing to the lameness.

What are the signs of acute fluorosis?

Approximately 30 minutes following accidental ingestion of large amounts of fluoride, an animal may show signs of excitement, colic, diarrhea, stiffness, excessive salivation and incontinence. Alternate muscle spasms and relaxation (clonic convulsions), weakness and severe depression are seen before death follows from heart failure. Fluoride (in large amounts) forms a strong acid when it reaches the stomach and causes extensive damage to the intestinal mucosa. This allows toxins from the digestive tract to attack body tissues which causes shock and depression of normal body functions.

Can fluorosis be treated?

Acute fluorosis may be treated with gastrointestinal sedatives, substances to neutralize the fluorine in the digestive tract and calcium salts administered intravenously. Aluminum salts have been found to be effective in neutralizing the acid formed in the stomach. Treatment often has to be repeated for satisfactory results. Glucose is often administered to offset the effects of fluoride on glucose metabolism.

Chronic fluorosis may be treated by removing the animals from contaminated areas while teeth are forming or by preventing ingestion of contaminated feed and water. Since fluoride may be passed through the placenta, mature broodmares should be protected from excessive levels of fluoride in food and water. Bone and tooth lesions cannot be corrected by any means, but good quality feed should be supplied to horses with affected teeth. Due to difficulties in chewing and digestion caused by malformed teeth, hay may need to be chopped or pelleted for affected horses.

25

WOUNDS, DRUGS, AND TREATMENTS

WOUNDS AND TREATMENTS

What is a wound?

Technically any bodily injury caused by physical means that results in disruption of the continuity of structures or tissues is called a wound. There are several types of wounds, however.

What are the different types of wounds?

Wounds are classified as being (1) incised, (2) abrasions, (3) contusions, (4) lacerations, (5) punctures and (6) burns. Each type of wound varies in severity according to the location and degree of its damage.

How are wounds treated?

Most wounds can be treated by the horseman if they do not involve the eye or deep structures such as muscles, tendons, bones or joints. Involvement of these structures can cause permanent disability if they are not treated properly, so a veterinarian should be called.

Fig. 25-1. This wound of the lower leg involved the extensor tendon. Such wounds should not be treated without the supervision of a veterinarian.

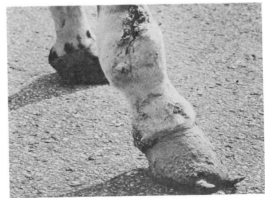

What is the first concern in wound treatment?

The most alarming aspect of some wounds is the copious bleeding that occurs. Bleeding may be controlled by tourniquets, if the wound is on a limb, by ice packs or by pressure bandages. It must be remembered, though, that a moderate amount of bleeding is useful in cleansing wounds of debris. If bleeding cannot be controlled within a few minutes, or if the blood is spurting from a wound, a veterinarian should be called immediately.

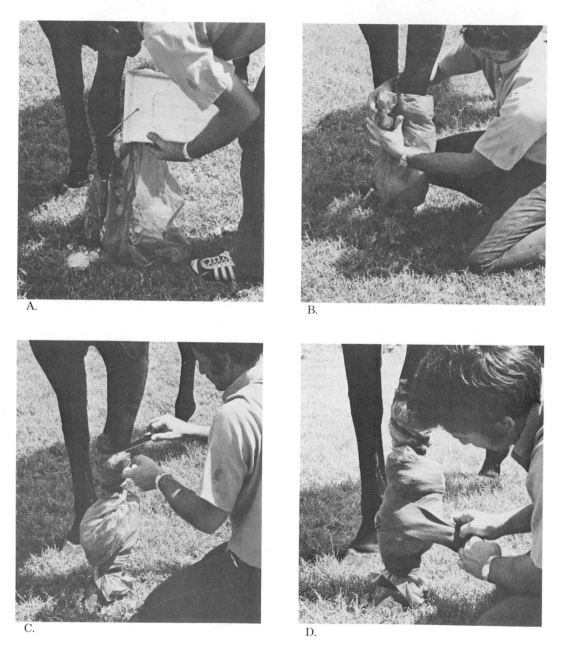

Fig. 25-2. Figures A-D show the application of an emergency ice pack. Ice is placed in a plastic bag, which is taped in place. A stretch bandage is then applied to keep the ice close to the leg.

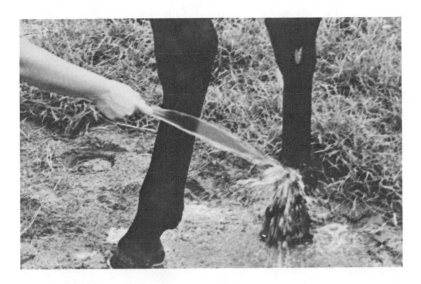

Fig. 25-3. Cleaning a wound with a gentle stream of water prevents grinding foreign matter into the damaged tissues.

When the bleeding is controlled, what next?

When the bleeding has stopped, the next concern is to remove all foreign particles from the wound. In most cases, a hose with a slight stream of water works very well. Harsh antiseptics are useless, and may cause more damage to the injured tissues. (see Drugs and Their Actions, p. 659.) Rinsing with clear water may be accompanied by washing with a mild soap and water, if the wound exudate has caked or dirt has been ground into the injury. Once the wound is clean, evaluation can be made of its severity. If it appears that the bone or tendon sheath is involved, the veterinarian should be called before any further treatment is given. It is a good idea to have the veterinarian stop by with some tetanus antitoxin, especially if the wound is caused by objects around the barn.

What should be done after the wound is cleaned?

Once the wound is clean, very little needs to be done. Efforts to aid healing may include a *clean* bandage to protect the wound from flies and dirt. Dry powders may interfere with granulation, so do not apply dusts or powders to a *fresh* wound. If there has been a loss of tissue (a gouge or hole in the skin), granulation must fill in the gap before it can heal over. A saline solution (one teaspoon salt to one pint sterile water) can be used to keep the area free of accumulated exudates and restore the normal salt balance around the damaged tissues.

Should clean wounds be bandaged?

The bandaging of wounds depends upon their location. Bandaging often helps leg wounds heal and fill in lost tissue without constant fly irritation or contamination. A properly applied bandage can reduce the movement of the injured area, often enough to promote healing. Wounds that are very extensive (of the forearm, for example) often heal better if they are bandaged because the edges of the skin are brought closer together and the open surface of the wound is reduced. Many wounds of the upper body are difficult to bandage and do not benefit greatly by the restriction of movement that bandaging can accomplish. These types of wounds should be gently cleaned every day and protected from flies.

What medication, if any, does a wounded horse require?

Many horses benefit from antibiotics, but the veterinarian must prescribe the proper ones for the type of infection that may be present. Tetanus antitoxin is advisable as a preventative, however, if the horse is on a regular schedule of tetanus toxoid injections a toxoid booster should be given instead. Besides preventing new infection in the wound, the horseman can ensure proper healing if the horse is eating good quality feed. A balanced diet is always important, but even more so when the body is being stressed by inflammation and healing processes (see page 2). Hydrotherapy (a fairly strong stream of water from a hose) often stimulates the healing process and also keeps the wound free of exudate and debris, especially if it is not bandaged. Hydrotherapy should normally be done once or twice daily for about twenty minutes during the granulation phase of wound healing. Restraint may sometimes be necessary to keep the horse from chewing on, or rubbing, a healing wound. Cross ties, neck cradles, and side sticks can sometimes prevent further damage to healing tissues. Fly control is very important, to prevent wound infection and irritation to the horse.

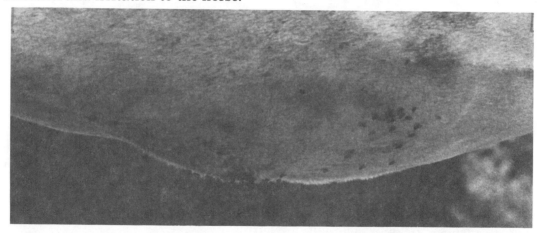

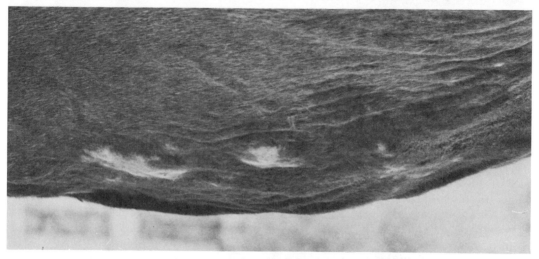

Fig. 25-4. Lack of proper fly control (top photo) can result in the formation of excessive fibrous tissue (bottom photo).

Can anything be done to prevent wounds?

A serious wound often prompts clean-up operations around a barn. Old boards can be replaced in fences, and loose nails, wires that project and broken boards can be removed. Jagged pieces of tin, bent metal buckets, baling wire, and trash should be repaired, replaced and picked up. It may seem strange, but veterinarians comment that few injuries occur around clean, well-kept barns and fences. Fencing does not have to be fancy, but it should be maintained tight and strong.

What is an incision?

An incision is the ideal wound, in many respects. Caused by very sharp objects (like a surgical scalpel or a piece of sharp metal, glass, etc.) the edges of the wound are cleanly cut, with a minimum of crushing or tearing and bleed freely. Incisions frequently heal very well if they do not become infected. However, due to the sharp edge that causes incisions, underlying muscle and nerves are likely to be cut, especially if the incision is accidental.

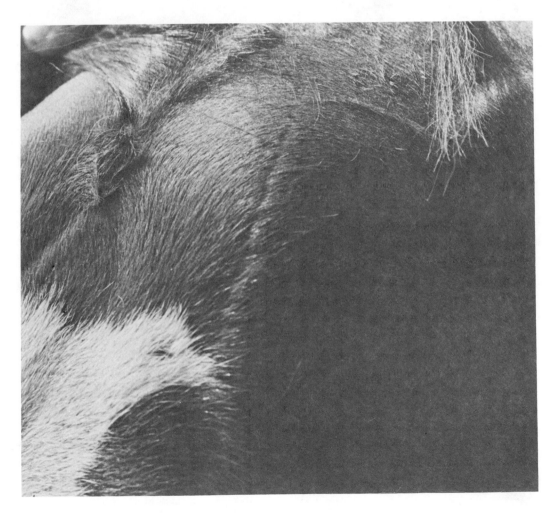

Fig. 25-5. This accidental incision healed with only a fine, hairline scar. Ideally, all wounds would heal this way. Head wounds like this often heal very well because there is a minimum of movement in this area.

How are incisions treated?

Treatment of an incision is determined by the amount of tissue damage it causes. This is the best type of wound to suture, if it is not infected. If incisions occur on the lower leg, suturing is often not recommended because the skin is not loose and the sutures would probably be under too much tension to heal properly. Shallow incisions should be gently cleaned (see general treatment of wounds) and bandaged if they are on the lower leg. Incisions often heal with minimal scars if they are protected and do not become infected or torn open again.

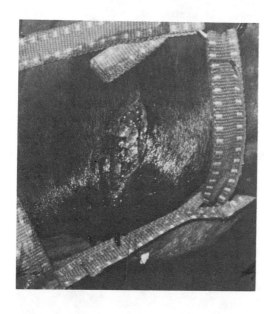
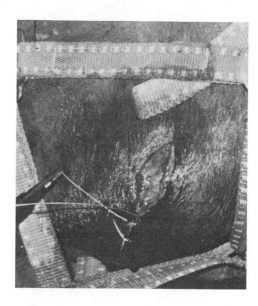
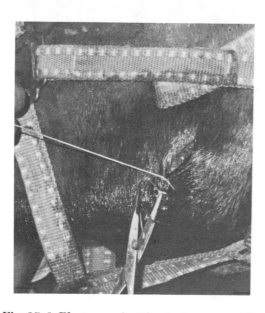
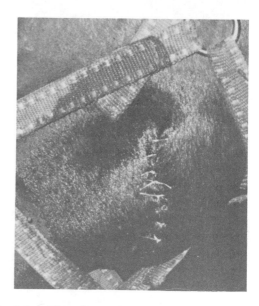

Fig. 25-6. Photographs of suturing an accidental incision. The edges of this wound were even enough that no trimming was required before they were sutured. Also, this wound is on the cheek, an ideal location for suturing.

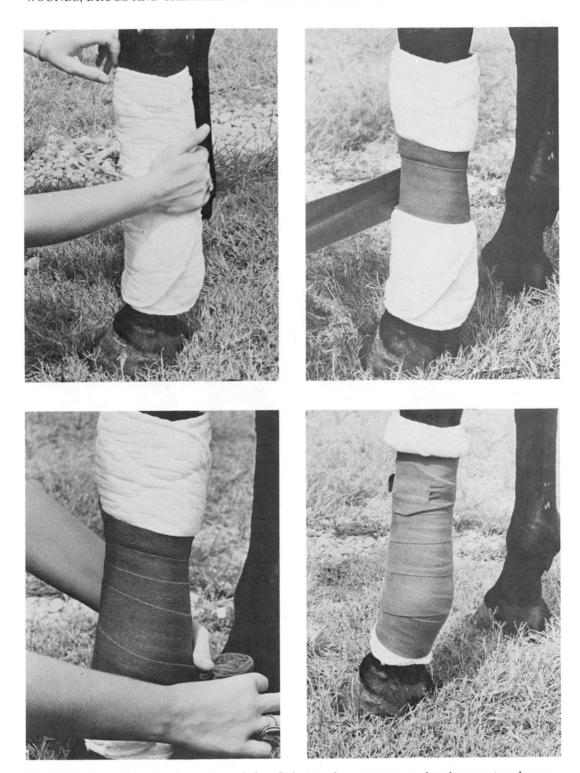

Fig. 25-7. Steps in bandaging a horse's leg. It is very important to maintain even tension on the wrap. A loose wrap or an excessively-tight segment could cause a disruption of circulation to a small segment of tissue, commonly referred to as a "wrap bump."

What is an abrasion?

An abrasion is a wound caused by rubbing or friction (rope burns are typical abrasions). Characteristically, only the top layer of skin and hair are rubbed off, but sometimes deeper tissues are involved. Abrasions usually seep serum or blood and tend to stay moist and messy.

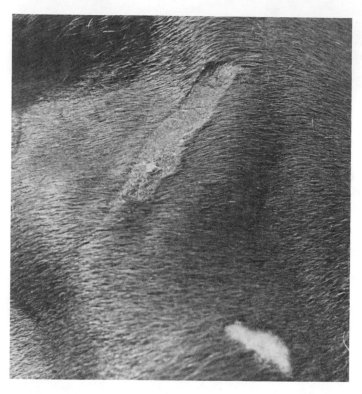

Fig. 25-8. Above, simple abrasions that involve the loss of hair and the top layers of skin. The noticeable "scab" on the upper wound is formed of dried serum, which protects the growing tissue underneath.

Fig. 25-9. Below, a rope burn that was not treated resulted in the formation of "proud flesh".

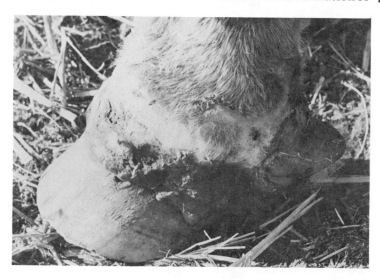

What treatment is used with abrasions?

Abrasions are usually washed gently and treated with a soothing gel (tannic jelly, panalog). Bandages keep the bare area clean and help the area to form a scab. Rope burns of the lower leg frequently form excessive granulation tissue, which can be prevented by a snug bandage or removed with the use of escharotics like "Granulex" or butter of antimony, under the supervision of a veterinarian.

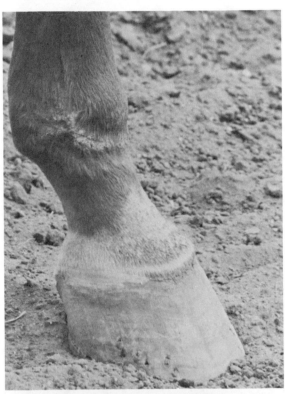

Fig. 25-10. The closer a wound is to the hoof, the more likely it is to form excessive granulation tissue. This abrasion healed with a great deal of fibrous tissue because harsh antiseptics were used excessively.

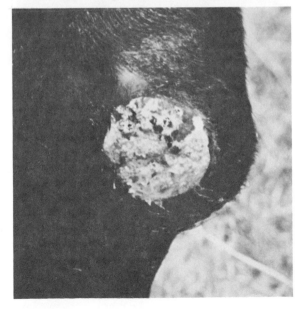

Fig. 25-11. Excessive granulation tissue is being removed from this abrasion. Butter of antimony (an escharotic) causes the tissue to turn white when it is burned off by the destructive action of the medication.

What is a contusion?

A contusion is a bruise, a wound that does not involve a break in the skin. They usually are characterized by swelling and bleeding beneath the skin. Contusions may mask fractures and tears of ligaments, in which case they should be referred to a veterinarian. Kicks, blows and falls are the usual causes of contusions.

How are contusions treated?

Contusions can cause a great deal of pain, due to the movement of bruised tissues and the pressure of the accompanying swellings. Ice packs can constrict blood vessels and slow down hemorrhage, and often prevent lameness in contusions of the lower leg. Application of heat after the bleeding has stopped, either from heat packs or rubbing with liniments, helps the body to reabsorb the fluid and aids circulation in the bruised area. Blows to the eye should always be treated by a veterinarian, due to the possibility of blindness.

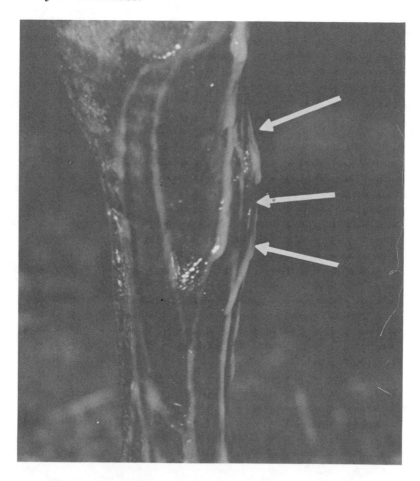

Fig. 25-12. This contusion on the outside of the cannon is about 48 hours old. Most contusions, if they do not involve the bone, reach the height of their heat and swelling when they are 48 to 72 hours old. They begin to slow down on the inflammatory process when 7 days have passed, and most contusions start to resolve when they have had 2 weeks of treatment. The veterinarian has applied an antiphlogistic dressing to this wound, which will then be bandaged. Treatment with cold water and rubbing will help the inflammatory swelling recede with a minimum of adhesions left to cause a fibrous "bump". Wrapping the injury and giving the horse light exercise will also increase the circulation to the damaged tissues.

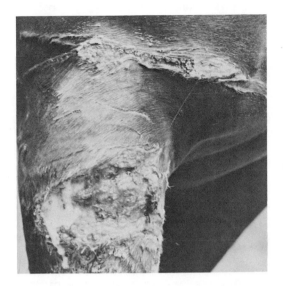

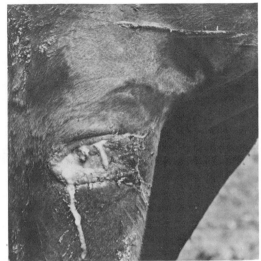

Fig. 25-13. Extensive lacerations like this one cannot be sutured because of the large area of tissue avulsion. This one was able to heal with very little scarring, which often happens with wounds of the forearm. Even without bandaging this wound healed very rapidly, due to the care it received and the fly control that was exercised.

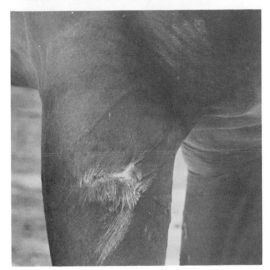

What is a laceration?

A laceration is a wound in which the edges are torn and irregular. If tissue is torn away, the wound is called an avulsion. The most frequent cause of lacerations is barbed wire. These wounds do not bleed as freely as incisions, and are likely to undergo a period of sloughing, during which damaged tissues, or those with an inadequate blood supply, are separated from healthy tissue.

How are lacerations treated?

Lacerations should be carefully cleaned and treated with a non-irritating dressing. If lacerations are deep, the veterinarian should be called in to administer antibiotics and prevent infection of the wound. Most lacerations of the lower body benefit from snug bandaging; in fact, severe lacerations of the hoof should be completely bandaged. Healing of a large laceration will seem to be very slow for the first week, but keeping the wound clean and free from fly irritation is the most important part of treatment. The veterinarian may decide to trim the torn edges of the laceration to obtain a good blood supply at the healing surface and reduce the size of the scar that will be formed.

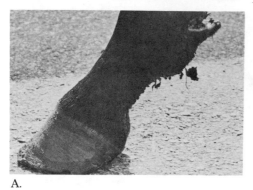 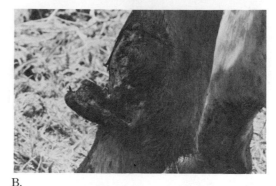

A.　　　　　　　　　　　　　　　　　　　　　　　　B.

Fig. 25-14. Figures A & B. Lacerations often need to be trimmed by the veterinarian. These will not drain properly because the loose skin is attached at the lower portion of the wound. The veterinarian will either remove the skin flaps (if they do not have a good blood supply), or he will freshen the edges of the torn flaps and open a drainage area at the lowest point of the wound.

What are punctures?

Punctures are small surface wounds that are deeper than they are wide. Typical punctures occur when a horse steps on a nail. Especially if they are located on the lower body, punctures are prone to infection. Debris and bacteria are usually deposited in the deepest part of the wound, often causing abscesses to form. These wounds are often overlooked until the spreading infection causes the horse to go lame or to show signs of fever and lack of appetite.

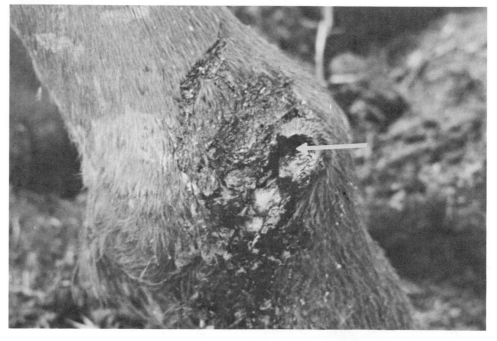

Fig. 25-15. The arrow points to the deepest point of this puncture wound. Since this wound is on the fetlock, it will be necessary to bandage it to keep the wound clean.

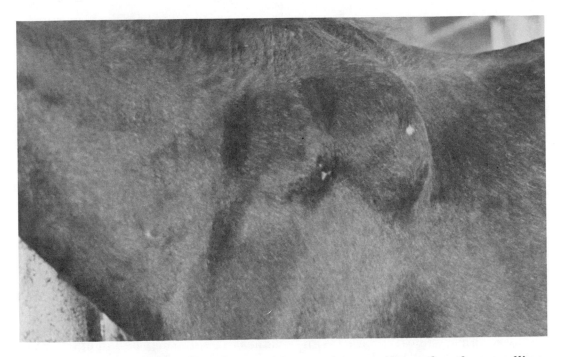

Fig. 25-16. Punctures caused by thorns or stickers can become abscessed, as these swellings illustrate.

What is the treatment for puncture wounds?

Puncture wounds should be treated as soon as possible after they occur. Hydrogen peroxide may be used to irrigate the puncture, which accomplishes both cleaning and the introduction of air into the wound. Many bacteria that are carried into puncture wounds do not multiply well in the presence of air. Tetanus antitoxin should always be given to a horse with a puncture wound, regardless of when it is discovered. Since puncture wounds often do not drain well, the veterinarian may want to increase the size of the external opening, to make sure that the wound heals from the inside out. Antibiotics are a good idea for treatment of puncture wounds; the veterinarian may suggest their use in the wound and systemically for four or five days.

Fig. 25-17. Puncture wounds of the foot are often treated with iodine, after the wound has been cut down and enlarged for drainage.

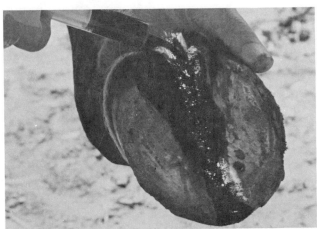

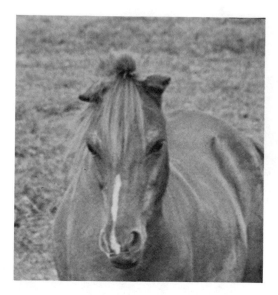

Fig. 25-18. The "cropped" or frostbitten ears on this mare were caused by cold "burns".

What is a burn?

Burns are caused by excessive heat, excessive cold (frostbite), electric currents and by certain chemicals (like acids and alkalies). The skin may be damaged, or the underlying bone and muscle may also be involved. Large surface burns are more serious than small, deep ones because a larger area is involved and the fluid loss will be greater. Severe burns and scalds may cause shock, toxemia and infection, and death. The veterinarian should supervise the treatment of most burns because shock is often present.

How are burns treated?

Burns should not be treated by the horseman with oil, grease, baking soda, iodine or any other irritating substance. Chemical burns should first be neutralized, then cleaned and treated as for other burns. Acids should be neutralized with an alkaline solution (one tablespoon of baking soda to one pint warm water). Corrosive alkalies (like quicklime) may be neutralized with an acid solution (half vinegar, half warm water). After burns have been cleaned with mild soap and water, they may be soaked with a warm saline solution (one teaspoon salt to one pint warm water) and dressed with tannic acid jelly, or an acriflavine (1 to 1,000) solution. Light gauze dressings can be bandaged in place to avoid contamination of the open wound. Burns caused by electric shock are usually secondary in importance to the systemic shock which usually accompanies them, and require the treatment of a veterinarian (see Shock, page 1).

DRUGS AND THEIR ACTIONS

What actions can drugs perform?

Drugs are organic or chemical substances used in or on the body of the horse in order to maintain its health. Some of them act by altering natural body processes of inflammation, edema, the sensation of pain, the functioning of the various organs, or the build-up of immunity to disease. Other drugs act upon the infectious organisms and parasites that can attack and harm the body.

What drugs alter inflammation?

While many drugs change the course of inflammation indirectly, there are drugs which serve the primary purpose of reducing it. Adrenocorticotropic hormone (ACTH), which is manufactured naturally by the pituitary gland, suppresses this normal tissue response to injury and infection by a mechanism which is not well understood. ACTH and similar drugs (such as cortisone and hydrocortisone) are now made synthetically for this purpose.

In the natural state, though, the body evidently uses these hormones for purposes other than controlling inflammation, so their effect on the body may not be totally desirable. It is known, for instance, that they can produce edema (watery swelling). To avoid these difficulties, non-hormonal substances such as phenylbutazone have come into use. In milder cases of inflammation, the effects can sometimes be reduced externally.

Are there drugs which reduce inflammation externally?

If the inflammation is non-infectious (resulting, for instance, from a "clean" injury or wound), a poultice applied to the site can be of tremendous help in reducing it. Denver Mud and Unna's Paste may be applied directly to the skin, but other antiphlogistic (anti-inflammatory) preparations such as magnesium sulfate or boric acid paste are usually too irritating to the tissues for direct use. Veterinarians sometimes recommend the use of a specific antiphlogistic following surgery.

Recently, enzymes such as streptodornase, streptokinase, and trypsin have been applied directly in the treatment of wounds. Their function is to remove fibrin and other body products from the site of the injury, which allows other drugs to fight the infection. This procedure has been reported to be quite successful, and some dressings (bandages) are now available impregnated with enzymes. Sprays are also available with enzymes (Granulex) which remove or prevent the build-up of wound secretions.

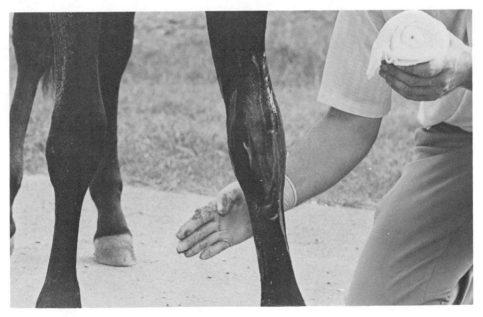

Fig. 25-19. Some antiphlogistic dressings may be applied directly to the skin, as the veterinarian is doing here.

Are there drugs that deliberately produce inflammation?

Inflammation is generally a beneficial process. This fact has led to the development of drugs that can cause inflammation in order to speed up healing. The inflammation may be produced by a rubefacient (liniment), which causes only redness and swelling, a resciant, which results in blisters, or a caustic which burns, corrodes and kills skin and underlying tissue. Generally one substance such as iodine, mercury or an aromatic oil, mixed in varying strength, can produce any or all of these reactions. Familiar liniments (like Medi-Kool and Absorbine) can be applied with greater frequency, which increases their effect. An example of their use would be the application of a resciant to a non-strangulated, reducible umbilical hernia (see Umbilical Hernia, page 277). This method usually causes a healing of the rupture which allowed the hernia to descend.

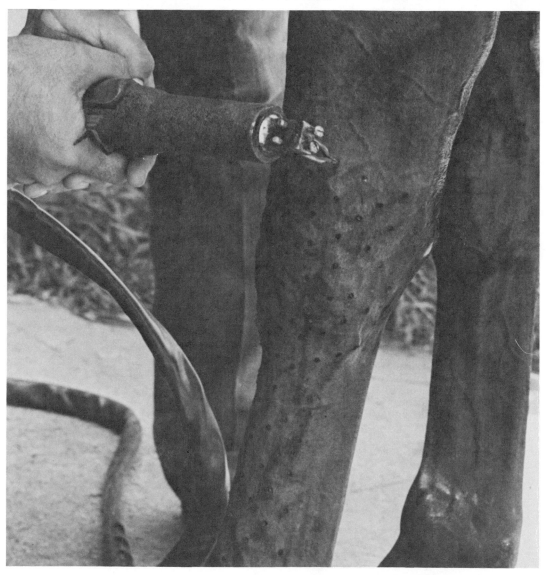

Fig. 25-20. The procedure of "firing" is the most common artificial use of the process of inflammation.

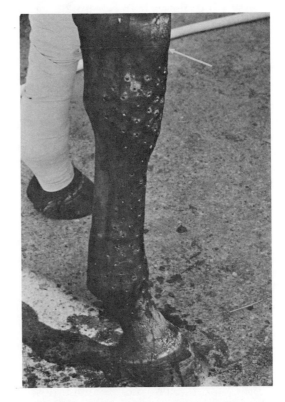

Fig. 25-21. The appearance of the leg after it has been fired. Notice the ring of swelling (arrow) where the nerve block was injected.

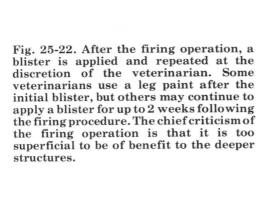

Fig. 25-22. After the firing operation, a blister is applied and repeated at the discretion of the veterinarian. Some veterinarians use a leg paint after the initial blister, but others may continue to apply a blister for up to 2 weeks following the firing procedure. The chief criticism of the firing operation is that it is too superficial to be of benefit to the deeper structures.

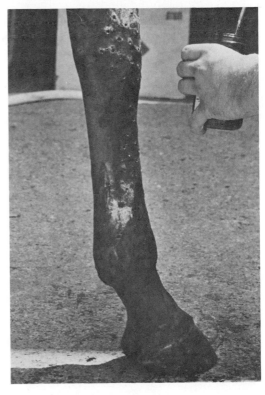

How do drugs alter edema?

Edema is usually limited or reduced by use of a diuretic. These drugs act upon the system in such a way that excess fluids are removed through increased urine production. Some compounds containing mercury, such as mellauride sodium are effective for this purpose, or drugs like theobromide, which contain xanthine, may be used. Supportive bandages are also used to prevent edema of the legs.

How do drugs alter the sensation of pain?

The discovery of effective pain killers has made surgery possible for horses. In fact, a large number of drugs used in veterinary medicine have been developed to help in surgery. Probably the first of these were ether and chloroform, which are general anesthetics. This group of drugs serves to limit the perception of pain by rendering the patient unconscious. The patient is usually administered the drug as an inhalant, through a device called a closed-system gas machine. Chloroform and ether were found to have some bad side effects (particularly respiratory damage), and have been largely replaced by a more refined "new generation" of inhalant gases, like halothane and methoxyflurane.

Amytal sodium, nembutal and pentothal sodium also induce unconsciousness, but they are given intravenously.

If surgery is not major, a veterinarian may frequently choose a local anesthetic. Most of these drugs were originally derived from cocaine, and it was discovered that injecting then under the skin prevented nerves from sending bio-electric impulses back to the central nervous system. Although strict regulation has limited the use of cocaine, synthetic substances such as procaine and lidocaine are widely used in the same manner. The pain which follows surgery can be treated locally by these same drugs, but longer lasting relief may be had from systemic treatment with phenylbutazone.

Severe pain following surgery or injury, or pain which accompanies some kinds of illness, may call for more general relief. This can be afforded by synthetic narcotics such as Demerol® or Talwin®. Pain relief can also be obtained (in some cases) by simply relaxing the smooth muscles, which can be done by administering dipyrone, for example.

Much of the time effective medical attention calls for the use of a drug to make the horse more cooperative. A horse that becomes excited, for instance, prior to medical attention, can be calmed through the use of a tranquilizer like Acepromazine. If, on the other hand, a horse has difficulty regaining consciousness at a desirable rate after surgery, stimulants like amphetamine may be administered. In recent years, there have been abuses of tranquilizers by trainers who could not handle fully conscious horses, and "uppers" have been used to win races on unsupervised tracks. There is, of course, no substitute for good training and management, and drugs should be left to the realm of medicine. Most of these drugs are legal only when they are used by or under the strict supervision of a veterinarian.

How can drugs alter the functioning of the organs?

The actions of the organs are mostly controlled by the autonomic nervous system (see Autonomic Nervous System, page 552). It may be helpful to intervene in their natural action when, for instance, the horse is having spasms of the intestinal tract. The administration of atropine has the effect of calming the smooth muscles of the intestine, which would stop the spasms. On the other hand, if evacuation of the intestines was desired, their digestive movements could be "stepped up" with carbachol. Constriction of the pupil of the eye is also controlled through the autonomic nervous system, and if it needs to be constricted (as it does, for example, in the treatment of glaucoma), this end may be accomplished by applying pilocarpine directly to the surface of the eye.

Can drugs build up immunity to disease in a horse?

Each species has certain diseases that it simply does not get, almost without exception. There are no known cases, for instance, of a horse getting hoof and mouth disease. This quality is known as "natural immunity," and no known medical procedure can provide protection from disease that is quite so certain. Immunization that can be stimulated is based upon the body's "antigen-antibody" reaction and is done with products formed by biological means. In other words, the immunizing agent is "grown" in a laboratory rather than manufactured in a chemical plant. For this reason, immunizing agents are called biologicals, not drugs, even though some drugs are produced in a "biological" manner, such as penicillin. This means that the horse is injected with a substance containing small amounts of an organism that causes disease (the antigen). The body's reaction is to become mildly infected, and to form cells (antibodies) which combat the infection and remain in the blood to fight future infections. The antigen may consist of fully virulent (live) bacteria or virus, organisms of reduced strength, or dead organisms.

LEVEL OF IMMUNITY CHART

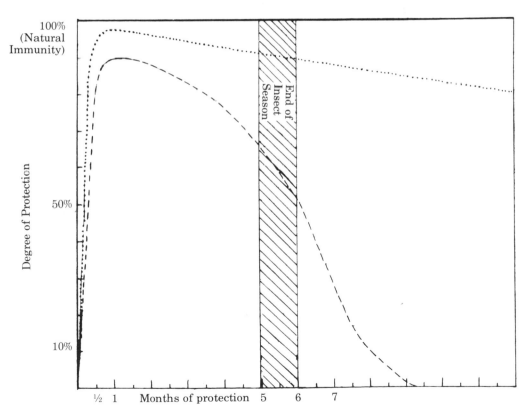

... Protection given by VEE immunization
— — — Protection given by EEE & WEE immunization

IMMUNIZATION TABLE

Disease	Product	Initial Immunization	Annual Booster
Strangles	bacterin	1st dose; 2nd dose in 7 days, 3rd dose in 7 days	single dose annually
Tetanus	bacterial toxoid	1st dose; 2nd in 4-8 weeks	single dose annually
Influenza	killed virus vaccine	1st dose; 2nd dose in 6-12 weeks	single dose annually
Encephalomyelitis (Eastern & Western)	killed virus vaccine	1st dose; 2nd dose in 7-10 days	repeat series annually
VEE	live virus vaccine	1 dose	single dose annually
Viral Rhino-pneumonitis	intramuscular type live virus	(a) Pregnant mares: 1st dose after 2nd month of pregnancy & again at the 5th-7th month. (b) all other horses: 1st dose; 2nd dose in 4 weeks	single dose annually

Date derived from proceedings of Horse Production Short Course, Texas A&M University, January, 1974.

What immunizations are needed?

Some immunizations are needed only in certain areas. The presence of African horsesickness in Africa and parts of Europe, for instance, makes immunization against it necessary in those areas, but not in the United States. Some illnesses, though, occur in widespread areas, and regular immunization against them is standard practice. Equine encephalomyelitis and Venezuelan equine encephalomyelitis immunizations can now be given together, which is usually done annually. Equine rhinopneumonitis vaccinations are given once a year. Equine influenza protection is usually given annually before the onset of cold weather, and repeated if the disease is reported in the area. Strangles immunization is usually given about two weeks before weaning, but veterinarians may hesitate to introduce the antigen into the foal's system if the disease is reported in the area, since this might leave the animal more vulnerable to the disease for a short period immediately after the injection.

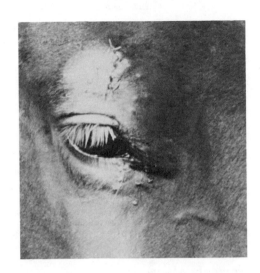

Fig. 25-23. A powdered sulfonamide has been dusted on this eye wound because fly infection is frequent with this type of injury.

What drugs act upon infectious organisms?

A group of drugs known as antibiotics are now widely used to fight infection.

The oldest and probably best known antibiotic is penicillin, which is, like several other antibiotics, organic. That is, it is a naturally grown substance, as opposed to a synthetic or manufactured substance.

Penicillin has the ability to inhibit bacterial growth, a quality which is called bacteriostatic. Unlike many antibiotics, which can act in only one way, it also has the capacity to be bactericidal, which means that it can kill bacteria. This is an ability possessed by certain molds growing in the soil, and is called antibiosis. The substance called penicillin is the agent which performs antibiosis in *Penicillium* molds. Penicillin is effective against many strains of *Clostridium* and *Streptococcus* bacteria, and against some strains of many other kinds of bacteria. The need for antibiotics to combat other organisms has led to the development of other organic antibiotics such as streptomycin and terramycin, and the synthetic production of chloramphenicol, erythromycin and others.

Sulfonamides fight infection on a bacteriostatic level, which they do by causing a "growth lag" in the development of the bacteria. They are particularly effective against *Streptococcus* infections, and some compounds are used against enteritis. The strongest sulfonamide, in compound, is sulfathiazole; least potent is sulfaguanidine.

Powered sulfonamides are sometimes applied to wounds or incisions to control infection. However, an entire range of products is also available to perform this task, called antiseptics and disinfectants.

An antiseptic is a substance which is bacteriostatic, as long as it remains in contact with the bacteria. Usually it is applied directly to the site of the wound. Antiseptics are made in varying degrees of strength, and a stronger antiseptic normally is more irritating to the patient's tissues. A disinfectant is bactericidal, but can cause necrosis of the tissue as well. Not infrequently, one compound can be used in varying strengths to serve as an antiseptic and a disinfectant. Zephiran chloride may be varied in this manner, and to a lesser degree, phemerol chloride. Probably the best known antiseptic-disinfectant compounds are alcohols.

RECOMMENDED WORMING PROGRAM

Age	Schedule of Administration	Parasites to Control
FOALS:		
60 days	60 days	Strongyles and Ascarids
120 days	60 days	Strongyles and Ascarids
180 days	60 days	Strongyles and Ascarids
220 days	40 days (Weaned)	Strongyles, Ascarids and Bots
December	Weanlings	Strongyles, Ascarids and Bots
February-March	Yearlings	Strongyles, Ascarids and Bots
November-December		Strongyles, Ascarids and Bots
MARES: (Brood and/or Barren)		
Pregnant	December, January or February (one month before foaling)	Strongyles and Bots
Lactating	August 1	Strongyles and Bots
Post Weaning	October 15	Strongyles and Bots
STALLIONS:	On fecal examination every 60 days. A count of 50 eggs/gm. or more indicates need for reworming.	Strongyles and Bots

STRONGYLES: Relatively safe and effective Strongyle wormers:
   (1) Thiabendazole, (2) Mebendazole, (3) Cambendazole,
   (4) Pyrantle Tartrate, (5) Dichlorvos, (6) Phenothiazine*

ASCARIDS: Relatively safe and effective Ascarid wormers:
   (1) Piperazine, (2) Butonate, (3) Neguvon, (4) Dichlorvos,
   (5) Cambendazole

BOTS: Relatively safe and effective Bot wormers:
   (1) Carbon Disulfide*, (2) Neguvon, (3) Dichlorvos,
   (4) Butonate

These compounds are found in many commercial (brand name) wormers. The horseman is urged to read all labels on commercial products, to determine if they are effective against the parasites present in his horse. Many of these compounds are available only to a veterinarian. However, they are reported to be the most effective means of controlling the various parasites.

---

*Not as safe and effective as other compounds, but are used.

What drugs are used against internal parasites?

The majority of internal parasites in horses are nematodes (roundworms). They belong to the phylum *Nemathelminthes,* and drugs used against them are called anthelmintics. Great care must be taken in using these drugs, first of all because they may be toxic to the horse in large amounts, and secondly because most of them work on only one or two types of parasites. It is important to remember that the brand name of a product has nothing to do with its effectiveness. Only the proper amount of a chemical which is designed to eliminate the specific parasite troubling the horse will get rid of the problem. Trichlorfon and butonate are effective against bots, thiabendazole and pyrantel against strongyles, and dichlorvos kills both. Ascarids may be eliminated with piperazine. Strongyles and ascarids are also killed by phenothiazine, but its overuse can cause anemia.

BIBLIOGRAPHY

Adams, O. R., D.V.M., M.S., **Lameness in Horses.** Lea & Febiger, Philadelphia, Pennsylvania (1962).

Adams, O. R., D.V.M., M.S., **Lameness in Horses.** Lea & Febiger, Philadelphia, Pennsylvania (Second Edition, 1966).

Adams, O. R., D.V.M., M.S., **Lameness in Horses.** Lea & Febiger, Philadelphia, Pennsylvania (Third Edition, 1974).

Adams, O. R., "Surgical Arthrodesis for Treatment of Bone Spavin," **Journal of the American Veterinary Medical Association.** Vol. 157 (11): 1480-1485 (1970).

Adams, O. R., "Vascular Changes in Experimental Laminitis," **Proceedings of the Eighteenth Annual Convention of the American Association of Equine Practitioners.** San Francisco, California (1972): 359-374.

Baker, Henry J., and J. Russell Lindsey, "Equine Goiter Due to Excess Dietary Iodide," **Journal of the American Veterinary Medical Association.** Vol. 153 (12): 1616-1630 (1968).

Bennett, D. G., "Predisposition to Abdominal Crisis in the Horse," **Journal of the American Veterinary Medical Association.** Vol. 161 (11): 1189-1194 (1972).

Berman, David T., "Some Basic Aspects of the Immune Response," **Journal of the American Veterinary Medical Association.** Vol. 155, Part 2 (2): 250-255 (1969).

Blood, D. C., B.V.Sc., and J. A. Henderson, D.V.M., M.S., **Veterinary Medicine.** The Williams and Wilkins Company, Baltimore, Maryland (Second Edition, 1963).

Blood, D.C., B.V.Sc., F.A.C.V.Sc., and J. A. Henderson, D.V.M., M.S., **Veterinary Medicine.** The Williams and Wilkins Company, Baltimore, Maryland (Fourth Edition, 1974).

Bone, J. F., B.A., B.S., D.V.M, M.S., E. J. Catcott, D.V.M., Ph.D., A. A. Gabel, D.V.M., M.Sc., L. E. Johnson, D.V.M., M.Sc., and W. F. Riley, Jr., D.V.M., M.S., Editors, **Equine Medicine & Surgery.** American Veterinary Publications, Inc., Wheaton, Illinois (First Edition, 1963).

Breazile, James E., D.V.M., Ph.D., Editor, **Textbook of Veterinary Physiology.** Lea & Febiger, Philadelphia, Pennsylvania (1971).

Burns, S. J., "Equine Infectious Anemia: Plasma Clearance Times of Passively Transferred Antibody in Foals," **Journal of the American Veterinary Medical Association.** Vol. 164 (1): 64-65 (1974).

Byrne, Robert J., "Immunity Against Eastern and Western (Equine) Encephalomyelitis Viruses," **Journal of the American Veterinary Medical Association.** Vol. 155, Part 2 (2): 365-368 (1969).

Calislar, T., and L. E. St. Clair, "Observations on the Navicular Bursa and the Distal Interphalangeal Joint Cavity of the Horse," **Journal of the American Veterinary Medical Association.** Vol. 154 (4): 410-412 (1969).

Catcott, E. J., D.V.M., Ph.D., and J. F. Smithcors, D.V.M., Ph.D., Editors, **Equine Medicine & Surgery.** American Veterinary Publications, Inc., Wheaton, Illinois (Second Edition, 1972).

Catcott, E. J., D.V.M., Ph.D., and J. F. Smithcors, D.V.M., Ph.D., Editors, **Progress in Equine Practice.** American Veterinary Publications, Inc., Wheaton, Illinois (Book One, 1966).

Catcott, E. J., D.V.M., Ph.D., and J. F. Smithcors, D.V.M., Ph.D., Editors, **Progress in Equine Practice.** American Veterinary Publications, Inc., Wheaton, Illinois (Vol. II, 1970).

Coffman, James R., and Harold E. Garner, "Acute Abdominal Diseases of the Horse," **Journal of the American Veterinary Medical Association.** Vol. 161 (11): 1195-1198 (1972).

Coffman, James R., Harold E. Garner, Allen W. Hahn and Jess Hartley, "Characterization of Refractory Laminitis," **Proceedings of the Eighteenth Annual Convention of the American Association of Equine Practitioners.** San Francisco, California (1972): 351-358.

Coffman, James R., Jerry H. Johnson, Mary M. Guffy, and Ernest J. Finocchio, "Hoof Circulation in Equine Laminitis," **Journal of The American Veterinary Medical Association.** Vol. 156 (1): 76-83 (1970).

Coggins, L., H. Adldinger, M. J. Kemen, Jr., N. L. Norcross, F. Noronha, S. R. Nusbaum, and C. G. Rickard, "Equine Infectious Anemia: Reports of Progress in Research," **Journal of the American Veterinary Medical Association.** Vol. 155, Part 2 (2): 344-345 (1969).

Coles, Embert H., D.V.M., M.S., Ph.D., **Veterinary Clinical Pathology.** W. B. Saunders Company, Philadelphia, Pennsylvania (1967).

Dakin, M. V., "Some Causes of Lameness Correctable Through Shoeing and Nutrition," **Proceedings of the Seventeenth Annual Convention of the American Association of Equine Practitioners.** Chicago, Illinois (1971): 247-251.

Delahanty, D. D., "Surgical Correction of Contributory Causes of Uterine Disease in the Mare," **Journal of the American Veterinary Medical Association.** Vol. 153 (12): 1563-1566 (1968).

Dorland's Illustrated Medical Dictionary. W. B. Saunders Company, Philadelphia, Pennsylvania (Twenty-fifth Edition, 1974).

Dunn, Angus M., Ph.D., M.R.C.V.S., **Veterinary Helminthology.** Lea & Febiger, Philadelphia, Pennsylvania (1969).

Edwards, Gladys Brown, **Anatomy and Conformation of the Horse.** Dreenan Press Ltd., Croton-on-Hudson, New York (1973).

Fallon, E. H., "The Clinical Aspects of Streptococcic Infections of Horses," **Journal of the American Veterinary Medical Association.** Vol. 155, Part 2 (2): 413-414 (1969).

Frandson, R. D., B.S., D.V.M., M.S., **Anatomy and Physiology of Farm Animals.** Lea & Febiger, Philadelphia, Pennsylvania (1965).

Frank, E. R., B.S.A., D.V.M., M.S., **Veterinary Surgery.** Burgess Publishing Company, Minneapolis, Minnesota (Sixth Edition, 1959).

Frank, E. R., B.S.A., D.V.M., M.S., **Veterinary Surgery.** Burgess Publishing Company, Minneapolis, Minnesota (Seventh Edition, 1964).

Garner, Harold E., James R. Coffman, Allen W. Hahn and Jess Hartley, "Indirect Blood Pressure Measurement in the Horse," **Proceedings of the Eighteenth Annual Convention of the American Association of Equine Practitioners.** San Francisco, California (1972): 343-349.

Gibbons, W. J., **Clinical Diagnosis of Diseases of Large Animals.** Lea & Febiger, Philadelphia, Pennsylvania (1966).

Gilman, M. A., "Horses in Motion," **Proceedings of the Eighteenth Annual Convention of the American Association of Equine Practitioners.** San Francisco, California (1972): 17-18.

Greeley, R. Gordon, B.S., M.S., D.V.M., **The Art and Science of Horseshoeing.** J. B. Lippincott Company, Philadelphia, Pennsylvania (1970).

Green, Ben K., **Horse Conformation as to Soundness and Performance.** Ben K. Green, Greenville, Texas (1969).

Gribble, David H., "Equine Ehrlichiosis," **Journal of the American Veterinary Medical Association.** Vol. 155, Part 2 (2): 462-469 (1969).

Halterman, Lemuel G., and James L. McQueen, "A Serologic Study of Equine Influenza," **Journal of the American Veterinary Medical Association.** Vol. 153 (8): 1069-1073 (1968).

Ham, Arthur W., M.B., F.R.S.C., and Thomas Sydney Leeson, M.A., M.D., B.Ch., **Histology.** J. B. Lippincott Company, Philadelphia, Pennsylvania (1961).

Hansen, Jay C. (Moderator), and Gerald E. Frey, D. D. Farmer, Thomas A. Hackathorn, and Alan R. Raun (Panelists), "Panel—Chronic Lameness," **Proceedings of the**

Seventeenth Annual Convention of the American Association of Equine Practitioners. Chicago, Illinois (1971): 279-292.

Haugh, C. G., E. H. Page and W. W. Kirkham, "The Effect of Diet and an Anabolic Agent on the Strength of Bone and Tendon," **Proceedings of the Seventeenth Annual Convention of the American Association of Equine Practitioners.** Chicago, Illinois (1971): 237-246.

Hawkins, J. A., et al., "Role of Horse Fly and Stable Fly in Transmission of Equine Infectious Anemia to Ponies in Louisiana," **Journal of the American Veterinary Medical Association.** Vol. 164 (1): 65 (1974).

Hayes, M. Horace, F.R.C.V.S., **Veterinary Notes For Horse Owners.** Arco Publishing Company, Inc., New York, New York (1968).

Haynes, P. F., and O. R. Adams, "Internal Fixation of Fractured Extensor Process of Third Phalanx in a Horse," **Journal of the American Veterinary Medical Association.** Vol. 164 (1): 61-63 (1974).

Hickman, John, M.A., F.R.C.V.S., and Robert G. Walker, M.A., M.R.C.V.S., **An Atlas of Veterinary Surgery.** J. B. Lippincott Company, Philadelphia, Pennsylvania (1973).

Holbrook, A. A., "Biology of Equine Piroplasmosis," **Journal of the American Veterinary Medical Association.** Vol. 155, Part 2 (2): 453-454 (1969).

Hughes, John P., George H. Stabenfeldt and J. Warren Evans, "Clinical and Endocrine Aspects of the Estrous Cycle of the Mare," **Proceedings of the Eighteenth Annual Convention of the American Association of Equine Practitioners.** San Francisco, California (1972): 119-151.

Johnson, Jerry H., H. E. Garner, D. P. Hutcheson and J. G. Merriam, "Epistaxis," **Proceedings of the Nineteenth Annual Convention of the American Association of Equine Practitioners.** Atlanta, Georgia (1973): 115-121.

Jones, L. Meyer, A.B., D.V.M., M.S., Ph.D., **Veterinary Pharmacology and Therapeutics.** Iowa State University Press, Ames, Iowa (1957).

Jones, T. C., "Clinical and Pathologic Features of Equine Viral Arteritis," **Journal of the American Veterinary Medical Association.** Vol. 155, Part 2 (2): 315-317 (1969).

Jones, William E., D.V.M., Ph.D., and Ralph Bogart, Ph.D., **Genetics of the Horse.** Caballus Publishers, East Lansing, Michigan (1971).

Kester, Wayne O., "Concern of the Equine Industry About Infectious Diseases," **Journal of the American Veterinary Medical Association.** Vol. 155, Part 2 (2): 242-244 (1969).

Kirkham, W. W., "The Treatment of Equine Babesiosis," **Journal of the American Veterinary Medical Association.** Vol. 155, Part 2 (2): 457-460 (1969).

Knight, H. D., "Corynebacterial Infections in the Horse: Problems of Prevention," **Journal of the American Veterinary Medical Association.** Vol. 155, Part 2 (2): 446-452 (1969).

Knowles, Ralph C., "Equine Infectious Anemia (EIA): The Facts Before The Furor," **Journal of the American Veterinary Medical Association.** Vol. 155, Part 2 (2): 327-331 (1969).

Laufenstein-Duffy, Helga, "The Daily Variation of the Resting Packed Cell Volume in the Racing Thoroughbred and the Difficulty in Evaluating the Effectiveness of Hematinic Drugs," **Proceedings of the Seventeenth Annual Convention of the American Association of Equine Practitioners.** Chicago, Illinois (1971): 151-154.

Lieux, Pierre, Robert H. Baker, Alice DeGroot, Herbert H. Laskey, Robert E. Raynor, John G. Simpson, and Earl Tobler, "Results of a Survey on Bacteriologic Culturing of Broodmares," **Journal of the American Veterinary Medical Association.** Vol. 157 (11): 1460-1464 (1970).

Lindeman, **The Quarter Horse Breeder.** Quarter Horse Breeders Publishing Company (1959).

Lindholm, Arne, Hans-Erik Johansson and Per Kjaersgaard, "Acute Rhabdomyolysis ('Tying-Up') In Standardbred Horses," From the Department of Clinical Biochemistry and the Department of Pathology, Royal Veterinary College, Stockholm, Sweden, the Department of Normal Anatomy, Royal Veterinary and Agricultural University, Copenhagen, Denmark, and the Equine Hospital, Solvalla, Stockholm, Sweden. **Acta Vet. Scand.** 1974, 15.

Merchant, I. A., D.V.M., Ph.D., M.P.H., and R. A. Packer, B.S., D.V.M., Ph.D., **Veterinary Bacteriology and Virology,** Iowa State University Press, Ames, Iowa (1961).

Meyerholz, G. W., D.V.M., William J. Lee, Jr., D.V.M., and Carl J. Meyer, D.V.M., "Limb Edema Associated with Ingestion of Moldy Hay by Horses," **Journal of the American Veterinary Medical Association.** Vol. 164 (1): 41 (1974).

Miller, Albert B., Publisher, **Physicians' Desk Reference to Pharmaceutical Specialties and Biologicals.** Medical Economics, Inc., Oradell, New Jersey (1969).

Morgan, Banner Bill, B.S., M.S., Ph.D., and Philip A. Hawkins, A.B., M.A., Ph.D., D.V.M., **Veterinary Helminthology.** Burgess Publishing Company, Minneapolis, Minn. (1949).

Morter, R. L., R. D. Williams, H. Bolte, and M. J. Freeman, "Equine Leptospirosis," **Journal of the American Veterinary Medical Association.** Vol. 155, Part 2 (2): 436-442 (1969).

O'Conner, James T., Jr., "The Treatment of Fatigue in Trail Ride Horses," **Proceedings of the Seventeenth Annual Convention of the American Association of Equine Practitioners.** Chicago, Illinois (1971): 39-43.

O'Connor, James T., Jr., "The Untoward Effects of the Corticosteroids In Equine Practice," **Journal of the American Veterinary Medical Association.** Vol. 153 (12): 1614-1617 (1968).

Panciera, Roger J., "Serum Hepatitis in the Horse," **Journal of the American Veterinary Medical Association.** Vol. 155, Part 2 (2): 408-410 (1969).

Pickett, B. W., and J. L. Voss, "Reproductive Management of the Stallion," **Proceedings of the Eighteenth Annual Convention of the American Association of Equine Practitioners.** San Francisco, California (1972): 501-531.

Prickett, M. E., "Abortion and Placental Lesions in the Mare," **Journal of the American Veterinary Medical Association.** Vol. 157 (11): 1465-1470 (1970).

Prickett, Milton E., "The Untoward Reaction of the Horse to Injection of Antigenic Substances," **Journal of the American Veterinary Medical Association.** Vol. 155, Part 2 (2): 258-262 (1969).

Purvis, Alan D., "Elective Induction of Labor and Parturition in the Mare," **Proceedings of the Eighteenth Annual Convention of the American Association of Equine Practitioners.** San Francisco, California (1972): 113-118.

Riddle, W. E., Jr., "Healing of Articular Cartilage in the Horse," **Journal of the American Veterinary Medical Association.** Vol. 157 (11): 1471-1479 (1970).

Roberts, Stephen J., D.V.M., M.S., **Veterinary Obstetrics and Genital Diseases.** Stephen J. Roberts, Ithaca, New York (1956).

Rooney, James R., D.V.M., **Autopsy of the Horse.** The Williams & Wilkins Co., Baltimore, Maryland (1970).

Rooney, James R., D.V.M., **Biomechanics of Lameness in Horses.** The Williams & Wilkins Company, Baltimore, Maryland (1969).

Rooney, James R., D.V.M., **Clinical Neurology of the Horse.** KNA Press Inc., Kennett Square, Pennsylvania (1971).

Rossdale, Peter D., M.A., F.R.C.V.S., **The Horse.** The California Thoroughbred Breeders Association, Arcadia, California (1972).

Sager, Floyd C., "Management and Medical Treatment of Uterine Disease," **Journal of the American Veterinary Medical Association.** Vol. 153 (12): 1567-1569 (1968).

Schlam, Oscar W., D.V.M., Ph.D., **Veterinary Hematology.** Lea & Febiger, Philadelphia, Pennsylvania (1961).

Siegmund, O. H., Editor, **The Merck Veterinary Manual.** Merck & Co., Inc., Rahway, New Jersey (1973).

Sippel, William L., Eldred E. Keahey, and Tommy L. Bullard, "Corynebacterium Infection in Foals: Etiology, Pathogenesis, and Laboratory Diagnosis," **Journal of the American Veterinary Medical Association.** Vol. 153 (12): 1610-1613 (1968).

Sisson, Septimus, S.B., V.S., D.V.Sc., **The Anatomy of the Domestic Animals.** Revised by James Daniels Grossman, G.PH., D.V.M., W. B. Saunders Company, Philadelphia, Pennsylvania (Fourth Edition, Revised 1953).

Smith, Hilton Atmore, D.V.M., M.S., Ph.D., Thomas Carlyle Jones, B.S., D.V.M., D.Sc. (Hon.), and Ronald Duncan Hunt, B.S., D.V.M., **Veterinary Pathology.** Lea & Febiger, Philadelphia, Pennsylvania (1972).

Solomon, Wm. J., R. H. Schultz and M. L. Fanning, "A Study of Chronic Infertility in the Mare Utilizing Uterine Biopsy, Cytology and Cultural Methods," **Proceedings of the Eighteenth Annual Convention of the American Association of Equine Practitioners.** San Francisco, California (1972): 55-68.

Stormont, Clyde, "Current Status of Equine Blood Groups and Their Applications," **Proceedings of the Eighteenth Annual Convention of the American Association of Equine Practitioners.** San Francisco, California (1972): 401-410.

Stromberg, Berndt, Gunnar Tufvesson, and Gunnar Nilsson, "Effect of Surgical Splitting on Vascular Reactions in the Superficial Flexor Tendon of the Horse," **Journal of the American Veterinary Medical Association.** Vol. 164 (1): 57-60 (1974).

Swenson, Melvin J., D.V.M., M.S., Ph.D., Editor, **Dukes' Physiology of Domestic Animals.** Comstock Publishing Associates, Ithaca, New York (1970).

Vaughan, J. T., "Surgical Management of Abdominal Crisis in the Horse," **Journal of the American Veterinary Medical Association.** Vol. 161 (11): 1199-1212 (1972).

Way, Robert F., V.M.D., M.S., and Donald G. Lee, V.M.D., **The Anatomy of the Horse.** J. B. Lippincott Company, Philadelphia, Pennsylvania (1965).

Wearly, W. K., P. W. Murdick and J. D. Hensel, "A Five Year Study of the Use of Post-Breeding Treatment in Mares in a Standardbred Stud," **Proceedings of the Seventeenth Annual Convention of the American Association of Equine Practitioners.** Chicago, Illinois (1971): 89-96.

Wheat, J. D., "Sinus Drainage and Tooth Repulsion in the Horse," **Proceedings of the Nineteenth Annual Convention of the American Association of Equine Practitioners.** Atlanta, Georgia (1973): 171-176.

White, N. A., and E. A. Rhode, "Correlation of Electrocardiographic Findings to Clinical Disease in the Horse," **Journal of the American Veterinary Medical Association.** Vol. 164 (1): 46-56 (1974).

Willcox, Sheila, **The Event Horse.** Pelham Books Ltd, London (1973).

Witherspoon, Don M., and R. B. Talbot, "Ovulation Site in the Mare," **Journal of the American Veterinary Medical Association.** Vol. 157 (11): 1452-1459 (1970).

Zinn, Roy S., III, Albert A. Gabel, and R. B. Heath, "Effects of Succinylcholine and Promazine on the Cardiovascular and Respiratory Systems of Horses," **Journal of the American Veterinary Medical Association.** Vol. 157 (11): 1495-1499 (1970).

668

APPENDIX

VITAL FUNCTION NORMS OF THE HORSE

HEMATOLOGY:		BLOODED*		CROSSBRED	
		Range	Average	Range	Average
Erythrocytes (RBC)	[millions/cu. mm.]	7.0-13.0	9.75	5.5-09.5	7.5
Leukocytes (WBC)	[thousands/cu. mm.]	7.0-14.0	10.00	6.0-12.0	8.5
Packed Cell Volume (PCV)	[volume per cent]	32.0-55.0	42.00	24.0-44.0	35.0
Hemoglobin	[gm/100 ml.]	10.0-18.0	13.40	8.0-14.0	11.5

PULSE RATE, NORMAL RESTING:

Horses	30-40 pulses/ min.
Foals up to 2 weeks old	100
Foals 4 weeks old	70
Colts and fillies 6 to 12 months old	45-60
2 year-olds	40-50

RESPIRATION RATE AT REST: 8-16 breaths/min.

TEMPERATURE (RECTAL):   Normal 99.5°-101.5°F [100.5°F (38.0°C) average]

FEVER:		
	mild	100.5-102.5°F
	moderate	102.5-104.0
	high	104.0-106.5
	very high	above 106.5

NORMAL RANGES OF REPRODUCTIVE PHENOMENA:

Age at puberty: 10-24 months (18 mo. average).

Length of estrous cycle (from beginning of one heat period to beginning of next): 19-23 days (21 days average).

Length of heat period (estrus): 4.5-7.5 days (5.5 days average).

Time of ovulation: 1 to 2 days before end of estrus.

Optimum time for service: 3 to 4 days before end of estrus. Service every other day starting on second day of estrus usually assures service at optimum time.

Length of pregnancy: 330-345 days (336 days average).

Blooded usually refers to horses with considerable Arabian ancestry such as Arabians and Thoroughbreds. American Saddle horses, Morgan horses and Standardbreds may also be included in this category.

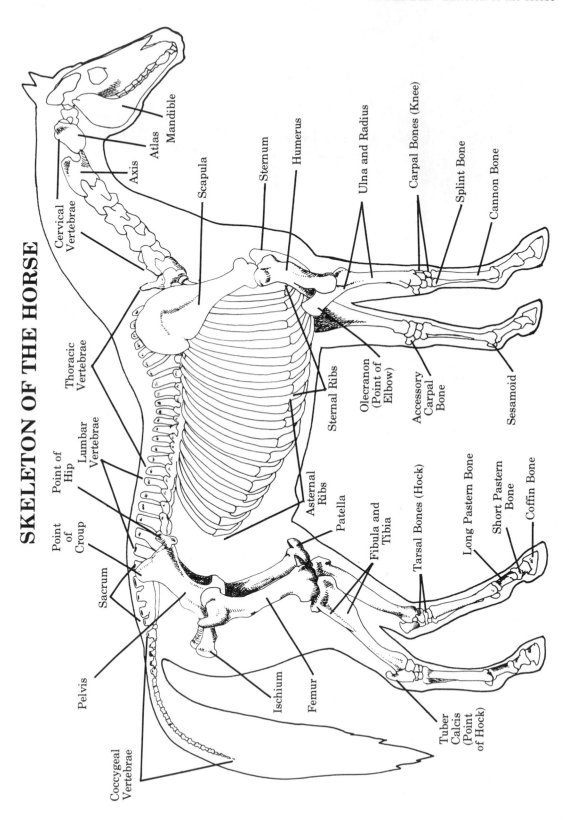

SKELETON OF THE HORSE

PARTS OF THE HORSE

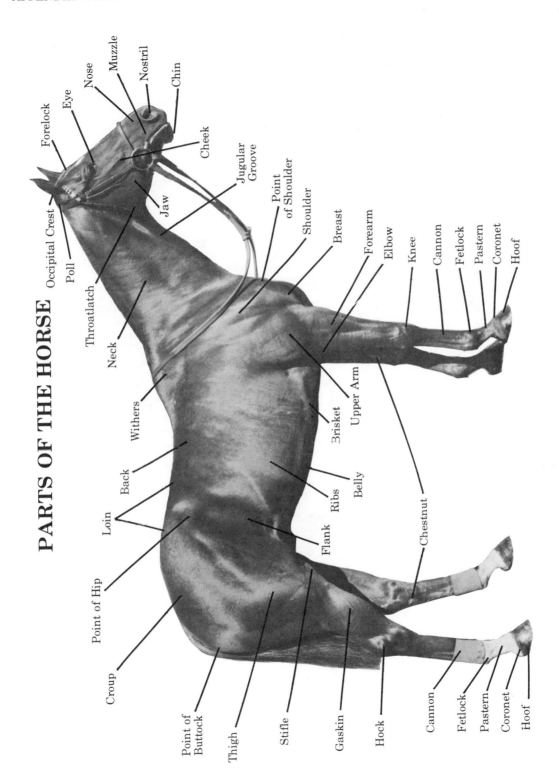

Occipital Crest
Forelock
Eye
Nose
Muzzle
Nostril
Chin
Cheek
Jugular Groove
Point of Shoulder
Shoulder
Breast
Forearm
Elbow
Knee
Cannon
Fetlock
Pastern
Coronet
Hoof
Poll
Jaw
Throatlatch
Neck
Withers
Back
Loin
Point of Hip
Croup
Point of Buttock
Thigh
Stifle
Gaskin
Hock
Flank
Ribs
Belly
Brisket
Upper Arm
Chestnut
Cannon
Fetlock
Pastern
Coronet
Hoof

PLANES OF REFERENCE

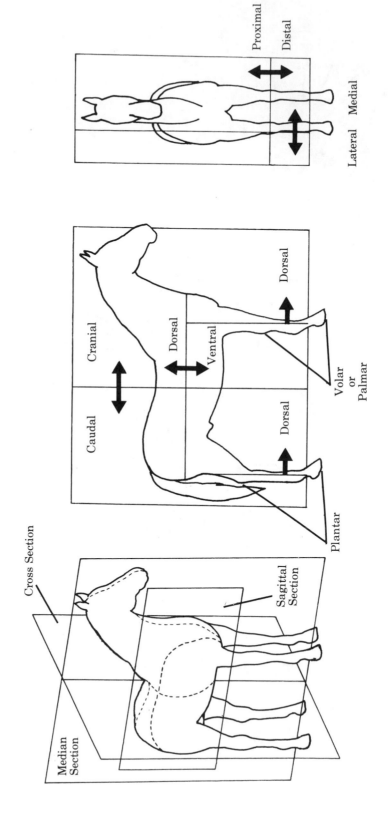

GLOSSARY

Abdomen: That portion of the body which lies between the chest and the pelvis.

Abduction: A drawing away from the median plane of the body.

Abortion: The premature expulsion from the uterus of the embryo or fetus.

Abrasion: A wound caused by the wearing away of the top layer of skin and hair by friction.

Abscess: A localized collection of pus in a cavity formed by the disintegration of tissues.

Absorption: The uptake of substances into or across tissues.

Acoustic: Pertaining to sound or to the sense of hearing.

Acute: Having a short and relatively severe course.

Adduction: A drawing toward the median plane of the body.

Adenoma: A benign epithelial tumor in which the cells are derived from granular epithelium or form granular structures.

Adhesion: A fibrous band abnormally joining tissues together.

Adjunct: An accessory agent or measure.

Adrenocortical: Pertaining to the cortex of the adrenal gland.

Aerobe: A microoganism that can live and grow in the presence of oxygen.

Aerobic: Growing in the presence of oxygen.

Afferent: Carrying toward a center.

African Horsesickness: A highly fatal viral infection transmitted by flying insects.

Agent: Any substance or principle capable of producing a physical, chemical or biological effect.

Agglutination titer: The highest dilution of a serum that causes clumping of bacteria or other particulate antigens.

Albino: An individual suffering from albinism, which is the congenital absence of pigment in the skin, hair and eyes.

Albuginea: A tough, whitish layer of fibrous tissue covering a part.

Alkaloid: A very bitter, basic organic substance found in plants, such as atropine, morphine, or nicotine.

Allergen: A protein or non-protein substance capable of inducing allergy or hypersensitivity.

Allergy: A hypersensitive state acquired through exposure to a particular allergen, reexposure resulting in an altered capacity to react to the substance.

Alopecia: A lack of hair in areas where it is normally present.

Alternative Inflammation: An inflammation in which cell changes caused by bacterial toxins lead to tissue necrosis.

Alveolar Periostitis: An inflammation of the periosteum of the alveoli due to infection, and marked by supperation and pain.

Alveolus, Alveoli: A small cavity or pit, as a socket for a tooth; air cell of the lungs.

Ambient: Surrounding, encompassing, prevailing.

Ameboid: Moving or changing shape by protoplasmic flow, thereby resembling an ameba.

Amino Acid: Any of a class of organic compounds containing nitrogen and forming the building blocks of proteins.

Anaerobe: An organism capable of growing in the complete, or almost complete, absence of oxygen.

Analgesic: A drug that relieves pain without causing a loss of consciousness.

Anaphylaxis: An unusual allergic reaction to a foreign protein or drug.

Anaplasia: A loss of differentiation of cells.

Anastomose: To create a connection between two vessels through a channel.

Anemia: A below normal number of erythrocytes per cubic mm., or in the quantity of hemoglobin, which occurs when the equlibrium between blood loss and blood production is disturbed.

Anesthetic: A drug or agent that is used to abolish the sensation of pain.

Anesthetize: To cause a loss of sensation of pain with or without a loss of consciousness.

Anestrus: A period of sexual inactivity between cycles.

Aneurysm: A blood-filled sac formed by an abnormal dilatation of the wall of an artery, a vein, or the heart.

Anhidrosis: An abnormal deficiency of sweat.

Aniridia: Absence of the iris.

Ankylosis: Immobilization and consolidation of a joint due to disease, injury, or surgical procedure.

Annular: Shaped like a ring.

Anomaly: A marked deviation from the normal, particularly as a result of a congenital defect.

Anoxia: Lack of oxygen.

Anterior: Situated in front of, or in the forward part of, an organ; toward the head end of the body.

Anthelmintic: A drug that destroys or removes parasitic worms.

Anthrax: An infectious disease resulting from the injestion of spores in the soil, leading to acute septicemia in the horse, and rapid death.

Antibiotic: A chemical substance produced by a microorganism that has the ability to kill or inhibit the growth of other microorganisms.

Antibody: A protein in the blood or other body fluid that interacts with a specific antigen to neutralize toxins and break down bacteria or cells.

Antidote: A remedy for counteracting a poison.

Antiferment: An agent which prevents fermentation.

Antigen: Any substance such as a toxin, foreign protein, bacteria, or tissue cells, which enters the body and causes the formation of an antibody.

Antihistamine: A drug which counteracts the action of histamine. Histamine is a powerful dilator of capillaries and stimulator of gastric secretions.

Anti-inflammatory: An agent that counteracts or suppresses the inflammatory response.

Antiphlogistic: An agent that counteracts fever and inflammation.

Antiseptic: An agent that prevents the decay or decomposition of tissue by inhibiting the growth and development of microorganisms.

Antiserum: A serum that contains antibodies.

Antitoxin: An antibody to the toxin of a microorganism, to a zootoxin, or to a phytotoxin, that combines with the toxin, causing its neutralization.

Antitussive: An agent that prevents or relieves coughing.

Antivenin: A proteinaceous material used in the treatment of poisoning caused by animal venom.

Anus: The external opening of the rectum.

Aorta: The main artery of the arterial system which carries blood away from the heart.

Apathy: Lack of feeling or emotion; indifference.

Apical: Pertaining to the top or tip of a structure.

Aplastic: Pertaining to the lack of development of an organ or tissue.

Apocrine: A type of granular secretion that contains part of the secreting cell.

Aponeurosis: A flattened tendinous expansion which connects a muscle with the parts that it moves.

Aqueous humor: The fluid produced in the eye, occupying the anterior and posterior chambers, and diffusing out of the eye into the blood. It is considered the lymph of the eye, although its composition varies from that of the body's lymph.

Arcade: An anatomical structure resembling a series of arches, usually referring to the surface of the jaws that holds the teeth.

Arrythmia: Any variation from the normal heart beat.

Arteriole: A minute arterial branch, especially one near a capillary.

Arteritis: Inflammation of an artery.

Artery: Vessel through which blood passes away from the heart toward the various parts of the body.

Arthritis: Inflammation of joints.

Arthrodial: Pertaining to a gliding joint.

Articular: Pertaining to, divided by, or united by joints.

Articulate: Divided into or united by joints.

Artifical Insemination: Depositing semen in the vagina or cervix by artificial means.

Aspect: The part of a surface facing in any designated direction.

Aspergillosis: A disease caused by Aspergillus and marked by inflammatory granular lesions in the skin, ear, orbit, nasal sinuses, and sometimes in the bones and meninges.

Asphyxiation: Suffocation.

Aspirate: The act of inhaling, or the withdrawal of fluids or gases from a cavity by suction.

Assimilation: The transformation of food into living tissue.

Asternal: Not joined to the sternum.

Ataxia: An inability to coordinate voluntary muscular movements.

Atrophy: A decrease in size or wasting away of a body part or tissue.

Atropine: A drug used to relax smooth muscles in various organs, to increase heart rate, and to dilate the pupil when applied to the eye.

Attentuate: To render thin or less virulent.

Auditory: Pertaining to the sense of hearing.

Aural Plaques: Small grey or white spots found on the inner surface of the pinna.

Auscultation: The act of listening for sounds within the body, chiefly for determining the condition of the lungs, heart, pleura, abdomen, and other organs.

Autonomic Nervous System: The part of the nervous system that regulates the internal environment of the body.

Autopsy: The postmortem examination of a body.

Avascular: Not supplied with blood vessels.

Avulsion: The tearing away of part of a structure.

Axis: A line around which part of the body is arranged or is symmetrical.

Axon: The process of a nerve cell by which the impulses travel away from the cell body.

Azoturia: A disease of horses marked by a sudden attack of perspiration and paralysis of the hindquarters, and by the passing of light red to dark brown urine. It occurs in horses that, after being engaged in continuous work, are rested and well-fed and then returned to work.

Babesiasis: An infection of Babesia, usually transmitted by ticks.

Bacteria: Any microorganism of the class Schizomycetes.

Bactericidal: Destructive to bacteria.

Bacteriostatic: An agent that inhibits the growth or action of bacteria.

Ball and Socket Joint: Enarthrodial joint.

Bandy Legs: A conformation defect in which the hocks are set too far apart, frequently resulting in interference between the hindfeet as they pass one another in travel. Also called Bow Legs.

Barker Foal: A foal suffering from convulsive syndrome, thought to be caused by a lack of oxygen at birth. The foal will bark like a small dog, have convulsions, and be blind and weak.

Bar Shoe: A therapeutic shoe in which the heels are joined by a bar, allowing greater pressure on the bar and frog of the foot.

Base Narrow: A conformation fault in which there is greater distance between the horse's legs at the top than at the bottom, caused by an improper positioning at the elbow.

Base Wide: A conformation fault in which there is greater distance between the horse's legs at the bottom than at the top, caused by an improper positioning at the elbow.

Basophil: A structure cell that stains easily with basic dyes.

Bean: A putty-like mass of smegma that collects in the diverticulum.

Bench Knees: The conformation fault in which the leg does not follow a straight line through the radius and cannon bone. Instead, the cannon is offset to the outside of the knee.

Benign: Not malignant or recurrable, with a favorable outlook for recovery.

Besnoitiosis: An infectious disease caused by protozoa that involves the skin, sucutaneous tissue, blood vessels, and other tissues.

Biceps: A muscle having two heads or parts.

Bifurcation: The site where a single structure divides into two branches.

Big Knees: Abnormal growth caused by epiphysitis resulting from concussion.

Bilateral: Having two sides or pertaining to both sides.

Bilirubin: A bile pigment formed from the breakdown of hemoglobin.

Bio-electric Impulse: An electrical impulse generated by living tissue such as muscle or nerve cells.

Bipartite: Having two parts or divisions.

Blastoma: A neoplasm composed of embryonic cells derived from the blastema of an organ or tissue.

Blemish: A minor conformation fault, either occurring congenitally or caused by an injury, that is considered undesirable, but does not interfere with the horse's soundness.

Blind Spavin: A spavin where the bone has degenerated but there is no visible exostosis. A horse suffering from this condition will be lame without showing external signs of spavin.

Blister: A counterirritant agent applied to the skin to cause blistering and inflammation, used to treat chronic or subacute inflammation of joints, tendons, and bones.

Blistering: Applying an agent to the skin to produce blistering and inflammation of the skin, used to treat chronic or subacute inflammation of joints, tendons, and bones.

Blood Blister: A hemotoma, which is a collection of usually clotted blood caused by a break in the wall of a blood vessel.

Blood Pressure: The pressure of blood on the walls of the arteries, dependent on the energy of the heart action, the elasticity of the walls of the arteries, and the volume and viscosity of the blood.

Blow: Greatly increased force of respiration, as after hard exercise.

Blue Nose: Photosensitization occurring on the nostrils.

Bog Spavin: A chronic distension of the joint capsule of the hock with synovial fluid.

Bolet, Bolus: A rounded mass of food or medicine which is given orally.

Bone Marrow: The soft material filling the cavities of the bones, made up of a meshwork of connective tissue containing branching fibers, the meshes being filled with marrow cells.

Bone Spavin: A lameness originating in the hock which is characterized by either exostosis or bone destruction on the inner surface of the hock.

Borna: A meningoencephalitis caused by a virus found in food and water. The disease is highly fatal and has signs resembling those of WEE.

Bots: The larvae of botflies, which are parasitic in the stomach.

Botulism: A type of food poisoning caused by a neurotoxin, characterized by abdominal pain, nervous symptoms, secretion disturbances, and mydriasis.

Bow Legs: A conformation fault in which the hocks are set too far apart, frequently causing interference between the hind feet as they pass each other in travel. Also called Bandy Legs.

Bowed Tendon: Damage to the tendon that results in inflammation.

Bradykinin: Factors formed by a group of enzymes produced by the body that maintain dilatation of the blood vessels in the inflammatory process.

Breeding Roll: A roll placed between the stallion and mare at the time of breeding to prevent the stallion from penetrating too far into the vagina and injuring the mare.

Broad Spectrum: A wide range of activity, as in a wide range of bacteria affected by a broad spectrum antibiotic.

Broken Wind: An inability to empty the lungs of air, caused by the rupture of some alveoli, and characterized by difficult breathing, a chronic cough, and generally poor condition.

Bronchial: Pertaining to either or both of the two main branches of the trachea, one going to each lung.

Bronchitis: An inflammation of one or more bronchi, often marked by fever, coughing, and dyspnea.

Bronchopneumonia: An inflammation of the lungs that begins in the terminal bronchioles, which become clogged with mucopurulent exudate.

Bronchus, Bronchi: Either or both of the two main branches of the trachea, one going to each lung.

Brucellosis: The infection found in the lesions of poll evil and fistulous withers, which causes variable temperature, stiffness, and bursa enlargement.

Bruise: A contusion caused by impact without laceration.

Brushing: Limb contact during movement, in which a foot lightly strikes another foot.

Buck Knees: Sprung over at the knees.

Bucked Shins: A periostitis of the front side of the cannon bone, usually occurring on the forelegs of young horses that are strenuously exercised.

Bursa: A sac or sac-like cavity filled with fluid and situated at places in the tissues at which friction would otherwise develop.

Bursitis: An inflammation of the bursa, occasionally accompanied by the formation of a calcific deposit in the underlying tendon.

Buttress Foot: A form of low ringbone in which the horse's hoof becomes pyramidal in shape.

Calcification: The process of tissue becoming hardened by a deposit of calcium salts.

Calf Knees: A conformation fault in which the knees deviate towards the back, or the front leg bends back at the knees.

Callus: Localized hyperplasia of the epidermis due to friction or pressure; an unorganized woven meshwork of bone which forms at the site of a fracture and is eventually replaced by hard adult bone.

Camped: A conformation fault in which the hind legs are too far behind the horse. A straight line from the point of the hip to the ground, perpendicular to the ground, will not touch the point of the hock, and will end forward of the middle of the hoof.

Cancer: An anaplastic cellular tumor that will metastasize and which has a naturally fatal course.

Canker: An ulceration; a disease of the keratogenous membrane, beginning at the frog and extending to the sole and wall, characterized by a serous discharge and the loss of function of the horn-producing cells.

Cantharidin: An agent occurring in crystal form that has a bitter taste. It has been given as a diuretic, and applied externally to produce blistering as a rubefacient.

Capillaries: Minute vessels that connect the arterioles and venules, forming a network in nearly all parts of the body. Their walls act as semipermeable membranes for the interchange of various substances between the blood and tissue fluid.

Capped Elbow: A soft, flabby swelling over the point of the elbow due to trauma.

Capped Hock: An inflammation of the bursa over the point of the hock caused by trauma.

Carbohydrate: Starches and sugar; the chief source of nutrients.

Carbuncle: A necrotizing infection of skin and subcutaneous tissue composed of a cluster of boils.

Carcinoma: A malignant new growth of epithelial cells that tends to metastasize.

Cardiac: Pertaining to the heart.

Cardiac cycle: The actions of the heart during one complete heart beat.

Cardiovascular: Pertaining to the heart and blood vessels.

Carpal: Pertaining to the knee.

Carpitis: Inflammation of the synovial membranes of the bones of the knees, causing swelling, pain, and lameness.

Carrier: An animal that carries a recessive gene or the organisms of a disease without showing signs of the condition. The animal may then transmit the gene to offspring or the disease to another animal.

Cartilage: A specialized type of fibrous connective tissue.

Caruncle: A small, fleshy outgrowth.

Caseous: Resembling cheese or curd.

Caslick's Operation: An operation to correct pneumovagina that involves suturing the upper vulvar lips together.

Cast: A stiff casing made of bandages impregnated with plaster of paris or another hardening material that is used to immobilize a part of the body in cases of fractures, dislocations, or infected wounds.

Cataract: An opacity of the lens of the eye.

Catheter: A flexible tubular instrument for withdrawing fluids from or introducing fluids to a body cavity.

Caudal: Referring to a position near the tail.

Caustic: Burning, corrosive, and destructive to living tissue.

Cautery: The application of a caustic substance, a hot iron, or an electric current to destroy living tissue.

Caverna: A general term used to designate a hollow place within the body or an organ.

Cavity: A real or potential hollow space within the body or an organ.

Cecum: The first part of the large intestine which is in the form of a blind pouch.

Cellulitis: Purulent inflammation of the loose subcutaneous tissue.

Cellulose: A carbohydrate that appears only in plants and cannot be digested by horses; also referred to as fiber.

Cervical: Pertaining to the neck, or to the neck of any organ or structure, such as the cervix of the uterus.

Cervicitis: An inflammation of the cervix.

Chadwick Spring: A V-shaped steel spring, fitted to the bottom of the foot, which keeps constant pressure on the bars of the foot.

Chemotherapy: The treatment of disease by chemical agents.

Chlorophyll: The green coloring of plants by which photosynthesis is accomplished.

Choke: A partial or complete esophageal obstruction that may cause death through perforation of the esophagus or degeneration and death of the tissue due to pressure.

Chondroid: Resembling cartilage.

Chondromalacia: Softening of the articular cartilage, especially in the patella.

Chorioptic Mange: A skin disease caused by mite infection on the legs of the horse, frequently resulting in secondary infection and grease.

Chorioretinitis: An inflammation of the choroid and the retina.

Chronic: Long term, continued, not acute.

Chyme: The semi-fluid, creamy or gruel-like material produced by gastric digestion of food.

Cilia: Minute hair-like processes that move in a swaying motion.

Circumduction: The circular movement of an eye or leg.

Cirrhosis: A liver disease characterized by loss of the normal lobe structure and fibrous regeneration.

Clinical Diagnosis: Diagnosis based on signs shown during life.

Clip: A thin metal projection on the outside of a shoe that lies against the hoof to give support to the shoe.

Close-coupled: Short and strong; undesirable in a neck, but often considered an advantage in a back.

Clot: A semi-solidified mass of blood.

Coagulate: To cause to clot, forming an insoluble fibrin clot.

Coccidiodomycosis: A fungus disease that has two forms, primary and secondary. The primary form is an acute respiratory infection from inhalation of spores, while the secondary type is a virulent granulomatous disease that involves the viscera, central nervous system, lungs, etc.

Coggins Test: A test used to determine the presence of EIA antibodies in a blood sample.

Coital Exanthema: A contagious disease, carried by a herpes virus, which results in temporary sterility in mares, and is characterized by the development of many small blisters on the mucous membranes of the vulva and vagina.

Coitus: Sexual intercourse.

Cold Lameness: Incapable of normal movement on first starting exercise.

Colic: Acute abdominal pain corresponding to smooth muscle peristalsis.

Colitis X: A highly fatal, noncontagious disease that causes death within 3 to 48 hours. It is believed to be related to stress, and the horse will suffer from diarrhea and shock.

Collagen: A main fibrous protein of skin, bone, tendon, cartilage and connective tissue.

Collateral: Secondary or accessory; a small side branch, as of a blood vessel or nerve.

Colloid Goiter: A swelling of the thyroid gland in which the acini contain excessive amounts of colloid.

Colon: The part of the large intestine extending from the cecum to the rectum.

Colostrum: The milky fluid from the mammary glands of the mare, with high protein and antibody content, secreted shortly before and for a few days after delivery of a foal.

Coma: A state of unconsciousness from which the animal cannot be aroused.

Comminute: To break or crush into small pieces.

Compound Fracture: A comminuted fracture that has broken the skin.

Compression Screw: A special kind of screw used to fix bone fragments together that has the property of compressing the fragments together.

Concave: Hollowed or rounded inward like the inside of a bowl.

Conchal Sinus: A Dentigerous Cyst.

Concurrent: Acting in conjunction.

Concussion: A violent jar or shock.

Condyle: A rounded projection on a bone.

Conformation: The shape or contour of the body or body structures.

Congenital: Existing at and usually before birth; referring to conditions that may or may not be inherited.

Conjestion: Excessive abnormal accumulation of blood in a part of the body.

Conjunctivitis: Inflammation of the membrane that lines the eyelid and covers part of the eyeball.

Connective Tissue: The tissue which binds together and is the support of the various structures of the body, made up of fibroblasts, fibroglia, collagen fibrils, and elastin fibrils.

Consolidation: The process of becoming solid, as when, in pneumonia, the lung becoms firm as the air spaces fill with exudate.

Constipation: Infrequent or difficult evacuation of the feces.

Constriction: An area of compression and of drawing together; a stricture.

Contagious Acne: An infection, caused by a small intra-cellular parasite, that is usually limited to areas in contact with harness or tack. Lesions are small, painful, and take a week to heal.

Contaminant: Something that causes the introduction of foreign material by contact, as with the introduction of microorganisms into a wound through a dirty bandage.

Contracted Heels: A condition in which the foot is contracted and narrowed, caused by lack of frog pressure and moisture.

Contusion: A bruise or injury incurred without breaking the skin.

Convalescence: Period of recovery from surgery or injury.

Convex: Curved or rounded like the outside of a sphere.

Coon-footed: A conformation fault in which the hoof and pastern angles are not identical.

Copulation: Sexual intercourse.

Corium: The layer of skin below the epidermis (hoof or skin), consisting of a dense bed of vascular connective tissue.

Corn: A swelling on the sole of a horse's foot between the wall and the bar caused by pressure.

Cornify: To convert to keratin.

Coronary: Pertaining to the heart; encircling in the manner of a crown, as applied to blood vessels, ligaments, or nerves (coronary band encircles the hoof).

Corrective Shoeing: The practice of trimming and shoeing a horse's hoofs in such a way as to correct a defect in the way of traveling or to reduce pain.

Corticosteroids: A term applied to hormones of the adrenal cortex or to any other natural or synthetic compounds having a similar activity. They have a systemic and metabolic effect and inhibit the inflammatory process.

Counterirritant: An agent that produces a superficial irritation to relieve another irritation.

Cow Hocks: A conformation fault in which the hocks are pointed inward when viewed from behind.

Coxitis: Inflammation of the hip joint.

Coxofemoral: Pertaining to the hip and thigh.

Cranial: Pertaining to the cranium (skull), or the anterior end of the body.

Cranium: Skull; may refer to all the bones of the head, all of them except the mandible, or the eight bones which form the vault that contains the brain.

Crepitation: The noise made by rubbing together the ends of a fractured bone. A sound like that made by rubbing the hair between the fingers.

Cretinism: A form of idiocy present at birth, caused by thyroid deficiency and characterized by stunted mental and physical growth.

Cribbing: A vice of horses in which the animal chews wood.

Cross-ties: A form of restraint in which short lead ropes are attached to each cheek ring of the horse's halter and then to eyes set into posts or the stall. This restraint is used to keep a horse from bandage chewing.

Croup: Top line of hindquarters (rump).

Crura: Pertaining to the legs, from knee to foot.

Cryptococcosis: An infection caused by a yeast-like fungus that results in lesions in the nasal cavity and lips, in the lungs, and in the meninges; it is usually fatal.

Cryptorchidism: A development defect marked by the failure of the testes to descend into the scrotum.

Culture: A growth of microorganisms or living tissue cells.

Curb: A thickening of the plantar tarsal ligament, resulting in an enlargement below the point of the hock, and marked by inflammation and lameness.

Curettage: The removal of growths or other material from the wall of a cavity, usually by scraping.

Cuticle: A layer of more or less solid substance that covers the free surface of an epithelial cell.

Cut out under the knee: A conformation fault in which there is an indentation just below the knee on the front of the cannon bone.

Cyanosis: A bluish discoloration of skin and mucous membranes due to deficient oxygenation of the blood.

Cyst: Any normal or abnormal closed cavity or sac, lined by epithelium, particularly one that contains a liquid or semi-solid substance.

Cystitis: Inflammation of the urinary bladder.

Dam: The female parent of an animal.

Debilitate: To weaken.

Deciduous Teeth: The teeth which are shed at maturity.

Degenerative: Pertaining to deterioration and change of a tissue to a less functional form.

Dehydration: Condition resulting from excessive loss of body water.

Demineralize: To excessively eliminate mineral or organic salts, as in tuberculosis, cancer, and osteomalacia.

Demodectic Mange: A skin disease caused by demodectic mites living in hair follicles and sebaceous glands, causing tissue damage through the production of toxins.

Dendrite: The part of a nerve that carries the nerve impulse toward the cell body.

Dentigerous Cyst: A tumor containing different types of material such as hair or tooth tissue. Also known as an Ear Fistula or Conchal Sinus.

Denude: To make bare by removing the epithelial covering from a surface.

Depression: A lowering of functional activity.

Dermatitis: Inflammation of the skin.

Dermographism: Pertaining to urticaria due to physical allergy, in which moderately firm stroking or scratching of the skin with a dull instrument produces a pale, raised welt or wheal.

Dermoid: Resembling the skin.

Desmitis: Inflammation of a ligament.

Desmotomy: The cutting or division of ligaments.

Dextrose: Glucose; a monosaccharide that is widely distributed in nature, and is the carbohydrate found in the blood of animals where it is an immediate source of fuel or energy.

Diagnosis: Distinguishing one disease from another, or identifying a disease from its characteristics and/or causative agent.

Diaphragm: The muscular membrane separating the abdominal and chest cavities.

Diaphysis: The portion of a long bone between the ends (shaft of long bone).

Diarrhea: Abnormal frequency and liquidity of fecal dischages.

Diastole: The period of dilatation of the heart, coinciding with the interval between the first and second heart sounds.

Diestrus: A short period of sexual quiescence between metestrus and proestrus.

Differentiation: The distinguishing of one disease or thing from another; the process of acquiring completely individual character as occurs in the diversification of cells and tissues of an embryo.

Diffusion: The non-energy-requiring process of widely spreading throughout a system.

Digital: Pertaining to the long and short pastern bones and the coffin bone.

Dilatation: The condition of being dilated or stretched beyond normal dimensions.

Dilation: A stretching or expansion.

Dimple: A slight depression.

Dipping: The soaking of an animal's entire body in a solution. A dip of lindane, for example, could be used on a horse with ringworm.

Dish: The indentation below the bulging forehead of an Arabian horse.

Dislocation: The displacement of any part, usually referring to a bone.

Distal: Remote; farther from the point of attachment or any other point of reference.

Distemper: Strangles, an infectious disease characterized by a mucopurulent inflammation of the respiratory mucous membrane.

Distension: The state of being swollen or enlarged from internal pressure.

Diuretic: An agent that increases the secretion of urine.

Diverticulum: A pouch or sac of variable size confined to a limited space occurring normally or created by herniation.

Dormant: Sleeping, inactive.

Dorsal: Pertaining to the back or denoting a position more toward the back surface than some other point of reference.

Doughnut: A roll placed around a horse's pastern to prevent Capped Elbow or Shoe Boil.

Dourine: A contagious disease marked by lymph gland swelling, genital inflammation, and paralysis of the hind limbs.

Dropped Elbow: Loss of control of the forelimb because of radial nerve paralysis.

Dry Coat: Anhidrosis, the lack of the ability to sweat.

Dry Rale: A rale produced by the presence of sticky secretion in the bronchial tubes or by spastic contraction of the walls of the tubes; heard in asthma or bronchitis, it has a squeaky sound.

Duct: A passage with definite walls.

Dummy Foal: A foal suffering from convulsive syndrome caused by lack of oxygen at birth; also called a Barker Foal.

Duodenum: The proximal portion of the small intestine, extending from the stomach to the jejenum.

Dynamic: Pertaining to or manifesting force; moving.

Dysentery: A disorder characterized by inflammation of the intestines and abdominal pain. There will be blood and mucus in the frequent stools, and it can be caused by chemical irritants, bacteria, protoza, or parasitic worms.

Dysfunction: Disturbance or impairing of the function of an organ.

Dysphagia: Difficulty in swallowing.

Dyspnea: Difficulty in breathing.

Dystrophy: Any disorder, particularly a muscle disorder, resulting from poor nutrition.

Ear Fistula: See Dentigerous Cyst.

Ecchymosis: A discoloration of the skin or mucous membranes caused by the escape of blood from vessels into the tissue.

Eccrine: The type of outward secretion from the sweat glands.

Eclampsia: Convulsions and coma.

Eczema: An inflammation of the outermost layer of skin.

Edema: An accumulation of abnormally large amounts of fluid between cells in the tissues.

Efferent: Carrying away from a center.

Electrocardiogram: A graphic tracing of the electric current produced by the heart muscle.

Electrocution: The taking of life by the passing of electric current through the body.

Electrolyte: A substance present in body fluids which is capable of conducting electricity in various body functions such as nerve impulses, oxygen and carbon dioxide transport, and muscle contraction.

Elongate: To increase in length.

Emaciated: The condition of being excessively thin, in a wasted condition.

Embolism: The sudden blocking of an artery by a clot or foreign material carried by the blood.

Embryonic: Pertaining to the offspring during its period of most rapid development before birth.

Emollient: Softening or soothing.

Emphysema: An abnormal accumulation of air in tissues or organs.

Empirical: Based on experience.

Enarthrodial: Pertaining to a ball and socket type of joint.

Encephalitis: Inflammation of the brain.

Encephalomalacia: Softening of the brain.

Encephalomyelitis: Inflammation of the brain and spinal cord.

Encystation: The process or condition of being or becoming enclosed in a sac, bladder, or cyst.

Endocarditis: Inflammation of the endocardium.

Endocrine: Secreting internally; applied to various organs and structures which secrete hormones into the blood or lymph and have an effect on other parts of the body.

Endometritis: Inflammation of the endometrium.

Endopyrogen: A substance released from the infection-fighting cells of the body which stimulates the hypothalamus to cause a fever.

Endoscope: An instrument for the examination of the interior of a hollow organ such as the bladder.

Endothelial: The layer of epithelial cells lining the cavities of the heart and of the blood and lymph vessels, and the serous cavities of the body.

Endotoxin: A heat-stable toxin present in the bacterial cell.

Enema: A liquid injection into the rectum.

Engorgement: Hyperemia; local congestion; excessive fullness of any organ or vessel.

Enteric: Pertaining to the intestines.

Enteritis: Inflammation of the intestine, particularly the small intestine.

Enterotoxemia: A condition characterized by the presence in the blood of toxins produced in the intestines.

Enzootic: A disease present in an animal community at all times but occurring only in small numbers of cases.

Enzyme: A protein which catalyzes (helps cause or accelerate) a chemical reaction, as in digestion of feed, without being consumed in the process.

Eosinophil: A structure, cell, or histological element readily stained by the dye eosin.

Epicondyle: A projection on a bone above its condyle.

Epidermis: The outermost layer of skin which is not supplied with blood vessels.

Epiglottis: The thin plate of cartilage in front of the entrance to the larynx that prevents food from entering the larynx and trachea while swallowing.

Epilepsy: Transient disturbances of brain function that may show as a loss of consciousness, seizures, etc.

Epinephrine: A hormone secreted by the adrenal gland which stimulates the sympathetic nervous system, causing contraction of the capillaries and arteries, an increase in blood pressure and heart rate, and stimulation of the heart muscle.

Epiphysis: A part of a bone, especially at the end of a long bone, which develops separately from the shaft of the bone during the growth period. During this time it is separated from the main portion of the bone by cartilage.

Epiphysitis: Inflammation of the end of a long bone or of the cartilage that separates it from the long bone.

Epistaxis: Nosebleed.

Epithelial: Pertaining to the epithelium, which is the covering of the internal and external surfaces of the body, including the lining of vessels and other small cavities.

Epithelium: The covering of internal and external surfaces of the body, including the lining of vessels and other small cavities. It consists of cells joined together by small amounts of cementing substances.

Epizootic: Attacking many animals in any region at the same time; rapidly spreading.

Erosion: An eating away; a kind of ulceration.

Erupt: The act of breaking out, appearing, becoming visible.

Erythrocytes: Red blood cells which transport oxygen.

Escharotic: A corrosive or caustic agent, such as butter of antimony, used to remove granulation tissue.

Estrous: Pertaining to estrus.

Estrus: A period of sexual receptivity in the female when she is able to conceive; heat.

Etiologic: Pertaining to the causes of disease.

Eustachian Tube: A channel between the tympanic cavity of the ear and the nasopharynx which makes possible adjustment of the pressure of air in the cavity to equal the outside air pressure.

Euthanasia: An easy or painless death; mercy killing.

Evacuation: An emptying, as of the bowels.

Ewe Neck: A conformation fault in which the neck is put on upside down. Instead of a crest, the horse has a dip in the neck.

Excision: Removal of an organ or structure by cutting.

Excretion: The act of eliminating the body's waste materials.

Exercise Bandage: A bandage applied to a horse's legs before exercising to provide support to the tendons and ligaments.

Exopthalmus: Protruding eyeball.

Exostosis: A benign bony growth projecting outward from the surface of a bone.

Expectorant: Promoting the ejection, by spitting, of mucus or other fluids from the lungs and trachea.

Expiration: The act of exhaling or expelling air from the lungs.

Extension: A movement that brings a limb into a straight line.

Extensor: Any muscle that extends a joint.

Extravasation: A discharge or escape of blood or other substance from a vessel into the tissues.

Exudate: Fluid or cells which have escaped from blood vessels into tissues or onto tissue surfaces, usually as a result of inflammation.

Facet: A small plane or surface on a hard body, as on a bone.

False Distemper: Abscesses resulting fron contagious acne and related disorders.

Fascia: A sheet or band of fibrous tissue lying below the skin or surrounding muscles and various organs of the body.

Fasciculation: A small, local contraction of muscles, visible through the skin, representing a spontaneous discharge of a number of fibers innervated by a single motor nerve filament.

Feathering: Long hair on the back of the fetlocks of cold-blooded horses.

Febrile: Relating to fever.

Fecal: Relating to the bodily waste discharged from the intestines, consisting of bacteria, cells from the intestines, secretions (mainly of the liver), and food residue.

Fenestration: To pierce with one or more openings.

Fermentation: Enzymatic decomposition.

Fetid: Having a rank or disagreeable smell.

Fetlock: The area or joint of the lower leg above the pastern and below the cannon.

Fever: Elevation of body temperature above the normal.

Fibrin: The essential fibrous protein portion of the blood.

Fibrinogen: A protein in the blood essential to the clotting process.

Fibrinous Inflammation: Inflammation characterized by a fibrin exudate.

Fibrosis: The formation of fibrous tissue.

Fibrous Adhesion: A fibrous band or structure by which parts abnormally adhere.

Filing: The act of filing down the teeth to remove sharp edges; also referred to as Floating.

Firing: Applying a heated firing iron to a leg to produce a severe inflammation, used to treat chronic or subacute inflammations of the joints, tendons, and bones.

Fissure: Any normal or abnormal cleft or groove.

Fistula: An abnormal passage between two organs or from an internal organ to the surface of the body.

Fistulous Withers: A condition in which an infection of the withers leads to an abscess.

Flatulence: Pertaining to excessive amounts of air or gases in the stomach or intestine which may be expelled through the anus.

Flexion: The act of bending.

Floating: The act of filing a horse's teeth to remove the sharp edges.

Fluorosis: A condition in which the teeth deteriorate because of an excess of flouride.

Foal Heat: The heat period that occurs approximately nine days after a mare has foaled; also called Nine-day Heat.

Follicle: A small sac or a cavity.

Foramina: Natural openings or passages in the body.

Forging: A type of limb contact during movement, in which the toe of the hindfoot hits the bottom of the forefoot on the same side.

Fossa: A hollow or depressed area.

Founder: The crippled condition caused by laminitis.

Founder Ring: A ring around the hoof that results from mal keratin synthesis during an attack of laminitis.

Founder Stance: The typical stance of a horse with founder in which the animal will try to take as much weight as possible off his feet. For example, if the forefeet are affected, the horse will bring them forward in front of his body, and move his hind feet up under his body.

Fracture: The breaking of a part, especially a bone.

Frog: The band of horny substance in the middle of the sole of a horse's foot, dividing into two branches and running toward the heel in the shape of a "V."

Fungus: A general term used to designate a group of eukaryotic protists.

Fusion: The abnormal coherence of adjoining parts of bodies.

Gamma-ray Therapy: A type of radiation therapy using gamma rays to treat such conditions as neoplasms.

Gangrene: Death of tissue, usually due to loss of blood supply.

Gaseous: Of the nature of a gas.

Gaskin: The thigh of a horse.

Gastric: Pertaining to the stomach.

Gastric Dilatation: Excessive distension of the intestines, as in colic.

Gastrorrhagia: Hemorrhage from the stomach.

Gene: The self-reproducing biologic unit of heredity located on a chromosome.

Generalized: Having spread throughout the body; not local.

Genitalia: The organs of the reproductive system, especially the external organs.

Genotype: The hereditary make up of an animal.

Germ: A pathogenic organism.

Ginglymus: A type of synovial joint that allows movement in only one plane, forward and backward, as the hinge of a door.

Glanders: A contagious disease characterized by purulent inflammation of the mucous membranes and an eruption of nodules on the skin which form deep ulcers, possibly causing bone and cartilage necrosis.

Glands: Aggregation of cells, specialized to secrete and excrete materials not needed in their normal metabolic process.

Glass Eye: An eye without pigment, often present in horses with white face markings.

Glaucoma: Eye disease marked by an increase in the intraocular pressure which causes changes in the optic disk.

Glioma: A tumor composed of tissue that represents neuroglia in one of its stages of development.

Glomerulonephritis: An inflammation of the capillary loops of the glomeruli of the kidneys.

Glucose: A sugar which is a principal source of energy.

Goiter: An enlargement of the thyroid gland.

Gonitis: Inflammation of the knee.

Grand Mal: Epilepsy in which a sudden loss of consciousness is immediately followed by convulsions.

Granulation: The formation in wounds of small rounded masses of tissue, composed of capillaries and connective tissue cells.

Granules: Small particles or grains.

Gravel: An infection in the hoof resulting from the penetration of the white line which drains at the coronet.

Green Osselet: Inflammation of the joint capsule of the fetlock joint.

Guttural Pouch: A large mucous sac near the base of the skull which is an outpocketing of the eustachian tube.

Hair Follicle: A flask-like depression from which a hair grows.

Halitosis: Bad breath.

Heart Block: Impairment of conduction in heart excitation.

Heat Exhaustion: Hyperthermia; circulatory collapse and shock caused by high environmental temperature, high humidity, and poor ventilation.

Heat Stroke: Hyperthermia; caused by the same situations as heat exhaustion but is more serious. Sweating usually stops, and heat stroke is often fatal.

Heaves: A respiratory ailment, characterized by forced expiration and dyspnea, resulting from the rupture of alveoli in the lungs, and caused by such things as allergies and dust.

Heel Crack: A sand crack located in the heel of the hoof that can involve the sensitive lamina.

Hematinic: An agent which improves the quality of the blood, increasing the hemoglobin level and the number of erythrocytes.

Hematoma: A localized collection of blood, usually clotted, in an organ, space, or tissue, due to a break in the wall of a blood vessel.

Hemoglobin: The oxygen-carrying protein pigment of the red blood cells.

Hemoglobinuria: The presence of free hemoglobin in the urine.

Hemolysis: The release of hemoglobin by the destruction of red blood cells.

Hemophilia: A hereditary deficiency of a clotting factor in the blood.

Hemoptysis: The exporation of blood or blood stained sputum.

Hemorrhage: The escape of blood from the vessels; bleeding.

Hemorrhagic Inflammation: An inflammation characterized by an exudate containing large numbers of erythrocytes.

Hemothorax: A collection of blood in the pleural cavity.

Hepatic: Pertaining to the liver.

Hepatitis: Inflammation of the liver.

Hernia: The protrusion of a loop of an organ or tissue through an abnormal opening.

Heterochromia: A diversity of color in a part or parts that should normally be of one color.

Hirsutism: Abnormal hairiness.

Histamine: A chemical compound which dilates capillaries, constricts the smooth muscle of the lungs, and increases secretions of the stomach; may be used to reduce sensitivity to allergens.

Hives: Urticaria.

Homeostasis: A tendency to stability in the normal internal environment of an organism.

Hoof Tester: A pincer-like instrument used to gently squeeze the hoofs to find any sore areas. If this is done in an area of inflammation the horse will flinch.

Hormone: A chemical substance produced in the body by an organ which regulates the activity of a specific organ.

Horse Pox: A mild form of smallpox affecting horses, marked by a pustular eruption of the skin.

Host: An animal or plant that harbors or nourishes another organism.

Humerus: The bone that extends from the shoulder to the elbow.

Husbandry: The scientific management of domestic animals.

Hyaloid Vessel: An artery present in the eye of the fetus which is commonly present at birth and usually disintegrates within the first two weeks of life.

Hydrocephalus: An abnormal amount of fluid beneath the skull, resulting in an enlarged head, brain atrophy, and mental deterioration.

Hydrolysis: The splitting of a compound into fragments by the addition of water.

Hydrothorax: A collection of watery fluid in the pleural cavity.

Hygroma: A sac distended with fluid.

Hymen: A fold of mucous membrane which partially or completely covers the opening of the vagina.

Hyperemia: An excess of blood in a part.

Hyperexcitability: Abnormal excitation of the nervous system.

Hyperextend: Extreme or excessive extension of a limb.

Hyperflexion: Forcible overflexion of a limb or part.

Hyperirritability: Pathological responsiveness to slight stimuli.

Hyperparathyroidism: Abnormally increased activity of the parathyroid gland.

Hyperpigmentation: Abnormally increased pigmentation.

Hyperplasia: An abnormal increase in the normal number of cells in a tissue.

Hyperresonance: An exaggerated resonance (intensification of sound produced by the transmission of vibrations to a cavity).

Hypersensitivity: A state of altered activity in which the body reacts with an exaggerated response to a foreign agent.

Hyperthermia: Heat stroke or heat exhaustion.

Hyperthyroidism: Excessive functional activity of the thyroid gland.

Hypertrophy: The enlargement or overgrowth of an organ or part due to an increase in size of its constituent cells.

Hyphema: Hemorrhage within the anterior chamber of the eye.

Hypoglycemia: An abnormally diminished level of glucose in the body.

Hypopigmentation: Abnormally diminished pigmentation.

Hypoplasia: Incomplete development of an organ so that it fails to reach adult size.

Hypopyon: An accumulation of pus in the anterior chamber of the eye.

Hypothalamus: The part of the brain which regulates part of the nervous system, hormone activity, and many body functions.

Hypothyroidism: A deficiency of thyroid activity.

Ileum: The distal portion of the small intestine, extending from the jejunum to the cecum.

Ilium: The expansive cranial (front) portion of the hip bone.

Impaction: The condition of being firmly lodged or wedged.

Incidence: An expression of the rate at which a certain event occurs, as the number of new cases of a specific disease occurring during a certain period.

Incised: Cut, made by cutting.

Incompetence: Physical or mental inadequacy or insufficiency, as in cardiac insufficiency (incompetence), the regurgitation of blood.

Incubation: The period of development of an infectious disease from the time the disease-producing organism enters the body until signs of the disease appear.

Infarction: The formation of an area of dead tissue resulting from obstruction of circulation to the area by a clot.

Inflammation: A condition of tissues characterized by pain, heat, redness, swelling and various exudations as a reaction to injury. It serves to eliminate harmful substances and damaged tissue.

Influenza: An acute viral infection involving the respiratory tract, occuring in isolated cases or in epidemics, striking many continents simultaneously or in sequence. It is marked by inflammation of the nasal mucosa, the pharynx, and conjunctiva.

Ingestion: The act of taking food, medicines, etc., into the body by mouth.

Inhalation: The act of drawing air or other substances into the lungs.

Injection: The act of forcing a liquid into a part, as into the subcutaneous tissues, the blood vessels, or an organ; a substance so forced or administered.

Innervation: The distribution or supply of nerves to a part; the supply of nervous energy or of nerve stimulus sent to a part.

Inoculate: The introduction of a vaccine or disease-producing organism into the body.

Inspiration: The act of inhaling or drawing air into the lungs.

Integument: A covering, as the skin.

Intercostal: Between ribs.

Interosseous: Between bones.

Intersesamoidean: Between the sesamoids.

Interventricular Septal Defect: A condition arising from the failure of the septum to develop completely in the fetus, causing an opening between the ventricles of the heart at birth.

Intestinal: Pertaining to the intestines.

Intestinal Flora: The bacteria normally present within the intestine.

Intima: A general term denoting an innermost structure, as the inner lining of a blood vessel.

Intravenous: Within a vein.

Intussusception: The prolapse of one part of the intestine into the lumen of an immediately adjoining part.

Involuntary: Performed independently of the will, contravolitional; as in an involuntary muscle.

Irritant: An agent that produces irritation.

Ischial: Pertaining to the caudal part of the hip bone.

Isoimmunization: Development of antibodies against an antigen derived from a genetically dissimilar individual of the same species.

Jacksonian Epilepsy: Epilepsy characterized by unilatral clonic movements that start in one group of muscles and spread systematically to adjacent groups, reflecting the march of the epileptic activity through the motor cortex.

Jack Spavin: An exceptionally large bone spavin.

Jaundice: A syndrome characterized by hyperbilirubinemia and deposition of bile pigment in the skin and mucous membranes with resulting yellow appearance of the patient.

Jejunum: The middle portion of the small intestine, extending from the duodenum to the ileum.

Joint: An articulation; the place of union or junction between two or more bones of the skeleton.

Joint Mouse: A small chip of bone enclosed in the joint capsule.

Jugular Pulse: The rhythmic expansion of an artery of the neck that may be felt with the finger.

Kallidin: Factors formed by a group of enzymes produced by the body that maintain dilation of the blood vessels in the inflammatory process.

Keratin: An insoluble protein which is the principal constituent of epidermis, hair, nails, horny tissues, and the enamel of teeth.

Keratoma: A horny tumor on the inner surface of the wall of a horse's hoof.

Knock Knee: Epiphysitis occuring in foals (sometimes because of diet deficiency).

Laboratory Diagnosis: Diagnosis based on the finding of various laboratory tests.

Laceration: A torn, ragged wound.

Lacrimation: The secretion and discharge of tears.

Lactation: The secretion of milk.

Lactic Acid: An organic acid normally present in muscle tissue, produced by anaerobic muscle metabolism. It may also be produced in carbohydrate matter, usually by bacterial fermentation.

Lamella: A thin plate, as of bone.

Laminae: Thin, flat plates or layers.

Laminitis: Inflammation of a lamina, especially the laminae of a horse's foot.

Lampas: A swelling and hardening of the mucosa of the hard palate, immediately behind the upper incisors in horses.

Larva: An early developmental stage, usually the feeding form of an animal such as an insect or worm.

Laryngitis: Inflammation of the larynx, a condition attended with dryness and soreness of the throat, cough, and dysphagia.

Larynx: The structure of muscle and cartilage located at the top of the trachea and below the root of the tongue; "voice box."

Latent: Concealed, not manifest; potential.

Lateral: Pertaining to a side or outer surface, a portion further from the midline of the body or of a structure.

Lathyrism: A morbid condition resulting from ingestion of the seeds of leguminous plants.

Laxative: An agent that acts to promote evacuation of the bowl; a cathartic or purgative.

Leg Swing: An outward swing of the foreleg due to popped knee or arthritis. Due to the pain involved, the horse swings his leg out and around instead of bending the knee as he walks.

Leptospirosis: Infection by Leptospira.

Lesion: An abnormal change in the structure of a part due to injury or disease.

Lethargy: Condition of drowsiness or indifference.

Leukocytes: White blood cells or corpuscles.

Leukoderma: An acquired type of localized loss of melanin pigmentation of the skin.

Libido: Sexual drive.

Ligament: A band of fibrous tissue that connects bones or cartilages.

Lipid: An organic substance containing fat which is an important component of living cells.

Lipoid: Fatlike, resembling fat.

Liquefaction: The conversion of material into a liquid form.

Listeriosis: Infection caused by organisms of the genus Listeria. An infectious disease, though not very pathogenic.

Lobe: A well-defined portion of any organ.

Lockjaw: A common term for Tetanus. See also Tetanus.

Lopped Ears: Ears which are placed too far apart.

Lumbar: Pertaining to the loins, the part of the back between the thorax and pelvis.

Lumen: The cavity or channel within a tube or tubular organ.

Luxation: Dislocation.

Lymph: A transparent yellowish liquid containing mostly white blood cells and derived from tissue fluids.

Lymphosarcoma: A general term applied to malignant neoplastic disorders of lymphoid tissue.

Malignant: Tending to become progressively worse and to result in death.

Malleolus: A rounded process of a bone.

Mammillary: Pertaining to, or resembling a nipple.

Mange: A contagious skin disease caused by various types of mites.

Mania: Aiphase of mental disorder characterized by an expansive emotional state and increased motor activity.

March Fracture: Fracture of a bone of the lower extremity, developing after repeated stresses.

Mastitis: Inflammation of the mammary gland.

Mastocytosis: An accumulation, either local or systemic, of mast cells in the tissue. Characterized by the appearance of nodules under the skin.

Matrix: The basic material from which a structure develops, the substance between cells.

Meconium: A dark green, adhesive material in the intestine of the full-term fetus, being a mixture of the secretions of the intestinal glands and some amniotic fluid.

Medial: Pertaining to the middle or inner surface; a position closer to the midline of the body or of a structure.

Melanin: The dark pigment of the body.

Melanocytes: Cells responsible for the synthesis of melanin.

Melanoma: A tumor made up of melanin-pigmented cells. When used alone, the term refers to a malignant melanoma.

Melioidosis: A bacterial infection occurring mainly in tropical countries, and transmitted by rodents. The bacteria live in the soil and infect the horse through skin abrasions, inhalation, or insect bite. Similar to Glanders, symptoms include high fever, nasal discharge, and a slight cough.

Membrane: A thin layer of tissue which covers a surface, lines a cavity, or divides a space or organ.

Meninges: The three membranes that envelop the brain and spinal cord.

Meningitis: Inflammation of the meninges, usually a complication of a pre-existing disease. Generally characterized by incoordination, compulsive movement, convulsions, and a high but fluctuating body temperature.

Mesentery: A fold or membrane attaching various organs to the body wall.

Mesothelium: The layer of flat cells, derived from the mesoderm, which lines the coelom or body cavity of the embryo.

Metabolism: The sum of physical and chemical activities of an animal.

Metacarpal: Cannon; the area between the knee and fetlock joint of the foreleg.

Metastasis: The transfer of disease from one organ or part of the body to another not directly connected to it, due to transfer of disease-causing microorganisms or of cells through blood or lymph.

Metatarsal: Cannon; the area between the hock and fetlock joint of the hindleg.

Metestrus: The period of rest following estrus in female mammals.

Microcornea: A congenital condition characterized by an abnormally small (sometimes less than 10 mm) cornea.

Microorganisms: Minute, microscopic organisms such as bacteria, viruses, molds, yeasts, and protozoa.

Microphthalmia: Congenital condition characterized by the presence of an abnormally small eyeball.

Mineral Deposits: Extraneous inorganic matter collected in the tissues or in a cavity.

Miotic: Any drug that causes the pupil to contract.

Modified Live Virus: A virus that has been taken from the natural state and raised in a laboratory under somewhat unnatural conditions. Because of the unnatural conditions in which it was raised, the virus does not have the disease-causing abilities of a virus in the natural state, but it still has the properties of stimulating the production of antibodies when injected into an animal. The stimulation of antibody production makes it valuable as a vaccine.

Monday Morning Sickness: A condition associated with forced exercise after a period of rest during which feed has not been reduced. Characterized by painful movement and "tying up." Also known as Azoturia.

Monocytes: White blood cells active in fighting subacute infections.

Morbid: Pertaining to or affected with disease, diseased.

Morphology: The science of the forms and structure of organized beings.

Motility: The ability to move.

Mucopurulent: Containing both mucus and pus.

Mucosa: A mucous membrane.

Mucus: The free slime of the mucous membrane, composed of secretion of the glands.

Mule Ears: Ears which are abnormally long.

Multiple Exostosis: Benign bony growths projecting outward from the surface of bones, characteristically capped by cartilage.

Murmur: A periodic sound of short duration of cardiac or vacular origin.

Muscle: An organ which by contraction produces the movements of an animal organism.

Muscle Relaxant: An agent that specifically aids in reducing muscle tension.

Muscle Tremor: An involuntary trembling or quivering of a muscle.

Mydriatic: Any drug that dilates the pupil.

Myelin Sheath: The lipid substance forming around certain nerve fibers.

Myocarditis: Inflammation of the muscular walls of the heart.

Myoglobin: A ferrous complex contributing to the color of muscle and acting as a store of oxygen.

Myopathy: Any disease of a muscle.

Myositis: Inflammation of a voluntary muscle.

Myotonia: Increased muscular irritation and contraction with decreased power of relaxation, tonic spasm of muscle.

Navicular: A small bone in the foot of a horse; common term to designate pathology of the navicular bone.

Neck cradle: A wooden collar used as a restraint to prevent the horse from bending his neck.

Necropsy: Examination of a body after death, an autopsy.

Necrosis: Death of a cell or group of cells which is in contact with living tissue.

Nematode: Any of a group of roundworms which are mainly internal parasites.

Nematodosis: A nervous disorder characterized by incoordination, caused by one of the Nematodes. Also known as kumri.

Neonatal: Pertaining to the first month after birth.

Neonatal Isoerythrolysis: A severe red blood cell destroying disease of newborn foals, often called foal jaundice.

Neoplasm: A new and abnormal growth of tissue in which the growth is uncontrolled and progressive; a tumor.

Nephritis: Inflammation of the kidneys.

Nephrons: The anatomical and functional units of the kidneys.

Nephrosis: Any disease of the kidneys.

Nerves: Cordlike structures, visible to the naked eye, comprising a collection of nerve fibers which convey impulses between a part of the central nervous system and some other region of the body.

Neural: Pertaining to a nerve or to the nerves.

Neurectomy: The excision of part of a nerve.

Neuroglia: The supporting structure of nervous tissue.

Neuroma: A tumor or new growth largely made up of nerve cells and nerve fibers; a tumor growing from a nerve.

Neuron: Any of the conducting cells of the nervous system.

Neurotoxic: Poisonous or destructive to nerve tissue.

Neutrophil: Any cell or structure readily stainable by neutral dyes.

Nictitating Membrane: A fold of mucous membrane at the inside corner of the eye; the third eyelid.

Nine-day Heat: Also called Foal Heat, the period (usually 9-11 days after foaling) during which mares show signs of heat.

Nodules: Small nodes, or knots, which are solid and can be detected by touch.

Nonvascular: Not supplied with blood vessels.

Norepinephrine: A hormone secreted by neurons which acts as a transmitter substance of the peripheral sympathetic nerve endings.

Occlude: To fit close together, or to obstruct or close off.

Occult Spavin: A term for typical spavin lameness without external signs.

Olecranon: The point of the elbow, formed by the bony projection of the ulna.

Olfactory: Pertaining to the sense of smell.

Onochoerciasis: A general term applied to several disorders which involve the larvae of a certain parasitic Nematode. These disorders are characterized by redness, swelling, the formation of lesions, and eventual drying of the skin.

Opacity: An opaque area, as in the eye, which does not allow light to pass through; neither transparent nor translucent.

Opaque: Not allow light to pass through.

Open knee: A condition, usually the result of a mineral imbalance, wherein the profile of the knee is irregular due to the enlarged epiphysis of the lower end of the radius and the carpal bone deviation toward the back.

Opthalmology: That branch of medicine dealing with the eye, its anatomy and physiology, etc.

Opthalmoscope: An instrument containing a perforated mirror and lenses used to examine the interior of the eye.

Optic: Pertaining to the eye.

Orbital Cellulitis: Inflammation of the tissue surrounding the eyeball.

Orchitis: Inflammation of the testes.

Organ: A somewhat independent part of the body that performs a special function or functions.

Organization: The replacement of blood clots by fibrous tissue.

Organophosphate: A phosphorus-containing organic pesticide.

Orifice: The entrance or outlet of any cavity in the body.

Osmosis: Diffusion through a semipermeable membrane (as of a living cell) typically separating a solvent and a solution that tends to equalize their concentrations.

Osselet: A bony growth on the inner aspect of a horse's knee or on the lateral aspect of the fetlock.

Ossify: To change or develop into bone.

Osteitis: Inflammation of a bone.

Osteochondrosis: Disease of a growth center in a bone.

Osteodystrophy: Defective bone formation.

Osteomyelitis: Inflammation of bone caused by a pyogenic (pus producing) organism.

Ovoid: Egg-shaped.

Oxidant: Substance that combines another substance with oxygen.

Oxyhemoglobin: A compound formed from hemoglobin on exposure to atmospheric conditions.

Pain Receptors: Sensory nerve terminals which respond to stimuli of various kinds.

Palliative Treatment: Care which is designed to relieve pain and distress, but which does not attempt a cure.

Pallor: Paleness, absence of skin coloration.

Palpation: The act of feeling with the hand.

Papilla: A small, nipple-shaped projection.

Papilloma: A growth of epithelial tissue (wart).

Paralysis: Loss or impairment of motor function in a part.

Paraphimosis: Retraction of phimotic foreskin, causing a painful swelling of the glans that, if severe, may cause dry gangrene unless corrected.

Parasite: A plant or animal which lives upon or within another living organism at whose expense it obtains some advantage.

Parasympathetic: A substance of the nervous system that soothes and is constantly active when the animal is at rest.

Parathormome: Hormone secreted by the parathyroid glands, instrumental in maintaining proper calcium levels in the body.

Parenchymal: The essential elements of an organ; used as a general term to designate the functional elements of an organ, as in parenchyma of the liver.

Parenteral: Administration of medication through some other route than the alimentary canal, such as subcutaneous, intramuscular, etc.

Parietal: Pertaining to the walls of a cavity.

Parrot Mouth: A congenital defect of imperfectly meshed teeth, similar to buck teeth in humans.

Particulate: Composed of separate particles.

Pastern: The area between the fetlock joint and the coronary band.

Pasturellosis: Infection by microorganisms of the genus Pasteurella. An acute septicemia that may be associated with pneumonia and other upper respiratory tract infections.

Patella: A triangular sesamoid bone situated at the front of the stifle. Also called knee cap.

Patent Ductus Arteriosis: The abnormal persistence of an open lumen in the ductus arteriosus after birth, with the direction of flow being from the aorta to the pulmonary artery, resulting in recirculation of arterial blood through the lungs.

Pathogen: Any microorganism or material.

Pathological: A diseased condition.

Pectoral: Pertaining to the chest.

Pelvis: The rear portion of the trunk of the body, bounded by the hip bones.

Pendular: Having a pendulum-like movement.

Pepsin: An enzyme of the stomach that breaks down most proteins to polypeptides, aiding in digestion.

Peracute: Excessively acute or sharp.

Percussion: The act of striking a part with short, sharp blows as an aid in diagnosing the condition of the parts beneath by the sound obtained.

Periarticular: Situated around a joint.

Pericarditis: Inflammation of the pericardium, the fibroserous sac that surrounds the heart.

Perilymph: The fluid contained within the space separating the membranous from the osseous labyrinth of the ear.

Perineal: Pertaining to the pelvic floor and the structures of the pelvic outlet.

Periodic Ophthalmia: An inflammatory disease of the eye which is the most common cause of blindness in the horse. Also known as "moon blindness."

Periople: The layer of soft, light-colored horn covering the outer aspect of the hoof.

Periosteitis: Inflammation of the periosteum (bone covering).

Periosteum: A specialized connective tissue covering all bones of the body, which is capable of forming bone.

Peripheral Circulatory System: The part of the circulatory system that carries blood to the outer parts of the body such as the legs.

Peristalsis: Waves of contraction along the muscular walls of the intestine and other hollow organs which propel the contents.

Peritoneum: The serous membrane lining the walls of the abdominal and pelvic cavities and surrounding the internal organs.

Peritonitis: Inflammation of the peritoneum; a condition marked by exudations in the peritoneum of serum, fibrin, cells, and pus.

Permeate: To spread through or penetrate.

Pervious Urachus: A condition that develops when the urachus, a small ureter-like structure within the umbilical cord, fails to close when the umbilical cord is severed.

Pessary: An instrument placed in the vagina to support the uterus or rectum or as a contraceptive device.

Petechia: A small, round purplish-red spot caused by hemorrhage which later turns blue or yellow.

Petit Mal: Epilepsy, characterized by mild convulsive seizures.

Phagocyte: Any cell that ingests microorganisms or other cells and foreign particles.

Phagocytosis: The engulfing of microorganisms and foreign particles.

Phalanx: Any of the three bones below the fetlock: the long pastern bone, short pastern bone, and coffin bone.

Pharyngitis: Inflammation of the pharynx.

Pharynx: The sac between the mouth and the esophagus. It communicates above with the larynx, mouth, nasal passages, and eustachian tubes and below with the esophagus.

Phlegmon: Inflammation of the connective tissues.

Photophobia: An abnormal aversion to light.

Photosensitization: An excessive reaction of the skin to sunlight, resulting in swelling and inflammation.

Phycomycosis: An infection caused by any of several fungi in the class Phycomycetes; the most common type of internal disease affecting the horse. The first signs of the infection may be swellings on the skin with discharges of clear fluids.

Physiology: The branch of biology which deals with the functions and activities of life or living matter (cells, organs, tissues), and of the chemical and physical phenomena involved.

Phytotoxin: In the broadest sense, any toxic substance of plant origin.

Pigeon-toed: Condition in which a horse's feet point in, because the legs are turned inward from their origin down.

Pig-eye: An eye which is considered too small.

Pigment: Any coloring matter of the body.

Pin-firing: Using a firing mechanism to artificially introduce inflammation to an area (especially the lower leg) for therapeutic purposes.

Piroplasmosis: Also called Texas Fever, a term describing Babesiasis, a protozoal disease carried by blood-sucking ticks which infect the horse.

Pit: The imprint retained by an edematous swelling after pressure has been applied (by the finger) and released.

Pituitary Gland: A body at the base of the brain which secretes and stores hormones that regulate most of the basic body functions.

Placenta: An organ which joins the fetus to the uterus of the mare and allows for the exchange of substances through the blood.

Plantar: Pertaining to the sole of the foot.

Plaque: Any patch or flat area.

Plasma: The liquid portion of the blood, containing the suspended particulate components.

Plasma Extenders: Substances which can be transfused to maintain plasma volume of the blood.

Platelets: Disk-shaped structures found in the blood of all mammals and chiefly known for their role in blood coagulation; also called blood platelets. See also Thrombocytes.

Pleura: The serous membrane enclosing the lungs and lining the thoracic cavity.

Pleurisy: Inflammation of the pleura with exudation into its cavity and upon its surface. Also called pleuritis.

Plexus: A network of lymphatic vessels, nerves, veins, or arteries.

Pneumovagina: Infection due to the presence of air in the vagina; the single most common cause of female infertility in mares.

Polyarthritis: An inflammation of several joints together.

Polycythemia: An increase in the total red blood cell mass of the body.

Polyp: A protruding growth from mucous membrane.

Polyuria: Passage of an abnormally large volume of urine in a given period, characterized by frequent urination.

Posterior: Situated in back of, or in the back of, a structure; toward the rear end of the body.

Postmortem: After death.

Postpartum: Occurring after delivery, with reference to the mother.

Postparturient: Occurring after delivery.

Poultice: A soft, moist, mass of the consistency of cooked cereal, spread between layers of muslin, linen, gauze, or towels, and applied hot to a given area in order to create moist local heat or counterirritation.

Presumptive Diagnosis: Expected diagnosis.

Primary Treatment: First treatment in order, or in time of development. The principle treatment.

Process: A projection, as of bone.

Prognosis: The prospect of recovery from a disease or injury.

Progressive: Advancing, going from bad to worse; advancing in severity.

Prolapse: The falling down, or sinking, of a part of an interior organ.

Proliferate: To multiply; to grow by reproducing similar cells.

Propulsion: The tendency to fall forward in walking.

Protein: Any of a group of complex compounds which contain nitrogen and are composed of amino acids.

Proteinaceous: Pertaining to, or of the nature of protein.

Protozoa: One-celled organisms, the simplest organisms of the animal kingdom.

Proud Flesh: Excessive granulation tissue.

Proximal: Nearest, closer to the point of attachment or any point of reference.

Psoroptic Mange: Mange caused by a species of the genus Psoroptes. It occurs mainly on sheltered parts of the body, as on areas covered with long hair.

Pulmonary: Pertaining to the lungs.

Pulmonary Emphysema: Also know as broken wind, a condition of abnormal distention and inability to empty the lungs of air, caused by the rupture of some alveoli. See also Heaves.

Pulse: Rhythmic throbbing of an artery which may be felt with the finger; caused by blood forced through the vessel by contractions of the heart.

Puncture: A wound that is deeper than it is wide.

Purgative: An agent that causes a cleansing or evacuation of the bowels.

Purpura Hemorrhagica: A disease of the horse characterized by extensive collections of fluid and blood in tissues beneath the skin, occuring primarily on the head and legs.

Purulent: Consisting of or containing pus; associated with the formation of, or caused by pus.

Purulent Inflammation: An inflammation associated with the formation of pus.

Pus: A liquid inflammation product made up of leukocytes and a thin fluid called liquor puris.

Pustules: Visible collections of pus within or beneath the epidermis.

Putrid: Rotten or decomposed

Pyometra: An accumulation of pus within the uterus.

Pyramidal: Shaped like a pyramid, cone-shaped; referring to a cone-shaped structure or part.

Pyramidal Disease: A form of low ringbone, a new abnormal bone growth which may be due to fracture or periostitis or osteitis of extensor process of the coffin bone. Also known as Buttress Foot.

Pyrogen: A fever-producing substance.

Quarantine: Restrictions placed on the entrance to and exit from the place or premises where a case of communicable disease exists.

Quidding: A habit in which the horse rolls his food into a ball and drops it on the ground.

Quittor: A chronic, deep-seated inflammation of the lateral cartilages characterized by necrosis of the inflamed part.

Rabies: An acute infectious disease of the central nervous system, usually fatal in mammal species.

Rachitic: Pertaining to or affected with rickets.

Radiation Therapy: Treatment using x-rays, beta rays, and gamma rays to destroy or retard the growth of tumors, and to treat certain areas with artificial inflammation.

Radiational Irritant: An agent that is used in radiation therapy to cause counterirritation.

Radiograph: A film of internal structures of the body produced by the action of x-rays or gamma rays on a specially sensitized film.

Rales: Any abnormal respiratory sound.

Rarefaction: Also called rarification, denotes becoming less dense; a decrease in density and weight but not in volume.

Rasping: Filing the teeth with a rasp to provide dental care.

Recessive: Tending to recede; not exerting a ruling or controlling influence. A recessive gene in genetics.

Reciprocal Action: The complementary interaction of two distant entities.

Recumbency: A lying down position.

Red Blood Cells: Hemoglobin carrying corpuscles in the blood that transport oxygen. See also Erythrocytes.

Reflex Arc: The neural arc used in a reflex action.

Regeneration: The natural renewal of a structure, as of a tissue or part.

Regurgitation: A backward flowing, as of undigested food from the stomach, or of blood through the heart.

Resciant: A counterirritant agent which produces blistering and scurfing of the skin.

Resilient: Elastic, returning to its former shape after distortion.

Resolution: The subsidence of an inflammation, or the softening and disappearance of a swelling.

Resonance: The prolongation and intensification of sound produced by the transmission of its vibrations to a cavity, especially a sound elicited by percussion; a vocal sound as heard in auscultation.

Retention: A process of keeping a fluid or secretion within the body which is normally excreted.

Reticuloendothelial Tissue: Tissue having both reticular (net-like) and endothelial attributes.

Retinal Detachment: A condition associated with periodic ophthalmia or injuries that may affect the eye. May cause blindness in the eye affected.

Rhinitis: Inflammation of the mucous membrane of the nose.

Rhinopneumonitis: Inflammation of the nasal and pulmonary mucous membranes.

Rhinosporidiosis: A nonfatal fungal infection characterized by growths on the mucous membrane of the nasal cavity.

Ricin: A poisonous substance found in the seeds of the castor oil plant.

Ringbone: A general term that applies to bony enlargments and areas of new bone growth below the fetlock.

Roach Back: A conformation fault in which the back is arched and convex. This fault predisposes a horse to forging and shortens the gait of the animal.

Roaring: The common whistling or roaring sound that is a characteristic sign of paralysis of one or both intrinsic muscles of the larynx.

Rotation: The process of turning around an axis.

Route of Treatment: The path in, or part of, the body through which a remedy is administered.

Rubefacient: An agent that reddens the skin, and produces a mild irritation.

Rupture: A breaking or tearing of tissue.

Saccule: A small bag or sac.

Sacroiliac: Pertaining to the sacrum and ilium, denoting the joint or articulation between the sacrum and ilium and associated ligaments.
known as equine incoordination and jinxed back.

Sacrum: The triangular bone just below the lumbar vertebrae, wedged dorsally between the two wings of the hip bone.

Saddle Sore: A simple inflammation of hair follicles (usually on the withers) caused by friction between the horse and the saddle.

Saline Solution: A salt-containing solution.

Saliva: The clear, alkaline, somewhat sticky secretion from various glands of the mouth; it serves to moisten and soften food for digestion.

Salmonellosis: Infection with certain species of the genus Salmonella, usually caused by the ingestion of food containing the organisms, and marked by violent diarrhea and cramps. Fever is usually present in this inflammation of the intestines.

Salve: A thick ointment.

Sand Cracks: Cracks in the hoof wall.

Saprophytic: Organisms, such as bacteria, which live on dead or decaying organic matter.

Sarcoid: Tumor composed mainly of connective tissue which appears on the skin as the most common tumor of the horse.

Sarcoma: An often highly-malignant tumor made up of a substance similar to embryonic connective tissue.

Sarcoptic mange: The most serious type of mange usually affecting areas where the hair is thin (head, neck, and shoulders).

Scab: A crust or covering.

Scar Tissue: Tissue remaining after the healing of a wound or other morbid process.

Sebaceous: A thick, fatty semifluid substance secreted by the skin.

Seborrhea: A skin disease, probably the result of an abnormal production of keratin. Normally a secondary disease in horses following dermatitis or eczema.

Sebum (Sebaceous): A thick, fatty, semifluid substance secreted by the skin.

Secondary: A condition derived from or consequent to a primary condition.

Secrete: To produce and give off cell products.

Sedative: An agent that reduces and controls excitement.

Seedy Toe: A disease of the hoof wall in the toe region in which the hoof wall is separated from the white line.

Semilunar: Resembling a crescent, or half-moon.

Semipermeable: Permitting the passage of certain molecules and hindering the passage of others.

Sensitization: The initial exposure of an individual to a specific antigen, resulting in an immune response.

Septic: A state of decomposition produced by microorganisms.

Septicemia: Disease associated with disease-producing microorganisms or their poisons in the blood; blood poisoning.

Septum: A dividing wall or partition.

Sequestra: Pieces of dead bone that have been broken off or become separated, during the process of necrosis, from the sound bone.

Serous: The clear liquid portion of the blood or any body fluid that separates after complete clotting; blood plasma with the fibrinogen removed.

Sesamoid: A small nodular bone embedded in a tendon or joint capsule.

Sesamoiditis: An inflammation of the proximal sesamoid bones, usually involving both osteitis and periostitis.

Sheath: A tubular structure enclosing or surrounding an organ or part.

Shigellosis: An acute, highly fatal septicemia, also called navel ill, joint ill, and sleepy foal disease. Symptoms include sudden fever, diarrhea, rapid respiration, and lethargy.

Shin Buck: Inflammation of the bone covering of the front side of the cannon bone. Often seen in young horses that have been strenuously exercised.

Shivering: A disease of horses characterized by trembling or quivering of various muscles.

Shock: A condition of acute peripheral circulatory failure due to derangement of circulatory control or loss of circulating fluid.

Shoe Boil: A soft, flabby swelling over the point of the elbow. See also Capped Elbow.

Sickle Hocks: Deviations in the angle of the hock as seen from the side. The cannon slopes forward due to excessive angulation of the hock.

Sidebones: Ossification of the two lateral cartilages of the wings of the coffin bone.

Sign: Evidence of a disease, as observed by someone other than the patient.

Sinking Vagina: A condition, particularly found in older mares, in which the cervix end of the vagina has dropped down and become filled with urine.

Sinusitis: Inflammation of a sinus, marked by discharge of pus from one or both nostrils.

Sitfast: An area of dry dead skin on the neck or back; caused by pressure which stops the blood supply to the area.

Slough: Dead tissue in the process of separating from the body.

Smegma: The secretion of sebaceous glands, especially the cheesy secretion.

Solution: The homogeneous mixture of one or more substances dispersed in a sufficient quantity of dissolving medium.

Spasm: A sudden, involuntary contraction of a muscle or constriction of a passage.

Spasmolytic: Checking spasms, anti-spasmodic.

Spasticity: Increase in the normal tone of a muscle.

Spavin: An exostosis, usually medial, of the tarsus of equines.

Spavin Test: A test in which the affected leg is held acutely flexed for about two minutes, then released immediately before the horse is trotted. The test is considered positive for bone spavin if lameness is markedly increased for the horse's first few steps.

Spermatozoa: Mature male germ cells, the specific output of the testes; sperm.

Sphincter: A ringlike band of muscle fibers that constricts a passage or closes an opening.

Splay-footed: A condition in which the feet turn outward because the legs turn out through their entire length.

Splints: Rigid or flexible appliances for the fixation of displaced or movable parts.

Spores: The reproductive elements of one of the lower organisms, such as protozoa, fungi, algae, etc.

Sporotrichosis: A mildly contagious disease causing nodules in the subcutaneous lymph nodes; a chronic fungal infection.

Sprain: A joint injury in which some of the fibers of a ligament are ruptured.

Standing Under: Description of a limb that is placed too far beneath the horse, when viewed from the side.

Stapling: A process used to join the epiphyses to encourage even growth.

Stenosis: Narrowing or stricture of a duct or canal.

Sterile Abscess: One which contains no microorganisms.

Sterilization: Any procedure by which an individual is made incapable of reproduction, as by castration.

Sternum: The bone connecting the cartilages cf the ribs; the breastbone.

Stifling: Upward fixation of the patella, occurring when the stifle joint is fully extended.

Stimulant: Any agent or remedy that produces stimulation.

Stock Up: Swelling of the horse's lower legs due to restricted exercise.

Stones: Masses of extremely hard and unyielding material.

Straight Behind: Excessively straight legs as viewed from the side.

Strain: An overstretching or overexertion of some part of the musculature.

Strangles: An infectious disease of horses, characterized by a mucopurulent inflammation of the respiratory mucous membrane.

Strangulated: Overloaded with blood due to constriction.

Strangulated Hernia: One in which the hernial ring has narrowed, trapping a piece of intestine. This affects the circulation, and may cause hemorrhage and death of the tissue.

Stress: Forcibly exerted influence or pressure.

Strongyles: Various parasitic roundworms (family *Strongylidae)* commonly called bloodworms.

Subacute: Somewhat acute, between acute and chronic.

Subcutaneous: Beneath the skin.

Subcuticular: Situated beneath the epidermis.

Subluxation: An incomplete or partial dislocation.

Submucous: Situated beneath the mucous membrane.

Subscapular: Beneath the scapula.

Sulci: Grooves, trenches, or furrows.

Summer Sores: Wounds which do not heal during the summertime because of larvae infestation.

Supportive Treatment: That which is mainly directed at sustaining the strength of the patient.

Suppurative: Producing pus.

Supraspinous: Above a spine or spinous process.

Suspension: A condition of temporary cessation, as of animation, of pain, or of any vital process; or a preparation of a finely divided drug intended to be incorporated (suspended) in some suitable liquid before it is used.

Suspensory: A ligament, bone, muscle, sling or bandage which holds up a part.

Suture: A stitch used to close a wound. (2) A type of fibrous immovable joint in which the edges of the bones are closely united, as in the bones of the skull.

Swan Neck: A term denoting the downward arch of the upper and lower sides of the neck.

Sweeney: A condition involving shrinkage of the supraspinatus and infraspinatus muscles in the shoulder of the horse. Also called slipped shoulder and shoulder atrophy.

Sympathetic: Existing or operating through an interdependence or mutual association.

Symptom: Evidence of a disease, as perceived and described by the patient. (By definition, symptoms of a disease can only be found in humans.)

Symptomatic: Pertaining to or of the nature of a symptom.

Syndrome: A set of symptoms which occur together usually indicating a particular type of disease process.

Synovial Fluid: A transparent fluid, resembling the white of an egg, secreted by the synovial membrane and contained in joint cavities, bursae and tendon sheaths for lubrication.

Synthesis: The production or building up of a substance by combining its elements or compounds.

Systemic: Pertaining to or affecting the body as a whole.

Systemic Treatment: Care affecting the whole body directed to the cure of a disease or injury.

Systole: The contraction or period of contraction of the heart.

Tarsus: The region of articulation between the gaskin and lower hindleg; the hock.

T-bar Shoe: A corrective shoe that applies constant pressure on the frog.

Teasing: A method used to test mares in estrus for heat. Especially useful when the mare exhibits no visible signs of heat.

Tectorial: The nature of a roof or covering, as with the tectorial membrane.

Tendinitis: Inflammation of tendons and tendon-muscle attachments.

Tendon: A fibrous cord of connective tissue which attaches muscle to bone or other structures.

Tenectomy: The cutting out of a lesion of a tendon or of a tendon sheath.

Tenosynovitis: Inflammation of the tendon sheath.

Tenotomy: The cutting of a tendon.

Teratoma: A true neoplasm made up of a number of different types of tissue.

Terminal: Forming or pertaining to an end or ending; the conclusion.

Tetanus: An infectious disease in which tonic muscle spasm and hyperreflexia result in lockjaw and generalized muscle spasm. Caused by toxin of anaerobic Clostridium tetani.

Tetany: Grass and lactation tetany; disorders probably related to the high crude protein content of certain pasturage. A diet lacking in magnesium and calcium is associated with the condition.

Therapy: The treatment of disease.

Thoracentesis: Surgical puncture of the chest wall for draining fluid.

Thorax, Thoracic: The chest; the part of the body between the neck and the diaphragm, encased by the ribs.

Thoroughpin: A distention of the synovial sheath of the flexor perforans tendon of the horse at the hock joint.

Thrombin: The enzyme derived from prothrombin which converts fibrinogen to fibrin.

Thrombocytes: Blood platelets.

Thromboplastin: A substance having procoagulant properties or activity.

Thrombosis: The formation of a blood clot which remains attached at the point of formation in the blood vessel, causing an obstruction.

Thrush: A disease of the horse's foot, characterized by a fetid discharge.

Tied in at the knee: A condition occurring when the flexor tendons appear to be too close to the cannon bone just below the knee.

Tissue: An aggregation of similarly specialized cells united in the performance of a particular function.

Toe Crack: Term for a sand crack located specifically at the toe of the horse's foot.

Topical: Pertaining to a particular surface area, as in Topical Treatment (treatment applied to and affecting a particular location.)

Topical Treatment: Care affecting a particular spot on the surface of the body directed to the cure of a disease or injury.

Torticollis: A condition marked by contracted neck muscles, producing twisting of the neck and an unnatural position of the head.

Tourniquet: An instrument for the compression of a blood vessel by application around an extremity to control the circulation and prevent the flow of blood to or from the distal area.

Toxemia: A general intoxication or poisoning sometimes due to the absorption of bacterial products (toxins) formed at a local source of infection.

Toxic: Pertaining to, due to, or of the nature of a poison.

Toxin: An organic poison, usually a protein produced by a living organism.

Trachea: The windpipe, descending from the larynx to the bronchi.

Tracheitis: Inflammation of the trachea.

Tracheotomy: The formation of an artificial opening into the trachea.

Tranquilizer: An agent that produces a quietening or calming effect, without changing the level of consciousness.

Transfusion: The introduction of whole blood or blood component directly into the blood stream.

Transmission: A transfer of a disease or nerve impulse or inheritable characteristics.

Transplacental: Through the placenta.

Transudate: A fluid substance that has passed through a membrane or has been forced out of a tissue, sometimes as a result of inflammation.

Transverse: Placed crosswise, at right angles to the long axis of a body part.

Trauma: A wound or injury.

Trephine: A crown saw for removing a circular area of bone, chiefly from the skull.

Triceps: A muscle having three heads or parts.

Trichomoniasis: An infectious intestinal disease characterized by sudden severe diarrhea.

Trocar: A sharp-pointed, hollow instrument for piercing the wall of a cavity.

Trochanteric Bursitis: Inflammation of the bursa of the trochanter.

True Osselet: The chronic abnormal growth of new bone in the fetlock joint.

Trypanosomiasis: A general term for the diseases Nagana, Surra, Mal de Caderas, and Murrina, all caused by various Trypanosomes.

Tuberculosis: Any of the infectious diseases of men and animals caused by species of Mycobacterium and characterized by the formation of tubercles and caseous necrosis in the tissues.

Tuberosity: A large prominence on a bone, usually for the attachment of muscles or ligaments.

Tubule: A small tube.

Tularemia: A disease of rodents, resembling plague, which is transmitted by the bites of flies, fleas, ticks, and lice, and which may be contracted in horses by the bite of a tick. It is highly contagious.

Tumor: A mass of new tissue which persists and grows independently of its surrounding structures and which has no useful function.

Tunica: A covering or coat; a general term for a membrane or other structure covering or lining a body part or organ.

Turbulence: Departure in a fluid from a smooth flow.

Turgid: Swollen and congested.

Tympany: Distension due to the presence of gas or air, as in the abdomen or guttural pouch.

Type A knee: Relating to the lower epiphysis of the radius. Mature, completely closed.

Type B knee: Relating to the lower epiphysis of the radius. In the process of closing, slightly open.

Type C knee: Relating to the lower epiphysis of the radius. Open, immature.

Ulcer: A hollowed-out space on the surface of an organ or tissue due to the sloughing of dead tissue.

Ulcerated: Affected with or of the condition of an ulcer.

Ultrasonics: The use of controlled doses of high-frequency sound (radiation) for therapeutic treatment.

Ultra-violet Rays: Light rays beyond the violet end of the spectrum, having powerful chemical properties, and used in radiation treatment.

Umbilical Hernia: The protusion of contents of the abdomen through an opening in the muscles, forming a swelling or lump in the area of the navel.

Unilateral: Affecting one side.

Urethra: The membranous canal for conveying urine from the bladder to the exterior of the body; also carries semen in the male.

Urinalysis: A physical, chemical, or microscopic analysis or examination of urine.

Urinary Calci: See Urolithiasis.

Urine: The fluid excreted by the kidneys, passed through the ureters, stored in the bladder, and discharged through the urethra. Healthy urine is of a slight amber color.

Urolithiasis: The formation of urinary stones, solid masses of mineral substances, somewhere in the urinary tract.

Uroliths: Urinary stones.

Urticaria: An allergic condition characterized by the appearance of wheals on the skin surface. Also known as Hives.

Vaccine: A suspension of attenuated or killed microorganisms administered for the prevention or treatment of infectious diseases.

Vaginitis: Inflammation of the vagina, marked by pain and by a purulent discharge.

Vascular: Pertaining to blood vessels or indicative of an abundant blood supply.

Vaso Constrictor Muscles: Muscles that constrict the flow of blood vessels.

Vector: An animal that transmits a disease-producing organism.

Vein: A vessel through which the blood passes from various organs or parts back to the heart.

Venom: A poison, specifically, a toxic substance normally secreted by a snake, insect, or other animal.

Venous: Pertaining to the veins.

Ventral: Denoting a position more toward the belly surface than some other object of reference.

Venule: Any of the small vessels that collect blood from the capillaries and join to form veins.

Vesicle: A small sac containing fluid, as a blister.

Vesicular Stomatitis: A localized inflammation of the soft tissues of the mouth, containing blisters or other lesions.

Vesiculitis: Inflammation of a vesicle, especially a seminal vesicle.

Vessel: Any channel for carrying a fluid.

Vestigial: Pertaining to a remnant of a structure which functioned at an early stage of development, rudimentary.

Viable: Alive or capable of living.

Villi: Tiny, finger-like extensions of a membrane.

Virulent: Characterized by being exceedingly pathogenic or noxious.

Virus: One of a group of minute infectious agents, usually not seen in a light microscope, and characterized by a lack of independent metabolism and by the ability to replicate only within living host cells.

Visceral: Pertaining to the large internal organs in the thoracic, abdominal and pelvic cavities, especially those in the abdomen.

Vitiligo: Condition characterized by destruction of melanocytes in small or large circumscribed areas of the skin.

Vitreous Humor: The clear, gelatinous substance filling the area behind the lens in the eye.

Volar: Indicating the back or bottom surface of the forearm, knee, fetlock, pastern, or hoof.

Voluntary: Accomplished in accordance with the will.

Wall: A layer enclosing a space (such as the chest, abdomen, or hollow organ) or mass of material (such as the hoof wall).

Wanderer Foal: A foal suffering from convulsive syndromes caused by lack of oxygen at birth.

Warts: Epidermal tumors caused by a papilloma virus.

Wave Mouth: A condition of uneven teeth wear found mainly in older horses.

Weaving: A nervous condition or habit affecting horses suffering from boredom, in which the horse continually shifts his weight from one leg to another.

Wheals: Smooth, slightly raised areas of the skin surface which are redder or paler than the surrounding areas.

Windgalls: Also called windpuffs; a distention (overfilling) of the synovial sheath between the suspensory ligament and the cannon bone, or of the synovial sheath between the long pastern and the middle inferior sesamoidean ligament.

Windsucking: An undesirable habit of some horses in which the animal grasps the manger or other object with the incisor teeth, arches the neck, makes peculiar movements with the head, and swallows quantities of air. This condition is closely associated with Cribbing.

Wobbles: A disease that affects the cervical spinal cord and vertebrae of young horses; it is a sporadic, nonparalytic condition marked by incoordination. Also known as equine incoordination and jinxed back.

Zootoxin: A toxic substance of animal origin.

PREFIXES AND SUFFIXES

Centesis: Suffix indicating the part on which an operation is performed.

Dys: Prefix or combining form signifying painful, bad, or abnormal.

Emia: Suffix donating condition of having a specific substance in the blood.

Epi: Prefix denoting on, upon, or over.

Hemo: Combining form denoting relationship to the blood.

Hydro: Combining form denoting relationship to water.

Hyper: Prefix signifying above, beyond, or excessive.

Hypo: Prefix meaning beneath, under, or deficient.

Iso: Prefix or combining form meaning equal, alike, or the same.

Itis: Suffix denoting inflammation of the part indicated by the root word.

Oma: Suffix denoting a tumor or neoplasm.

Osis: Suffix denoting a process, especially a disease or morbid process.

Osteo: Prefix referring to bone or bones.

Para: Prefix meaning beside, beyond, apart from.

Peri: Prefix meaning around.

Rhino: Combining form denoting relationship to the nose.

Supra: Prefix meaning above or over.

Tomy: Suffix meaning cutting or incision.

Trans: Prefix denoting across or through.